INTEGRATED TREATMENT FOR DUAL DISORDERS

Treatment Manuals for Practitioners

David H. Barlow, *Editor*

Recent Volumes

INTEGRATED TREATMENT FOR DUAL DISORDERS

A Guide to Effective Practice

KIM T. MUESER
DOUGLAS L. NOORDSY
ROBERT E. DRAKE
LINDY FOX

Series Editor's Note by David H. Barlow

Foreword by Kenneth Minkoff

THE GUILFORD PRESS
New York　London

© 2003 The Guilford Press
A Division of Guilford Publications, Inc.
72 Spring Street, New York, NY 10012
www.guilford.com

Printed in Canada

This book is printed on acid-free paper.

Last digit is print number: 9 8 7 6

Library of Congress Cataloging-in-Publication Data

Integrated treatment for dual disorders : a guide to effective practice / by Kim T. Mueser . . . [et al.].
        p. cm.—(Treatment manuals for practitioners)
Includes bibliographical references and index.
    ISBN 1-57230-850-8 (pbk.)
    1. Dual diagnosis—Handbooks, manuals, etc.   2. Dual diagnosis—Treatment—Planning.
I. Mueser, Kim Tornvall.   II. Series.
RC564.68.I684 2003
616.86′ 06—dc21

                                                                            2002151260

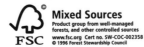

We dedicate this book to the memory of Carolyn Mercer and Tom Fox, who were friends, colleagues, and teachers. Tom and Carolyn's compassion, sense of humor, insight, and spirit have been an inspiration to us all, both personally and professionally, instilling hope and a sense of purpose. Among the many things we learned from Carolyn and Tom, one of the most important was that we receive more than we give in our work with clients and their families, and that we are privileged to be let into their lives.

About the Authors

Kim T. Mueser, PhD, is a clinical psychologist and Professor of Psychiatry at Dartmouth Medical School. His clinical and research interests include the psychosocial treatment of severe mental illnesses, dual disorders, and posttraumatic stress disorder. Dr. Mueser has published extensively and has given numerous lectures and workshops on psychiatric rehabilitation. He is the coauthor of several books, including *Social Skills Training for Psychiatric Patients* (1989), *Coping with Schizophrenia: A Guide for Families* (1994), *Social Skills Training for Schizophrenia: A Step-by-Step Guide* (1997), and *Behavioral Family Therapy for Psychiatric Disorders, Second Edition* (1999).

Douglas L. Noordsy, MD, is Associate Professor of Psychiatry and Associate Director of Education and Training in the Department of Psychiatry, Dartmouth Medical School. He is also Chief of Clinical Research at the Mental Health Center of Greater Manchester and Medical Director of Westbridge, Inc., a private, nonprofit organization providing services to individuals with dual disorders and their families. Dr. Noordsy has provided clinical care and leadership across the New Hampshire community mental health system, including active work with dual-diagnosis treatment teams, since 1990. He has lectured and published extensively, especially in the areas of comorbid substance abuse and mental illness and recovery-oriented treatment for people with severe mental illness.

Robert E. Drake, MD, PhD, is a community psychiatrist, Professor of Psychiatry at Dartmouth Medical School, and Director of the New Hampshire–Dartmouth Psychiatric Research Center. He has worked with community mental health teams developing and refining approaches to integrated dual-disorder treatments for over 20 years.

Lindy Fox, MA, LADC, is a Research Associate at the New Hampshire–Dartmouth Psychiatric Research Center. She has worked extensively on research projects examining the effectiveness of integrated treatment for people with serious mental illnesses and substance use disorders, including involvement in assessments, treatment, and clinical teaching. Ms. Fox's expertise has been gained through a combination of formal education, personal experience, and professional focus. She has been a recipient of the services she now participates in designing and evaluating. Ms. Fox has consulted throughout the United States and in other countries including Australia, Canada, England, and Sweden. She has also coauthored several articles, and is on the faculty at Dartmouth College in the Department of Family and Community Medicine.

Series Editor's Note

In the ongoing battle against mental illness, some of our most valiant warriors are on the front lines working with dually diagnosed, seriously mentally ill individuals—that is, individuals who present not only with chronic and severe mental illness such as schizophrenia or bipolar disorder, but also with substance abuse. These patients confound the best efforts of public mental health systems and networks of treatment programs for addiction. As the authors of this book point out, the traditional approach has been to choose one diagnosis and focus treatment efforts on that before moving on to treat the second diagnosis. Typically and tragically, these efforts have most often been futile. Now Kim Mueser and his coauthors describe in this groundbreaking work a treatment for these difficult patients that provides a "seamless integration of psychiatric and substance abuse interventions in order to form a more cohesive unitary system of care." This program, because of its success and empirical support, has been widely adopted in state mental health systems and other service delivery settings across the full range of mental health providers. Everyone involved with this very needy population will want to be aware of this important new approach to severe mental illness.

DAVID H. BARLOW, PHD

Foreword

The publication of this comprehensive textbook on the integrated treatment of individuals with co-occurring severe mental illness and substance abuse represents a historic milestone in the evolution of mental health and substance abuse treatment in the United States. Twenty years ago, when the first reports emerged in the literature of prevalent substance abuse problems among new "young adult chronic patients" of the post-deinstitutionalization era, the concept of *dual diagnosis* more commonly related to the combinations of mental illness with medical illness or developmental disability, and the idea of integrated systems or integrated treatment for individuals with psychiatric and substance use disorders was simply nonexistent. During the last two decades, enormous changes have occurred—in both the mental health system and the addiction system—in our understanding of co-occurring disorders, as well as the system-level, program-level, and clinician-competency-level strategies required to address such disorders.

The first set of changes related to the emergence of research demonstration projects that began to identify evidence-based best practices for individuals with severe mental illness and co-occurring substance use disorders, particularly for those who were homeless or otherwise significantly disengaged from traditional treatment approaches. During the 1980s, the National Institute of Mental Health funded a series of such projects, focusing on implementation of integrated case management strategies within the context of a comprehensive community support system. The team of individuals who are the authors of this book, along with their many colleagues at the New Hampshire–Dartmouth Psychiatric Research Center (NHDPRC), have been in the forefront of this research from the very beginning. NHDPRC has an unmatched national reputation as a center for both clinical excellence and research leadership in those with co-occurring substance abuse and mental illness. This reputation derives from two important characteristics: first, an insistence on only disseminating research that is carefully designed according to the best practices of clinical research methodology; second, and more important, a firm ideology that the best clinical research is designed and implemented by individuals who continue to involve themselves as front-line clinicians with the types of clients they are researching. As a consequence, NHDPRC has developed clinical treatment models and interventions that make sense in real-world clinical situations, and has demonstrated the effectiveness of those interventions through high-quality research. This book reflects both the clinical acumen and the careful conceptual precision that characterize the work of this team.

As a result of these demonstration projects in the 1980s, NHDPRC developed and disseminated the continuous treatment team (CTT) model of intensive, integrated case management for individuals with co-occurring disorders, and began to identify and refine particular treatment principles and interventions. The principles include proactive empathic outreach, continued optimism, continuity, longitudinal perspective, integration of mental health and substance interventions, small-step objectives, and stage-specific treatment. From these principles have been developed well-designed programmatic components for individualized case management, stage-specific group interventions, engagement and education of family members and other collateral individuals, contingency management strategies, treatment manuals for staff training, and strategies for program implementation in mental health settings. All of this expertise, developed over 20 years, is reflected in the content of this book.

During the last decade, as experience with integrated treatment demonstration projects has widened and treatment technology has been increasingly refined, broad changes have been occurring at the system level. Continued research on the epidemiology and outcome of co-occurring disorders has demonstrated powerfully that in both mental health and addiction treatment settings, comorbidity is sufficiently prevalent for dual diagnosis to be considered an expectation rather than an exception. In addition, it is becoming clearer that in all treatment environments and in multiple service systems (including primary health care, corrections, protective services, shelters, and managed care), comorbidity is associated with poorer outcomes and higher costs. Increasingly, it is clear that people with co-occurring disorders represent the same faces in different places throughout our service system, yet they have remained system misfits in all places. As the high prevalence of comorbidity has become more widely recognized, it has become increasingly apparent that system-level changes are necessary to address the extent of the problem; small numbers of transiently funded demonstration projects can address neither the magnitude nor the persistence of the need for integrated service interventions throughout the system. As a consequence, growing numbers of state and national systems have begun large-scale initiatives to identify best practices that result in more comprehensive, continuous, integrated systems of care for individuals with co-occurring disorders. These efforts have been stimulated by the development of an unprecedented national consensus of state mental health program directors and substance abuse system directors on an integrated conceptual framework for system-level planning for individuals with co-occurring disorders. State and local initiatives in turn have incorporated a wide range of specific strategies, including system-level consensus building, widespread implementation of evidence-based models, regulatory and reimbursement changes, collaboration with correctional and protective service systems, managed care quality and financial incentives, implementation of practice guidelines or standards, and systematic training initiatives to achieve widespread competency.

A key concept that underlies system-level efforts is that because comorbidity is an expectation, and is so strongly associated with poor outcome and high costs, *all* programs need to achieve a certain level of dual-diagnosis capability, and *all* staff members need to demonstrate basic competency in integrated treatment—not just those working in specialized dual-diagnosis programs.

Within this context, this book becomes particularly valuable. For many years, the field of dual-diagnosis treatment has been plagued by a dramatic lack of comprehensive training materials accessible to the average clinician. This volume specifically addresses that need. In clear, straightforward language, complemented by well-designed clinical examples, every aspect of integrated treatment is systematically addressed—ranging from assessment, through various group treatment strategies, to family involvement, to program and system design. The appendices are replete with instruments, forms, and tools that can be adapted to real-world clinical use. Consequently, as more and more large systems move to require basic competency for large numbers of clinicians, this book stands out as the obvious resource for any clinician whose competency domain will include working with individuals with serious mental illness and substance use disorders.

More important, however, this book conveys a powerful clinical message of empathy, hope, and respect. In my work as a trainer and consultant on developing services for individuals with co-occurring disorders, I have found consistently that these individuals are commonly experienced as system misfits, often acquiring negative labels (e.g., "antisocial, manipulative, med-seeking borderline") that interfere with clinicians' ability to engage them in positive treatment relationships. Yet the research clearly indicates the importance of empathic, hopeful, continuous, and integrated relationships in promoting successful outcome. This book's most significant accomplishment is that it helps to make individuals with co-occurring disorders into real people, with real feelings, and provides clinicians with useful skills with which to help these individuals grow and change in a caring context. In so doing, this book inspires all of us to grow and change as well, as we integrate new competencies into our existing repertoire of skills.

KENNETH MINKOFF, MD
Harvard Medical School

Preface

This book is about how to help people with comorbid psychiatric and substance use disorders manage their illnesses, develop and pursue personal goals, and get on with the business of their lives. In short, this book provides guidance for professionals about facilitating the recovery process in persons with *dual disorders* (or with a *dual diagnosis*).

Mental health and substance abuse treatment professionals frequently encounter clients with prominent psychiatric symptoms and problems related to their use of alcohol or drugs. For example, a client with a history of schizophrenia is admitted to a psychiatric hospital for the treatment of an acute exacerbation of psychotic symptoms, and a routine urine screen tests positive for the presence of cocaine and marijuana. During subsequent assessment, the client reveals that he uses crack cocaine whenever he can afford it, and smokes marijuana and drinks alcohol when he is coming down from crack or cannot obtain it. This combination of problems is not unusual.

As another example, a client with alcoholism who has had several prior episodes of inpatient detoxification calls her substance abuse counselor in the midst of a relapse, and describes struggling with suicidal thoughts and feelings. After steps have been taken to assure her safety, a closer examination of her mental health indicates that she has been struggling with mood problems for many years, and that her emotions fluctuate from the depths of despair to the elation, overconfidence, and euphoria of mania. Again, both substance abuse problems and mental health symptoms are present in a client seeking treatment for one of the disorders.

Traditionally, the most common approach to treating such clients with dual disorders has been to identify one disorder as "primary" and the other as "secondary," and to focus attention first on treating the primary disorder. Treatment of the other disorder is only attempted when the primary disorder has been successfully managed. Alternatively, sometimes clients with dual disorders are referred to different clinicians (and different agencies) to be given simultaneous treatment of their substance abuse and mental health problems.

Sadly, these traditional approaches to treating dual disorders have been shown to be ineffective for the care of either psychiatric or substance use disorders. Most often, efforts to treat one disorder without attending to the other have been unsuccessful; invariably, clients relapse in one disorder and then the other. On the rare occasions when clients receive treatment for both disorders in separate systems, differences between mental health and substance abuse treatment philosophies and the lack of coordination between different clinicians have doomed these efforts to failure.

The key to effective treatment for clients with dual disorders is the seamless integration of psychiatric and substance abuse interventions in order to form a cohesive, unitary system of care. In this book, we provide a blueprint for creating, organizing, delivering, and evaluating the effectiveness of these integrated services. Our work in developing integrated dual-disorder treatment programs has been conducted in a wide variety of places, including urban and rural locations, in New Hampshire, other states, and in other countries. A wide variety of professionals have been involved in providing integrated dual-disorder services, ranging from psychiatrists to doctoral and master's-level psychologists to nurses, substance abuse counselors, social workers, case managers, rehabilitation counselors, and occupational therapists, within both mental health and substance abuse agencies. We are confident, therefore, that the principles of integrated dual-disorder treatment outlined here can be implemented successfully in typical public or private community treatment settings.

Although we describe the essential components of integrated dual-disorder treatment in this book, we also recognize that no two programs are identical, nor should they be. Integrated treatment programs differ from one another, depending on client needs and characteristics; the setting; and the background, training, and personal philosophies of the professional staff. In order for an integrated program to be effective, it must be capable of performing state-of-the-art assessment, and at least some individual, group, and family treatment modalities should be available. To determine specific dual-disorder programming needs, administrators or clinicians are encouraged to conduct an analysis of their own agencies, using the Dual-Disorder Treatment Fidelity Scale contained in Appendix A.

This book is designed to be a guide to clinicians in providing the critical interventions, and to administrators in creating dual-disorder programs. We also expect that some clients and family members will find the guidelines useful in seeking and advocating for the services they need. We provide literature reviews of pertinent information concerning the treatment of dual disorders; tools for assessment and for tracking clients' progress; educational handouts on topics related to dual disorders; and clinical guidelines for implementing specific individual, group, family, and other interventions.

Part I provides background information about the nature of dual disorders, integrated treatment, and organizational factors for developing effective programs. Chapter 1 summarizes the prevalence of substance use disorders in persons with severe mental illness, demographic and clinical correlates, and theories about the high rates of dual disorders. In Chapter 2 we describe the problems with traditional, nonintegrated approaches to treatment. We then provide an overview of the integrated treatment model, and specify the principles of integrated care upon which the Dual-Disorder Treatment Fidelity Scale is based. Effective programs require well-organized agencies with leadership that is supportive of integrated services, and that builds ongoing evaluation and accountability into its structures. Chapter 3 describes the necessary organizational factors for establishing effective integrated dual-disorder treatment programs, including infrastructure, training, identifying the target population, assessment, array of services (fundamental mental health services and specialized dual-disorder services), levels of care (e.g., inpatient, outpatient), program monitoring, and financing mechanisms.

Part II provides information to clinicians about the process of assessment for substance use disorders in clients with severe mental illness. Chapter 4 describes how to detect substance abuse in the psychiatric population, how to classify substance use disorders, how to assess clients' functioning in different domains of their lives, and how to understand the role that substance use plays in the clients' lives. In Chapter 5 we provide guidance for conducting a functional analysis of substance use behavior, which is aimed at identifying factors that maintain substance abuse and, if not otherwise addressed, that may interfere with achieving sobriety. Based on the functional analysis and clients' motivation to change their substance use behavior, this chapter also provides guidance for developing integrated treatment plans that attend to substance abuse, mental illness, and their interactions.

Parts III, IV, and V describe specific treatment approaches for conducting individual, group, and family interventions. In Part III, Chapter 6 addresses the elements of stage-wise case management for clients with dual disorders, in which services are provided in a manner consistent with clients' motivation to change their substance use behavior (i.e., their stage of treatment). These case management services include psychotherapeutic work, advocacy and clinical coordination, and promoting rehabilitation and recovery. Chapter 7 covers the fundamentals of motivational interviewing, which involves helping clients develop an interest in and desire for working on their substance use problems by exploring and working toward personal goals, and evaluating whether substance abuse interferes with the attainment of these goals. Chapter 8 describes the use of cognitive-behavioral counseling to help clients reduce their use of substances or to maintain abstinence, with information also provided about the numerous cognitive-behavioral methods for treating psychiatric illnesses.

In Part IV, devoted to group intervention, Chapter 9 describes how to develop and run persuasion groups for clients with dual disorders who are engaged in treatment but who continue to experience problems related to their substance use. Persuasion groups are designed to help clients understand the effects of substances on their lives, and to motivate them to work on these problems in a supportive, nonconfrontational group milieu. Chapter 10 describes how to conduct active treatment groups, which are aimed at helping motivated clients to reduce their use of substances or to achieve abstinence. In Chapter 11 we review the fundamentals of social skills training for clients with dual disorders, including how to develop more effective skills for establishing and deepening interpersonal relationships, managing negative emotions, and dealing with social situations involving substance use. Chapter 12 addresses the role of self-help groups, such as Alcoholics Anonymous and Dual Recovery Anonymous, in helping clients with dual disorders on the road to recovery.

In Part V, dedicated to family work, Chapter 13 outlines the importance of collaboration with families, including reaching out and engaging them in treatment. Chapter 14 describes a specific model, behavioral family therapy (BFT), for working with families with a dually disordered member. BFT includes the following components: connecting with the family, assessment, psychoeducation about dual disorders, communication skills training, and problem-solving training. Chapter 15 contains guidelines for conducting multiple-family groups aimed at providing education about dual disorders and their management, and generating social support among relatives and clients.

Part VI addresses other treatment approaches for integrated treatment programs. Chapter 16 focuses on residential programs and other housing options. Chapter 17 deals with the use of coerced or involuntary interventions, such as payeeships, involuntary hospitalization, inpatient treatment, and work with clients involved in the criminal justice system (including both offenders on probation or parole and those in correctional settings). Chapter 18 provides guidance regarding the role of vocational rehabilitation in the process of recovery from dual disorders, including the benefits of work for clients early in treatment, as well as for clients whose substance abuse is in remission and who are active participants in their own mental health treatment. Chapter 19 describes the principles of psychopharmacology for dual disorders, including medications for the treatment of specific psychiatric disorders; medications for substance abuse; and interactions between and among medications, alcohol, and commonly abused drugs.

In recent years there has been an accelerated movement toward identifying and implementing evidence-based practices for the treatment of psychiatric disorders and substance abuse. Clinicians and administrators need to understand and evaluate the empirical support for specific treatments, and clients and families have a right to know which interventions are effective. To meet this demand, Part VII, Chapter 20, provides a review of the research on integrated treatment. Because of the importance of this chapter to all stakeholders, including professionals, clients, and families, we have avoided (or explained) technical language or jargon in order to make it accessible to all readers.

The book concludes with a brief Epilogue. In contrast to the other chapters, which focus on establishing and delivering dual-disorder treatment services, the Epilogue shifts attention away from the clients to the clinicians themselves. Providing dual-disorder services can be taxing work that takes an emotional toll on clinicians, compromising their effectiveness in working with clients. In the Epilogue we address this potential strain; we provide clinicians with strategies for minimizing burnout and demoralization, and for remaining energized, hopeful, creative, and successful in their work with this challenging population.

This book provides a very comprehensive guide to developing and implementing integrated dual-disorder services. We realize that some clinicians and program administrators may find its sheer size daunting, so we offer some suggestions here on how to use the book. Readers can use it as a reference guide by selecting chapters of particular interest. To help readers find the information they need, the introductory section to each chapter reviews its scope, and the summary at the end of each chapter highlights the main points covered. Following the introductory section of each treatment chapter, we also provide a brief section in which we highlight the role of that treatment approach in the overall integrated treatment of dual disorders.

To achieve minimum competence, we recommend that all clinicians working with dually disordered clients read Chapters 1, 4, 5, 6, 7, 8, 13, 16, 18, and the Epilogue, and that they peruse the educational handouts contained in Appendix B. We recommend that clinicians whose caseloads are composed of at least 50% of clients with dual disorders—as well as directors of dual-disorder services at agencies, who need to develop a thorough understanding of integrated dual-disorder treatment—read the entire book.

Individuals responsible for developing dual-disorder services, including directors of state and local mental health services, administrators, and program managers, need to have a basic understanding of the impact of substance abuse on severe mental illness, the fundamentals of integrated treatment, options for organizing and maintaining high-quality programs, and what the research shows about the effects of integrated treatment programs. This information is contained in Chapters 1, 2, 3, and 20. As clients with dual disorders often have multiple problems and needs, potentially involving different systems, agencies, or service providers, familiarity with Chapters 16, 17, and 18 may also prove useful to persons with administrative responsibility.

On a final note, we point out that the primary psychiatric disorders focused on in this book are those generally subsumed under the rubric of *severe mental illness*. Psychiatric disorders are considered *severe* if they result in persistent impairments in role functioning (e.g., work, school, parenting), social relationships, or the ability to care for oneself. Persistent impairments in these areas frequently result in clients being eligible for disability benefits. The most common types of severe mental illness are schizophrenia, schizoaffective disorder, bipolar disorder, and major depression, but other disorders may also be severe and persistent, such as posttraumatic stress disorder, obsessive–compulsive disorder, other anxiety disorders, and personality disorders. We recognize that there is no precise demarcation between severe mental illnesses and other psychiatric disorders. Thus, while our emphasis is on the integration of substance abuse and psychiatric treatment in persons with severe mental illness, clinicians treating substance abuse in clients with less severe psychiatric disorders will also benefit from these guidelines.

Dual disorders are pervasive in mental health and substance abuse treatment settings, and there is an urgent need to develop integrated services that address both problem areas. Despite this, there has been a lack of cohesive, articulated models for providing integrated dual-disorder services. We believe that the model described here, and the detailed guidelines for delivering specific services, will provide program administrators and clinicians with the necessary tools for developing and implementing integrated treatment for this important population.

Acknowledgments

This book would not have been possible without the help of numerous people—too many to mention, including colleagues, clinicians, program administrators, clients, and their families. Among the many colleagues who have contributed to our thinking about dual disorders and the development of our approach, we extend our thanks to the following people: Tim Ackerson, Stephanie Acquilano, Arthur Alterman, Hoyt and Marianne Alverson, Steve Bartels, Richard Bebout, Debbie Becker, Mary Brunette, Gary Bond, Kate Carey, Robin Clark, Lisa Dixon, Ted Eckman, Susan Essock, Tom Fox, Linda Frisman, Shirley Glynn, Paul Gorman, Alan Green, Maxine Harris, James Herbert, David Kavanagh, Jack Kline, Anthony Lehman, Robert Paul Liberman, Greg McHugo, Shery Mead, Tom Mellman, Alexander Miller, Ken Minkoff, Fred Osher, Roger Peters, Ernest Quimby, Stan and Harriet Rosenberg, Andrew Shaner, Donald Shumway, Nick Tarrier, Greg Teague, Will Torrey, George Vaillant, Robert Vidaver, and Roberto Zarate.

Among the many clinicians and program administrators with whom we have worked and from whom we have learned, we particularly appreciate the contributions of the following persons: Carmen Abraham, Gordon Archambault, Debra Bailey, Deborah Clement, Marty Connarton, Harry Cunningham, Peter Delfaus, A. J. Ernst, Perry Edson, Linda Freisinger-Baird, Brad Geltz, Patrick Haney, Tim Hartnet, Chris Hatala, Eva Issavi, David Johnson, Linda Kennison, Nannette Latremouille, Judy Magnon, David Macey, Kathy Moffitt, Bob Murray, Bill Naughton, Linda Neily, Chris O'Keefe, Steve Pierce, Dan Potenza, Maggie Pritchard, Nydia Rios-Benitez, Jonathon Routhier, Gary Savill, Ed Schlaeger, Sean Shea, Peggy Sherrer, Lou Tuffano, Jude Turner, Deborah Webb, Mary Woods, and Deb Wooster.

We appreciate the tireless efforts of Kathy Luger and Linda LaRose for their role in preparing countless drafts of chapters, forms, and handouts. We thank John Sklader for the artwork that appears in the book. We also thank our editor at The Guilford Press, Barbara Watkins, for her patience, help, encouragement, editing prowess, and overall role in ushering this book into publication. Finally, we thank our families for their love, support, and willingness to put up with our hectic work schedules.

Terminology

We have adopted a number of conventions for the terms used throughout this book. For the sake of clarity, we describe these conventions here.

The term *substance use disorder* is used to refer to individuals who meet diagnostic criteria for either *substance abuse* or *substance dependence*. When referring to the pattern of problems associated with substance use, we use the terms *substance use disorder* and *substance abuse* interchangeably.

Dual diagnosis and *dual disorders* are terms we use interchangeably to describe individuals who have both a severe mental illness and a substance use disorder. The term *co-occurring disorders* is occasionally used to refer to dual disorders as well.

As noted in the Preface, *severe mental illnesses* refer to psychiatric disorders with a severe and persistent impact on a person's psychosocial functioning, including the ability to work, maintain interpersonal relationships, and care for oneself. These illnesses often include psychotic symptoms, such as hallucinations or delusions. The most common severe mental illnesses include schizophrenia, schizoaffective disorder, bipolar disorder, and major depression with psychotic symptoms; other disorders may also be severe, such as anxiety disorders (e.g., posttraumatic stress disorder) and personality disorders (e.g., borderline personality disorder).

Following standard convention in the substance abuse field, we distinguish between drugs and alcohol, while referring to both types as *substances. Drugs* refer to commonly abused illicit substances, such as cannabis, cocaine, amphetamines, hallucinogens, opiates, and inhalants, as well as misused over-the-counter medications or prescription medications. Although *alcohol* is also a drug, the distinction between *alcohol* and *drugs* recognizes the legal status of alcohol in the United States, and the fact that most surveys indicate that alcohol consumption and alcohol use disorders far exceed all types of drug use and drug disorders. Although nicotine and caffeine have effects on mental processes and are addictive, we do not focus on their treatment, because of a lack of evidence suggesting negative effects on psychosocial functioning or the course of severe mental illness. However, we note that as clients with dual disorders make progress toward recovery, and succeed in reducing and stopping the negative effects of substances on their lives, they often turn their attention to other addictions—including stopping smoking, as well as making other changes in health behaviors (e.g., exercise, diet).

We refer to individuals with dual disorders as *clients*. A survey we conducted among people using mental health services indicated that most preferred the term *client*, followed by the term *patient*, followed by the term *consumer* (Mueser, Glynn, Corrigan, & Baber, 1996).

Contents

I

Basics

1

Substance Abuse and Severe Mental Illness

The use of psychoactive substances, such as alcohol, cannabis, cocaine, and opiates (or narcotics), dates back almost as far as civilization itself (Rudgley, 1998). In many societies, the use of sanctioned substances for ceremonial, celebratory, or mood-enhancing purposes is normative behavior. At times or within certain subgroups, even the use of illicit substances may be normative. For example, alcohol use was common in the general population in the United States during Prohibition in the 1920s, and during the height of the counterculture in the late 1960s, the majority of persons between 16 and 30 years old had at least tried marijuana. In the late 1980s and 1990s, crack cocaine overtook marijuana as the most popular drug among some inner-city subgroups.

The widespread use of alcohol and drugs is associated with a number of negative consequences, including interpersonal difficulties, interference with work or school, and health and legal problems. Despite the common and profound effects of substance abuse on the day-to-day functioning of some people, their impact on persons with severe and persistent mental illness, such as schizophrenia or bipolar disorder, has often been overlooked. Although recognition of the problem of substance abuse in clients with severe mental illness (i.e., dual diagnosis) grew in the late 1980s and 1990s, substance use disorders continue to be underdiagnosed in the psychiatric population. Even when substance abuse is correctly identified by treatment providers, its effects on the course of psychiatric disorders are often misunderstood. And to make matters worse, ineffective or inappropriate treatments, such as the use of strong interpersonal confrontation, are often provided to clients with dual disorders. The net result of inadequate assessment and ineffective treatment of dual disorders is that

clients are frequently doomed to a poor course of their illnesses, including more frequent relapses and rehospitalizations, with the increased costs of care and containment borne by families, clinicians, law enforcement, and society.

In order to treat clients with dual disorders effectively, and therefore to improve their long-term prognosis, clinicians need to be familiar with current knowledge about substance use in the psychiatric population. This chapter provides an overview of the necessary information. Specifically, we begin with a review of the prevalence of substance use disorders among persons with severe psychiatric illness, followed by a discussion of the demographic and clinical correlates of substance abuse in this population. Next, we summarize the impact of substance use on psychiatric disorders, including effects on symptoms, social functioning and family relationships, legal consequences, and health. This is followed by considering different theories that have been proposed to explain the high rate of substance use disorders among clients with severe psychiatric disorders. We conclude by providing a summary of the natural course of dual disorders, and underscoring the need for effective treatment of these conditions.

PREVALENCE OF SUBSTANCE ABUSE

Studies of the prevalence of substance use disorders in psychiatric clients have shown significant variations from one sample to the next (Cuffel, 1996; Mueser, Bennett, & Kushner, 1995). For example, rates of these disorders in clients with severe mental illness have been reported to be as low as under 20% (Hall, Popkin, & DeVaul, 1977; Whitlock & Lowrey, 1967) and as high as over 65% (Ananth et al., 1989; Safer, 1987). Several factors may contribute to the variability in estimates of substance abuse.

Factors Affecting Prevalence Estimates

The most important factors that can affect estimates of substance use disorders in the psychiatric population include the methods used to assess substance abuse, the diagnostic criteria used to define substance abuse and dependence, the setting where a sample is obtained, and the demographic characteristics of the sample. These different factors are briefly discussed below.

Assessment Methods

A variety of strategies can be used to assess substance use disorders, including chart reviews, laboratory tests, direct client interviews (using either structured or unstructured formats), information from informants such as family members, and clinician-based reports. Each of these assessment methods has both advantages and disadvantages (see Chapter 4). To the extent that a single assessment method is used to the exclusion of others, the resulting estimate will tend to be lower than the true prevalence of substance use disorders (Drake, Rosenberg, & Mueser, 1996).

Diagnostic Criteria

Another factor that can contribute to differences in estimates of the prevalence of substance use disorders is the way in which these disorders are classified and diagnosed. Diagnostic systems for classifying psychiatric and substance use disorders, such as the *Diagnostic and Statistical Manual of Mental Disorders* (DSM) series and the *International Classification of Diseases* (ICD) series, differ in the criteria used to define substance use disorders; they also change slightly over time. Both factors lead to variations in estimated prevalence rates.

Setting

The setting in which a substance abuse assessment takes place can also influence prevalence estimates (Galanter, Castaneda, & Ferman, 1988). Clients with dual disorders tend to use numerous high-cost services, such as emergency room visits and acute inpatient hospital treatment (Bartels et al., 1993; Dickey & Azeni, 1996). In addition, clients with dual disorders often experience legal repercussions of their involvement in substance abuse, resulting in time spent in jails and prisons (Drake & Brunette, 1998). Finally, as substance abuse often interferes with clients' natural support systems (especially with family members), and may also make clients less desirable tenants, clients with dual disorders often have housing problems, leading to housing instability and homelessness (Drake, Wallach, & Hoffman, 1989).

Therefore, clients who are assessed in emergency rooms or acute inpatient settings, who are in jail or prison, or who are homeless are more likely to have substance use disorders than are similar clients receiving outpatient treatment at a local community mental health center or community-based samples. In fact, clients who are in any type of institutional setting, whether clinical or legal, are more likely to have a substance use disorder than clients not in such a setting (Regier et al., 1990).

Demographic Characteristics

A final factor related to substance abuse among persons with severe mental illness is that of client demographics. As we discuss later in this chapter, demographic characteristics such as age and sex are related to substance use disorders, both in the general population and among persons with psychiatric disorders. Depending on the nature of the population served in a particular area, rates of substance abuse may be higher or lower than in populations served by other providers. For example, a mental health center serving an urban population of mainly young men with severe mental illness will have higher rates of substance abuse than another center serving a more heterogeneous population will have. Thus the particular demographics of the client population can influence the estimated prevalence of substance use disorders.

Lifetime Prevalence of Substance Abuse in Severe Mental Illness

Numerous studies have evaluated the prevalence of substance abuse in persons with severe mental illness (Cuffel, 1996). The most extensive study to examine the prevalence of dual disorders is the Epidemologic Catchment Area (ECA) study (Regier et al., 1990). The ECA study involved a comprehensive diagnostic assessment of both psychiatric and substance use disorders, via structured interviews with over 20,000 randomly selected people living throughout the United States. In order to ensure that sufficient numbers of psychiatric clients were included, persons who were living in institutional settings were oversampled, including state and private psychiatric hospitals, general hospitals, nursing homes, and jails or prisons.

The ECA prevalence rates of substance use disorders in the general population and among clients with severe mental illness are summarized in Table 1.1. The

TABLE 1.1. Lifetime Prevalence (%) and Odds Ratios (ORs) of Substance Use Disorders for Various DSM-III Psychiatric Disorders

Group	Any substance abuse or dependence		Any alcohol diagnosis		Any drug diagnosis	
	%	OR	%	OR	%	OR
General population	16.7	—	13.5	—	6.1	—
Schizophrenia	47.0	4.6	33.7	3.3	27.5	6.2
Any mood disorder	32.0	2.6	21.8	1.9	19.4	4.7
Any bipolar disorder	56.1	6.6	43.6	5.1	33.6	8.3
Major depression	27.2	1.9	16.5	1.3	18.0	3.8
Dysthymia	31.4	2.4	20.9	1.7	18.9	3.9
Any anxiety disorder	23.7	1.7	17.9	1.5	11.9	2.5
Obsessive–compulsive disorder	32.8	2.5	24.0	2.1	18.4	3.7
Phobia	22.9	1.6	17.3	1.4	11.2	2.2
Panic disorder	35.8	2.9	28.7	2.6	16.7	3.2

Note. An odds ratio (OR) is the ratio of the odds of having a substance use disorder in the psychiatric diagnostic group to the odds of the disorder in the remaining population. The data are from the National Institute of Mental Health Epidemiologic Catchment Area (ECA) study (Regier et al., 1990).

data show that clients with a variety of different DSM-III psychiatric disorders were significantly more likely to have a substance use disorder than individuals with no psychiatric illness. For example, the lifetime prevalence of alcohol use disorders in the general population was 13.5%, and the lifetime rate of drug use disorders was 6.1%. For individuals with schizophrenia, these rates increased to 33.7% for alcohol use disorders and 27.5% for drug use disorders. For respondents with bipolar disorder, the rates were even higher, with 43.6% having a lifetime prevalence of alcohol use disorders and 33.6% having drug use disorders. The rates of substance abuse for individuals with other psychiatric disorders were also higher than in the general population, but tended to be lower than the rates for schizophrenia and bipolar disorder. Two other large epidemiological studies of psychiatric–substance abuse comorbidity—the National Comorbidity Survey (NCS) in the United States (Kessler et al., 1996), and the National Survey of Mental Health and Wellbeing (NSMHW) in Australia (Teeson, Hall, Lynskey, & Degenhardt, 2000)—have yielded similar findings. In addition, numerous other studies report similarly high rates of substance abuse among clients in treatment for severe psychiatric disorders (e.g., Duke, Pantelis, & Barnes, 1994; Fowler, Carr, Carter, & Lewin, 1998; Mueser, Yarnold, & Bellack, 1992; Mueser et al., 1990, 2000; Rosenthal, Hellerstein, & Miner, 1992; Stone, Greenstein, Gamble, & McLellan, 1993; Ziedonis & Trudeau, 1997).

The question of whether people diagnosed with certain psychiatric disorders are more prone to abusing particular types of substances has been the topic of much debate. Early reviews suggested that people with

schizophrenia were more likely to abuse stimulants than clients with other diagnoses (e.g., Schneier & Siris, 1987). However, more recent and larger studies of the prevalence of specific types of substance abuse in clients with a variety of severe psychiatric illnesses, including the ECA, NCS, and NSMHW studies, have failed to replicate this finding (Kessler et al., 1996; Regier et al., 1990; Teeson et al., 2000). The evidence suggests that the availability of different types of substances, rather than their subjective effects, is the primary determinant of which specific substances are abused (Mueser, Yarnold, & Bellack, 1992).

Research on substance abuse in clients with severe mental illness has mainly examined the most commonly abused types of substances, including alcohol, cannabis, stimulants (cocaine and amphetamines), sedatives, hallucinogens, and narcotics. In practically all studies, history of alcohol abuse is most common, followed by either cannabis or cocaine abuse. Clients with psychiatric disorders may also abuse other types of substances, such as inhalants (e.g., aerosols, gas fumes, glue, amyl nitrate), over-the-counter pills, and anticholinergic medications (e.g., benztropine). In addition, a very high proportion of clients with psychiatric disorders smoke or chew tobacco (de Leon et al., 1995; Hall et al., 1995; Hughes, Hatsukami, Mitchell, & Dahlgren, 1986) and consume large quantities of caffeine (Hughes & Howard, 1997). Much less is known about the interactions between tobacco, caffeine, and psychiatric disorders or their treatment than alcohol or drugs such as marijuana, stimulants, and hallucinogens. Therefore, we do not focus on the treatment of tobacco or caffeine problems in this book.

In summary, the lifetime prevalence of substance use disorders is higher in clients with a psychiatric illness than in the general population, particularly if that illness is severe and persistent, such as schizophrenia or bipolar disorder. Alcohol is usually the most commonly abused substance, followed by cannabis and cocaine. Diagnostic groups do not tend to differ in their preference for one type of substance over another, with availability the most important determinant of which substances are abused.

Prevalence of Recent Substance Abuse

The lifetime prevalence of substance abuse in persons with severe mental illness is generally between 40% and 60%. However, at any one point in time, the rate of recent substance abuse is lower. Most surveys suggest that the rate of recent (i.e., in the past 6 months) substance abuse in this population is 25–35% (Graham et al., 2001; Mueser et al., 1990; Rosenberg et al., 1998). This lower recent rate indicates that some clients with substance use disorders experience periods of remission, although they remain at risk for relapse of their substance abuse.

DEMOGRAPHIC, CLINICAL, AND HISTORICAL CORRELATES OF SUBSTANCE ABUSE

Understanding which clients with severe mental illness are most likely to have substance use disorders can facilitate the recognition and treatment of these clients. We review the demographic, clinical, and historical correlates of substance use disorders below, focusing on findings that have been obtained across multiple studies (for reviews, see Cantor-Graae, Nordström, & McNeil, 2001; Drake & Brunette, 1998; Mueser, Bennett, & Kushner, 1995; RachBeisel, Scott, & Dixon, 1999).

Demographic Correlates

A number of different demographic characteristics are correlated with substance abuse. In general, the same characteristics that are related to substance abuse in the general population are also related to it in persons with severe mental illness.

Gender

Men are consistently more likely to develop alcohol and drug use disorders than women. However, despite this difference, significant numbers of women experience problems related to substance abuse, and it is important not to neglect the assessment of these disorders in women. For example, in a study of 325 psychiatric admissions to New Hampshire Hospital, 50% of the women had a lifetime alcohol use disorder, 30% had a lifetime cannabis use disorder, and 15% had a lifetime cocaine use disorder (Mueser et al., 2000).

Age

Younger individuals are more likely than older ones to abuse substances, especially such drugs as cocaine and cannabis. Substance abuse often begins at a relatively early age and may precede the onset of the psychiatric disorder. In addition, substance abuse may precipitate an earlier onset of psychiatric illness (Addington & Addington, 1998; Breakey, Goodell, Lorenz, & McHugh, 1974; Mueser et al., 1990), propelling a person into treatment at an earlier age.

Education

Clients with dual disorders often have lower levels of educational attainment than other clients with severe mental illness. This may reflect either the effects of substance abuse problems that develop at an early age, or premorbid or prepsychotic cognitive symptoms of severe mental illness that interfere with the completion of secondary education. The relationship between substance abuse and lower levels of education tends to be stronger for drugs than for alcohol.

Marital Status

Marital status has often been found to be related to drug abuse, with clients with severe mental illness who have never married more likely to develop drug abuse or dependence than clients who have married.

Race

Race has been found to be related to the type of substance abused, although the specific correlates vary, depending on location and time. For example, in a study conducted in Philadelphia from 1984 to 1988, Mueser and colleagues (1990) reported that African American clients were more likely to have abused cannabis, whereas European American clients were more likely to have abused sedatives. In a follow-up study covering the years 1988 to 1990 in the same location, Mueser, Yarnold, and Bellack (1992) reported that African American clients were more likely to have abused cocaine than European American clients. Over this time period in Philadelphia, cocaine overtook cannabis as the most popular type of illicit drug abuse. Racial differences in the abuse of particular substances appear to reflect their availability, rather than specific preferences that are a function of race.

Rural–Urban Differences

Another characteristic related to substance abuse is whether the client lives in an urban or rural setting. Some drugs, such as cocaine, may be more difficult to obtain in rural settings, resulting in lower rates of abuse in rural than in urban settings (Mueser, Essock, Drake, Wolfe, & Frisman, 2001). However, the rates of alcohol abuse and cannabis abuse are quite consistent across rural and urban settings. Like racial differences, geographical differences in drug abuse probably reflect the market availability of different types of substances.

Clinical Correlates

Two clinical correlates are related to substance abuse in clients with severe mental illness: antisocial personality disorder (ASPD) and treatment nonadherence. We describe the evidence for these correlates below.

Antisocial Personality Disorder

Adult ASPD and its childhood precursor, conduct disorder, are important clinical correlates of substance abuse. Conduct disorder (according to DSM-IV criteria; American Psychiatric Association, 1994) refers to a pattern of behavior present before the age of 15, characterized by such behaviors as cruelty to animals, repeated truancy, lying, and frequent initiation of fights. ASPD, according to DSM-IV criteria, requires the presence of conduct disorder before the age of 15 as well as other behavior problems in adulthood, such as blatant disregard for the truth, initiation of fights, and lack of empathy for others. Both conduct disorder and ASPD are important predictors of substance abuse in the general population (Alterman & Cacciola, 1991; Robins, 1966).

As in the general population, ASPD has been found to be related to substance use disorders in clients with severe psychiatric illness (Caton et al., 1994, 1995; Mueser et al., 1999). Furthermore, among individuals with dual disorders, clients with ASPD tend to have an earlier age at onset of both psychiatric illness and substance use disorders, tend to have more severe substance abuse problems, are more likely to abuse a wide range of drugs, are more symptomatic, are more likely to have been arrested and spent time in jail, and have greater impairment in their independent living skills than are clients with dual disorders who do not have ASPD (Mueser, Drake, et al., 1997). Because of the severity of their substance abuse combined with vulnerability to numerous consequences, clients with dual dis-

orders and ASPD represent a high-need subgroup that may require more intensive monitoring and treatment in order to optimize outcomes.

Treatment Nonadherence

Poor adherence to recommended treatments is a common problem in clients with dual disorders (Coldham, Addington, & Addington, 2002; Miner, Rosenthal, Hellerstein, & Muenz, 1997; Weiss, Smith, Hull, Piper, & Hubbert, 2002), and medication nonadherence combined with substance abuse often results in relapses and rehospitalizations (Swartz et al., 1998b). Some clients report that they stop taking medications when they use drugs or alcohol, because they are concerned about interactions between their medications and substances. Others complain about the side effects of medication, and some studies have suggested that clients with dual disorders are more likely to experience medication side effects (Dixon, Weiden, Haas, Sweeney, & Frances, 1992; Salyers & Mueser, 2001; Voruganti, Heslegrave, & Awad, 1997). Similarly, many clients with a dual diagnosis have a checkered history of compliance with outpatient treatment programs, and are especially vulnerable to dropping out when their substance abuse is more severe. As we discuss in the next chapter, problems with adherence to pharmacological and psychosocial treatments in clients with dual disorders mean that outreach is often necessary to reengage such clients in treatment.

Historical Factors

Three aspects of client history are related to substance abuse: client premorbid social functioning, family history of substance use disorders, and exposure to intrapersonal trauma. We describe each of these factors below.

Premorbid Social Functioning

Premorbid social functioning refers to both the quantity and quality of social relationships a person achieved before developing a psychiatric illness—that is, the number of close friends, as well as depth and intimacy in close relationships. Psychiatric clients with drug use disorders tend to have had *better* premorbid social functioning than similar clients without drug abuse (Arndt, Tyrrell, Flaum, & Andreasen, 1992; Breakey et al., 1974; Cohen & Klein, 1970; Dixon, Haas, Weiden, Sweeney, & Frances, 1991; Tsuang, Simpson, & Kronfol, 1982). However, the evidence is mixed (e.g., Salyers & Mueser, 2001), and certainly some clients with dual disorders have poor premorbid social functioning.

The key to understanding the association between premorbid functioning and drug abuse in persons with severe mental illness may lie in understanding how people learn to use alcohol and drugs. Most individuals are introduced to different substances in social situations, by friends or family members; ongoing substance use also primarily occurs with other people. Indeed, learning to use drugs is a social process that develops gradually over time and with exposure to peer groups of users (Becker, 1953). Clients with poor premorbid social functioning are less likely to be exposed to substances (especially drugs) through peers, because of their lack of friendships. Consequently, these clients are less likely to develop substance use disorders than clients with better premorbid social functioning.

It should be noted that poor premorbid social functioning is an important predictor of a worse outcome in severe psychiatric disorders (Zigler & Glick, 1986). On the other hand, substance abuse can also worsen the course of mental illness, despite the good premorbid adjustment of some clients. This means that helping clients cut down on or stop using alcohol and drugs can substantially improve their prognosis (Zisook et al., 1992).

Family History of Substance Use Disorder

In the general population, there is abundant evidence showing that genetic factors play a role in vulnerability to substance use disorders (Anthenelli & Schuckit, 1992). Similarly, among clients with a severe mental illness, family history of substance use disorder is related to an increased risk of substance abuse (Gershon et al., 1988; Munsey, Galanter, Lifshutz, & Franco, 1992; Noordsy, Drake, Biesanz, & McHugo, 1994; Pulver, Wolyniec, Wagner, Moorman, & McGrath, 1989; Tsuang et al., 1982). In addition, among clients with dual disorders, family history of substance use disorder is related to more severe substance abuse problems (Noordsy et al., 1994). Thus family history is an important risk factor for substance abuse among clients with a severe and persistent mental illness.

Trauma and Posttraumatic Stress Disorder

Within the general population, prior exposure to trauma, including physical and sexual abuse in childhood and adulthood, is strongly related to substance use disorders (Dansky, Saladin, Brady, Kilpatrick, & Resnick, 1995; Deykin & Buka, 1997; Miller, Downs, & Testa, 1993; Triffleman, Marmar, Delucchi, & Ronfeldt, 1995; Wasserman, Havassy, & Boles, 1997; Yandow, 1989). Furthermore, the most common consequence of trauma, posttraumatic stress disorder (PTSD), is also related

to substance abuse in the general population (Kessler et al., 1997; Stewart, 1996). Similarly, among persons with severe mental illness, both a history of trauma and PTSD are strongly linked to substance use disorders (Briere, Woo, McRae, Foltz, & Sitzman, 1997; Carmen, Rieker, & Mills, 1984; Craine, Henson, Colliver, & MacLean, 1988; Goodman et al., 1999; Rose, Peabody, & Stratigeas, 1991; Rosenberg, Trumbetta, et al., 2001). This association is of particular concern, considering the high rate of trauma in the lives of people with severe psychiatric disorders (Carmen et al., 1984; Greenfield, Strakowski, Tohen, Batson, & Kolbrener, 1994; Hutchings & Dutton, 1993; Jacobson, 1989; Jacobson & Herald, 1990; Mueser, Goodman, et al., 1998; Rose et al., 1991; Ross, Anderson, & Clark, 1994) and the high rate of PTSD in this population (Cascardi, Mueser, DeGiralomo, & Murrin, 1996; Craine et al., 1988; McFarlane, Bookless, & Air, 2001; Mueser, Goodman, et al., 1998; Mueser, Salyers, et al., 2001; Neria, Bromet, Sievers, Lavelle, & Fochtmann, 2002; Switzer et al., 1999).

Although evidence indicates that PTSD often precedes the onset of substance use disorders (Chilcoat & Breslau, 1998; McFarlane, 1998; Stewart, 1996), research also suggests that substance abuse may lead to subsequent retraumatization (Hiday, Swartz, Swanson, Borum, & Wagner, 1999; Kilpatrick, Acierno, Resnick, Saunders, & Best, 1997; Lam & Rosenheck, 1998). Trauma related to substance abuse may occur for such reasons as use in unsafe situations, decreased inhibitions or impaired judgment, or trading sex for drugs. Persons with severe mental illness may be especially sensitive to these effects of substances, due to their substandard living conditions and relationships with marginalized persons, cognitive deficits, or lack of economic resources. The net result of this trauma may be a vicious cycle in which retraumatization due to substance abuse worsens PTSD, leading to more severe substance abuse and further retraumatization (Mueser, Rosenberg, Goodman, & Trumbetta, 2002).

THE IMPACT OF SUBSTANCE ABUSE ON PSYCHIATRIC ILLNESS

Substance abuse can produce a wide range of negative effects on persons with a major mental illness (Drake & Brunette, 1998). Clinically, substance abuse can lead to an increased risk of relapse and rehospitalizations (Hunt, Bergen, & Bashir, 2002; Linszen et al., 1996; Swofford, Kasckow, Scheller-Gilkey, & Inderbitzin, 1996). The strongest evidence linking symptom severity and substance use is the effect of alcohol on worsening depression. Risk of suicide is significantly increased in persons with a primary substance use disorder (Meyer, Babor, & Hesselbrock, 1988), as well as in individuals with schizophrenia, bipolar disorder, and major depression (Drake, Gates, Whitaker, & Cotton, 1985; Roy, 1986). This risk is compounded in persons who are dually diagnosed (Bartels, Drake, & McHugo, 1992; Torrey, Drake, & Bartels, 1996).

Dual disorders are associated with increased burden on family members, as well as interpersonal conflicts with relatives and friends (Dixon, McNary, & Lehman, 1995; Kashner et al., 1991; Salyers & Mueser, 2001). Financial problems often accompany substance abuse, as clients spend their money on drugs and alcohol rather than such essentials as food, clothing, and rent. In addition, substances or craving for substances can have disinhibitory effects that result in aggression and violence toward family, friends, treatment providers, and strangers (Rägänen et al., 1998; Steadman et al., 1998; Swartz et al., 1998b; Yesavage & Zarcone, 1983). The combined effects of substance abuse on family burden, interpersonal conflict, financial problems, and aggression and violence render clients with dual disorders highly vulnerable to housing instability and homelessness (Drake et al., 1989b; Goldfinger et al., 1999). Furthermore, substance abuse can result in legal encounters, for such reasons as possession of illegal drugs, disorderly conduct secondary to drug use, or theft or assault resulting from efforts to obtain drugs (Mueser, Essock, et al., 2001).

In addition to the clinical, social, and legal consequences of substance abuse, severe health consequences are also common. Substance abuse may contribute to risky behaviors, such as unprotected sex and sharing needles, that are associated with HIV and hepatitis infections (Cournos et al., 1991; Rosenberg, Goodman, et al., 2001; Rosenberg, Trumbetta, et al., 2001). As discussed above, clients with dual disorders are also more prone to victimization, as their judgment may be impaired by substances or their craving for them, and they are more likely to be exposed to others who may take advantage of them sexually or financially (Goodman et al., 2001). Last, alcohol and drug use may have direct effects on health (e.g., liver, heart, and lung damage), and can increase vulnerability to accidents. The net consequence of the negative effects of substance abuse on health are that, like individuals with primary substance use disorders, clients with dual disorders are vulnerable to early mortality and considerable morbidity as long as they continue to abuse substances.

In summary, substance abuse in clients with severe mental illness worsens a wide range of outcomes, including psychiatric outcomes, social functioning, and health. The effects of severe psychiatric disorders and substance abuse on overall functioning appear to be additive, and underscore the importance of reducing substance abuse in order to improve clients' long-term prognosis.

MODELS OF COMORBIDITY

As we have previously reviewed, persons with severe psychiatric illness are at much greater risk for developing a substance use disorder than people in the general population. What accounts for the very high rate of comorbidity of the psychiatric and substance use disorders? Understanding the factors that contribute to the high rate of comorbidity may provide clues useful in the treatment of dual disorders.

Kushner and Mueser (1993) have described four general types of models that might account for the high rate of comorbidity between substance abuse and psychiatric illness: *common-factor* models, *secondary substance abuse* models, *secondary psychopathology* models, and *bidirectional* models. These models are summarized in Figure 1.1. We briefly review the evidence supporting different models of comorbidity below. For a more in-depth reviews, see Mueser, Drake, and Wallach (1998) and Phillips and Johnson (2001). For disorder-specific reviews, see Blanchard, Brown, Horan, and Sherwood (2000) on schizophrenia; Kushner, Abrams, and Borchardt (2000) on anxiety disorders; Strakowski and DelBello (2000) on bipolar disorder; Swendsen and Merikangas (2000) on depression; and Trull, Sher, Minks-Brown, Durbin, and Burr (2000) on borderline personality disorder.

Common-Factor Models

Common-factor models propose that one or more factors independently increase the risk of both psychiatric illness and substance abuse. Three potential common factors have been the focus of some research—familial (genetic) factors, ASPD, and common neurobiological dysfunction—although many other factors are possible. If genetic factors, ASPD, or some other factor were found to independently increase the risk of both psychiatric and substance use disorders, this would support that particular common-factor model.

Familial (Genetic) Factors

One strategy for testing the role of familial (genetic) factors has been to examine family history of psychiatric illness and substance abuse in clients with dual disorders, clients with only a psychiatric disorder, clients with only a substance use disorder, and people with no psychiatric or substance use disorders. If genetic factors contribute

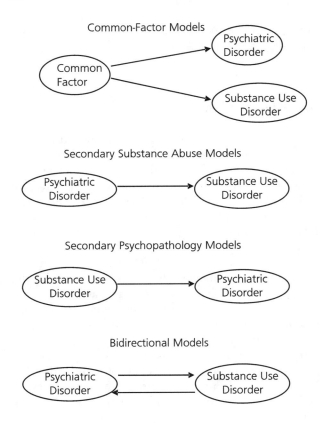

Common-Factor Models

Secondary Substance Abuse Models

Secondary Psychopathology Models

Bidirectional Models

FIGURE 1.1. Four types of theoretical models accounting for increased rates of comorbidity between psychiatric disorders and substance use disorders: common-factor models, secondary substance abuse models, secondary psychiatric disorder models, and bidirectional models.

to the increased comorbidity of psychiatric and substance use disorders, clients with a psychiatric disorder would be expected to have more relatives with substance use disorders than persons in the general population would be. Similarly, if genetic vulnerability is a common contributing factor, clients with a substance use disorder would be expected to have more relatives with psychiatric illnesses than people in the general population would be.

However, research has consistently failed to find this association. That is, clients with a psychiatric illness are *not* more likely than persons in the general population to have relatives with a substance use disorder, and likewise, clients with a substance use diagnosis are *not* more likely than persons in the general population to have relatives with psychiatric illness (Bidaut-Russell, Bradford, & Smith, 1994; Gershon et al., 1988; Maier, Lichtermann, Minges, Delmo, & Heun, 1995; Rimmer & Jacobsen, 1977). As previously mentioned, clients with dual disorders are more likely than individuals in

the general population to have relatives with either psychiatric illness or substance use disorders. These findings indicate that genetic vulnerabilities to psychiatric illness and substance use disorders are independent of each other and do not account for the increased rate of comorbidity between the two disorders.

Antisocial Personality Disorder

As noted earlier, ASPD is strongly linked to increased rates of substance use disorders (Kessler et al., 1997; Regier et al., 1990). Similarly, conduct disorder, the childhood precursor to ASPD, is a common antecedent problem in persons who later develop severe mental illness (Cannon et al., 1993; Robins, 1966). Furthermore, ASPD is more prevalent in clients with severe mental illness than in the general population (Bland, Newman, & Orn, 1987; Hodgins, Toupin, & Côté, 1996; Jackson, Whiteside, Bates, Rudd, & Edwards, 1991). Thus evidence suggests that ASPD is a common factor that may account for at least some of the excess in rates of comorbid substance abuse in clients with severe mental illness. These findings are also consistent with the observation that ASPD is more common in clients with dual disorders than in clients with severe mental illness and no substance abuse problems (Caton et al., 1994, 1995; Mueser et al., 1999).

Common Neurobiological Dysfunction

One common factor that could simultaneously increase risk of both psychiatric and substance use disorders is shared neurobiological dysfunction. All commonly abused substances exert their euphoric effects through stimulation of a dopamine-mediated reward system in the mesolimbic tract of the brain (Galanter & Kleber, 1999). Vulnerability to addiction is thought to be based in impaired activity in this reward system, leading individuals to use substances in order to stimulate positive feelings in which they are otherwise deficient. Psychotic symptoms, such as hallucinations and delusions, are thought to be based in excessive activity in the mesolimbic dopamine tracts (Stahl, 1996). This anatomical confluence suggests that a common factor leading to disordered mesolimbic activity could contribute to both disorders (Green, Zimmet, Strous, & Schildkraut, 1999). Chambers, Krystal, and Self (2001) have recently described a neurobiological basis for this model, hypothesizing that abnormalities in the hippocampus and frontal cortex not only create symptoms of schizophrenia, but facilitate positive reinforcing effects of drug reward and reduce inhibitory control over drug seeking.

Other Factors

Another example of a possible common factor is cognitive impairment. Individuals with mild cognitive impairments or "soft" neurological signs have been found to be more vulnerable both to psychiatric illnesses (Jones, Guth, Lewis, & Murray, 1994) and to substance use disorders (Berman & Noble, 1993). Yet another example is poverty, which is a well-established risk factor for the development of psychiatric disorders (Bruce, Takeuchi, & Leaf, 1991; Keith, Regier, & Rae, 1991) as well as substance abuse (Anthony & Helzer, 1991; Hawkins, Catalano, & Miller, 1992). Although these common factors are compelling, systematic research has not yet examined whether they can account for some of the high rate of comorbidity.

Secondary Substance Abuse Models

Secondary substance abuse models posit that high rates of comorbidity are the consequence of primary psychiatric illnesses leading to substance use disorders. Within this general model, three different models have been suggested: *psychosocial risk factor* models, the *supersensitivity* model, and *iatrogenic vulnerability to substance abuse*. These models are described below.

Psychosocial Risk Factor Models

Within general risk factor models, there are several different hypotheses to explain excess comorbidity. Perhaps the most widely known model is the *self-medication* hypothesis. According to this model (Khantzian, 1985, 1997), people with psychiatric disorders are more prone to substance abuse because they use drugs and alcohol to self-medicate disturbing psychiatric symptoms. For example, high levels of anxiety, depression, hallucinations, or apathy may lead someone to use substances in an effort to reduce these symptoms or cope with them more effectively.

The self-medication hypothesis has tremendous appeal. Almost all clients with dual disorders are able to point to some symptoms or negative emotional states that they report using drugs or alcohol to modify (Addington & Duchak, 1997; Carey & Carey, 1995; Dixon, Haas, Weiden, Sweeney, & Frances, 1990; Mueser, Nishith, Tracy, DeGirolamo, & Molinaro, 1995; Noordsy et al., 1991). However, these subjective reports provide only weak support for the hypothesis. Three types of evidence would provide stronger support for the self-medication hypothesis: (1) if clients with dual disorders described beneficial effects of substance use on symptoms; (2) if epidemiological studies suggested that clients with

particular psychiatric diagnoses were more prone to abusing specific types of substances; or (3) if psychiatric clients with more severe symptoms were more likely than less symptomatic clients to abuse substances.

Research does not provide support for any of these possibilities. In self-report studies, clients with dual disorders tend to report that substance use reduces social problems, insomnia, depressed mood, apathy/anhedonia, and a variety of other conditions, but they rarely report that specific substances alleviate specific symptoms of a particular mental disorder (e.g., Dixon et al., 1990; Noordsy et al., 1991). As reviewed earlier in this chapter (see section on "Lifetime Prevalence of Substance Abuse in Severe Mental Illness"), epidemiological studies do not suggest that different diagnostic groups prefer different types of substances; rather, they indicate that individuals with severe mental illness abuse the same substances as others in society, but at higher rates. Finally, amount or type of substance use does not appear to be related to severity or type of symptoms for clients with psychiatric disorders (Bernadt & Murray, 1986; Brunette, Mueser, Xie, & Drake, 1997; Hamera, Schneider, & Deviney, 1995; Mueser et al., 1990; Noordsy et al., 1991). Thus very limited research supports the self-medication hypothesis as an explanation for the increased comorbidity of substance use disorders in persons with severe mental illness.

These findings do not mean that the self-reports of clients with severe mental illness about why they use substances are unimportant. As we discuss in Chapter 5, clients' perceptions of the roles and effects of substance use, including coping motives, are important to assess and address in treatment (see also Graham, 1998). The cause of each individual client's substance use may vary. However, the available research on self-medication suggests that it alone does not account for the increased comorbidity of substance abuse in clients with severe mental illness.

A second type of psychosocial risk factor model is the *alleviation-of-dysphoria* hypothesis. This model is similar to the self-medication hypothesis, except that it states that substance use is motivated by (or correlated with) dysphoria, rather than specific symptoms. As severe mental illness is often associated with anxiety and depression related to symptoms, loss of functional abilities, support, financial well-being, and social stigma, an increased vulnerability to substance abuse would be an expected corollary. Some evidence provides support for this hypothesis. Client self-reports indicate that substance use often provides temporary relief from dysphoria (Addington & Duchak, 1997; Baigent, Holme, & Hafner, 1995; Spencer, Castle, & Michie, 2002; Warner et al., 1994). In addition, some research has reported that clients with schizophrenia and substance use disorders report higher levels of dysphoria than clients with schizophrenia but no substance use disorder (Blanchard et al., 1999; Scheller-Gilkey, Thomas, Woolwine, & Miller, 2002). Furthermore, children and adolescents with mood and anxiety disorders are at increased risk for the later development of substance use disorders (Birmaher et al., 1996). More research is needed to determine whether dysphoria is related to increased rates of dual disorders in other psychiatric illnesses.

Various other psychosocial risk factors due to severe mental illness may also contribute to vulnerability to substance use disorders. The *multiple-risk-factor* model subsumes the alleviation-of-dysphoria model, but also incorporates other risk factors as well. Examples of risk factors include poor interpersonal skills, cognitive impairment, school and vocational failure, lack of well-developed leisure and recreational activities, poverty, lack of adult role responsibilities, lack of structured and meaningful daily activities, association with deviant subgroups, and living in neighborhoods with high rates of drug availability. For example, individuals with severe mental illness often have poor social competence (Bellack, Morrison, Wixted, & Mueser, 1990) and perceive the social stigma of their mental illness (Corrigan & Penn, 1999). In order to gain social acceptance and to escape the effects of labeling, these individuals may gravitate toward other deviant groups in which alcohol and drug use is the norm (Dusenbury, Botvin, & James-Ortiz, 1989; Pandina, Labouvie, Johnson, & White, 1990). Indeed, many clients with dual disorders report that they use substances to facilitate social interactions with peers (Drake, Brunette, & Mueser, 1998).

Little direct research addresses the more general multiple-risk-factor model of comorbidity. However, it has important clinical implications. If the cognitive, emotional, interpersonal, vocational, societal, and financial consequences of severe mental illness can increase clients' risk for developing or sustaining substance use disorders, effective treatment of dual disorders may require clinicians to address those risk factors in order to successfully reduce or eliminate substance abuse.

The Supersensitivity Model

The supersensitivity model is an extension of the stress–vulnerability model of severe mental illness (Liberman et al., 1986; Nuechterlein & Dawson, 1984; Zubin & Spring, 1977). According to this model, biological vulnerability, determined by a combination of genetic and early environmental (e.g., perinatal) events, interacts with environmental stress either to precipitate the onset of a psychiatric disorder or to trigger relapses. In addi-

tion to the effects of stress on biological vulnerability, medications can decrease vulnerability, while use of alcohol or drugs may increase it. This sensitivity to the effects of substances may render clients with severe mental illness more likely to experience negative consequences from using relatively small amounts of alcohol or drugs. Thus this model suggests that what differentiate most clients with dual disorders from the general population are the negative consequences they experience from moderate amounts of substance use, rather than their use of excessive amounts of substances.

Several avenues of research support the supersensitivity model. First, clients with dual disorders tend to abuse lower quantities of substances than individuals with primary substance use disorders (Cohen & Klein, 1970; Crowley, Chesluck, Dilts, & Hart, 1974; Lehman, Myers, Corty, & Thompson, 1994), and consequently are less likely to develop physical dependence on substances (Corse, Hirschinger, & Zanis, 1995; Drake et al., 1990; Test, Wallish, Allness, & Ripp, 1989). Second, very small amounts of psychoactive substances have been found to provoke symptoms in clients with severe mental illness (Drake, Osher, & Wallach, 1989; Janowsky & Davis, 1976; Treffert, 1978). Third, as a result of this increased sensitivity to small amounts of substances, relatively few clients with severe mental illness are able to sustain moderate substance use over time without experiencing negative consequences. For example, in a longitudinal study of clients with schizophrenia, Drake and Wallach (1993) reported that fewer than 5% were able to sustain symptom-free drinking over time without experiencing negative consequences, in marked contrast to approximately 50% of the general population who drink alcohol over time without developing a disorder.

Thus, research provides support for the supersensitivity model, which hypothesizes that some excess comorbidity of severe psychiatric and substance use disorders can be accounted for by increased biological vulnerability to the effects of alcohol and drugs. An important clinical implication of this model is that relatively few clients with dual disorders may be able to sustain controlled substance use, because moderate use may either result in negative consequences or escalate into more severe substance abuse. Educating clients about their biological sensitivity to the effects of alcohol and drugs is an important component of integrated dual-diagnosis treatment.

Iatrogenic Vulnerability

As mentioned above, addictions are thought to be based in impaired activity in dopaminergic reward systems in the mesolimbic tract in the brain (Galanter & Kleber,

1999). Antipsychotic medications block some types of dopamine receptors in the brain in order to control psychotic symptoms (Stahl, 1996). Theoretically, this could accidentally lead to an underactive dopamine reward system and increased vulnerability to substance abuse. All conventional antipsychotic medications block dopamine type 2 (D2) receptors (Stahl, 1996). Some newer antipsychotic medications (e.g., clozapine, quetiapine, and olanzapine) bind to D2 receptors less powerfully, so that these medications do not completely block D2 receptors at therapeutic concentrations (Mansour, Meador-Woodruff, López, & Watson, 1998). This is thought to underlie the lower likelihood of dopamine-mediated movement disorders seen with these medications. If blockade of D2 receptors increases vulnerability to addictions, clients treated with newer antipsychotic agents should demonstrate lower rates of substance abuse. There is some evidence to suggest that this is the case (Drake, Xie, McHugo, & Green, 2000; Noordsy & O'Keefe, 1999; Noordsy, O'Keefe, Mueser, & Xie, 2001).

This model would also imply that clients with severe mental illness who are unmedicated should have lower rates of substance abuse. The fact that clients with bipolar disorder have high rates of substance abuse, but are less likely to be treated with dopamine-blocking (antipsychotic) medication than clients with psychotic disorders, suggests that this model alone cannot explain the excess comorbidity of substance abuse among clients with severe mental illness. We are not aware of any studies that address this question.

Secondary Psychopathology Models

Secondary psychopathology models of comorbidity are the exact opposite of secondary substance abuse models. That is, they posit that substance abuse leads to or triggers a long-term psychiatric disturbance that would not otherwise have developed. These models are difficult to test directly, because it is almost impossible to determine which individuals would have developed psychiatric illness had they not abused substances.

Research comparing clients who develop severe mental illness following substance abuse to clients with mental illness only or substance use disorders only reveals two general findings (Tsuang et al., 1982; Vardy & Kay, 1983). First, like clients with mental illness but no substance use disorder, individuals whose onset of mental illness follows substance abuse are more likely than clients with only substance abuse to have family members with psychiatric illness. This suggests that clients who use alcohol and drugs and then develop psychiatric disorders are biologically (genetically) vulnerable to mental illness. Second, clients who develop severe psy-

chiatric disorders after substance abuse are quite similar in their clinical presentation and course of illness to clients with severe mental illness but no substance abuse. This trend indicates that substance abuse does not precipitate a different or unique form of severe mental illness.

Thus severe psychiatric disorders tend to develop in substance-abusing individuals who are biologically vulnerable to mental illness, and once the psychiatric illness develops, these clients are indistinguishable from non-substance-abusing psychiatric clients. It is possible that substance abuse triggers mental illness in some individuals who, while biologically vulnerable to mental illness, would not have otherwise developed the disorder (Bühler, Hambrecht, Löffler, An der Heiden, & Häfner, 2002). The psychiatric illness could be precipitated by substance use, and maintained through the process of neuronal kindling or behavioral sensitization in the absence of subsequent substance abuse (Lieberman, Kinon, & Loebel, 1990; Sonne, Brady, & Morton, 1994; Strakowski, Sax, Setters, & Keck, 1996).

There are only limited data bearing on the theory. Some research does suggest that substance abuse, especially drug abuse, precipitates an earlier age at onset of severe mental illness (e.g., Addington & Addington, 1998; Mueser et al., 1990; Salyers & Mueser, 2001), although findings are not consistent on this relationship (see Drake & Brunette, 1998). Regarding bipolar disorder, clients whose alcohol use disorder came first have been found to have a later age of onset of bipolar disorder than those whose alcoholism came second (Strakowski, McElroy, Keck, & West, 1996; Winokur et al., 1995). In addition, lower familial rates of bipolar disorder have been found in clients whose alcoholism antedated their bipolar disorder (DelBello et al., 1999), as well as fewer mood episodes and a more rapid recovery, compared to clients with a first onset of bipolar disorder (Winokur et al., 1994, 1995). These findings may suggest that alcohol abuse can precipitate first episodes of mania in some persons who might not otherwise develop the disorder (Strakowski, DelBello, Fleck, & Arndt, 2000). More research is needed to evaluate this intriguing hypothesis.

Bidirectional Models

Bidirectional models stipulate that different factors may be involved in initiating and maintaining dual disorders. For example, a person who is biologically vulnerable to psychiatric illness may begin using substances while socializing with peers. This substance abuse could trigger the person's psychiatric disorder. Once the psychiatric illness has begun, the individual may continue to use substances as a strategy for coping with dysphoria, gaining social approval, and engaging in recreation, resulting in an intensification of the psychiatric disorder. Bidirectional models have not been directly examined in research, but are consistent with clinical observations that multiple factors are associated with the development and maintenance of dual disorders.

Summary of Comorbidity Models

There are many possible explanations for why clients with severe psychiatric disorders are so vulnerable to substance use disorders. No single model can explain all such comorbidity, and it is likely that multiple models contribute to comorbidity, both within and across clients. Research provides the strongest support for the supersensitivity model (i.e., biological vulnerability due to mental illness increases sensitivity to low quantities of alcohol and drugs) and the ASPD common-factor model (i.e., ASPD simultaneously increases risk for both mental illness and substance abuse). Multiple risk factors related to mental illness, such as dysphoria and unemployment, may contribute to comorbidity with substance abuse. Self-medication of symptoms does not appear to account for the high rates of comorbidity, although problems with dysphoria do appear to be more common in clients with dual disorders.

THE NATURAL HISTORY OF DUAL DISORDERS

Substance abuse is common among persons with a major mental illness, but what is the natural course of dual disorders in traditional mental health and substance abuse treatment systems? We begin this section with a brief review of what is known about the course of primary alcohol and drug use disorders. We then address research examining the longitudinal course of clients with dual disorders.

Course of Primary Substance Use Disorders

Vaillant's (1995) seminal work on the natural history of alcohol use disorders provides compelling evidence that for most clients, alcoholism is lifelong and is associated with a substantial risk for early mortality. Despite the overall negative (and often progressively deteriorating) long-term outlook for alcoholics, a cumulative proportion of individuals achieve abstinence, even in the absence of professional treatment. Vaillant estimated that approximately 3% of individuals with alcoholism stop abusing alcohol each year without the benefit of formal treatment programs, and that 1–2% of such individuals who are abstinent or who drink socially relapse back

into alcoholism. Among those who receive treatment, the estimated rate of recovery increases from approximately 3% to 6% yearly.

Less is known about the longitudinal course of primary drug use disorders (Simpson, Joe, Lehman, & Sells, 1986; Vaillant, 1983, 1988), although in general, the findings are compatible with those reported by Vaillant (1995) for alcoholism. In one of the largest and longest longitudinal studies published to date, Hser and colleagues (Hser, Anglin, & Powers, 1993; Hser, Hoffman, Grella, & Anglin, 2001) reported 24- and 33-year outcomes for 581 clients with narcotics addiction who had been admitted to the California Civil Addict Program between 1962 and 1964. The long-term outcome of these clients' drug use disorders revealed high mortality rates and a rate of spontaneous remission of drug abuse in the absence of treatment that was somewhat lower than that reported by Vaillant (1983) for individuals with alcoholism. At the end of the 24- and 33-year follow-up periods, 28% and 49% of the sample were dead, respectively, and only 19% and 22% had attained stable abstinence, respectively.

Interpretation of the negative long-term outcomes for the Hser and colleagues (1993, 2001) study needs to be tempered by recognition that the sample probably represented a more severely ill group than the persons studied by Vaillant (1983). For example, the clients studied by Hser and colleagues met criteria for a drug use disorder at an early age and were involved with the legal system. Despite differences across longitudinal studies in sample characteristics, research on the natural course of primary alcohol and drug use disorders indicates that these disorders are often chronic over a lifetime. There is considerable variation in clients' substance use behavior over time, but relatively few spontaneously attain stable abstinence, and clients are at increased risk of early mortality.

Course of Dual Disorders

Only limited research has examined the natural history of substance use disorders in people with severe mental illnesses. However, the available data suggest that the outcome of persons with dual disorders who receive services from the traditional, nonintegrated treatment system is bleak. Several prospective studies have shown increased rates of hospitalization over 1 year for psychiatric clients with a substance use disorder (Drake, Osher, & Wallach, 1989; Osher et al., 1994). Furthermore, even minimal levels of drinking (i.e., levels not considered alcohol abuse by clinicians) predicted rehospitalizations (Drake, Osher, & Wallach, 1989). One-year follow-up studies also show little remission of substance use disorders (Drake, Mueser, Clark, & Wallach,

1996). In line with the evidence indicating that substance abuse frequently precipitates disruptive behavior, symptom exacerbations, and rehospitalizations, the McKinney demonstration project on homeless mentally ill adults concluded that substance use disorders were the single most important factor contributing to housing instability in this population (Center for Mental Health Services, 1994).

Several longer-term studies also show low rates of spontaneous remission of substance abuse in clients with severe mental illness. Bartels, Drake, and Wallach (1995) conducted follow-up assessments 7 years after an initial evaluation on 148 out of 170 (86%) clients with severe mental illness. At baseline, 24% of the sample had an alcohol use disorder, and at follow-up 21% had such a disorder—a nonsignificant difference. Similarly, the rate of drug use disorder also did not change significantly from baseline (20%) to follow-up (17%). Despite these essentially negative findings, there was evidence that some clients were successful in recovering from substance use disorders. Over the 7 years, 25% of the clients with an alcohol use disorder at the initial evaluation (4% per year) and 35% of the clients with a drug use disorder (5% per year) experienced a remission of their substance use disorder. Furthermore, clients with substance abuse diagnoses were more likely to achieve a remission of their disorder than those with substance dependence diagnoses.

The lack of change in the overall rate of substance use disorders across the two assessments of the Bartels and colleagues (1995) study reflects the fact that some clients who did not meet criteria for a substance use disorder at the baseline assessment did so at the follow-up. Indeed, in two separate samples, Drake and Wallach (1993) found that clients with severe mental illness who appeared to be drinking moderately and nonabusively were likely to develop alcoholism over several years. This finding is also consistent with Cuffel and Chase's (1994) analysis of the stability of substance use disorders over 1 year in persons with schizophrenia, and with Chouljian and colleagues' (1995) results in a similar population tracked over a 1½-year period.

In summary, the information currently available about the natural history of dual disorders suggests a picture similar to that for persons with primary substance use disorders, but complicated by an increased risk for disruptive behavior, relapses and hospitalizations, and psychosocial problems. The relative stability of substance abuse over time in clients with dual disorders, coupled with the multitude of problems they typically experience in traditional treatment programs, underscores the importance of improving care through cohesive, integrative mental health and substance abuse treatment. In the next chapter, we discuss the limitations of traditional, nonintegrated treatment approaches for these clients. We also describe the core elements of integrated treatment programs, and introduce the concept of stages of treatment to guide clinicians in selecting and implementing interventions that are matched to clients' goals and motivational states, and therefore have the greatest promise for an optimal outcome.

SUMMARY

We have begun this chapter with a review of epidemiological research which documents that persons with severe psychiatric disorders are much more likely to also have substance use disorders than persons in the general population. Overall, approximately 50% of clients with severe mental illness have a lifetime substance use disorder, and 25–35% have an active substance abuse problem. Alcohol is the most commonly abused substance, followed by cannabis and cocaine. Higher rates of substance abuse tend to be found in clients who are male, young, less educated, and single. Substance abuse is more common in clients with better premorbid social functioning, ASPD, a family history of substance use disorders, and/or a history of trauma and PTSD. Substance abuse is associated with a wide range of negative outcomes, including relapses and rehospitalizations, violence, suicide, interpersonal problems, legal repercussions, health consequences, and higher treatment costs.

Different theories have been proposed to address the high comorbidity of severe mental illness and substance abuse. Two models have the greatest empirical support: the supersensitivity model (i.e., biological vulnerability due to mental illness lowers the threshold for experiencing negative consequences from relatively small quantities of substances), and the ASPD common-factor model (i.e., ASPD independently increases the risk of developing a severe mental illness and a substance use disorder). The self-medication model (i.e., high comorbidity is due to clients' attempts to treat their own symptoms with substances) does not appear to explain the high rate of substance use disorders in clients with severe psychiatric disorders.

The natural course of dual disorders in the traditional, nonintegrated treatment system is characterized by low rates of spontaneous remission of substance abuse. These findings, combined with the negative consequences of substance abuse, underscore the need for integrated mental health and substance abuse treatment services.

2

Principles of Integrated Treatment

In order to develop better treatment programs for persons with dual disorders, it is crucial first to understand the limitations of traditional approaches to the management of these disorders. Only then can clinicians and program developers appreciate the need for integrated mental health and substance abuse treatment, and the necessary ingredients of such programs. We begin this chapter with a review of the problems associated with traditional sequential or parallel treatment approaches to dual disorders, and address how these problems are overcome by the integration of mental health and substance abuse services.

Next, we address a core value that permeates the provision of all integrated treatment services: shared decision making. After reviewing the importance of developing a collaborative relationship with the client, we describe the principles of integrated treatment, including integration, comprehensiveness, assertiveness, reduction of negative consequences, a long-term perspective (time-unlimited service), motivation-based treatment, and multiple psychotherapeutic modalities. In our discussion of motivation-based treatment, we describe the stages of treatment for dual disorders, which provide a conceptual model for identifying clients' motivation to work on substance abuse and tailoring treatment based on their desire to change. We cite relevant research supporting the different components of integrated treatment for dual disorders. Chapter 20 contains a review of research on comprehensive integrated treatment programs. The principles of integrated treatment are included in a fidelity scale contained in Appendix A.

TRADITIONAL APPROACHES TO TREATING DUAL DISORDERS

There has been a historical division between mental health and substance abuse treatment services for many years. Consequently, two different treatment systems oversee and provide separate services for each type of disorder. Education, training, and credentialing procedures differ between the two systems, as do eligibility criteria for clients to receive services. As a result of the bureaucratic separation between mental health and substance abuse treatment services, two general approaches to the treatment of dual disorders have predominated until recently: the sequential treatment approach and the parallel treatment approach. Each of these approaches is associated with a variety of difficulties, including administrative and organizational problems, philosophical differences between providers, and clinical hurdles inherent to nonintegrated treatment, as summarized in Table 2.1 and discussed below.

Sequential Treatment

The *sequential treatment* approach is a common clinical justification for exclusion from treatment, rather than an explicit treatment model. In this approach, a client with dual disorders is not eligible for treatment in one part of a system until the other problem is resolved or suitably stabilized. This approach defends programmatic boundaries while ignoring individual clients' and larger systems' needs. For example, a man with schizophrenia and an alcohol use disorder is informed by a substance

TABLE 2.1. Disadvantages of Traditional Sequential and Parallel Treatment Approaches to Dual Disorders

Sequential treatment

- The untreated disorder worsens the treated disorder, making it impossible to stabilize one disorder without attending to the other.
- There is a lack of agreement as to which disorder should be treated first.
- It is unclear when one disorder has been "successfully treated" so that treatment of the other disorder can commence.
- The client is not referred for further treatment.

Parallel treatment

- Mental health and substance abuse treatments are not integrated into a cohesive treatment package.
- Treatment providers fail to communicate.
- Burden of integration falls on the client.
- Funding and eligibility barriers to accessing both treatments exist.
- Different treatment providers have incompatible treatment philosophies.
- A client "slips between the cracks" and receives no services, due to failure of either treatment provider to accept final responsibility for the client.
- Providers lack a common language and treatment methodology.

abuse counselor that his alcohol problem cannot be treated until his schizophrenia has been successfully stabilized, or that he cannot be treated with antipsychotic medication and participate in the substance abuse program. Alternatively, a woman with bipolar disorder and drug abuse who comes for treatment to a mental health professional is informed that mood-stabilizing medications for her bipolar disorder cannot be prescribed until her drug abuse ceases.

The most important problem with the sequential treatment approach is that it ignores the interactive and cyclical nature of dual disorders. Substance use disorders rarely remit spontaneously and often worsen the course of psychiatric illness. For example, stimulant abuse and heavy marijuana abuse can have potent effects on worsening the symptoms of schizophrenia (Serper et al., 1995; Treffert, 1978). Without attempts to address the substance abuse problem, successfully stabilizing these symptoms can be difficult or impossible. Furthermore, as psychiatric disorders become more severe, and clients experience greater amounts of distress, their substance abuse often worsens, leading to more substance abuse and even worse consequences. For example, acute mania is often associated with an increase in alcohol consumption (Bernadt & Murray, 1986), further worsening the manic episode. Unless the mania is

pharmacologically stabilized, the substance abuse may continue unabated.

In addition to clinical problems related to sequential treatment, there are organizational and administrative obstacles. The most common problem is that clients are never referred to other treatment, or when they are referred, they fail to follow through. Problems making referrals may be due to a clinician's belief that the "primary disorder" has not yet been sufficiently controlled, or lack of awareness of the other disorder's severity. Clients often do not follow through on treatment referrals for their other disorder because of lack of motivation, lack of awareness of the problem, or difficulties establishing new relationships with treatment providers.

Parallel Treatment

In the *parallel treatment* approach, mental health and substance use disorders are treated simultaneously by different professionals (often working for different agencies, but sometimes within the same agency). In theory, providers of separate services should attempt to coordinate care by making regular contacts and reaching consensus on the essential elements of the treatment plan. However, in practice, organizational and administrative problems usually preclude active collaboration between professionals (Kavanagh et al., 2000), and often there is little contact between mental health and substance abuse clinicians. Consequently, the burden of integration is placed on the client, who is usually ill equipped to handle this responsibility. Cognitive impairments associated with severe mental illness may make this task impossible for a client.

A variety of explanations can account for the poor integration of services in parallel treatment approaches. One important factor is that the mental health and substance abuse professions espouse different philosophies of treatment. Traditionally, in the United States, clinicians in the substance abuse treatment field have often employed emotionally charged, confrontational strategies in order to convince clients that they have a substance use disorder. These strategies include direct confrontation during individual and group sessions, as well as the practice of conducting an "intervention," in which various family members and friends are convened at a surprise meeting with the client to express their concern over his or her substance abuse and the importance of addressing this problem. In contrast, among mental health professionals there is widespread acceptance, supported by evidence (Butzlaff & Hooley, 1998), that emotionally charged, confrontational interactions can have deleterious effects on clients with severe mental disorders: They may precipitate social withdrawal, symptom relapses, rehospitalizations, and even violence.

Another difference between mental health and substance abuse treatment professionals lies in their attitudes toward "enabling behaviors." Mental health services attempt to help clients achieve and maintain stable housing, benefits, and social networks, whereas traditional substance abuse services often view such services as "enabling" clients by insulating them from the natural consequences of their substance abuse. These differences may make it more difficult for clinicians in different agencies who are attempting to provide parallel treatment to collaborate actively, as each group of clinicians retains an allegiance to its home agency. In addition, even well-intentioned efforts by clinicians to integrate mental health and substance abuse treatment within the same agency may by thwarted by differences in philosophy that translate into contradictory messages to clients, reducing the prospects of clinical improvement.

In addition to differences in philosophy, the parallel treatment approach often involves funding barriers that prevent access to treatment for one or the other of the disorders. For example, some treatment systems specifically prohibit clients from utilizing mental health and substance abuse services simultaneously. Furthermore, systems that employ parallel treatment methods often rely on the clients to seek services from both mental health and substance abuse treatment providers. As just discussed in the section on "Sequential Treatment," clients often fail to follow through on seeking treatment, due to poor motivation, lack of awareness, or difficulties establishing relationships with treatment providers. An unfortunate result of this policy is that some individuals fail to receive treatment for either disorder—"falling between the cracks" of mental health and substance abuse systems, as providers deem them inappropriate for their type of service. Thus many people with dual disorders fail to receive care for one or both of their disorders in systems that provide these services in a parallel fashion.

Poor Outcomes in Traditional Dual-Disorder Treatments

By the end of the 1980s, reviews of traditional dual-disorder treatment services had documented the problems described above and others (El-Guebaly, 1990; Polcin, 1992; Ridgely, Goldman, & Willenbring, 1990; Wallen & Weiner, 1989). In addition, there has been growing evidence showing a poor prognosis for clients with dual disorders treated with traditional sequential and parallel approaches (Drake, Mueser, et al., 1996;

Havassy, Shopshire, & Quigley, 2000), and suggesting higher rates of costly service utilization (Bartels et al., 1993; Dickey & Azeni, 1996). As these facts became more widely recognized, new programs began to be developed, with the primary aim of integrating mental health and substance abuse services in order to improve the long-term outcome of persons with dual disorders.

INTEGRATED MENTAL HEALTH AND SUBSTANCE ABUSE TREATMENT

Integrated treatment programs can overcome many of the disadvantages of traditional sequential and parallel approaches to dual disorders. First, organizational and administrative lapses are effectively eliminated with integrated treatment, because no coordination between different service providers is required; both mental health and substance abuse services are provided by the same team. Second, clinical problems related to treating one disorder first and the other disorder second are avoided with integrated treatment, as both disorders are viewed as "primary" and are targeted for concurrent treatment. Third, conflict over different philosophical perspectives of mental health and substance abuse professionals on treating dual disorders is minimized when the clinicians work side by side, on the same treatment team, and preferably for the same agency. Although philosophical differences between clinicians may exist, the need to work collaboratively as a team, and to present a consistent message to clients, often leads to compromises and gradual shifts toward shared perspectives and a unified treatment approach.

The health care delivery system has moved rapidly toward endorsing integrated treatment approaches for clients with dual disorders (Center for Mental Health Services, 1994; Osher & Drake, 1996; Smith & Burns, 1994; Woody, 1996). Various different integrated treatment programs have been developed to meet the needs of these clients (Brady et al., 1996; Carey, 1996; Drake, Antosca, Noordsy, Bartels, & Osher, 1991; Kavanagh, 1995; Minkoff, 1989; Osher & Kofoed, 1989; Rosenthal et al., 1992; Sitharthan et al., 1999; Ziedonis & Fisher, 1996). Many of these treatment programs share common values, as well as fundamental organizational, assessment, and treatment components. The balance of this chapter introduces and then reviews the essential components of integrated programs, based on our experiences and those of our colleagues (Drake, Bartels, Teague, Noordsy, & Clark, 1993; Drake, Osher, & Wallach, 1989; Drake, Wallach, & Hoffman, 1989; Mueser, Drake, & Noordsy, 1998).

THE COMPONENTS OF INTEGRATED TREATMENT AND HOW THEY WORK TOGETHER

As noted at the beginning of the chapter, effective treatment for dual disorders is based on the core value of shared decision making, and it incorporates the following core components: integration of services, comprehensiveness, assertiveness, the reduction of negative consequences, a long-term perspective (time-unlimited services), motivation-based treatment, and the availability of multiple psychotherapeutic modalities. Each of these components represents a different dimension of integrated treatment; together, they result in effective treatment for clients with dual disorders.

The *integration of services* represents the organizational dimension of treatment: Services for both mental illness and substance abuse need to be provided simultaneously by the same clinicians within the same organization, in order to avoid gaps in service delivery and to ensure that both types of disorders are treated effectively. *Comprehensiveness* addresses the scope of dual-disorder interventions: Services are directed not only at the problem of substance abuse, but at the broad array of other areas of functioning that are frequently impaired in clients with dual disorders, such as housing, vocational functioning, ability to manage the psychiatric illness, and family/social relationships. *Assertiveness* addresses the location of service provision and how clients are engaged in treatment: Effective treatment programs for clients with dual disorders do not wait for (often reluctant) clients to seek treatment on their own, but instead use assertive outreach and legal mechanisms to involve them in treatment. The *reduction of negative consequences* represents the philosophical dimension of integrated treatment: Given the damaging impact of dual disorders on the lives of clients, the first and foremost goal of clinicians is to reduce the harmful effects. This should be done without judging them or imposing clinicians' own personal values on them regarding causes or moral responsibility for these consequences.

The *long-term perspective* addresses the need for *time-unlimited services*: Artificial constraints on the duration of services can prematurely terminate intervention for clients with dual disorders who would otherwise improve with continued integrated treatment. The *motivation-based treatment* component orients interventions to the clients' desire to change their behavior. This needs to be done to avoid unnecessary and potentially destructive conflict, and to maximize treatment gains through collaborative work. *Multiple psychotherapeutic modalities* provide psychological treatment services for dual disorders in as many formats as needed (and several usually are). Individual, group, and family therapy modalities are all useful approaches to treating dual disorders, each with its own unique advantages.

The ability to incorporate each of these core components into treatment is critical for achieving the best possible outcomes for clients with dual disorders, and inattention to any one component can undermine the overall effectiveness of a treatment program. A narrow focus on substance abuse, and neglect of other important areas of functioning (e.g., housing, work, social relationships, quality of life), can make it difficult or impossible for clients to develop lifestyles worth living without alcohol and drugs. Lack of integration of treatment can result in clients' receiving services for one type of disorder but not the other, or receiving services from clinicians whose efforts are inconsistent with one another. Lack of assertiveness can make a program unable to engage clients, leading to continued substance abuse and dismal outcomes. Inattention to reducing the negative consequences of substance abuse can likewise condemn clients to poor outcomes (including victimization, disease, and mortality) and can squander important opportunities for engaging clients in treatment. Lack of a long-term perspective can result in premature termination of effective services and a consequent reversal of treatment gains. Poor attention to motivation-based treatment can lead to ineffective services as clinicians attempt to change the substance use behavior of clients who are not yet motivated to address those problems. Unavailability of multiple treatment modalities can limit the flexibility of a treatment program for using different strategies to help clients understand the effects of substances on their lives, reduce their substance use, and make progress in other important life areas.

Thus the different components of treatment work in harmony by addressing different dimensions of service delivery, including organization, focus, locus, philosophy, and specific treatment modalities. Because integrated treatment programs are flexible, with treatment planning and intervention based on clients' unique needs, effective programs may differ in the specific array of services they offer. However, organization commitment and resources, quality assessment, and an adequate range of services (including all different treatment modalities) are required to optimize client functioning. This means that while integrated programs will differ, the more components of integrated treatment that are incorporated into a program, the better the outcomes are likely to be. We now focus in more detail on each of these dimensions of integrated treatment, starting with the core value of shared decision making.

SHARED DECISION MAKING

At the core of integrated treatment is *shared decision making* among all critical stakeholders. A major premise of integrated treatment is that clients with dual disorders, like those with either severe mental illness or substance use disorders, are capable of playing a vital role in the management of their disorders and in making progress toward achieving their goals. Such a philosophy is consistent with an emphasis on consumerism, illness self-management, community integration, quality of life, rehabilitation, and recovery for persons with severe mental illness (Anthony, 1993; Copeland, 1997; Deegan, 1992; Fisher, 1992). In addition, the emphasis on self-help is consistent with a long tradition in the substance abuse field.

Shared decision making also recognizes the critical role that many families play in the lives of persons with dual disorders. Since family members are often involved as caregivers for clients with severe mental illness, and serve to buffer them from many of the negative effects of stress, families also need to be engaged and involved in making decisions (Clark, 1996). Family members may also suffer the negative effects of dual disorders in a loved one, and decreasing this stress and tension is often critical to maintaining their support and involvement with the client (Hatfield & Lefley, 1987, 1993).

For a number of medical illnesses, shared decision making has resulted in better educated clients, greater treatment adherence, higher satisfaction with care, and improved biomedical outcomes (Wennberg, 1991). Similar benefits occur in mental health care. Making decisions collaboratively requires that clients and their families have as much information as possible about illnesses and their treatment to facilitate better decision making. Providers accept the responsibility of getting information to clients and their families so that they can become more effective participants in the treatment process.

Shared decision making maximizes the chances that treatment plans will be followed up, as different stakeholders are involved in selecting and implementing solutions to identified problems that they believe will work. Over the long run, clients and families become more able to advocate for themselves and to work collaboratively with professionals. The goal is for people with dual disorders to become responsible for recognizing and managing their own illnesses, using their family members for support and professionals for specific consultations and treatment. Clients and families are more satisfied with care as they learn more and take responsibility for implementing treatment plans that they understand and have chosen. Shared decision making assumes that more knowledge, greater choice of treatment, increased responsibility for self-management, and

higher satisfaction with care will produce better outcomes, including less severe symptoms, better social and vocational functioning, and a better quality of life.

CASE EXAMPLE

Sharon was a 30-year-old woman with bipolar disorder and alcohol dependence. She had been in treatment for 5 years, and although she took her prescribed medications, she continued to drink and was repeatedly hospitalized for both severe depression and mania. Her case manager recognized that alcohol was a problem for her, and transferred her to the dual-diagnosis treatment team at the agency. Sharon's new case manager began to conduct outreach with Sharon at her home, where she lived with her parents. He spent several meetings educating her family about alcoholism and describing how substances like alcohol interact with mental illness. Over time, Sharon and her parents were able to see that her frequent hospitalizations were related to her drinking. Sharon planned with her case manager to attend Alcoholics Anonymous (AA) meetings and a substance abuse group at the agency. After a few months of regular attendance and some reductions in her alcohol use, Sharon was ready to try a period of abstinence. She worked collaboratively with her case manager to develop a treatment plan that focused on maintaining her abstinence and included obtaining a part-time job.

In addition to the overriding value of shared decision making, effective integrated intervention for dual disorders requires attention to the core set of treatment components introduced earlier. Each of these components is operationalized in a behaviorally anchored fidelity scale, which is included in Appendix A. We discuss these components in more detail below.

Integration

An *integrated* treatment program is a program in which the same clinician (or team of clinicians) provides treatment for mental illness and substance use disorders at the same time. As treatment for severe mental illness is typically provided by multidisciplinary treatment teams that include a range of different professionals (e.g., psychiatrist, nurse, master's-level clinicians, case managers), treatment for dual disorders will also most often be given by teams of professionals rather than a single clinician (see Chapter 3 for a discussion of the composition and staffing of dual-disorder treatment teams). Clinicians on these teams assume the responsibility of integrating the treatments so that interventions are selected, modified, combined, and tailored for each specific client. Because the educational and prescriptive message is integrated, there is no need for the client to reconcile two messages, and the approach is seamless. There is ample evidence supporting the effects of integrated over nonintegrated dual-disorder treatment (Barrowclough et al., 2001; Carmichael et al., 1998; Drake, Yovetich, Bebout, Harris, & McHugo, 1997).

In addition to the integration of services, it is important to integrate several other aspects of treatment, including assessment, treatment planning, and crisis planning. *Integrated* assessment is critical to understanding the interactions between mental illness and substance abuse. Substance abuse worsens the outcome of severe mental illness; yet clients often continue using substances for other reasons related to their mental illness, such as coping with symptoms or increasing social contact and acceptance. Identifying how substance abuse and mental illness interact can lead to treatment plans that specifically address these areas. For example, clients whose substance abuse is related to coping with persistent symptoms or facilitating social opportunities may benefit from learning more effective coping strategies or developing other social outlets.

People with dual disorders are at increased risk for experiencing crises, such as substance abuse or mental health relapses, housing instability and homelessness, and legal problems. Assessment and treatment planning needs to take these increased risks into account, and develop crisis plans for responding to problems of either disorder. At a minimum, such plans should identify the early warning sings of relapse for any disorder in remission, should consider the interactions between the client's disorders, and should specify the steps to be taken in the event of a crisis (such as whom to contact and where to go).

Comprehensiveness

Although a major goal of integrated treatment is to decrease or altogether eliminate substance abuse, achieving this goal usually involves more than changing behaviors directly related to substance use. To reduce substance abuse or to achieve the long-term goal of abstinence, individuals must not only decrease or stop using alcohol and other drugs, but must also develop a lifestyle that is no longer centered around substance use. Decreasing or eliminating one's involvement in substance use for more than a few days is difficult precisely because this involves changing habits, activities, expectations, beliefs, friendships, and ways of dealing with internal distress—indeed, almost everything about one's life.

Individuals with dual disorders typically have a wide range of needs, such as finding work or other meaningful activity; improving the quality of family and social relationships; developing a capacity for independent living, leisure, and recreation; and developing skills for managing anxiety, depression, and other negative moods. Integrated treatment programs need to be *comprehensive*, because the recovery process occurs longitudinally in the context of making many life changes. In addition, even before clients have acknowledged their substance abuse or developed motivation to reduce alcohol and drug use, they can make progress by improving their skills and supports. These improvements can increase clients' hopefulness about making positive changes and facilitate their subsequent efforts to change their destructive involvement with substances.

Comprehensive treatment requires comprehensive assessment that spans the range of areas affected by mental illness and substance abuse. Such assessment requires the evaluation of psychosocial history; symptoms; history of psychiatric and other emergency/crisis services; social and vocational functioning; leisure and recreational activities; family contact and other social supports; housing and safety, independent living skills; medical needs; and insight into/understanding of the mental illness. It also involves the evaluation of history of substance use and abuse; treatment history; current/recent use of alcohol and specific drugs (including patterns and amounts of use); social context, motives, and consequences of use; insight into substance abuse problems; and motivation to address substance abuse.

Seven types of services need to be considered to determine the comprehensiveness of a treatment program: residential services, an appropriate model of case management, supported employment, family psychoeducation, social skills training, training in illness management, and pharmacological treatment. The rationale for including each type of these services is provided below.

Residential Services

Clients living in environments replete with substance use and abuse face special challenges in achieving sobriety (Trumbetta, Mueser, Quimby, Bebout, & Teague, 1999). As elaborated in Chapter 16, in order to protect clients from either street life or substance-abusing social networks, residential services are needed that do not exclude clients with ongoing substance abuse (Osher & Dixon, 1996). Research indicates that integrated dual-disorder services attending to the residential needs of clients result in better housing and substance abuse outcomes than traditional, nonintegrated services do (Drake et al., 1997). Furthermore, there is evidence that long-term residential treatment for clients with dual disorders improves substance abuse outcomes more than short-term programs do (Brunette, Drake, Woods, & Hartnett, 2001).

Case Management: The Assertive Community Treatment Model

The *assertive community treatment (ACT) model* of case management was developed to meet the needs of clients with severe mental illness who have histories of very high service utilization (e.g., multiple or prolonged psychiatric hospitalizations) or extremely impaired psychosocial functioning. The essence of the ACT model is that instead of waiting for clients to come to the clinic for treatment, most services are delivered to them in the community, in their natural living settings. The ACT model is characterized by the following: low clinician-to-client caseload ratios (1:10, rather than the usual 1:30 or higher in standard case management); shared caseloads across clinicians, rather than individual caseloads; most services provided in the community; most services provided directly by the ACT team and not brokered to other service providers; and 24-hour availability of the ACT team (Allness & Knoedler, 1998; Stein & Santos, 1998).

Extensive research on the ACT model documents that for clients who frequently utilize hospital and emergency services, it is effective at reducing hospitalizations, stabilizing housing, decreasing symptom severity, and improving quality of life (Bond, Drake, Mueser, & Latimer, 2001; Mueser, Bond, Drake, & Resick, 1998). Research on ACT-delivered integrated treatment for clients with dual disorders indicates modest benefits in terms of substance abuse and some quality-of-life outcomes, compared to integrated treatment provided by standard clinical case management (Drake, McHugo, et al., 1998). Clients with dual disorders who have frequent hospitalizations or severe psychosocial impairments may benefit from ACT-level case management.

Supported Employment

Helping clients with dual disorders develop meaningful lives is an important goal of treatment. One common goal of clients is to obtain competitive work. The approach to vocational rehabilitation for clients with severe mental illness that has the strongest evidence is *supported employment*. As elaborated in Chapter 18, supported employment programs emphasize helping clients obtain competitive jobs in the community (working alongside nondisabled workers) by minimizing prevocational assessment and training, emphasizing rapid job search based on client preferences, and providing follow-along supports to help clients maintain jobs or move on to other jobs (Becker & Drake, 1993). Multiple controlled studies show that supported employment is more effective at improving vocational outcomes in clients with severe mental illness than other approaches

are (Bond, Becker, et al., 2001; Bond, Drake, Mueser, & Becker, 1997). Furthermore, even clients with dual disorders are capable of getting and keeping jobs in supported employment programs (Sengupta, Drake, & McHugo, 1998).

Family Psychoeducation

Families play a crucial role in providing support to clients with dual disorders (Clark, 1996), and such support is associated with improvements in substance abuse outcomes (Clark, 2001). *Family psychoeducation* for severe mental illness has been shown to improve outcomes (Dixon et al., 2001), and family intervention is associated with better outcomes for substance use disorders as well (Stanton & Shadish, 1997). As described in Chapters 13–15, family psychoeducation is aimed at teaching families (including clients) basic information about dual disorders and the principles of their treatment, as well as reducing stress and improving coping. Psychoeducational handouts for families are included in Appendix B.

CASE EXAMPLE

Sandy, a 35-year-old married woman with diagnoses of major depression with psychotic features and posttraumatic stress disorder, had a long history of alcohol abuse with occasional suicide attempts. Sandy's episodes of drinking were usually precipitated by exacerbations of her depression and anxiety, interpersonal conflicts with her husband, or both. In addition to providing Sandy and her husband with information about the interactions among alcohol abuse, depression, and anxiety, her comprehensive treatment also involved teaching her cognitive-behavioral strategies for managing her anxiety and depression (e.g., relaxation strategies, challenging self-defeating thoughts that led to depression) and engaging her and her husband in couple counseling to help them develop more effective skills for handling their conflicts. This approach to treatment was successful in decreasing Sandy's reliance on alcohol during times of distress and conflict, and enlisting her husband's support in her pursuit of treatment goals.

Social Skills Training

As described in detail in Chapter 11, *social skills training* involves teaching new interpersonal skills through the systematic application of social learning theory (e.g., modeling, role playing, positive feedback, etc.). Research indicates that such training for clients with severe mental illness is effective at improving social functioning (Dilk & Bond, 1996; Heinssen, Liberman, & Kopelowicz, 2000). This is of crucial importance, considering that impairments in social functioning are defining characteristics of some severe mental illnesses (e.g., schizophrenia; American Psychiatric Association, 1994), and that poor social functioning predicts a worse course of mental illness (Rajkumar & Thara, 1989; Strauss & Carpenter, 1977). Furthermore, social skills training has been found to be an effective intervention for persons with substance use disorders (Miller et al., 1995; Monti, Abrams, Kadden, & Cooney, 2002). Skills training may be an especially important treatment strategy for clients with dual disorders, because of the important role social relationships play in maintaining ongoing substance abuse (Trumbetta et al., 1999), and clients' need to develop new relationships with persons who do not abuse substances if they are to be successful in achieving sobriety.

Training in Illness Management

Illness management programs have been developed to teach clients with severe mental illness strategies for managing their disorders in collaboration with others and getting on with their lives (Ascher-Svanum & Krause, 1991; Copeland, 1997; Weiden, 1999). This training typically incorporates a variety of methods, including psychoeducation about the mental illness and its management; teaching the recognition of early warning signs of relapse and the development of a relapse prevention plan; coaching in methods for taking medication as prescribed; and teaching strategies for coping with persistent symptoms and pursuing personal goals. Research on teaching illness management skills indicates that it is effective at improving clients' knowledge about mental illness, improving medication adherence, and reducing relapses and symptom severity (Mueser, Corrigan, et al., 2002). A central goal of treating clients with dual disorders is to improve their ability to manage their psychiatric disorder through such strategies as training in illness management.

Pharmacological Treatment

Antipsychotic, antidepressant, and mood-stabilizing medications continue to be mainstays in the treatment of severe mental illness, with more effective and more benign new medications becoming available every year. Abundant research documents the effects of psychotropic medications on reducing symptom severity and relapses in clients with severe mental illness (Schatzberg & Nemeroff, 1998). As described in Chapter 19, it is crucial that clients with dual disorders (including those clients with active substance abuse) have access to pharmacological treatment for their mental illness. Furthermore, clients with dual disorders may ben-

efit from trials of medications that decrease substance abuse, such as disulfiram for alcoholism and naltrexone for alcoholism or opiate abuse.

Assertiveness

Clients with dual disorders often drop out of treatment, due to the chaos in their lives, cognitive impairment, low motivation, and hopelessness (Miner et al., 1997; Swartz et al., 1998a). An *assertive* approach to treatment recognizes that clinicians cannot passively wait for clients to demonstrate the initiative and motivation to seek out dual-disorder treatment on their own; rather, clinicians must make every effort possible to actively engage reluctant clients in the process of treatment. One important assertive strategy is to reach out to clients and provide them with services in their natural living environments—such as their homes, local parks, restaurants, or homeless shelters—rather than in the clinic. By connecting with clients in their natural environments and providing practical assistance with immediate goals defined by the clients (such as housing, medical care, crisis management, and legal aid), assertive outreach is a means of developing trust and a working alliance between clinicians and clients.

In addition to facilitating engagement, assertive outreach is helpful in monitoring and improving the course of dual disorders. By meeting with clients regularly in their own natural environments, clinicians are able to obtain more information about their day-to-day functioning, and about the social and environmental factors that may influence the outcome of dual disorders. Furthermore, assertive outreach can provide clinicians with an important opportunity to enhance clients' adherence to their prescribed medications. Medication is important in stabilizing the psychiatric symptoms of clients with dual disorders, but many clients have difficulty following through on taking prescribed medications. Rather than relying on clients' going to a pharmacy for medication and taking it, clinicians can deliver medications to the homes of clients, watch them take some or all doses, and teach them how to incorporate taking medication into their usual routines (Mueser, Corrigan, et al., 2002). Without assertive outreach, many clients are never effectively engaged in integrated treatment and continue to suffer severe symptoms due to poor medication adherence. Assertive outreach is a core component of several dual-disorder programs supported by research (Drake et al., 1997; Drake, McHugo, et al., 1998).

Assertive outreach to clients with dual disorders requires sufficient staffing to account for clinicians' increased travel time. The average staffing required to accomplish these tasks is a ratio of 1 clinician to 30 clients.

Lower clinician-to-client ratios may be required (e.g., 1:15 or lower) if the clients are extremely impaired, or if they have been experiencing especially problematic consequences of their substance abuse (e.g., involvement with the criminal justice system or homelessness). Further consideration of the staffing required to deliver integrated dual-disorder services is provided in Chapters 3 and 6.

CASE EXAMPLE

Jerome, a 23-year-old client with a diagnosis of schizophrenia and severe cocaine and marijuana abuse, took his antipsychotic medication inconsistently and refused to come to the mental health center for appointments other than with his psychiatrist; he frequently missed even these meetings. His substance abuse, compounded by medication nonadherence, resulted both in housing instability and in multiple relapses and rehospitalizations. Soon after Jerome was assigned to an integrated dual-disorder program, members of his treatment team began to conduct brief daily visits to his residence. During these visits, clinicians spent time getting to know Jerome better, assessing his immediate needs, and providing him with medication that he took during the visit. These visits helped to engage Jerome in treatment, while stabilizing some of his most severe symptoms.

Although the term *assertiveness* frequently refers to outreach for the purposes of treatment engagement and service provision, the term may also be applied to the use of other legal mechanisms for involving clients in treatment. Clients with dual disorders often experience money problems, legal problems, and frequent hospitalizations, which may meet criteria for using coerced or involuntary interventions to involve them in treatment. As addressed in Chapter 17, thoughtful coerced or involuntary interventions can make a critical difference in engaging clients with dual disorders in treatment and ensuring ongoing access to them. A variety of such interventions may be available to clinicians, and effective treatment involves using those interventions appropriate to each client's needs. In addition to the use of civil commitment to the hospital when clients present a grave danger to themselves or others, the most common types of involuntary or coerced interventions include outpatient commitment to treatment (or, alternatively, discharge from a hospital that is conditional upon participation in outpatient treatment); payeeships; coordination with child welfare and protective services; and coordination with parole or probation officers. Though research on the effects of involuntary interventions on clients with dual disorders is limited, evidence suggests that outpatient commitment can increase treatment adherence and reduce rehospitalizations, vio-

lence, and victimization in clients with severe mental illness (Hiday, Swartz, Swanson, Borum, & Wagner, 2002; Swanson et al., 2000; Swartz et al., 1999, 2001).

Reduction of Negative Consequences

An important goal in the treatment of persons with dual disorders is to *reduce the negative consequences* of their substance abuse. This goal is based on the fact that many people with addictions lack the motivation to endorse abstinence early in treatment, or even to decrease their use of alcohol or drugs; yet significant gains can be made initially by focusing treatment on reducing the negative consequences of alcohol and drug use (Denning, 2000; Des Jarlais, 1995; Marlatt, 1998). Furthermore, in the absence of motivation to work on substance abuse, clients' continued use of alcohol and drugs may pose serious threats to their physical and psychological well-being. The essence of focusing on reducing the harmful effects of substance abuse is to protect clients from the most dire consequences of their substance use, while developing a good working alliance with them that can ultimately help them perceive the negative effects of substance abuse and develop the motivation to address it (Marlatt & Witkiewitz, 2002).

Reducing the negative effects of substance abuse is especially important early in treatment with clients with dual disorders, when substance abuse tends to be most destructive and may impair insight, and clients are least motivated to reduce their use of substances. Examples of strategies for reducing the negative effects of substances include supplying clean needles to a client who shares needles when using drugs with others; securing stable housing; limiting access to money for purchasing substances; accessing food or vitamins; teaching safe-sex methods for persons who exchange sex for money or drugs; and obtaining needed medical treatment (e.g., for infectious diseases, such as hepatitis C).

Attempting to reduce the negative consequences of substance abuse sometimes leads to debate among clinicians about whether such efforts protect clients from the natural consequences of their substance abuse, and actually impede the long-term goal of encouraging clients to address their substance abuse. Sometimes it is argued that people with substance use disorders need to "hit rock-bottom" before they become truly motivated to work on their substance abuse problems. However, considering the negative consequences of substance abuse, delaying until clients with dual disorders "hit rock-bottom" is tantamount to sitting back and watching as they experience relapses and rehospitalizations, contract infectious diseases, fail to receive proper attention for medical conditions, become violent, are victimized, become homeless or imprisoned, or even die. In addition, exacerbations of symptoms and cognitive impairment from excessive use of substances may impair clients' ability to perceive and learn from the negative consequences of their substance use behavior. The effects of unchecked substance abuse on clients with severe mental illness are so drastic that methods for reducing the negative consequences of substance abuse at the earliest possible time are essential to achieving positive outcomes in this population.

CASE EXAMPLE

Angela was a 23-year-old woman with schizoaffective disorder who was addicted to crack cocaine. To support her habit, she often prostituted herself—either exchanging sex for money from customers she met walking the street, or trading sex for cocaine with other addicted individuals at crack houses. Although Angela knew that her behavior increased her risk for HIV and other infectious diseases, she incorrectly believed that her chances of contracting these diseases were small because she used the "withdrawal method" when having sexual intercourse, and because she did not engage in anal sex. Angela's clinician provided her with more accurate information about risk behaviors for infectious diseases. Angela said that she was not ready to give up crack cocaine at that time; however, she expressed an interest in learning how to reduce her risk of contracting infectious diseases through sex. Her clinician discussed with Angela the use of condoms as an effective strategy for reducing risk. Angela said that when she had mentioned condoms to men before, they usually did not have one, and nearly always complained that they did not want to wear one. Angela's clinician talked over the importance of carrying condoms with her. To help her be more successful in getting her partners to wear condoms, Angela's clinician did several role plays with her of the skill "requesting that your partner use a condom" (Bellack, Mueser, Gingerich, & Agresta, 1997). Angela began using this skill, and reported feeling good about reducing her sexual risk behaviors. As Angela and her clinician continued to work together, they began exploring the effects of her cocaine addiction on her life.

A Long-Term Perspective (Time-Unlimited Services)

As we have reviewed in Chapter 1, when clients with dual disorders are not treated, or they are treated via traditional parallel or sequential service approaches, the longitudinal course of the disorders is both chronic and severe, with fewer than 5% of clients achieving stable remission of their substance use disorders each year. Available research on integrated treatment programs suggests that such programs have a beneficial effect on decreasing substance abuse and related negative outcomes in clients with dual disorders (Drake, Mercer-McFadden, Mueser, McHugo, & Bond, 1998). However, research also suggests that integrated treatment programs do not produce dramatic changes in most clients over short periods of time; rather, clients gradually improve over time, with approximately 10–20% achieving stable remission of their substance use disorders per year.

Adopting a healthier lifestyle—just like developing the skills and supports needed to manage one's illnesses, to work, and to attain satisfaction with activities and relationships—requires major life changes over months and years. It makes no sense to believe that recovery from two intertwined disorders might be faster than from either disorder alone. Thus effective integrated programs for dual disorders provide *time-unlimited services*, recognizing that each individual recovers at his or her own pace, given sufficient time and support. Furthermore, clinicians have good justification for being optimistic that in the long run, most clients with dual disorders respond to treatment, get better, and achieve stable remissions of their substance use disorders.

CASE EXAMPLE

Maria, a 49-year-old remarried mother of five, struggled for many years with her bipolar disorder and polysubstance abuse. During her 20s, Maria experienced over 25 hospitalizations, was divorced, and lost custody of her children, due largely to the effects of substance abuse on worsening her bipolar disorder. For many of these years, her substance abuse was ignored by her mental health providers, and she did not perceive it to be a significant problem. In her 30s, Maria began to receive integrated treatment for her dual disorders. Over a period of 4–6 years that involved many setbacks, Maria gradually began to achieve her goals of abstinence from alcohol and putting her life together. Ten years later, Maria had remarried, was working full time, had rekindled her relationships with her children, and had not had a major relapse of her alcoholism.

Motivation-based Treatment

In order to treat dual disorders most effectively, interventions must be *motivation-based*—that is, adapted to clients' motivation for change. The concept of *stages of treatment* is central to integrated dual-disorder treatment, as it provides a framework for assessing clients' motivational states, setting goals, and selecting interventions appropriate to achieving those goals. For many years, clinicians and researchers have proposed that changes in maladaptive behavior occur over a series of stages (DiClemente & Prochaska, 1998; Mahoney, 1991;

Prochaska, 1984). These stages differ in terms of clients' motivational states, orientation toward change, goals, and interventions most likely to be effective. Recognition of the stages of treatment can provide clinicians with valuable information about the immediate goals that need to be the focus of collaborative work, and therefore which interventions are most likely to be successful at a particular point in the course of recovery from dual disorders.

The stages of treatment for dual disorders reviewed here were first described by Osher and Kofoed (1989). Osher and Kofoed observed that clients who recover from dual disorders by participating in treatment progress through a series of four stages: *engagement, persuasion, active treatment*, and *relapse prevention* (although relapses and returns to prior stages are common). Each stage can be defined in terms of a client's abuse of alcohol or drugs and the nature of his or her relationship with a dual-diagnosis clinician. When a client's stage of treatment is determined, appropriate goals can be identified and a treatment plan formulated. Clinicians have a wide variety of treatment options they can use at each stage to help clients progress through the stages.

The concept of stages of treatment is closely related to that of *stages of change* (Connors, Donovan, & DiClemente, 2001; Prochaska, 1984). The latter concept is based on the observation that people who change maladaptive behaviors progress through a series of distinct stages, including *precontemplation, contemplation, preparation, action*, and *maintenance*, each characterized by different motivational states. The stages of change differ from the stages of treatment mainly in that the former are not specific to the change process that occurs in the context of a helping (therapeutic) relationship, whereas the latter are specific to changes that occur over the course of dual-disorder treatment. The overlap between the stages of treatment and the stages of change is summarized in Table 2.2.

We describe each stage of treatment below, including characteristic behaviors and treatment goals, and provide examples of interventions that can be used to achieve those goals. Table 2.3 summarizes the definitions and goals of each stage. Following this, we highlight the clinical utility of the stages concept.

Engagement

Definition and Goals. The *engagement* stage is defined by the lack of a working alliance between the client and the dual-diagnosis clinician. Without first establishing a therapeutic relationship, the clinician cannot help the client to modify his or her substance use behavior. Therefore, the goal of the engagement stage is to establish a working alliance between the clinician and the client.

The terms *working alliance* and *therapeutic relationship* are used widely in the psychotherapy literature, and have recently been adapted to address the relationship between the client and a case manager. For example, Bordin (1976) provides a broad definition of these terms as including (1) the perceived relevance of the cognitive-behavioral tasks involved in collaborative work; (2) agreement as to the goals of the intervention; and (3) the strength of the interpersonal bonds between the clinician and client (e.g., mutual trust and acceptance). Although a long-term goal of integrated treatment is to establish a close working relationship between the clinician(s) and the client, as described by Bordin and exemplified by the importance of shared decision making previously discussed in this chapter, for the purposes of engagement in dual-disorder treatment, we adopt a simpler and more behaviorally specific definition of a working alliance. We define a client as *engaged in treatment* (and hence as having a working relationship with the clinician) if he or she is seeing the clinician on a regular (e.g., weekly) basis.

There are two reasons for defining a working relationship in terms of regular contact between the client and the clinician, rather than the richer and more complex definition of Bordin (1976). First, it is easier for clinicians to agree with each other about the frequency of contact between a clinician and a client than about the level of agreement, trust, and acceptance between the two. Therefore, a simpler definition is less likely to result in disagreement between clinicians about a client's stage of treatment, reducing the possibility of inconsistencies in how different clinicians work with a client. This is especially important, considering that much of dual-disorder treatment is provided by multidisciplinary treatment teams. Second, the willingness of the client to see the clinician on a regular basis indicates a level of interpersonal or therapeutic involvement that is sufficiently robust and stable to begin exploring goals related to substance abuse, and thus to begin work on the next stage of treatment—the persuasion stage.

TABLE 2.2. Overlap between Stages of Treatment and Stages of Change

Stages of treatment	Stages of change
Engagement	Precontemplation
Persuasion	Contemplation
	Preparation
Active treatment	Action
Relapse prevention	Maintenance

TABLE 2.3. Stages of Treatment, Definitions, and Goals

Stage	Definition	Goal
Engagement	Client does not have regular contact with dual-diagnosis clinician.	To establish a working alliance with the client.
Persuasion	Client has regular contact with clinician, but does not want to work on reducing substance abuse.	To develop the client's awareness that substance use is a problem, and increase motivation to change.
Active treatment	Client is motivated to reduce substance use, as indicated by reduction for at least 1 month but less than 6 months.	To help the client further reduce substance use and, if possible, attain abstinence.
Relapse prevention	Client has not experienced problems related to substance use for at least 6 months (or is abstinent).	To maintain awareness that relapse can happen, and to extend recovery to other areas (e.g., social relationships, work).

Engagement Interventions. Clients who are not actively engaged in dual-disorder treatment often attend clinics on an inconsistent, sporadic basis and never establish a trusting relationship with a clinician. Therefore, in order to establish a therapeutic relationship with a client, outreach is often necessary.

The process of engagement typically begins with practical assistance related to securing food, clothing, shelter, crisis intervention, or support. While a clinician is rendering this assistance, sensitivity and skill are required to understand and respond to the client's language, behavior, and unspoken needs, so that some trust and openness develop. Most fundamentally, the clinician tries to make something positive (either tangible or emotional) happen in the client's life, or tries to lessen or remove something painful or unpleasant. As these changes are brought about by the clinician, the client begins to see him or her as potentially useful, and eventually as someone who cares about the client. This emerging therapeutic relationship serves as the critical bond through which all other integrated treatment becomes possible.

During the engagement stage, the clinician usually does not address substance use directly; instead, he or she focuses on learning about the client's experiences and developing a relationship that will later serve as a basis for modifying substance use behavior. Premature attempts to push clients toward substance use reduction or abstinence are often unsuccessful, because they fail to recognize that the client must first develop the motivation, skills, and supports to lead a healthier lifestyle free of substance abuse. The therapeutic alliance should allow discussion of the client's substance use and mental illness symptoms by the end of the engagement stage to facilitate persuasion-stage work.

Many different interventions are possible for achieving the goal of the engagement stage. Table 2.4 provides examples of interventions for this stage.

Persuasion

Definition and Goals. After establishing regular contact and a working relationship with a dual-disorder clinician, many clients fail to acknowledge the negative effects of their substance abuse and do not modify their substance use behavior. Recognizing the effects of substance abuse and trying to change one's own substance use behavior constitute motivation, and clients who are behaviorally unmotivated are in the *persuasion* stage. Clinically, it is not helpful to attempt to change a client's behavior before he or she views that behavior as undesirable or otherwise problematic. Therefore, the goals of persuasion are to help the client recognize the negative effects of substance abuse, to develop hope that his or her life can be improved by reducing substance use, and to demonstrate motivation to address substance abuse by attempting to change behavior. The tasks of persuasion are distinguished from directly helping the client acquire skills and supports for reducing substance use, which are the focus of the next stage of treatment.

Persuasion Interventions. A variety of different strategies can be used to help clients understand the problematic nature of their substance use. Active psy-

TABLE 2.4. Examples of Clinical Interventions for the Engagement Stage

- Outreach
- Practical assistance (e.g., food, clothing, housing, benefits, transportation, medical care)
- Crisis intervention
- Support and assistance to social networks
- Stabilization of psychiatric symptoms—medication management
- Help in avoiding legal penalties
- Help in arranging visitation with family
- Family meetings
- Close monitoring

chiatric symptoms need to be stabilized to the extent possible, in order to minimize impairment of insight and judgment due to grandiosity, psychosis, or thought disorder. Clients and family members often benefit from education about psychiatric illness, commonly abused substances, the interactions between psychiatric illness and substance use, and the principles of dual-disorder treatment. Individual counseling in the persuasion stage is based on *motivational interviewing* (Miller & Rollnick, 2002), which enables clients to identify their personal goals and to discover how their use of substances interferes with attaining those goals (see Chapter 7).

Group interventions help many clients develop the motivation to address substance-related problems. Persuasion groups are designed to provide an open forum for discussing experiences with alcohol and drugs among peers, including both positive and negative effects, in the absence of criticism (see Chapter 9). Social skills training groups (see Chapter 11) and individual cognitive-behavioral counseling (see Chapter 8) can help clients develop healthier skills for meeting needs that are otherwise met through substance use (such as socialization, coping with symptoms, and recreational/ leisure activities). As clients acquire these skills, their reliance on substance use for meeting their needs decreases; their awareness of the negative effects of substances on their lives increases; and, finally, their motivation to change increases. Family intervention (Chapters 13–15) is also frequently used during the persuasion stage.

Coercive interventions, such as involuntary hospitalizations, guardianship, or commitment to community treatment, are sometimes necessary to stabilize a dangerously ill client with dual disorders (see Chapter 17). It is important to recognize that the prevention of harm and compulsory compliance that involuntary measures may provide does not constitute treatment, and that such controls can only keep a client static at best (O'Keefe, Potenza, & Mueser, 1997). The most helpful aspects of involuntary measures may be increased access to the client and psychiatric stabilization. For the client to progress through the persuasion process, the clinician must still establish a therapeutic alliance and proceed with motivational development.

The term *persuasion* is sometimes misleading. The essence of persuasion is empowering the client to have the insight, courage, hope, and desire to change his or her substance use disorder—not forcing the client to decrease or eliminate substance use by persistent badgering or instituting behavioral controls. Motivation to reduce reliance on substances or to achieve abstinence must reside in the client, not in the clinician or family. This distinction is often misunderstood and frequently leads to frustration on the part of clinicians, who prema-

turely try to convince their clients with dual disorders to endorse abstinence as a goal before sufficient motivation has been developed.

Understanding that motivation must exist in the client helps providers to recognize that many other important changes may occur during the persuasion stage. For example, obtaining work, improving social skills, and enhancing social supports can be accomplished before there is any expressed motivation for abstinence; these changes help to instill hope and nurture motivation that will be needed by the client in developing a healthier lifestyle that is not dependent upon substance use. In order to empower clients to make changes based on their own desires, rather than on coercive or involuntary interventions, clinicians need to trust that if the clients' substance use is in fact problematic, it will do the work of persuading the clients to change. The job of clinicians is to create conditions that facilitate awareness of the consequences of continued substance use, and, most importantly, attractive alternatives for clients to move toward.

Examples of intervention strategies for the persuasion stage of treatment are provided in Table 2.5.

Active Treatment

Definition and Goals. A client is considered to be motivated to reduce substance use, and hence is in the *active treatment* stage, when he or she has significantly reduced substance use for more than 1 month and is actively seeking to sustain or enhance these reductions. It is critical that "motivation" to reduce or eliminate substance use is determined from clients' actual behavior (i.e., successful reduction of substance use), rather than from verbal reports. Client self-reports are fraught with social and contextual factors that severely limit their va-

TABLE 2.5. Examples of Clinical Interventions for the Persuasion Stage

- Individual and family education
- Motivational interviewing
- Peer groups (e.g., persuasion groups)
- Social skills training to address non-substance-related situations
- Structured activity (e.g., supported employment, volunteering, hobbies, church, social organizations, consumer committees, or task forces)
- Sampling constructive social and recreational activities
- Psychological preparation for lifestyle changes necessary to achieve remission
- Safe, "damp" housing (i.e., tolerant of some substance abuse)
- Use of medications to treat psychiatric illness that may have a secondary effect on craving/addiction (e.g., selective serotonin reuptake inhibitors [SSRIs], atypical antipsychotics, buspirone)

lidity in the absence of solid behavioral changes. Clients often verbally acknowledge the negative effects of substances on their lives and profess an interest in cutting down use or achieving abstinence in order to gain social acceptance or a clinician's support, or because they fear losing their benefits or other forms of assistance, rather than because they genuinely desire to work on their substance abuse problems. Defining motivation in terms of real behavior change, instead of verbal statements, avoids the unnecessary frustration of trying to change substance use behavior before a client is ready.

The goal of the active treatment stage is to help the client reduce substance use to the point of eliminating negative consequences, or to attain abstinence for a prolonged period of time. Although research data indicate that abstinence is a much more successful remission strategy than occasional or moderate use (Drake & Wallach, 1993), the decision to pursue abstinence must come from the client. Often clients begin the recovery process by gradually reducing their use of substances. As they emerge from their physical dependence on substances, or as they have difficulty limiting their substance use, the goal of abstinence develops as a more realistic approach to eliminating their substance abuse problems.

Active Treatment Interventions. A wide variety of different clinical strategies can be used to help clients reduce their substance use or attain abstinence. Traditional rehabilitation-based approaches are used to increase skills and improve supports, and these strategies can be implemented in a number of different treatment formats (individual, group, family) in a variety of settings. Individual cognitive-behavioral counseling employs techniques for decreasing substance use or enhancing abstinence, and for developing social networks that support a healthier lifestyle (Chapter 8). Supported employment can help clients obtain and keep competitive jobs (Chapter 18), thereby improving their self-esteem, financial standing, and investment in psychiatric stability, and decreasing their free time for using substances.

Active treatment groups (Chapter 10) and social skills training groups (Chapter 11) can help clients reduce their substance use by developing skills for dealing with high-risk situations (e.g., coping with boredom) or compensatory skills for meeting needs in ways other than using substances. Self-help groups, such as AA, can be useful for clients who endorse abstinence as a goal, and who wish to take advantage of the wide availability of such groups in most communities (Chapter 12). Clients may affiliate most readily with self-help groups tailored to the dually diagnosed population (e.g., Double Trouble in Recovery or Dual Recovery Anonymous).

Family problem solving, conducted either with individual families in behavioral family therapy or in multiple-family groups, can be used to identify possible triggers of substance use or urges to use substances. It can also help clients to get involved in alternative activities, to structure their time so as to decrease opportunities to use substances, and to provide behavioral rewards for achieving targeted goals (Chapters 14–15).

Although the explicit goal of the active treatment stage is to reduce substance use, clinicians must recognize that sustained behavioral change involves more than avoiding substances. It includes other lifestyle changes (such as work, social relationships, leisure and recreational activities, self-care skills, and housing), which reinforce sobriety and determine an individual's quality of life. Therefore, interventions during active treatment may need to address the broader changes needed to achieve a different lifestyle that does not rely on alcohol and drugs. Clinicians expand upon the persuasion process to develop clients' recognition and motivation for addressing these changes. This process determines which areas are addressed during active treatment and which are saved for future work.

Relapses or slips back into active substance abuse are common in the active treatment stage. Relapses are not viewed as failures, but rather as part of the course of a chronic illness. Relapses are used as opportunities to learn more about what the individual will need in order to achieve sustained remission of his or her substance use disorder. The client and clinician examine each relapse in microscopic detail, gleaning information about relapse triggers and the sequence of events leading to substance abuse. They use this information to refine their active treatment interventions and to identify new areas of lifestyle change that need attention.

If the client has a relapse into sustained substance abuse, the clinician shifts back into persuasion-stage work, only returning to active treatment interventions when the client again demonstrates motivation for abstinence or reduced substance use. As noted earlier, many clients choose to reduce their use of substances rather than to adopt abstinence during early active treatment. This strategy often fails to sustain remission, but the experience can be helpful in the long-term process of recovery as a client learns experientially that moderate use of alcohol or drugs is not viable, and thereby develops motivation to pursue abstinence.

Examples of intervention strategies for the active treatment stage are provided in Table 2.6.

Relapse Prevention

Definition and Goals. The client is defined as having reached *relapse prevention* when he or she has

TABLE 2.6. Examples of Clinical Interventions for the Active Treatment Stage

- Family and individual problem solving
- Peer groups (e.g., active treatment groups)
- Social skills training to address substance-related situations
- Self-help groups (e.g., Alcoholics Anonymous)
- Individual cognitive-behavioral counseling
- Substituting activities (e.g., work, sports)
- Pharmacological treatments to support abstinence (e.g., disulfiram, naltrexone)
- Safe, "dry" housing
- Psychoeducation
- Stress management and coping skills

not experienced negative consequences related to substance use (or has been abstinent) for at least 6 months. The goals of this stage are to maintain an awareness that relapse of the substance use disorder is possible; to prepare a plan for responding to a relapse should it occur; and to continue to expand the recovery to other areas of functioning, such as social relationships, work, and health. Clients who have achieved an extended period of abstinence often attempt to resume controlled use of substances, either because they believe they will have the self-control to prevent their substance use from escalating, or because of an impulsive, desperate wish to use "just once." These efforts at controlled use usually fail, resulting in partial or full-blown relapses. Therefore, helping clients maintain an awareness of their high vulnerability to relapse, and having them develop strategies for monitoring their inner dialogue as well as overt behaviors, are critical goals of the relapse prevention stage.

Relapse Prevention Interventions. As is true at every stage, the client's choices are paramount in accomplishing the goals of relapse prevention and expanded recovery. Some clients attend self-help groups; some continue in dual-disorder groups; some review their substance use status regularly with their clinicians; and some use other community-integrated support networks to maintain their sobriety and improve functioning in other areas. Usually several different strategies are employed with each client.

The overarching goal of this stage is to develop a meaningful recovery process. Clinicians facilitate a shift in focus from giving up substances to gaining a healthy life. The more clients are able to derive natural rewards from normative activities, such as work, social relationships, and leisure pursuits, the less susceptible they will be to relapses of their substance use disorders. Therefore, such strategies as supported employment (Chapter 18) and social skills training (Chapter 11) may be used to help clients achieve goals related to meaningful life

roles of employment and relationships. Clients in relapse prevention may benefit from serving as mentors for clients in earlier stages of treatment as well.

At the same time, preparing for relapses is also an important skill during this stage. A client must know how to expect relapses and begin working toward substance use reduction or abstinence immediately, rather than experiencing a prolonged relapse and accompanying sense of failure and hopelessness. Providing information to clients about the long-term process of recovery from dual disorders is often helpful in preparing them for the possibility of relapse, and formulating plans for either preventing relapses or minimizing their severity.

Examples of intervention for the relapse prevention stage of treatment are provided in Table 2.7.

Clinical Utility of the Stages of Treatment

The most important feature of the stages of treatment is that they provide a model for clinicians to identify appropriate goals and strategies at different points throughout the recovery process—especially early during intervention, when clients are often not engaged in treatment and fail to see their substance use as a significant problem. Attending to each client's stage of treatment ensures that interventions are appropriate to the individual's current motivational state, and avoids the negative effects of prematurely attempting to change behavior before the client is ready. For example, if a clinician attempts to help a client discover that his or her substance use is destructive (a goal of the persuasion stage) before a therapeutic relationship has been established (engagement stage), the client may be inadvertently driven away from treatment. Similarly, if the clinician tries to help the client reduce his or her substance use (a goal of the active treatment stage) before the client sees substance use as a problem (persuasion

TABLE 2.7. Examples of Clinical Interventions for the Relapse Prevention Stage

- Expanding involvement in supported or independent employment
- Peer groups (e.g., active treatment or relapse prevention groups)
- Self-help groups (e.g., Alcoholics Anonymous)
- Social skills training to address other areas
- Family problem solving
- Lifestyle improvements (e.g., smoking cessation, healthy diet, regular exercise, stress management techniques)
- Independent housing
- Becoming a role model for others (through group or individual peer counseling, mentoring or sponsor relationships, etc.)

stage), the client may become disenchanted and convinced that the clinician does not really understand him or her, and drop out of treatment. Therefore, the stages-of-treatment model helps clinicians increase the chances of selecting interventions that have the greatest immediate relevance for clients at particular points during their treatment.

Individual clinicians and treatment teams need to know each client's stage of treatment at all times, in order to treat the client's substance use disorder effectively. Stages of treatment should be discussed regularly at treatment team meetings; disagreements should be resolved based on consensus; and goals should be established that are consistent with each client's current stage of treatment. If clinicians are unaware of a client's stage of treatment, if there is significant and frequent disagreement among clinicians as to a client's current stage, or if discussion among treatment providers rarely alludes to a client's stage, then stage-wise treatment is probably not being provided. Consequently, treatment outcomes are not being optimized.

Multiple Psychotherapeutic Modalities

Within the field of substance abuse treatment, several different psychotherapeutic treatment modalities have been found to be effective in improving outcomes, including individual, group, and family approaches (Miller et al., 1995; Parks, Anderson, & Marlatt, 2001). Similarly, integrated dual-disorder treatment employing each of these therapeutic modalities has been found to be effective. Individual, group, and family approaches each have their own unique advantages. Individual work (described in Part III of this book) allows for the most attention to be focused on one person, with no distraction from others; it is thus especially conducive to developing a close working relationship, exploring personal motives and goals, and identifying individualized targets for intervention. Group approaches (described in Part IV of this book) offer the advantage of engendering social support among clients, providing positive role models for clients at earlier stages of treatment, and offering economy of teaching. Family intervention (described in Part V of this book) takes advantages of the natural supports available to clients, which can lead to creating an environment that is supportive of decreased substance use or abstinence. Although not all clients receive all treatment approaches, an array of different treatment modalities will optimize outcomes.

Individual Counseling

In addition to the informal counseling that takes place in the context of providing clinical case management to clients with dual disorders (see Chapter 6), two types of individual counseling are useful in the treatment of dual disorders: cognitive-behavioral counseling and motivational interviewing. Cognitive-behavioral counseling, as described in Chapter 8, involves using learning-based interventions to help clients develop more effective skills for achieving a variety of different goals—ranging from improved interpersonal relationships, to reducing or coping better with symptoms, to reducing substance use or avoiding relapses of substance abuse. Cognitive-behavioral approaches have a rich history of documented effectiveness in addressing both substance abuse (Heather, Peters, & Stockwell, 2001; Hester & Miller, 1995) and mental health problems (Caballo, 1998; Liberman, 1992).

As noted earlier in this chapter, motivational interviewing is a counseling approach designed to help clients become aware of their substance abuse problems and to develop motivation to overcome these problems through the process of articulating and pursuing their own personal goals. Motivational interviewing was originally developed for clients with substance abuse (Miller & Rollnick, 2002), and research supports its effectiveness both in this population (Foote et al., 1999; Miller, 1995; Project Matching Alcoholism Treatments to Client Heterogeneity [MATCH] Research Group, 1997) and in clients with dual disorders (Barrowclough et al., 2001). In addition to the use of motivational interviewing to address substance abuse in clients with dual disorders, as described in Chapter 7, motivational interviewing has been used successfully to improve attendance at aftercare appointments (Swanson, Pantalon, & Cohen, 1999), and to increase medication adherence in clients with severe mental illness (Kemp, Kirov, Everitt, Hayward, & David, 1998).

Integrated Group Treatment

There are several reasons for conducting group interventions for clients with dual disorders. First, there is a strong tradition of nonprofessional self-help groups, such as AA, in the primary addiction field. The group format is an ideal setting for capitalizing on the need for support and identification shared by persons with an addiction. Second, substance abuse among psychiatric clients frequently occurs in a social context (Dixon et al., 1991; Test et al., 1989). Addressing substance-use-related issues in a group setting makes it clear to clients that they are not alone, and provides an opportunity for the sharing of experiences and coping strategies. Third, there are economical advantages to offering group rather than individual therapy, because less clinician time is required.

Several different types of professional-based group

treatment for clients with dual disorders can be provided, including educational groups, stage-wise treatment groups (persuasion, active treatment, and relapse prevention groups), and social skills training groups. Although treatment settings may not provide all types of groups, effective programs offer several different options to ensure that some group interventions are available to all clients. In addition, self-help groups can provide another valuable source of social support to clients who recognize the destructive effects of substances on their lives, and who want to pursue an abstinent lifestyle. We briefly describe each of these types of groups here.

Educational Groups. Group-based educational interventions for clients with dual disorders are often time-limited (e.g., 4–8 weeks) and serve to inform clients about the nature of mental illness and its treatment, the interactions between substance abuse and psychiatric disorders, and strategies for addressing the problem of substance abuse (Alfs & McClellan, 1992; Kofoed & Keys, 1988). Although education groups are appropriate for clients at all stages of treatment, they often serve a primary function of educating clients at the earlier stages of treatment (e.g., engagement and persuasion), in order to motivate them to address their substance use problems. Longer-term programs often combine education with group support (Bond, McDonel, Miller, & Pensec, 1991; Hellerstein & Meehan, 1987; Hellerstein, Rosenthal, & Miner, 1995; Lehman, Herron, Schwartz, & Myers, 1993).

An alternative to educational groups that we have used in most of our clinical settings is to provide basic information about dual disorders that is interwoven into a longer-term group approach, such as stage-wise or social skills treatment groups. For this reason, we do not provide separate guidelines in this book for conducting educational groups. A curriculum for conducting such groups can be created from the educational handouts contained in Appendix B.

Stage-Wise Treatment Groups. Stage-wise treatment groups focus on helping clients progress from one stage of treatment to the next (Mueser & Noordsy, 1996). In the treatment programs in which we have worked, the most common stage-wise treatment groups are persuasion and active treatment groups, with relapse prevention groups less common. As described in Chapter 9, persuasion groups are focused on clients in the persuasion stage, although clients at later stages are typically included in these groups to serve as role models. The primary aim of persuasion groups is to explore the interactions between substance use and mental illness, and to instill motivation to address substance use problems.

Active treatment groups, described in Chapter 10, are targeted for clients at the active treatment (or, sometimes, relapse prevention) stage. They focus on supporting members' goals of reducing substance use or maintaining abstinence, through a combination of group support and teaching cognitive-behavioral strategies. Relapse prevention groups are similar to active treatment groups, but they include only clients who have attained sustained remission of their substance abuse, usually through abstinence. The principles for conducting relapse prevention groups are essentially the same as for active treatment groups, and we do not provide a separate chapter on them in this book. The clinical benefits of stage-wise treatment groups are supported by our research on integrated dual-disorder treatment programs conducted in New Hampshire (Drake, McHugo, & Noordsy, 1993; Drake, McHugo, et al., 1998).

Social Skills Training Groups. Although the availability of skills training groups is part of comprehensive treatment, social skills training groups that address the unique problems of clients with dual disorders can be especially useful (Bellack & DiClemente, 1999; Roberts, Shaner, & Eckman, 1999). As summarized in Chapter 11, such groups are appropriate for clients with dual disorders at the persuasion, active treatment, and relapse prevention stages of treatment. At the earlier stages of treatment, skills training aims to build clients' social competence, to make them less reliant on using substances to achieve their interpersonal needs. These same goals, as well as the goal of helping clients improve their skills for handling substance-use-related situations, apply to the later stages of treatment. Controlled research supports the effects of social skills training groups in integrated treatment for dual disorders (Jerrell & Ridgely, 1995a).

Self-Help Groups. Self-help groups, such as AA, Double Trouble in Recovery, or Dual Recovery Anonymous play an important role in recovery from substance abuse for many clients with dual disorders. Social contacts with other members of self-help groups is associated with better substance abuse outcome in clients with dual diagnoses (Trumbetta et al., 1999). As described in Chapter 12, clinicians can facilitate clients' exploration of self-help groups by recommending these groups to clients who are motivated to achieve or maintain abstinence, helping them identify and attend possible groups, and not pressuring reluctant clients to participate in self-help.

Family Intervention

Similar to the inclusion of family psychoeducation as a part of comprehensive treatment, family intervention that specifically targets dual disorders can be an especially powerful approach for improving substance abuse outcomes (Barrowclough et al., 2001; Mueser & Fox, 2002). Furthermore, the provision of different formats of family psychoeducation, including single-family and multiple-family group approaches, can increase access to family services for clients with dual disorders and their relatives (who may take advantage of either or both formats). The principles of collaborating with families are summarized in Chapter 13; guidelines for conducting single-family intervention (behavioral family therapy) are presented in Chapter 14; and multiple-family groups are covered in Chapter 15.

Selection of Treatment Modalities

The selection of which interventions should be provided to which clients is based on a combination of the nature of the treatment goals, the ease with which a client can be engaged in a treatment modality, and the unique advantages of each approach. For example, the goal of developing motivation to address substance abuse (a persuasion-stage goal) can be approached through motivational interviewing in an individual counseling format, through participation in stage-wise treatment groups, and/or through participating in psychoeducational and problem-solving family intervention. The selection of treatment modality can be influenced by such factors as the quality of the client's relationship with a primary clinician, the degree of social comfort the client experiences with peers, and the involvement of family members in the client's life and treatment. Thus different treatment modalities may be used to work with clients at the same motivational states to achieve similar goals. Multiple treatment modalities are frequently used simultaneously, to maximize clients' ability to benefit from treatment.

SUMMARY

We have begun this chapter by reviewing problems with traditional sequential or parallel treatment approaches to dual disorders. The most significant limitation of sequential treatment approaches is that they fail to account for the interactive nature of mental illness and substance use disorders, in which each untreated type of disorder contributes to and exacerbates the other. The greatest problems with parallel treatment methods are that mental health and substance abuse interventions are usually not integrated by the different providers, and treatments are sometimes incompatible with one another (e.g., use of strong, emotionally challenging methods in substance abuse treatment programs for persons with severe mental illness).

Integrated treatment programs for dual disorders embody the common value of shared decision making. In addition, integrated treatment is effective to the extent that it incorporates the core treatment components of integration, comprehensiveness, assertiveness, reduction of negative consequences, long-term commitment (time-unlimited services), motivation-based treatment (utilizing the stages-of-treatment concept), and multiple psychotherapeutic modalities. The more attention a treatment program gives to each of these components, the better the outcomes. The rationale, definition, and empirical support for each component of treatment have been described in this chapter. A fidelity scale is provided in Appendix A for assessing program adherence to the core components of integrated treatment.

3

Basic Organizational Factors

In Chapter 2, we have identified the need for integrated treatment and described the fundamentals of integrated treatment programs. In this chapter, we address organizational factors for creating and managing effective dual-disorder programs. This chapter is written primarily for individuals with administrative and leadership responsibilities for developing, financing, supervising, or coordinating services for clients with dual disorders, including state or local program directors, managers, or clinical supervisors. However, front-line clinicians may also benefit from understanding how organizational factors are related to the success of integrated dual-disorder treatment programs.

We begin the chapter with a discussion of different models for integrating mental health and substance abuse treatments. This is followed by considering how dual-disorder services can be adapted to the managed care environment that predominates in most U.S. treatment systems. We next consider different factors related to successful programs, such as leadership, infrastructure, array of services, and financing issues. We then highlight several controversies concerning the treatment of dual disorders that program leaders need to be prepared to address, such as violence, involuntary interventions, and testing for alcohol and drug use. We conclude with a discussion of different starting points for initiating dual-disorder services.

INTEGRATED DUAL-DISORDER SERVICE MODELS

Most individuals with severe mental illness and substance use disorders receive at least sporadic care from the mental health service system, with a minority also receiving services from substance abuse treatment providers. Comparatively few such individuals receive their primary treatment from the substance abuse service system (Ross, Glaser, & Germanson, 1988). Therefore, two approaches to integrating mental health and substance abuse services have predominated: importing substance abuse treatment expertise into existing mental health services, and forming new *blended services* that include clinicians from the mental health and substance abuse treatment agencies.

Incorporating substance abuse treatment into existing mental health treatment services involves broadening the traditional focus from psychiatric illness to problems related to substance use. This can be accomplished by a variety of strategies, including providing staff members with training in the recognition and treatment of substance abuse in persons with severe mental illness; forming specialized dual-diagnosis teams to treat clients with the most persistent substance use problems; and hiring new staff members with substance abuse treatment expertise (e.g., certified drug and alcohol abuse counselors) to work on treatment teams. When staffers with substance abuse expertise join mental health teams, their knowledge is often complemented by the experience of other staffers in the care of severe mental illness. The result is a new team that is capable of addressing substance use problems while maintaining awareness of the unique needs of persons with severe mental illness.

Adding new services to mental health treatment in order to address substance abuse has a number of advantages over the integration of the two service systems themselves. First, providing additional (or different) services to an existing agency requires changing only one system, not two, which is a simpler task. The mental health and substance abuse treatment systems have different ideologies, credentialing procedures, and funding streams. Integrating at the level of clinical care does not require direct attention to the many differences between the service systems. Second, as most clients with dual disorders already receive services in the mental health system, and most do not receive services in the substance abuse treatment system, access to the majority of such clients is gained when substance abuse services are added to existing mental health programs.

The advantages just outlined make this approach easier to implement, and it has been more widely adopted than integration at the system level. However, there are some disadvantages as well. Adding substance abuse treatment expertise to mental health services may fail to tap financial resources available within the substance abuse treatment system during times when the mental health system may already be overtaxed. In addition, a minority of clients with dual disorders do receive their primary services in the substance abuse treatment system, especially those with severe mood disorders (e.g., bipolar disorder, major depression with psychotic features). In the absence of integration at the system level, these clients' psychiatric illnesses go undetected and untreated; as a result, they experience a poor course of their dual disorders. The integration of mental health and substance abuse services in primary substance abuse treatment settings requires comprehensive training of clinicians in the recognition and treatment of psychiatric disorders (Maslin et al., 2001), as well as the development of an array of services necessary for the treatment of severe mental illness (see "Array of Services" in the section on "Organizational Factors," below).

The effort to integrate the mental health and substance abuse treatment systems needs to be distinguished from integration that occurs at the level of the clinical services themselves (Randolph et al., 1995). Some states have formally integrated mental health and substance abuse treatment services at an administrative level, but separate services continue to be provided. When integrated services by different systems are provided, it is most often in the form of blended teams of clinicians from both agencies. These blended teams may obtain specific dual-disorder training as they develop their own expertise, while serving as valuable resources to their parent organizations. Clients can be referred to these specialty teams from clinicians in either the mental health or substance abuse treatment agencies. However, it should be noted that blended teams still must be administratively placed within a single program. Otherwise, two sets of paperwork and other requirements are necessary, and the blended teams are vulnerable to being disowned by both programs when funds are short.

Blended dual-disorder teams take a longer time to create because of the need for change in both systems to facilitate the referral of eligible clients, to address funding barriers, and to determine the locus and staffing of services. In addition to logistical hurdles, there are further challenges imposed by the different philosophies and cultures of the two systems. K. Minkoff (personal communication, June 2002) has identified a number of barriers to integrating mental health and substance abuse services, which are summarized in Table 3.1. These barriers are not insurmountable, but awareness of them is critical if treatment providers are to develop a dialogue and seek common ground in providing services tailored to the needs of clients with dual disorders.

ADAPTING SERVICES TO THE MANAGED CARE ENVIRONMENT

Mental health and substance abuse treatment services are now delivered in the context of managed care. *Managed care* is an overarching concept that combines ways of organizing and financing services, and that now predominates in the U.S. health care system. Various strat-

---

TABLE 3.1. Philosophical and Clinical Differences between Traditional Systems of Care for Persons with Addictions Compared to Persons with Mental Health Disorders

Addictions treatment	Mental health treatment
Peer counselor model	Medical/professional model
Spiritual recovery	Scientific treatment
Self-help	Medication
Confrontation and expectation	Support and flexibility
Detachment/empowerment	Case management/care
Episodic treatment	Continuous treatment
Recovery ideology	Deinstitutionalization ideology
View of psychopathology as secondary to addiction	View of addiction as secondary to psychopathology

Note. From K. Minkoff (personal communication, June 2002). Adapted by permission.

egies are commonly used in managed care to maximize outcomes at the lowest possible cost. Case management, utilization review, prior authorization, and gatekeeping are employed to limit and monitor access to appropriate services. Costs are most often contained by *capitation* (i.e., a fixed per-person payment for a set period of time). Quality control and outcomes are addressed by quality indicators, practice profiles, provider qualifications, outcome measures, and report cards. In order to ensure that the special needs of clients with dual disorders are met, and to avoid the inappropriate inclusion or exclusion of clients from services, modifications in the service organization may be necessary.

The goal of responsible managed care—optimizing outcomes at the lowest possible cost—is consistent with the primary aim of dual-disorder programs. Effective managed care treatment systems can ensure the access of clients to needed treatments, while tracking the targeted outcomes over time. However, the problems of providing inappropriate services, cost shifting, and inadequate measurement of outcomes with instruments insensitive to change in this population can threaten the mission of treatment systems for clients with dual disorders. Mercer-McFadden and colleagues (1998) describe a variety of strategies for providing administrative and fiscal incentives to avoid these negative outcomes, including risk-adjusted payments, risk-adjusted premiums for high-cost groups, and careful management and monitoring of benefits to ensure that they are not manipulated in a way that results in exclusion of clients from services.

The measurement of outcomes is of critical importance for accurate tracking of systems' impact on substance abuse, and for demonstrations of their effectiveness and cost-effectiveness. As described in more detail in Chapter 4, measures of substance abuse developed in the general population tend to perform poorly in persons with severe mental illness. Such measures are also less sensitive in detecting the presence of substance use disorders or changes in these disorders over time in this population. Treatment systems need to employ outcome measures of substance abuse that have been developed and validated with persons with severe mental illness, and to train clinicians appropriately in the use of these instruments (see Chapters 4 and 5).

The ability of clinicians to provide the most effective interventions to clients with dual disorders is of critical importance. These strategies may differ from those used for other populations (e.g., clients with purely medical disorders). For example, most clients with dual disorders do not require prolonged inpatient treatment or intensive outpatient day programs, which, despite their lack of efficacy (see Chapter 20), are often funded by service providers. On the other hand, asser-

tive outreach, including meeting with clients in their natural environments, is crucial to successfully engaging clients and monitoring the course of dual disorders (see Chapter 2). Either providing ineffective treatments or using insensitive instruments to measure outcomes can result in conclusions that dual-disorder services are both costly and ineffective.

A fundamental concern when treating a vulnerable population in a competitive environment is the need for safeguards to ensure client access to services. The dual-disorder population is especially vulnerable to exclusion from services, for several reasons. They consume disproportionately large amounts of expensive services, making them unattractive clients in capitation funding schemes. Severe psychiatric illnesses also often impair clients' judgment and their ability to advocate for themselves—problems that are further exacerbated by substance abuse. Traditional treatment systems have assumed that mental health and substance use disorders are separable, and have used eligibility criteria to identify clients (and exclude others) deemed most appropriate for available services. The result is that many clients with dual disorders receive services from only one sector or none at all (Ridgely et al., 1990). Specific strategies for safeguarding clients with dual disorders from exclusion from treatment in the managed care environment are described in Table 3.2. Guidelines for services to clients with dual disorders served in a managed care environment have been developed by the Center for Mental Health Services to assist advocacy groups and policy makers (Minkoff, Rossi, Ajilore, & Cahill, 1997).

In the next section, we describe organizational factors relevant to integrating substance abuse services into existing programs for treating severe mental illness. However, many of these factors are also relevant to developing blended dual-disorder services through the integration of separate substance abuse and mental health programs.

ORGANIZATIONAL FACTORS

Leadership

Strong leadership is crucial for an effective program. Directors of mental health programs must embrace the mission to integrate substance abuse treatment into all aspects of their programs. Executive directors must set the tone for change by making clear the expectation that all clinicians need to acquire skills for assessing and treating substance use disorders; senior management must take responsibility for planning; middle managers must assure that training, supervision, and monitoring are in place; and medical directors must make certain that physicians also acquire the requisite skills. Moni-

TABLE 3.2. Safeguards for the Population of Clients with Dual Disorders

Arenas	Safeguards
Clinical programs	• Clear definition of the target population of clients with dual disorders • Requirements for screening, assessment, and treatment activities that are appropriate for the population • Clinical outcome measures that are appropriate for the population • Education to increase professional competencies and to reduce fears and stigma • Quality standards and quality assurance systems for dual-disorder services
Legal and administrative framework	• Laws and policies to prevent exclusion of the population from programs and services • Priority for the population within federal and state programs • Assignment to a lead agency with specific responsibility for population • Contract performance expectations linked with outcome measures that are appropriate for the population • Community-based planning for the population • Risk adjustments and/or other modifications in capitation payment systems • Financial incentives for providers to reach out, enroll, engage, treat, and follow clients with dual disorders
Societal and scientific context	• Advocacy by client and professional organizations • Social acceptance of people with dual disorders • Proven technologies for assessment, treatment, and service delivery • Scientific understanding of dual disorders and applications of new knowledge • Professional preparation that includes education about dual disorders and their treatment

toring should include not only reviews of records and management information system (MIS) data, but also a front-line presence—for example, attending intake conferences, treatment reviews, and team meetings to ensure that substance abuse is considered as a potential part of clients' problems and addressed when present.

One person should be designated the director of a dual-disorder program and charged with overseeing all dual-diagnosis services. The literature on program innovation indicates that major program change, and the maintenance of high-quality programming, require a director (often called a *champion*) who assumes primary responsibility for the overall quality of a new program (Backer, Liberman, & Kuehnel, 1986; Corrigan, 1995; Mueser & Fox, 2000; Spaniol, Zipple, & Cohen, 1991). The director of dual-disorder treatment need not hold a full-time position, but at least some of his or her time needs to be protected from other clinical or administrative responsibilities in order for effective services to be established and maintained.

The ongoing responsibilities of the director of a dual-disorder program include recruiting and training staff members; ensuring that services are being implemented with fidelity to the principles of integrated treatment (as described in Chapter 2 and operationalized in the Dual-Disorder Treatment Fidelity Scale in Appendix A); providing ongoing supervision of clinicians; monitoring substance abuse and other performance outcomes (e.g., utilization of inpatient services); and coordinating efforts across levels of care (e.g., inpatient, outpatient, residential) to make sure that appropriate clients are being identified and provided with dual-disorder treatment. The director evaluates all of these areas and, with other program directors, makes plans for development and for corrective actions when weaknesses are identified. The director also provides liaison with the substance abuse treatment agency and other agencies.

Staffing of Clinical Treatment Teams

Clients with severe mental illness, and likewise those with dual disorders, typically have a wide range of different treatment and living needs that cannot be met by a single clinician. To address these multiple needs, a team-based approach has become the dominant organizational model for treating clients with severe mental illness, and this approach is also recommended for the treatment of dual disorders. Multidisciplinary treatment teams for clients with dual disorders should include, at a minimum, a part-time psychiatrist and two or more case managers who develop experience in treating dual disorders. Early in the formation of such a team, it may be practical to include one or more case managers experienced in treating severe mental illness and one or more case managers experienced in treating addictions, with the expectation that these case managers' expertise in treating dual disorders will grow as a function of shared training and treatment experiences. Whenever possible, the team should also include a nurse and an employment specialist (see Chapter 18). Inclusion of one or more master's-level clinicians can be helpful for providing specialized treatment services, such as cognitive-behavioral substance abuse counseling (Chapter 8) and family work (Chapters 13–15).

Team leadership is important to effective team

functioning. The team leader is usually a clinician on the team who carries a caseload and is fully experienced in case management. The leader coordinates scheduling, assigns new cases, provides consultation on difficult cases, and presents the administrative concerns of the team to the management structure.

Dual-disorder treatment teams are most effective when they directly provide as many clinical services as possible, and avoid brokering services to other providers who are not team members (Drake & Noordsy, 1994; Noordsy & Drake, 1994). Such direct provision of services reduces the risk of nonintegrated treatment, which can lead to poor coordination of treatment, conflict among treatment providers, and counterproductive therapeutic efforts. Ideally, such services as residential support and vocational services are also provided by the team or are closely integrated with the treatment agency. When most treatment is provided directly, only a few services need to be brokered to other providers, such as general medical care, benefits, and highly specialized care (e.g., neurological testing).

Dual-disorder treatment teams are most effective when clinicians either partly or wholly share caseloads. Each client is assigned to a primary case manager on the team who takes responsibility for overseeing this client's care, coordinating his or her treatment, and completing necessary paperwork. However, all clinicians on the team are familiar with the entire caseload. Such services as crisis response, after-hours on-call duties, medication monitoring, and residential support may be provided to clients by different team members in a rotating fashion. At times a client may require a specific intervention from a team member who is not his or her primary case manager, but who has unique skills—for instance, family therapy, or dialectical behavior therapy for managing parasuicidal behaviors in a client with borderline personality disorder and alcohol dependence (Linehan, 1993). In these situations, the client may enter into a time-limited series of individual therapy sessions with another clinician on the team. The team nurse can provide nursing services for the whole caseload, including injections of depot medications and triage of general medical conditions. If in the course of treatment a client requests a different case manager, or it becomes clear that the client has a more effective therapeutic alliance with another member of the team, a change in the primary case manager can be made to achieve the best therapeutic fit.

The number of clients per clinician on the treatment team depends upon the severity of the dual disorders in the clients receiving treatment, the availability of ancillary supports within the agency, and the distance clinicians may be expected to travel to provide outreach

to clients in the community. The literature on case management services for clients with severe mental illness and clients with dual disorders has found that effective treatment teams employ caseloads ranging between 10 and 30 clients per clinician (Drake, Mercer-McFadden, et al., 1998; Rapp, 1998a). Therefore, treatment teams for clients with dual disorders should be designed with caseloads in this range. Lower caseloads are appropriate in situations where there are fewer ancillary support services (e.g., no discrete residential outreach service to assist the team in time-consuming, home-based services) or extremely impaired clients (e.g., clients with prolonged stays in state psychiatric hospitals, frequent or long-term homelessness, extensive involvement in the criminal justice system, or histories of significant violence). It is ideal for members of the treatment team to provide primary after-hours coverage for the clients on their team. At a minimum, a team member should always be available to an existing emergency services system for consultation, treatment planning, and direct client assessment, if required, to ensure that the team's treatment plan is followed during after-hours care.

Defining the Target Population

Some mental health agencies develop a special core of dual-disorder services for a targeted group of clients. Other agencies focus on a whole community and seek to identify clients who are at high risk for dual disorders. For example, programs that focus on engaging and treating homeless persons with dual disorders follow a community-based approach to defining the target population.

The terms *dual disorders*, *dual diagnosis*, or *co-occurring disorders* are generally used to define clients with severe mental illness (often meeting a state department of mental health's criteria for severe and persistent mental illness) and substance use disorders. In addition to diagnostic criteria for eligibility for dual-disorder programs, additional criteria may specify a pattern of service utilization, such as the number of inpatient hospitalizations, time spent in the hospital, or use of emergency services. When eligibility criteria for such programs include high utilization of acute care services, the treatment system must also offer some dual-disorder services for clients who do not meet criteria for these specialized programs. These services need to focus on preventing the emergence of substance use problems in vulnerable clients (e.g., psychoeducation concerning interactions between mental illness and substance abuse for clients with recent-onset mental illness), and on detecting and intervening with clients whose substance abuse is problematic but has not yet resulted in a pattern of costly service utilization. Addressing the needs of clients before their dual disorders become chronic may avert the need for long-term interventions.

The eligibility criteria for dual-disorder programs should avoid reference to the "primary–secondary" distinction between mental illness and substance use diagnoses. It is often difficult or impossible to distinguish which disorder is primary or secondary, especially because it is usually not possible to observe clients for prolonged periods of time when they are not under the influence of alcohol or drugs (Lehman et al., 1994). Moreover, eligibility criteria that require a primary diagnosis (or diagnoses) invariably result in the exclusion of some clients from needed services. It is preferable to assume that both disorders are primary, and to develop eligibility criteria that are not contingent on determining the primacy of one disorder (see Chapter 4 for more discussion of the issue of primary vs. secondary diagnoses).

Table 3.3 summarizes some options for defining the target population for dual-disorder services.

Infrastructure

Several organizational guidelines and structures are needed to launch and support a dual-diagnosis program. A peer review system for credentialing and privileging clinicians is important to ensure training and competence. Developing specific areas of competence for dual-disorder treatment providers, and recognizing

these skills in the form of credentials, acknowledge and value their expertise. As dual-disorder specialists are formally certified within an organization, these clinicians become empowered to undertake training of other clinicians within the same setting, and to serve as consultants in the management of related problems. The special "expert" status of trained dual-disorder clinicians within a treatment setting may facilitate the retention of people with unique skills in jobs as the system acknowledges their importance, thereby enabling the program to be more self-sufficient and less reliant on outside training to address dual disorders.

Practice guidelines provide clinicians with a consistent clinical framework and protocols. Although this book provides instruction on the delivery of a wide range of dual-disorder services, specific guidelines need to be developed for each treatment system, depending on the system's particular array of services and the characteristics of its client population. The MIS must track substance use diagnoses and treatments (see below). Clinical tools for record keeping are needed, many of which can be used directly or adapted from the instruments in Appendix C. Training programs for all clinicians are critical. Some of the individuals involved in providing treatment should participate in a quality improvement team to assess and, when necessary, improve the effectiveness of services. This effort should be tied to performance indicators that are consistent with practice guidelines (e.g., percentage remissions per year, engagement and retention in services). Finally, ongoing program planning, development, and evaluation are needed.

TABLE 3.3. Defining the Target Population for Dual-Disorder Services: Some Options

Severe mental disorder options
- DSM-IV diagnosis of schizophrenia, schizoaffective disorder, major mood disorder (major depressive disorder, bipolar disorder)
- State's definition of severe mental disorder
- Severe and persistent mental disorder with impaired role functioning

Substance abuse options
- Substance abuse history of at least 2 years' duration
- Active substance abuse during past 6 months
- Self-reported or recognized problem with substance abuse
- DSM-IV diagnosis of substance use disorder

Treatment history options
- Psychiatric hospitalization, incarceration, homelessness, or housing instability during last 6 months
- Extensive use of hospital and crisis services
- Not receiving adequate services
- Demonstrating a persistent pattern of nonengagement in mental health services, despite continuing outreach

Training

Since most clinicians come from either a mental health or a substance use disorder background, dual-diagnosis training must be the centerpiece of a new dual-disorder program. All clinicians should be trained in the fundamentals of assessing substance use disorders in clients with severe mental illness, as well as the basic principles of treatment. More in-depth training in specific interventions for dual disorders can be provided to a subset of clinicians who work with the most challenging clients; these clinicians can consult with and train others in work with clients with dual disorders. Substance abuse is both very common and episodic. The outmoded practice of referring clients with suspected substance abuse to a specialist for assessment frequently results in cases' being missed. Similarly, clinicians cannot count on a substance abuse specialist to provide treatment to all clients with a dual disorder. There are simply too many clients whose lives are affected by substance abuse to refer all of them to a specialist. Furthermore, substance abuse usually does not occur in single or discrete episodes; it is a chronic, relapsing condition that requires ongoing management woven into rehabilitation and lifestyle change efforts. It is more efficient for one set of clinicians to treat both types of disorders, as both benefit from the same treatment context. Therefore, all clinicians need to master certain basic skills, including assessment (Chapters 4 and 5), motivational interviewing (Chapter 7), and cognitive-behavioral substance abuse counseling (Chapter 8).

Changing clinical practices involves developing new attitudes, knowledge, and skills. Based on our experiences and those of others in creating innovative treatment programs (Becker, Torrey, Toscano, Wyzik, & Fox, 1998; Torrey et al., 2001), we believe that a realistic time frame for training and achieving adequate program implementation is approximately 1 year. During this year, the basic approach to training should be as follows. First, key clinicians and middle managers should participate in an intensive preliminary training experience, which optimally involves a combination of learning basic didactic material, visiting a mature program to shadow experienced clinicians, and discussing their observations with the experienced team. Second, clinicians and middle managers should have the opportunity to read and discuss clinical manuals, to observe training tapes, and to practice new skills with one another. Third, clinicians and middle managers should participate in weekly case-oriented supervision for at least 1 year. Cross-training within teams goes more smoothly when at least one clinician has experience in substance abuse counseling or dual-disorder treatment.

A dual-disorder specialist at the agency, such as the director of dual-disorder services, should provide group supervision. If the person designated by the agency to be the director of these services is him- or herself in the process of developing expertise in dual-disorder treatment, that person's supervision of other clinicians can be supplemented by teleconferencing and occasional visits from an expert outside the agency. However, it is important that an individual within the agency be identified as a supervisor of dual-disorder treatment, in order to prevent the agency from becoming dependent upon outside experts for providing this basic function. At the end of 1 year, some clinicians will have developed excellent skills, and the dual-disorder program leader can assess the need for further training. Training and supervision need to be continuous in order to incorporate new developments, to train new staff members, and to prevent experienced staffers' skills from atrophying.

A common mistake is to omit physicians from training efforts. Physicians must have the skills not only to recognize and diagnose substance use disorders in persons with severe mental illness and to develop effective treatment plans, but also to tailor medication management and medical care in light of substance abuse comorbidity (see Chapter 19). Physicians typically have the final say on critical treatment decisions, such as ordering involuntary hospitalization, drug screening tests, or medications. If a team physician is not intimately aware of the fundamentals of integrated dual-disorder treatment, he or she may inadvertently undermine the team's efforts to develop effective treatment plans. Ideally, a physician working on the dual-disorder specialty team should be an expert in dual-disorder treatment planning. Since many psychiatrists receive inadequate substance abuse training in their residencies and few will have direct dual-diagnosis training, they must be included in some of the general clinician training and must also master specific information and skills related to medications and medical care. For example, many psychiatrists do not understand the importance of treating psychiatric disorders when active substance abuse is present, and few have experience in using disulfiram or naltrexone to treat addictions. The medical director should be responsible for this training effort and should adjust the intensity of training to the medical staff's level of expertise.

Some clinicians naturally become dual-disorder specialists. This is a predictable and essential development, and these specialists can be counted on to help with training, to consult with other clinicians on difficult cases, and to provide treatment directly for individuals with the most difficult problems. Although natural leaders in dual-diagnosis treatment emerge over the course of developing special services, agencies can foster the development of these clinicians by recognizing their expertise and sponsoring their continued development in this area. In addition to establishing a credentialing procedure for formally recognizing dual-disorder specialists, providing an educational stipend to these clinicians for their professional development (e.g., so that they can purchase books, subscribe to journals, attend conferences, etc.) can result in both retention of these valued clinicians and continued training of other staff members in new developments in treatment.

Assessment

As described in the next two chapters (Chapters 4 and 5), the full assessment of substance use disorders in persons with severe mental illness includes detection, classification, functional assessment, functional analysis, and treatment planning. Detection procedures, including laboratory drug screens, should be routine for all new admissions, crises, hospitalizations, and failures to make progress. Full assessment, including all of the components mentioned above, should be part of the clinical record.

Routine utilization review should confirm adequate assessment procedures. Assessment should document the substances involved, patterns of use, and risk factors, as well as the client's stage of treatment. A functional analysis of the client's substance use behavior should be included in the record, to identify factors that may contribute to maintaining the client's use of substances or interfere with obtaining sobriety. The treatment plans should draw from the functional analysis and contain specific behavioral plans to address those factors. Functional analyses and treatment plans should be revised at least yearly and preferably every 6 months.

Array of Services

Many different treatments are available for clients with dual disorders. Individual clients may respond best to one or another of these treatments. Although the specific interventions may vary from one program to the next, an effective dual-disorder program requires a minimal set of treatments to improve the outcome of the disorders. A wide range of options increases the chances of good client–treatment fit. All dual-diagnosis programs should provide interventions at each of the four stages of treatment: engagement, persuasion, active treatment, and relapse prevention. The ability to provide assertive outreach to engage clients who are not actively receiving services is especially critical, as in the absence of such outreach, their outcomes tend to be very poor.

The types of services required for an integrated dual-disorder program are described in Chapter 2 and summarized in the fidelity scale in Appendix A. Briefly, two main types of treatment are needed: the foundations of mental health services, and specialized dual-disorder services (Table 3.4).

The *foundations of mental health services* are those interventions that form the core of all treatment for clients with severe mental illness, including individuals with no substance use problems. Many of these services involve substantial modification to address the problem of dual disorders, as described in this book—including case management (Chapter 6), family support and education (Chapters 13–15), housing (Chapter 16), involuntary and coerced interventions (Chapter 17), vocational rehabilitation (Chapter 18), and psychopharmacological treatment (Chapter 19). For example, the functions of clinical case management are informed by clients' motivation to change their substance use behavior, based on the concept of stages of treatment, in order to maximize treatment gains and minimize unnecessary confronta-

TABLE 3.4. Array of Services for Dual-Disorder Treatment

Foundations of mental health services (adapted for clients with dual disorders)

- Case management
- Family support and education
- Housing
- Involuntary and coerced interventions
- Vocational rehabilitation
- Training in illness management skills
- Crisis response services
- Inpatient psychiatric hospital services

Specialized dual-disorder services

- Dual-disorder assessment
- Motivational interviewing
- Cognitive-behavioral substance abuse counseling
- Dual-disorder groups

tion or dropout from treatment (see Chapter 6). In addition to these services, several other interventions are included as foundations of mental health treatment, including illness management training for clients, crisis response services, and inpatient treatment. As these latter three types of mental health services require coordination with the goals of substance abuse treatment, but do not involve major modifications for clients with dual disorders, we do not devote specific chapters in this book to each one.

Specialized dual-disorder services are interventions unique to this client population. These services include dual-disorder assessment (Chapters 4 and 5), motivational interviewing (Chapter 7), cognitive-behavioral substance abuse counseling (Chapter 8), and dual-disorder groups (Chapters 9–12). Effective programs need to provide both the foundations of mental health services and specialized dual-disorder services, and must be flexible and tailored to individual clients, in order to achieve the desired changes in outcomes. Individual program directors and the dual-diagnosis program director should monitor both types of services.

Self-Help Group Liaison

Most clients with dual disorders do not choose to participate in Alcoholics Anonymous (AA), Cocaine Anonymous, or other self-help groups in the community (Noordsy, Schwab, Fox, & Drake, 1996). Nevertheless, as we discuss in Chapter 12, many clients do participate in these programs when they reach the active treatment and relapse prevention stages, and find them helpful in remaining sober. A dual-disorder program should have at least one person who provides liaison with self-help groups in the community. This person can be the director of dual-disorder services or someone else. It is ideal if the liaison person is someone in recovery from substance use disorder (either a staff member or a client), but this is not mandatory. The person assesses the appropriateness of different self-help groups for clients with dual disorders, and helps them attend, understand, and fit into such groups. In addition, if sufficient numbers of clients are served, the liaison person can be instrumental in developing a self-help group that operates with support from the dual-disorder treatment program, such as a Double Trouble in Recovery or Dual Recovery Anonymous group.

Integrating Levels of Care

The continuum of dual-disorder services must involve vertical as well as horizontal integration. Clients with dual disorders need to receive care at all levels within a mental health program, including hospitalization, emergency, residential, and outpatient. All of these services need to be coordinated (for most clients, by their outpatient treatment team), so that the approach to substance abuse is consistent and continuous. For example, inpatient treatment should not be isolated from outpatient services, but should be linked with the overall program. Thus the focus of inpatient treatment should be on rapid stabilization, identification of substance abuse, thorough assessment, and linkage and coordination with outpatient services (Drake & Noordsy, 1995). Long-term substance abuse treatment should not usually be a goal of inpatient care. Similarly, when an individual with dual disorders becomes housed or receives treatment outside of the mental health center (e.g., during incarceration), the team should provide outreach and extend the treatment plan to these other settings.

Program Monitoring

Quality improvement committee members, clinicians, program managers, and the dual-disorder director should monitor program quality by direct mechanisms, such as reviewing records, attending case conferences, and attending team meetings. Based on prevalence estimates of lifetime substance abuse in clients with severe mental illness (see Chapter 1), for approximately half of these discussions comorbid substance abuse should be addressed in assessment and treatment as described above. Clinical records and the level of discussion should reflect treatment in stages, and can be used to monitor quality and to identify clinicians and programs needing extra training.

Program monitors depend on good data at the system level to assess implementation progress and quality.

Implementation can be measured quantitatively to reflect utilization and to identify areas for improvement. The fidelity of services to the principles of integrated dual-disorder treatment should be assessed at least annually, using the scale (or a modification thereof) provided in Appendix A.

MIS data should include rates of substance use diagnoses, rates of substance abuse treatment participation, and progress in substance abuse treatment. Based on estimates of recent substance use disorders in clients with severe mental illness (again, see Chapter 1), approximately 25–35% of a mental health agency's clients should be utilizing dual-disorder services. These estimates vary, depending on the demographic characteristics and the setting of the client population receiving treatment. For example, clients with recent histories of homelessness, males, and younger clients are all more likely to have comorbid substance abuse than other clients. If rates of substance abuse are remarkably lower than expected, it may indicate problems with identification and/or exclusion of clients with dual disorders.

Monitoring progress in treatment and recovery can be facilitated by the use of clinician rating scales (Chapters 4 and 5). In any cohort of clients with dual disorders, over 90% of such clients should be engaged in dual-disorder services within 6 months, and there should be a steady movement of clients through the persuasion and active treatment stages (McHugo, Drake, Burton, & Ackerson, 1995). The expected rate of stable remission (i.e., at least 6 months without evidence of abuse or dependence) is 10–15% per year cumulatively (Drake, Mercer-McFadden, et al., 1998; see Chapter 20).

Pharmacological interventions should be monitored in a similar fashion by the medical director. A significant proportion of clients who are not making progress in substance abuse treatment should be reviewed and given trials of interventions that are sometimes helpful, such as the second-generation ("atypical") antipsychotics, adjunctive antidepressants, disulfiram, or naltrexone (see Chapter 19).

Data from these various monitoring processes should be fed back to clinicians, so that they are aware of their own interventions and outcomes. Then they can participate in developing their own plans for learning and quality improvement.

Financing

Integrated treatment requires funding mechanisms that can be combined seamlessly at the program level. Mental health and substance abuse services are usually purchased by separate organizations or agencies. As every organization has its own rules about what services are reimbursable and who is eligible to receive them, combining different sources of funding can be a difficult task.

The advantages and disadvantages of integrating funding for dual disorders at the level of purchasers or government agencies have been debated, with no clear consensus about the best course of action. However, few would disagree that funding sources should support, not inhibit, integrated treatment. Practically speaking, this means that purchasers, administrators, and program staff members have to work together to ensure that reimbursement policies are supports rather than barriers to treatment.

Making treatment work in this context requires administrators who are well versed in the intricacies of reimbursement regulations, and who also understand the principles of effective dual-disorder treatment. Administrators may have to negotiate with purchasers to get reimbursement for substance abuse services provided in a mental health setting, or to cover the cost of services to families. In some cases, purchasers may provide incentives to engage and treat clients with dual disorders (Clark, Drake, McHugo, & Ackerson, 1995). Inducements like these may be necessary to offset the disincentives of capitated or case-based funding, which discourages enrollment of high-cost clients. Cutting through the complex, often competing interests embedded in substance abuse and mental health financing rules requires perseverance and a consistent commitment to placing clients first.

CLINICAL CONTROVERSIES AND CHALLENGES

Integrated treatment requires the recognition of clinical controversies that pose ethical dilemmas or that require professionals to change their normative behavior. If not attended to, these controversies can become a focus of conflict and distract providers from their primary goal of serving clients. Awareness of these challenges can promote open discussion among administrators and clinicians, leading to resolutions that are mutually accepted and form the basis for collaborative work. We highlight several prominent controversies below.

Violence and Criminality

The issues of violence and criminality need to be confronted by any program for dual disorders. Individuals with severe mental illness are at increased risk for violence, especially if they are not receiving treatment. Among persons with severe mental illness, the most im-

portant predictors of violence are a history of prior violence, including aggression dating back to before the onset of the psychiatric illness (Hodgins & Côté, 1993), and substance abuse (Swartz et al., 1998b). Integrated dual-disorder treatment systems can be effective in preventing and managing violence by employing (1) accurate assessment of past violence and risk assessment of potential for future violence; (2) treatment planning that takes into account risk factors for violence (including substance abuse); and (3) close monitoring (involving assertive outreach) of both psychiatric and substance use disorders. Assertive outreach to clients at high risk for violence requires careful attention to safety for the clinicians. Measures such as double staffing, cell phones, and personal emergency alarms can be useful. Close monitoring can ensure freedom from substance use and full compliance with treatment, which in turn will reduce risk of violence.

When clients' violence has had legal repercussions, close collaboration with the criminal justice system is crucial. Collaboration between administrators of dual-disorder treatment programs and the criminal justice system is necessary to avoid inappropriate incarceration (e.g., when a grossly psychotic client engages in an illegal behavior that is clearly due to impaired judgment), and to provide offenders who are in jail or prison with mental health consultation, prerelease planning, and postrelease supports. Dual-disorder treatment of clients who are on parole or probation needs to include persons from the criminal justice system, such as probation officers, in order to minimize the chances of reoffending and a return to prison (see Chapter 17).

Clients with active substance use disorders and antisocial traits may engage in dangerous or predatory behaviors that affect other clients served at a center. Clinicians and administrators should be prepared to take action to limit clients' access to the center when they exhibit such behaviors. This should not prevent treatment, however, and home- and community-based services should be substituted until such clients demonstrate improvement in problematic behaviors. Effective treatment will be the most effective means of reducing problematic behaviors in the long run.

Coerced and Involuntary Interventions

The use of coerced and involuntary interventions, such as inpatient hospitalization and conditional discharge, plays a critical role in the management of persons with severe mental illness. These interventions are part of the foundations of mental health services and ensure safety and access to clients for treatment, but are not treatment in and of themselves. Similarly, specialized dual-disorder services may occur in the context of co-erced or involuntary interventions to gain access to clients for treatment or as a result of legal consequences for possession of illicit substances or other criminal behavior. Integrated dual-disorder programs need to be comfortable with using involuntary interventions to protect clients or others after all voluntary interventions have been exhausted. The planning and evaluation of such interventions need to address several treatment objectives, including the development of client self-motivation and self-control, the delivery of effective treatment, and the assurance of safety. Specific guidelines for providing coerced and involuntary interventions are described in Chapter 17.

Drug and Alcohol Testing

Clients with dual disorders often deny substance abuse, for a variety of reasons. Legal sanctions prohibiting substance use, social stigma, and the fear of losing benefits are some of the most important reasons that clients do not accurately report their use of substances. Furthermore, although collateral reports of substance abuse are often useful, many informants do not know about clients' substance use, and many clients do not have family members or others who can provide information about their substance use.

Detecting and monitoring substance abuse in dual-disorder programs are facilitated by routine monitoring with alcohol and drug tests (Ananth et al., 1989). Agency policies need to outline clearly for both clients and staff members the purposes of testing, the methods employed, ways in which the results will be used, and methods for protecting client confidentiality. Staff members' willingness to employ alcohol and drug tests, and clients' cooperation with them and their continued involvement in treatment, will be best assured if sanctions or recriminations are not directly tied to test results. Agencies can reduce testing costs by ordering and contracting only for those tests that meet clinical needs (as distinguished from tests that meet forensic standards), and by making use of new technologies (e.g., saliva swab tests for alcohol).

Medication Issues

In some programs for clients with severe mental illness, there is controversy about whether to prescribe psychotropic medications for clients who also have substance use disorders. Although there is general consensus on the importance of pharmacologically treating psychiatric disorders in such clients (see Chapter 19), some physicians are nevertheless reluctant to do so. Objec-tions to providing pharmacological treatment include concerns over substance–medication interactions, questions about whether the psychiatric disorder is secondary to substance abuse, and the belief that pharmacological treatment may enable or facilitate continued substance abuse. However, the ability to treat substance abuse in clients who are not stabilized on medication and who display florid psychiatric symptoms is severely compromised and usually doomed to failure.

Dual-disorder agencies must equip their staff and facilities with expanded knowledge and tools for pharmacological treatment. Physicians and other clinicians need more information about psychopharmacology for people with dual disorders. For example, life-threatening interactions and adverse reactions between drugs or alcohol and specific psychotropic medications deserve utmost caution, but lethal combinations are rare. Agencies also need to have access to medical consultation from physicians skilled in addiction medicine.

In addition to expanding the knowledge base of clinicians about the pharmacology of dual disorders, clients need to be provided with correct information about substance–medication interactions, and help in complying with their medication regimens. For example, it is common in mental health settings to educate clients that it is unsafe to take alcohol or drugs when they are on psychotropic medications. Although such information is meant to discourage clients from using these substances, the unintended consequence is that they often stop taking their medication when they use substances because of their fear of these interactions. Adherence to medication can also be improved by educating clients about side effects and coping strategies for their management, developing behavioral prompts, delivering medications to clients in their natural home environments, and selectively using long-acting depot medications when required (Mueser, Corrigan, et al., 2002; Weiden, Mott, & Curcio, 1995). Chapter 19 addresses psychopharmacology issues in more detail.

Abstinence and Self-Help Programs

Traditional approaches to substance abuse need to be tempered by the realities of severe mental illness. Inflexible mandates for abstinence in housing programs, and requirements that clients attend AA or other self-help programs, may help some clients with dual disorders—but at the cost of failing to attend to the needs of many others. In order to engage and make progress with most clients with a dual disorder, it is necessary for clinicians to focus first on developing a working relationship with the clients and striving to minimize the immediate consequences of substance abuse. The majority of clients who successfully achieve abstinence do so through the gradual reduction of substance use rather than instantaneous cessation. Treatment programs need to accommodate this tendency.

Clients need decent, safe, and stable housing that supports their substance abuse treatment goals long before they achieve sobriety and abstinence (see Chapter 16). Hard-and-fast zero-tolerance rules are unrealistic for many clients and unnecessarily precipitate housing crises that can worsen their substance use disorders. Substance use reduction or abstinence can be encouraged by a well-trained housing support staff and can be cultivated at the individual planning level. In some settings, a continuum of housing options may be provided that varies with respect to tolerance of ongoing substance abuse (i.e., so-called "wet," "damp," or "dry" housing) (Osher & Dixon, 1996).

Self-help programs such as AA are helpful to some but not all clients with dual disorders (see Chapter 12). Participation in self-help is most likely to be beneficial in the later stages of treatment, such as active treatment or relapse prevention. By its very nature, involvement in self-help should be voluntary and never coerced, and clinicians need to respect clients' personal choices about participating in self-help. Clearly, other options need to be offered for clients who choose not to affiliate with self-help groups.

Therapeutic Boundaries

Dual-disorder services require clinical innovations, and these changes may run counter to some traditional professional roles. Although some boundaries remain the same (e.g., prohibitions against sexual contact, taking or using a client's money or possessions for personal gain, using a client for emotional support), others may be altered somewhat. As part of delivering services in clients' natural settings, the clinician may travel to a client's home; meet the client elsewhere in the community; travel around town with the client; transport the client in the clinician's vehicle; assist with shopping, laundry, or grooming tasks; and meet and talk with others in the client's support system, including family, friends, or an employer. This *in vivo* approach to service delivery is critical to establishing a working relationship with a client and monitoring the course of his or her disorders. However, it needs to be balanced against the fostering of dependency. Early in treatment dependency may be therapeutic, but decreasing dependency and increasing self-sufficiency become important goals later in treatment. It is helpful to review decisions with the dual-disorder team to provide protections against boundary violations.

GETTING STARTED

There are many different starting points for initiating new dual-disorder services. The decision to provide such services does not necessarily require creating a new department or new clinical positions. The willingness and readiness of staff members to innovate, the availability of financial resources, and strategic opportunities may also influence the organizing effort in a particular direction. Deciding where to focus the process of dual-disorder specialization and how to integrate services into an agency's structure demands consideration of the current needs and potential of the people who will be involved.

New dual-disorder services can be started through a gradual process of introducing training and forming work groups within an agency (or across agencies) to develop the program, or through creating a specialized service or pilot project. The critical ingredient to creating these new services is that there are leaders at the agency who are committed to improved treatment of dual disorders (including a designated director of dual-disorder services), who are willing to become involved in creating the new services, and who provide ongoing monitoring (and require accountability) of the providers themselves. Specific starting points for initiating dual-disorder services are presented in Table 3.5.

SUMMARY

Several different models exist for integrating mental health and substance abuse treatment services. The most common model involves the integration of substance abuse treatment into existing mental health services, while an alternative model is developing new service structures that include blended teams of mental

TABLE 3.5. Starting Points for Beginning Dual-Disorder Programs

- Establish a dual-disorder director position, with responsibility for organizing services, training staff, identifying clients, and tracking outcomes.
- Start a specialized service with several components to enhance the overall visibility and momentum of the effort.
- Start a single pilot project, to give staff and clients a chance to evaluate the new initiative and provide time for all concerned to learn.
- Develop a dual-disorder treatment team that obtains special training in dual-disorder treatment, and that serves to train other clinical staff members and can coordinate the development of new specialized services.

health and substance abuse professionals. Various organizational factors are critical to creating effective dual-disorder programs. These include multilevel leadership, infrastructure, specific training, widespread assessment and treatment, linkage with the self-help system, integration of expertise into all programs, coordination of levels of care, careful monitoring of clinical reviews and of program data, and financial mechanisms that support program development. High-quality implementation and program maintenance require that each of these areas be monitored, and that self-correcting feedback be built into the treatment center's program of supervision, training, and quality assurance.

Several controversies emerge in the development of dual-disorder programs, such as the management of violence, the use of involuntary and coerced interventions, drug and alcohol testing, the use of medications, abstinence and self-help groups, and therapeutic boundaries. Awareness of these issues, and a willingness to foster open discussion about them, are critical to preventing dissension and conflict among clinicians and will facilitate creating new services that meet clients' needs. A variety of different strategies can be used to start new dual-disorder services. Starting points include the development of a new program or specialized team, or the formation of special work groups aimed at incorporating new dual-disorder treatments into existing services. A new department or new staff positions are not required to initiate dual-disorder programs, although identifying a staff member who will be the director of dual-disorder services may be helpful. The starting points chosen by an organization depend on the financial resources available to it; the willingness of clinicians and leaders to innovate; and strategic opportunities, such as organizational change or state- or federal-sponsored initiatives.

II

The Assessment Process

4

Assessment I: Detection, Classification, and Functional Assessment

Assessment is the cornerstone of effective treatment. In order to treat clients with dual disorders, clinicians need first to be able to identify the possible signs of substance abuse, and to conduct more detailed follow-up assessments to determine whether these clients meet the diagnostic criteria for substance use disorders. Clinicians must have the tools for evaluating the specific nature of their clients' substance abuse, including their patterns of substance use, the context in which they occur, their functional significance, and the role that substances play in the clients' lives. Finally, clinicians need to be able to formulate coherent, specific, and realistic treatment plans based on these evaluations. The steps of assessment are not static activities that occur in a fixed sequence. Rather, the process of assessment is ongoing and continuous throughout the course of all work with clients with a dual disorder.

In this chapter and the next, we present the necessary ingredients for conducting a comprehensive assessment of substance abuse in clients with severe mental illness. We begin this chapter with an overview of the assessment process, which we organize into a model comprising five steps: detection, classification, functional assessment, functional analysis, and treatment planning. We next describe common problems clinicians encounter when assessing substance use disorders in clients with severe mental illness. Awareness of these potential obstacles, and of strategies for overcoming them, is critical to conducting an accurate assessment. We then provide a detailed description of the first three steps of assessment (detection, classification, and functional assessment), and introduce clinicians to specific

instruments and assessment forms that are contained in Appendix C. In Chapter 5, we complete the last two steps of assessment (functional analysis and treatment planning). Throughout both chapters, we make recommendations for how to integrate the assessment process into the ongoing day-to-day activities of individual clinicians and treatment teams caring for clients with dual disorders.

AN OVERVIEW OF THE ASSESSMENT PROCESS

Assessment is an ongoing process that is interwoven with treatment. Assessment begins at the earliest point of contact with the client, during the engagement stage, when a therapeutic relationship is being established between the client and clinician. It continues through the relapse prevention stage, when a sustained remission of substance abuse has been achieved and attention has turned to improving other areas of functioning. Information regarding a client's substance abuse and functional adjustment is gathered throughout the treatment process, along with evidence regarding the effects of interventions (or lack thereof). Treatment plans are then modified accordingly.

As mentioned above, the assessment of substance use disorders in persons with severe mental illness can be conceptualized as a five-step process (see Figure 4.1). Each step has a unique goal, specific assessment instruments, and various strategies available to clinicians for achieving that goal.

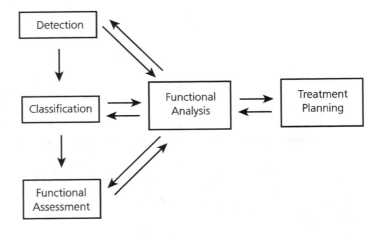

FIGURE 4.1. The five steps of assessing substance use disorders in clients with severe mental illness: detection, classification, functional assessment, functional analysis, and treatment planning. Treatment planning involves continuous feedback from the other four steps of assessment.

1. *Detection.* The first step of assessment is detection. Its goal is to identify clients who are experiencing problems related to substance abuse. Because the consequences of untreated substance abuse are so devastating, and because substance abuse is frequently unrecognized in clients with severe mental illness, it is preferable to "cast a wide net" and to be overinclusive rather than underinclusive in identifying these clients.

2. *Classification.* The second step is to classify the nature of those substance use problems by determining whether they meet *Diagnostic and Statistical Manual of Mental Disorders* (DSM) criteria for a substance use disorder. Classification involves evaluating whether clients' use of alcohol or drugs has led to *substance abuse* (i.e., substance use that results in negative social, role-related, or legal consequences) or *substance dependence*, including *nonphysiological (psychological) dependence* (i.e., excessive involvement in using substances to the point where other important activities are given up) or *physiological dependence* (i.e., development of physical tolerance to substances and/or withdrawal symptoms following cessation, leading to increased use to achieve desired effects). Clients who meet DSM criteria for a substance use disorder are in need of further dual-disorder assessment (described below); those who use substances without experiencing negative consequences should be educated and monitored, as their vulnerability to developing substance use problems in the future is high (Drake & Wallach, 1993).

3. *Functional assessment.* After a client has been determined to have a substance use disorder, the next step is to conduct a functional assessment of the client's adjustment, with a special focus on the role played by substance use in the client's life. The goal of the functional assessment is to obtain a comprehensive understanding of the client's adjustment across a range of different life domains, including psychiatric symptoms, physical health and safety, psychosocial functioning, and substance use. Specific needs related to substance abuse and other domains are identified during this assessment, as well as client strengths, which can be capitalized upon in developing treatment plans. As part of the functional assessment, the clinician obtains a thorough description of the client's pattern of substance use, including history of substance abuse and treatment, types, amounts, and situations in which substances are used, possible motives and consequences (both positive and negative) of substance use, and motivation to address substance abuse problems.

4. *Functional analysis.* When the clinician has obtained a description of the client's substance use behavior and functioning in other domains, the next step of assessment is to synthesize this information into a functional analysis. The goal of the functional analysis is to develop an understanding of the role played by substance use in the client's life, and to identify factors that may contribute to maintaining ongoing substance abuse and pose obstacles to achieving sobriety (or that pose a risk for relapse in clients not actively using substances). The functional analysis recognizes that a client often uses substances to meet particular needs (e.g., socialization, coping), even in the face of negative consequences, and that effective substance abuse treatment may require finding other ways for the client to meet these needs (e.g., improving social skills, finding alternative socialization outlets, developing better coping strategies).

5. *Treatment planning.* The final step in assess-

ment is to develop a treatment plan that addresses the problems and goals identified in the previous steps. In developing such a plan, the clinician needs to determine the client's most pressing needs and select strategies for addressing them (e.g., services to address housing and medical needs); the clinician must also articulate longer-range goals that are the major focus of treatment, and indicate the steps and methods for achieving these. Reducing substance use and achieving sobriety (or preventing relapses, for clients who have recently attained sobriety) are generally long-term goals in clients with dual disorders. Effective treatment plans for addressing these goals need to take into account clients' motivation to address their substance abuse, as well as factors identified in the functional analysis that may be obstacles to achieving or maintaining sobriety (e.g., a substance-abusing peer group, poor skills for coping with persistent symptoms). As treatment is provided, the success of interventions can be evaluated. Treatment plans are then modified in a continuous feedback loop based on ongoing assessment and refinements (or modifications) of the functional analysis.

The five steps of assessment, including their goals, instruments, and strategies, are summarized in Table 4.1. These steps are most effectively accomplished when they are the products of a team effort, involving all individuals who provide services to the client (e.g., case manager,

TABLE 4.1. Overview of the Five Steps of Assessment: Goals, Instruments, and Strategies

Step	Goals	Instruments	Strategies
Detection	To identify clients who may be experiencing problems related to substance abuse.	The Dartmouth Assessment of Lifestyle Instrument (DALI)	• Cast a wide net; assume that substance abuse is likely. • Explore past use of substances before current use. • Use lab tests to screen for substance use. • If use is detected, screen for presence of negative consequences.
Classification	To determine which, if any, DSM diagnoses apply to the client.	Alcohol Use Scale—Revised (AUS-R) Drug Use Scale—Revised (DUS-R)	• Complete AUS-R and DUS-R every 6 months. • Rate worst period of use. • Base ratings on team consensus. • Tap multiple sources of information. • Stick to evidence and get more information when needed.
Functional assessment	To gather information about the client's adjustment across different domains of functioning and his or her pattern of substance use.	Functional Assessment Interview Drug/Alcohol Time-Line Follow-Back Calendar (TLFBC)	• Obtain information about background, psychiatric illness and treatment, physical health and safety, psychosocial adjustment, substance use. • Use all sources of information. • Assess the client's range of different needs. • Identify client's strengths. • Update functional assessment every 6 months.
Functional analysis	To identify factors that maintain substance abuse, interfere with sobriety, or pose a risk of relapse.	Payoff Matrix Functional Analysis Summary	• Use information obtained from functional assessment. • Explore possible motives for using substances and costs of giving them up (e.g., reduced socialization, self-medication, pleasure/leisure, structure). • View identified motives and costs as working hypotheses, not facts. • Update/modify Payoff Matrix every 6 months.
Treatment planning	To develop an integrated treatment plan that addresses substance abuse and mental illness through concurrent treatment.	Substance Abuse Treatment Scale—Revised (SATS-R) Individual Dual-Disorder Treatment Plan Individual Treatment Review	• First address pressing needs. • Evaluate client motivation to address substance abuse. • Identify treatment goals and target behaviors. • Select interventions for achieving goals. • Choose measures to monitor outcomes of goal setting. • Follow up and modify treatment plans at least every 6 months.

psychiatrist, nurse, therapist), led by a single clinician. The clinician who takes the lead in conducting and coordinating the assessment obtains and consolidates information from all available sources (e.g., other team members, records, client self-reports, collateral reports); convenes regular meetings with the treatment team (or treatment providers) to discuss and reach a consensus regarding each step of assessment; documents each of the steps; and monitors follow-up of treatment plans, including periodic revision of the functional analysis and treatment plan. Although one individual is charged with spearheading the assessment process for a client, taking a team-based approach increases the likelihood that treatment providers will act in concert with one another, due to shared endorsement of the problems at hand and of the most promising treatment approach.

Assessment can take place anywhere, depending on where the client is and how involved the client is with the treatment team. At the engagement stage of treatment, assessment often begins in community locations convenient for the client, such as the home, a coffee shop, a local park, or a homeless shelter. For clients who have experienced psychiatric relapses, physical illnesses, or legal problems as a result of their dual disorders, the first steps of assessment may take place in an institutional setting (e.g., a psychiatric or general hospital, an emergency room, or a local jail or prison). For clients who are engaged in psychiatric services, but whose substance abuse has not been carefully evaluated, the earliest steps of assessment may occur at a mental health center, day treatment program, or vocational rehabilitation program.

The time required to complete the assessment process is partly dependent on the ease with which a client can be engaged by a clinician. For most clients, the detection and classification steps can be completed over 1–2 weeks. The functional assessment step often requires more time to complete—typically 2–3 weeks, although even longer periods may be required for clients who are minimally engaged in treatment and who have very limited contact with their primary clinician. The steps of functional analysis and treatment planning are less dependent upon client availability, and they can be completed in 1–2 weeks. Overall, it is best if the entire assessment process, including the treatment plan, can be completed within 4–6 weeks of initial contact with the client. Although the time required to complete this process is substantial, this investment is well spent, and it is an integral part of treatment. As clinicians spend time with clients learning about their substance use and abuse, functioning, and goals, clients become engaged in treatment, and a therapeutic relationship emerges. This relationship is critical to pursuing targeted goals, and thus serves the ends of treatment.

COMMON ASSESSMENT PROBLEMS

The assessment of substance use disorders in persons with severe mental illness is complicated by eight common problems (Carey & Correia, 1998; Drake, Rosenberg, & Mueser, 1996; Shaner et al., 1998). We highlight and discuss these problems here, and we suggest strategies for dealing with these issues. Awareness of these problems is helpful to clinicians in completing the detection and classification steps of assessment.

Failure to Take a Proper History

The most significant obstacle to assessing substance abuse in clients with psychiatric disorders is the failure to take a proper history of the clients' use of alcohol and drugs. Numerous studies have demonstrated that in routine clinical practice, clinicians are often unaware which of their clients use or abuse alcohol or drugs (Ananth et al., 1989; Barbee, Clark, Craqanzano, Heintz, & Kehoe, 1989; Drake et al., 1990; Galletly, Field, & Prior, 1993; Shaner et al., 1993). The most common reason for this is that clinicians simply fail to ask clients about their use of substances. Although not all clients are willing to discuss this subject freely, some are quite direct in acknowledging substance use and discussing the consequences of their use. It is often helpful to begin examining this topic with a discussion about a client's past substance use, and then to move gradually toward more recent use. Talking about past use first can help reduce client defensiveness, which is naturally likely to be greater when discussions focus immediately on current substance use. Of greatest importance, clinicians should know that if they do not ask their clients about substance use, most will not spontaneously divulge this information—and it may not otherwise emerge.

Denial and Minimization

It is common for individuals with substance use disorders to deny or minimize the negative effects of their substance use on their lives. In a similar fashion, individuals with severe mental illness often deny that they have an illness or minimize the extent of their disability. Therefore, it is not surprising that denial and minimization about both the amount of substance use and its consequences are pervasive in clients with dual disorders. Rather than directly confronting clients about denial or minimization, clinicians should expect these reactions, and strive toward the long-term goal of developing a trusting relationship with open, honest dialogue. In addition, clinicians must actively seek other sources of information about clients' substance use, such as reports of family members and significant others. Accurate assessment requires an ongoing process in order to overcome these barriers.

Confusion about the Effects of Substance Use

In the general population, substance abuse is defined in terms of its effects on a person's ability to work, the quality of social relationships, negative effects on health, and use of substances in dangerous situations (e.g., driving while intoxicated). However, even in the absence of active substance abuse, persons with severe mental illness are frequently underemployed or unemployed, experience significant problems with their interpersonal relationships, have health problems, and do not drive cars. The overlap between the core impairments of severe mental illness and the common consequences of substance abuse can make assessing the effects of substance use more difficult in the dual-diagnosis population.

Substance use disorders in clients with severe mental illness can be identified by exploring the interactions between substance use and the course of mental illness. Although mental illness may cause impairments in a number of different areas, substance use often exacerbates these problems, resulting in even worse functioning. Familiarity with a client's pattern of substance use and the course of severe mental illness can help a clinician discern the effects of substance use on the client's functioning. In addition, when active substance use coexists with a range of other psychosocial impairments, the clinician should assume that these impairments are related to the client's substance abuse until proven otherwise.

The Primary–Secondary Distinction

When working with clients with a dual diagnosis, clinicians often want to know which disorder is "primary" and which is "secondary." In discussions of substance use disorders and comorbid anxiety and depressive disorders, the primary–secondary distinction refers to the question of which disorder comes first, with the assumption that the earlier-onset disorder often causes the disorder that follows (Mueser, Drake, & Wallach, 1998; Schuckit, 1983; Schuckit, Zisook, & Mortola, 1985). Conventional wisdom holds that if the "primary" disorder is treated first, the "secondary" disorder will often go away automatically, and that it is futile to attempt to treat the secondary disorder until the primary one is successfully controlled.

There are several difficulties with attempting to distinguish which disorder is primary and which is secondary. First, it is notoriously difficult (and often impossible) to determine the effects of two mutually interacting disorders while both disorders are currently active (Lehman et al., 1994). Attempts to disentangle the causes and the effects of the different disorders are usually unsuccessful and frequently futile. Second, attempts to determine which disorder is primary or secondary often result in inadequate treatment of one or both disorders, resulting in poorer outcomes. For example, clinicians may decide to focus on treating the substance use disorder and to assume that the psychiatric disorder is secondary, with the belief that successful treatment will improve both disorders. As a result, the psychiatric disorder may be inadequately treated, interfering with effective treatment of the substance abuse as well (Cornelius et al., 1997; Mason, Kocsis, Ritvo, & Cutler, 1996; McGrath et al., 1996). Third, trying to disentangle primary from secondary disorders requires the assumption that, indeed, one disorder *is* primary and another *is* secondary. Such an assumption is often incorrect, and the designation of one disorder as primary and another as secondary is more of an arbitrary distinction than one based on their true causal relationships. Rather than attempting to determine which disorder is "primary" and which is "secondary," we encourage clinicians to view both disorders as primary, and to assess and treat both disorders simultaneously.

Cognitive, Psychotic, and Mood-Related Distortions

Severe mental illnesses are characterized by their effects on mental processes and mood. Cognitive impairments (e.g., poor attention and memory problems), hallucinations or delusions, and problems with moods (e.g., depression and mania) may compromise the validity of clients' self-reports about their substance use. However, clinicians' concerns over the validity of client self-reports often result in prematurely rejecting reports that are valid. In fact, there is abundant evidence that reliable and valid reports of substance abuse can be obtained from clients with severe mental illness (Mueser, Drake, & Wallach, 1998).

An individual client's cognitive impairments or psychiatric symptoms may interfere with his or her ability to report accurately about substance use and its consequences. However, the presence of symptoms or cognitive deficits alone does not mean that a client's self-reports are not valid. To evaluate the validity of a client's self-reports, a clinician needs to gather as much information as possible about substance use, its consequences, and other areas of functioning, in order to develop a comprehensive clinical picture of the client. The apparent consistency (or lack of it) among the client's reports of substance use, reports about other areas of functioning, and information obtained from other sources provides the necessary basis for judging whether cognitive, psychotic, or mood-related distortions are compromising the validity of the client's reports of substance use and its consequences.

History of Sanctions

Legal sanctions against drug use are a potent disincentive for persons with drug use disorders to provide an honest account of their use to treating clinicians. This obstacle to open dialogue also exists in persons with severe mental illness. In addition, efforts to restrict the access of clients with dual disorders to their disability income can act as a further deterrent to their willingness to talk about their substance use with clinicians. Clinicians need to be aware of these disincentives, in order to create a therapeutic relationship with their clients that is free of concerns over the legal sanctions associated with the clients' use of substances.

With respect to the abuse of illicit drugs, clients need to know when clinicians are, and when they are not, working in collaboration with law enforcement officials. Whether or not a clinician is actively working with people in the criminal justice system is usually determined by who employs the clinician and how a client has come into contact with dual-disorder treatment providers. When close collaboration with law enforcement authorities exists, clinicians may be required to report clients' use of substances to these authorities, and such reporting requirements need to be discussed openly with clients. In general, it is easier to develop an open and honest working relationship with a client when information about his or her substance abuse can be kept confidential and need not be reported to people other than the immediate treatment team. In such a therapeutic context, the client learns that he or she is free to discuss substance use without fear or sanctions; this permits a more open dialogue concerning the relative merits and disadvantages of continued substance use. However (as discussed in more detail in Chapter 17), even when a clinician does work for or in close collaboration with law enforcement, a strong working alliance can be formed with a client—provided that the clinician informs the client about the bounds of confidentiality.

A good relationship between the clinician and client also entails discussion of control over the client's finances, and the role of the clinician in determining the client's access to his or her money. Financial payeeships, in which a clinician or someone else controls the client's money, are useful early in dual-disorder treatment for limiting access to substances (Rosen et al., 2002), but they can also create tension in the therapeutic relationship. As discussed in Chapter 17, a clinician's honesty about the conditions under which a client can gain access to his or her money, and the steps necessary for the client to regain control over finances, are critical to establishing a good relationship in which the clinician can work together with the client toward the goal of removing these financial restrictions.

Premotivational State

As we discuss later in this chapter, many clients with dual disorders are not motivated to address their substance use problems and consequently are difficult to involve in the assessment process. It is helpful for clinicians to recognize that lack of motivation to work on substance abuse is common in the early stages of dual-diagnosis treatment, and that it need not be an obstacle to engaging clients and beginning the assessment process. Recognizing that most clients early in treatment are in a premotivational state can help clinicians lower their expectations for cooperation in the assessment process, and encourage them to work on understanding how clients perceive their own problems and goals. If assessment is approached as a desire to understand clients as they are, without prejudice or preconceived agendas for change, most clients will be able to participate with growing cooperation.

Different Norms for Substance Use Disorders

Clinicians often fail to recognize substance abuse in their clients with severe mental illness because of different norms for substance use disorders between these clients and the general population. Persons who develop substance use disorders in the general population frequently use large quantities of alcohol and drugs, leading to physiological dependence and health consequences (e.g., liver and circulatory problems due to alcohol abuse, or infections due to injection drug use). In contrast, individuals with severe mental illness frequently experience significant negative consequences with mild to moderate quantities of substance use (Cohen & Klein, 1970; Crowley et al., 1974; Lehman et al., 1994), and because of their moderate use, they are less likely to develop physical dependence (Corse et al., 1995; Drake et al., 1990; Test et al., 1989). Similarly, clients with dual disorders are less likely to use injection drugs on a regular basis than are individuals in the general population who develop drug use disorders. Therefore, applying the same standards for substance abuse from the general population to individuals with severe mental illness can result in failing to identify significant numbers of clients with dual disorders. To avoid this, clinicians need to be aware that persons with severe mental illness are likely to experience negative consequences from even low levels of alcohol or drug use.

We have now reviewed some of the most common problems associated with the assessment of substance use disorders in persons with severe mental illness. A summary of these problems and of strategies for overcoming them is provided in Table 4.2. We next describe the first three steps of assessment: detection, classification, and functional assessment.

DETECTION

The goal of detection is to identify clients with severe mental illness who may be experiencing problems related to substance use. At this step in the assessment process, it is important not to miss any such clients. Clinicians must "cast a wide net" and be willing to identify some clients for whom subsequent assessment will reveal that substance use is not currently a problem. Mistakenly identifying a client as experiencing negative consequences from substance use is a more acceptable error than failing to identify a client with an active substance use disorder.

During the detection step, clinicians need to maintain a high "index of suspicion"; that is, they must recognize that persons with severe mental illness are prone to substance use problems, and that it is possible for any such client to have a substance use disorder. This index of suspicion can be increased for the clients who are

most likely to develop such disorders. Table 4.3 provides a summary of the demographic, history, and clinical characteristics that increase the risk of substance use disorders in persons with severe mental illness. The presence of each of these factors increases the chances that the client has a substance use disorder in an additive fashion. See Chapter 1 for more information about these correlates.

Exploring past use of substances before discussing current use can help identify those clients most likely to have current problems. Use of laboratory tests, such as breath, saliva, urine, blood, or hair analysis, can aid in the identification of clients using different substances (Galletly et al., 1993; McPhillips et al., 1997), although such assessment methods can only be used effectively with clients who are engaged in treatment. Drug and alcohol screening should be performed during all hospital admissions and emergency room visits, and should be considered with other routine laboratory testing at times of concern about substance use.

One strategy for identifying clients with a dual disorder is to use a self-report screening instrument. Numerous screening instruments have been developed for the detection of alcohol and drug use disorders in the general population, such as the Michigan Alcoholism Screening Test (Selzer, 1971), the Drug Abuse Screening Test (Skinner, 1982), the Cut Down on Drinking, Annoyed, Guilt, and Eye-Opener Test (Mayfield, McCleod, & Hall, 1974), and the Tolerance, Worry, Eye-Opener, Amnesia, and Cut Down on Drinking Test (Russell, Martier, & Sokol, 1991). A common problem

TABLE 4.2. Common Obstacles to Assessment, and Solutions

Obstacle	Solution
Failure to take a proper history	Ask clients directly about substance use and its consequences, beginning with past use.
Denial and minimization	Expect denial and minimization, and tap additional sources of information about clients' substance abuse.
Confusion about effects of substance use	Explore associations between substance use and course of psychiatric illness; if a client uses substances, assume that problems in functioning are at least partly related to substance use.
The primary–secondary distinction	View both substance abuse and mental illness as "primary" disorders (and neither as "secondary").
Cognitive, psychotic, and mood-related distortions	Be aware of possible distortions without ruling out all client self-reports; seek out other sources of information about a client's substance abuse.
History of sanctions	Openly discuss the clinician's legal responsibilities, the client's concerns about legal issues, and control over the client's finances.
Premotivational state	Recognize that low motivation is common early in dual-diagnosis treatment, and actively seek to engage the client.
Different norms for substance use disorders	Remember that clients may experience adverse consequences to much lower amounts of alcohol and drug use than people with no psychiatric illness; the quantity of substance use is less important than the consequences of use.

TABLE 4.3. Demographic, History, and Clinical Correlates of Substance Abuse

Characteristic	Correlate with substance abuse
Demographic	
Gender	Male
Age	Young
Education	Low
Marital status	Not married
History	
Family history of substance use disorder	Present
Conduct disorder in childhood	Present
Premorbid social functioning	Good
Trauma and posttraumatic stress disorder	Present
Clinical	
Antisocial personality disorder in adulthood	Present
Medication and psychosocial treatment compliance	Poor
Violent/disruptive behavior	High
Depression	High
Suicidality	High
Legal system involvement	High
Homelessness	Present

with these instruments is that they were developed for the general population and often lack strong predictive utility for identifying substance use disorders in persons with severe mental illness (Dyson et al., 1998; Maisto, Carey, Carey, Gordon, & Gleason, 2000; Wolford et al., 1999). An exception to this is the Alcohol Use Disorders Identification Test (Saunders, Aasland, Babor, De La Fuente, & Grant, 1993), which has shown good sensitivity and specificity in detecting alcohol use disorders in persons with severe mental illness (Maisto et al., 2000; Seinen, Dawe, Kavanagh, & Bahr, 2000). However, most substance abuse screening instruments for the general population are of limited utility for a psychiatric population.

In order to facilitate substance abuse screening in persons with severe mental illness, we and our colleagues have developed an instrument tailored specifically to this population, the Dartmouth Assessment of Lifestyle Instrument (DALI; Rosenberg et al., 1998). The DALI is a brief, 18-item instrument that can be administered by interview, as a self-report questionnaire, or on computer; it requires less than 5 minutes to administer and score. A copy of the DALI and scoring instructions are provided in Appendix C (see Form C.1). Because the DALI was developed for a population of clients with severe mental illness, it has high sensitivity and specificity for the detection of recent substance use disorders, especially alcohol, cannabis, and cocaine use disorders. A positive score on the DALI indicates a high

probability (80–90%) that the client meets DSM criteria for a recent substance use disorder. The DALI can be very useful in detecting substance use disorders, especially if the clinician is not familiar with the client.

If clients have been identified as using alcohol or drugs, or if they score positive on the DALI, they should be further assessed for any of the common negative consequences of substance abuse in persons with severe mental illness. Clinicians should use all sources of information available in evaluating the presence of these negative consequences. A list of the common consequences of substance abuse in clients with psychiatric disorders is provided in Table 4.4.

TABLE 4.4. Common Consequences of Substance Use in Persons with Severe Mental Illness

- Relapse and rehospitalization
- Financial problems
- Family conflict
- Housing instability and homelessness
- Noncompliance with medication and psychosocial treatment
- Violence
- Victimization
- Suicide
- Legal problems and incarceration
- Trading sex for drugs or money
- Health problems
- Health risk behaviors for infectious diseases (e.g., exchanging needles, unprotected sex)

CLASSIFICATION

The goal of classification is to determine which, if any, specific DSM diagnoses for substance use disorders a client currently meets. Classifying substance use disorders is necessary for communicating the nature and severity of the disorders to other clinicians, and for monitoring the effects of treatment. Evaluating whether a client's substance use problem has improved over the course of treatment has important implications both for program evaluation and determining the need for, and nature of, subsequent treatment.

In classifying substance use disorders, the DSM distinguishes between substance abuse and substance dependence. *Substance abuse* refers to a pattern of substance use that results in significant problems in one or more areas of functioning (such as social relationships, legal status, or role functioning), or the use of substances in hazardous situations (such as driving). *Substance dependence* refers to the use of substances that meets the criteria for either nonphysiological (psychological) dependence or physiological dependence. *Nonphysiological (psychological) dependence* is a syndrome characterized by excessive involvement in using substances, as indicated by such behaviors as repeated unsuccessful attempts to cut down on substance use, giving up important activities to use substances, or spending large amounts of time obtaining and using substances. *Physiological dependence* is a syndrome in which persistent substance use results in the development of physical tolerance to the effects of the substance (requiring greater amounts of the substance to achieve the same desired effects), withdrawal symptoms following cessation of substance use, and substance use to decrease or avoid withdrawal symptoms. If a client meets criteria for either nonphysiological or physiological dependence, he or she is classified as having sub-

stance dependence. The specific signs and symptoms of DSM-defined substance abuse and dependence, including both nonphysiological and physiological dependence, are summarized in Table 4.5.

It is common for clients with dual disorders to develop nonphysiological (psychological) dependence on drugs or alcohol, despite relatively moderate amounts of use. Clients with severe mental illness often have limited social outlets and recreational activities, and substance use may fill a vacuum in this area, resulting in psychological dependence. As we have reviewed before, physical dependence on alcohol and drugs is less common among clients with dual disorders than among people in the general population with substance use disorders, due to the high sensitivity of clients with severe mental illness to the effects of psychoactive substances.

In order to classify substance use disorders in clients with dual disorders, we recommend the Alcohol Use Scale—Revised (AUS-R) and the Drug Use Scale—Revised (DUS-R) (Drake et al., 1990; Mueser, Drake, et al., 1995). These scales are provided in Appendix C. The AUS-R (Form C.2) and the DUS-R (Form C.3) both include a 5-point, behaviorally anchored scale that corresponds to the client's use of alcohol or drugs over the past 6 months. In each instrument, the 5-point rating scale is preceded by a number of items that reflect the DSM criteria for substance abuse and dependence, and/or that enable clinicians to identify specific negative consequences associated with clients' substance use. The answers to these items provide the basis for the 1–5 rating. A rating of 1 corresponds to no use of (abstinence from) that substance over the past 6 months. A rating of 2 corresponds to substance use over the past 6 months without evidence for substance abuse or dependence. A rating of 3 corresponds to meeting criteria for substance abuse, but not substance dependence. A rating of 4 means that the client meets DSM criteria for substance

TABLE 4.5. Signs and Symptoms of DSM-Defined Substance Abuse and Dependence

Substance abuse	Substance dependence

Substance use resulting in the following:
    Problems with social relationships
    Problems with role functioning
    Legal problems
Substance use in hazardous situations (e.g., driving)
	<u>Nonphysiological (psychological) dependence</u>
	Use of more of a substance than intended
	Repeated unsuccessful attempts to reduce use
	Giving up important activities to use substances
	Spending excessive time obtaining substances
	Continued substance use despite awareness of having a problem
	
	<u>Physiological dependence</u>
	Physical tolerance to substance (need for increased amounts, or lessened
	    effects with use of same amounts)
	Withdrawal symptoms after cessation of substance use
	Substance use to decrease withdrawal symptoms

dependence (either nonphysiological or physiological). Finally, a rating of 5 means that in addition to meeting criteria for substance dependence, the client's substance use has been so severe over the past 6 months that it has resulted in significant institutionalization, such as repeated hospitalizations, emergency room visits, or time spent incarcerated. Recommendations for completing the AUS-R and DUS-R are provided below.

1. *Complete the scales every 6 months*. We encourage clinicians to complete the AUS-R and DUS-R every 6 months on all of their clients, in order to track substance use disorders in those known to have them and to identify emergent cases of these as soon as possible. Periodic evaluations of substance use help clinicians to remember its importance and, when present, to incorporate dual-disorder treatment into service planning.

2. *Rate the worst period of substance use over the last 6 months*. Clinician ratings should correspond to the client's *worst* period of substance use over the last 6 months, rather than to the client's most recent use of substances or average substance use over the 6-month time period. Ratings are made of the most severe period of substance use for two reasons. First, clients often minimize their recent substance use problems, so that focusing on the past 1 or 2 months could lead to an overly optimistic assessment. Second, the worst period of substance use over the past 6 months has important clinical implications for the treatment of dual disorders. Clients who have met criteria for either substance abuse or substance dependence within the past 6 months, but who have recently experienced improvements in their substance use, remain at very high risk for relapse in the forthcoming months. Therefore, basing their substance use ratings on the worst period ensures that this high risk for relapse is taken into account in planning treatment.

3. *Base ratings on team consensus*. Rather than a client's primary clinician alone being responsible for rating the client's substance use, it is best if ratings are made following a discussion with the entire treatment team so that they reflect a consensus of team members, rather than the opinion of just one clinician. A major advantage of using team consensus is that it requires team members to share their views and to reach an agreement about the nature and extent of a client's substance use problems. Reaching a consensus about a client's substance abuse or dependence increases the team's ability to act in concert with one another in their work with the client, thereby minimizing possible conflicts and maximizing the chances that the substance use disorder will be an agreed-upon target of intervention.

4. *Tap multiple sources of information*. Clinician ratings of substance use should be based on all available sources of information, including client self-reports, direct observations of clinicians and other treatment providers, reports by significant others (e.g., family members), medical records, and laboratory tests (e.g., urine screens). These multiple sources of information are combined to arrive at substance use ratings that best summarize the accumulated evidence.

5. *Stick to the evidence and gather more information when needed*. Sometimes a clinician knows that a client uses substances, but the effects of this substance use are unclear. When classifying clients' substance use behavior, clinicians should not assume that clients experience negative consequences from their substance use when there is no supporting evidence. Rather, when clinicians are aware of clients' substance use but negative consequences are unknown, they need to gather additional information in order to arrive at an objective appraisal of the clients' substance use problems. In the absence of evidence indicating negative consequences, clinicians should not classify clients as meeting criteria for either substance abuse or substance dependence on the AUS-R or DUS-R.

FUNCTIONAL ASSESSMENT

The goals of the functional assessment are to develop an in-depth understanding of the client's adjustment across a broad range of life domains (e.g., living situation, social relationships), and to gather specific information about the client's substance use behavior (e.g., patterns of use, high-risk situations). The functional assessment is the most information-intensive part of the assessment process, since it involves gathering information not only about the client's substance use, but also about other areas of functioning. This is necessary because effective treatment of dual disorders requires a comprehensive assessment of needs related to both the mental illness and the substance use disorder. As the clinician gathers information about the client's functioning over multiple life domains, including a detailed description of the circumstances under which the client uses substances, he or she works like a detective to identify and evaluate the possible interactions between the two disorders, including how each disorder may worsen the other. This information plays a critical role in the next step of assessment, functional analysis (see Chapter 5), in which the clinician arrives at a formulation concerning the most important factors that contribute to the client's substance abuse or that pose a risk for relapse.

CASE EXAMPLE

Over the course of conducting the functional assessment of Jim, a 24-year-old man with schizoaffective disorder, the clinician learned that he drank large amounts of alcohol three to five times per week—typically averaging 10–15 drinks per episode and sometimes more, mostly with friends. According to Jim, his alcohol use helped him socialize with friends; in addition, drinking gave him temporary relief from his hallucinations, depression, and anxiety, and helped him get to sleep at night. However, Jim also indicated that although drinking gave him a temporary escape from his problems, he had struggled a great deal with depression since he began drinking heavily. He reported frequent suicidal ideation, several serious suicide attempts, and numerous hospitalizations. Jim said that he felt discouraged by his persistently depressed mood, and added that he hated going into the hospital, where he felt isolated from his friends and his inability to escape his painful feelings.

The functional assessment is best conducted over a series of meetings with the client, with additional information collected from family and friends, other treatment providers, and medical records. Information can be obtained during informal or formal meetings with the client, with discussion paced and intermingled with case management according to the client's comfort and need. When the clinician has recently established a relationship with the client, these discussions serve to develop and strengthen the therapeutic alliance between the two.

The Functional Assessment Interview is contained in Appendix C (Form C.4). The interview is divided into five main areas, as well as two sections titled "Goals" and "Strengths," covering the core topics of comprehensive assessment: background information, psychiatric illness, physical health and safety, psychosocial adjustment, and substance use. Guidelines for completing each section of the interview are provided below.

Background Information

The first section of the interview is straightforward and requires little elaboration. One area of potential importance in this section concerns clients who have children, especially women (Miller & Finnerty, 1996). Many such women experience difficulties managing their relationships and responsibilities with their mates and children. As a consequence of their dual disorders, these women often experience strained relationships with their partners and children, and lose custody of their children (Brunette & Dean, 2002). Issues of lost motherhood are

critical to these mothers (Fox, 1999). Helping mothers with dual disorders improve their relationships with their children, and potentially regain their parenting roles, are important goals that can contribute to their motivation to work on their substance abuse problems (Schwab, Clark, & Drake, 1991).

Psychiatric Illness

Information obtained about the client's psychiatric disorder includes the diagnosis, characteristic symptoms, and medication, as well as the client's understanding of the illness and its treatment. The purpose of this part of the evaluation is not to conduct a comprehensive assessment of the psychiatric disorder (which presumably has been conducted as part of the client's mental health treatment); rather, it is to summarize the information most critical to developing a treatment plan that addresses both the mental illness and the substance abuse. Some of the information in this section can be gleaned from the client's medical records (e.g., diagnosis, psychiatric history, medications), with other information obtained directly from the client (e.g., understanding of illness, symptoms).

When a clinician is inquiring about a client's understanding of the psychiatric illness, it is important not to attempt to persuade the client that he or she has a specific disorder. Many psychiatric clients deny having a specific psychiatric illness (e.g., schizophrenia), but are nevertheless willing to acknowledge some problem areas or difficulties in their lives. For example, some clients agree that they have problems with their "nerves" or that they are vulnerable to "stress," while resisting the idea that their problems are due to a diagnosable psychiatric condition. Other clients may even deny having any problems at all. Knowledge about and sensitivity to alternative cultural interpretations of mental illness are important. For example, *espiritsmo* in Puerto Rican culture is a system of beliefs involving the interactions between the invisible spirit world and the visible world, in which spirits can attach themselves to persons (Morales-Dorta, 1976). Spirits are hierarchically ordered in terms of their moral perfection, and the practice of espiritismo is guided by helping individuals who are spiritually ill achieve higher levels of this perfection. Troubled persons are not identified as "sick," nor are they blamed for their difficulties; in some cases, symptoms such as hallucinations may be interpreted favorably as signs that the person is advanced in his or her spiritual development, resulting in some prestige (Comas-Díaz, 1981).

Regardless of the client's level of insight into his or her psychiatric disorder, most clients can be engaged and helped to work on addressing problems or achieving goals, and (eventually) toward reducing substance abuse. Rather than trying to convince the client about having a psychiatric disorder, the clinician should seek to understand how the client perceives his or her own difficulties, and strive to emulate the client's language when discussing problems in order to develop and maximize rapport. Thus treatment plans need to correspond to the client's view of the world and personal goals.

Similarly, when exploring the client's understanding of medication and treatment of the psychiatric illness, the clinician should avoid attempting to correct or educate the client; the focus should be kept instead on evaluating the client's perceptions. Exploring the client's perceptions about the value of medication, problems with side effects, and concerns about the interactions between medication and substances can provide important information for treatment planning. For example, one side effect of antipsychotic medications is *akathisia*, an uncomfortable inner feeling of restlessness that is often accompanied by pacing (Bermanzohn & Siris, 1992; Raskin, 1972). Some clients do not take their medication regularly because of akathisia, while others may use alcohol and other substances to cope with this side effect (Duke et al., 1994). Recognition of akathisia as a troubling side effect in the functional assessment could result in modifications during treatment planning, such as changes in the dosage or type of medication used to treat the psychiatric disorder, or the development of more effective coping strategies for dealing with the side effect.

The clinician needs to have a detailed understanding of the client's primary psychiatric symptoms in order to effectively integrate treatment of mental health and substance abuse problems. The Functional Assessment Interview identifies the most common psychiatric symptoms in clients with severe mental illness, including mood problems (depression, anxiety, anger); sleep disturbances; cognitive impairment; apathy and anhedonia (lack of pleasure); and hallucinations and delusions. This list of symptoms is not comprehensive, and a more detailed assessment of particular symptoms can be useful.

There are numerous semistructured psychiatric rating scales for more comprehensively evaluating symptoms in persons with severe mental illness. These include the Brief Psychiatric Rating Scale (Lukoff, Nuechterlein, & Ventura, 1986), the Positive and Negative Syndrome Scale (Kay, Opler, & Fiszbein, 1987), and the Scale for the Assessment of Negative Symptoms (Andreasen, 1984; Mueser, Sayers, Schooler, Mance, & Haas, 1994). There are also self-report scales that can be administered to clients, such as the Brief Symptom Inventory (Derogatis, 1993), the Beck Depression Inventory (Beck, Steer, & Garbin, 1988), the Beck Anxiety In-

ventory (Beck & Steer, 1990), and the Posttraumatic Stress Disorder Checklist (Blanchard, Jones-Alexander, Buckley, & Forneris, 1996). If the clinician does not have expertise in the assessment of psychiatric symptoms, it may be helpful to work with other members of the client's treatment team who have more skills in this area, such as the client's psychiatrist. For example, the clinician can meet with the client and the psychiatrist to review the client's current symptoms.

Physical Health and Safety

A careful evaluation of physical health should be conducted, because clients with severe mental illness often neglect their health. In addition, the consequences of substance abuse, both direct and indirect, may include a range of health problems. Examples of the direct effects of substance abuse on health include the effects of alcohol on liver functioning (which in severe cases can interfere with the client's ability to metabolize psychotropic medications), and the risk of infectious diseases (e.g., hepatitis) resulting from injection or intranasal drug use with contaminated needles or straws. An example of the indirect effects of substance abuse on health is risky sexual behavior, such as unprotected sexual contact with multiple partners. Clients may engage in such behavior in exchange for drugs or money to support their substance use, because of lowered inhibitions and poor judgment following substance use, and/or because of increased vulnerability to victimization in substance abuse situations. Research indicates that clients with dual disorders are substantially vulnerable to such infectious diseases as hepatitis B, hepatitis C, sexually transmitted diseases, and HIV (M. P. Carey et al., 1999; Carey, Weinhardt, & Carey, 1995; Cournos & McKinnon, 1997; Grassi, Pavanati, Cardelli, Ferri, & Peron, 1999; Rosenberg, Goodman, et al., 2001; Rosenberg, Trumbetta, et al., 2001; see also Handout B.16 in Appendix B).

If health problems are not addressed, they can compromise the quality of the client's life and his or her ability to participate fully in treatment, as well as increase risk of premature mortality. Furthermore, failing to treat some health problems (such as sexually transmitted diseases) can have broader public health implications, including the spread of treatable and preventable diseases. Health issues are often some of the most pressing issues early in the treatment of clients with dual disorders. Diagnosing and treating diseases can help to solidify a good working alliance with a client. The clinician should be aware of the client's medical history from a chart review and available medical records. If the client has not had a physical examination conducted within the past year, one should be arranged.

Psychosocial Adjustment

Like the evaluation of the client's psychiatric illness, the assessment of psychosocial functioning is not intended to be comprehensive, but to provide an overview of the most critical components. Many different domains of functioning are covered in this section, including social relationships with family members and friends, leisure and recreational activities, work and education, financial matters, legal involvement, and spirituality. Much of the information about the client's psychosocial functioning may be available (or already known by the clinician) if the client is engaged and has been receiving treatment for his or her mental illness. In such cases, the assessment can be used to summarize information already collected and, if necessary, to update the most recent psychosocial assessment. If the client is new to the mental health system, has dropped out of treatment, or has received minimal services over the past several months, a more complete assessment should be undertaken.

There are several reasons why a careful assessment of clients' psychosocial adjustment may inform dual-diagnosis treatment planning. First, problems in functioning may be due to substance abuse. For example, conflict with family members is a common consequence of substance abuse (Dixon et al., 1995; Kashner et al., 1991), and clients may be motivated to reduce or stop using substances in order to improve their family relationships. Second, the evaluation of psychosocial adjustment may yield clues about motivational factors that maintain a client's current use of substances, or that threaten a relapse. For example, if the client reports spending a great deal of time with a close circle of friends, the clinician may explore whether drug or alcohol use is a shared activity among these friends, and whether ongoing substance use serves to maintain these relationships (see the section on "Substance Use," below, for more on assessing motivational factors).

Third, the evaluation of psychosocial adjustment may provide insights into the client's own strengths and into potential resources available in his or her social network. These strengths and resources can be capitalized upon when developing the treatment plan. For example, if a client expresses a strong desire to work, treatment can focus on securing competitive work and developing strategies for reducing the impact of substance use on getting or maintaining employment (see Chapter 18). If a client indicates strong religious or spiritual beliefs—as many clients with dual disorders do (McDowell, Galanter, Goldfarb, & Lifshutz, 1996)—it may be critical to incorporate these convictions into individual work (e.g., through motivational interviewing; see Chapter 7), and to identify others with similar beliefs in the community who may be sources of support and inspiration (e.g., members of churches or self-help groups; see Chapter 12). If a client's family ties are strong, involving the relatives at the earliest possible point will be an important part of the treatment plan (see Chapters 13–15).

Finally, comprehensive assessment of psychosocial functioning is critical if integrated treatment is to be successful in addressing the broad range of areas affected by mental illness, not only those affected by substance abuse. Improving psychosocial adjustment can help clients learn how to live a satisfying life without drugs or alcohol and build the foundation of recovery. This assessment serves to identify which areas need to be addressed in a client's treatment program.

Substance Use

The goals of the interview's fifth section are to obtain a detailed description of substance use behavior, to explore potential motivating factors for substance use, and to evaluate the client's insight and desire for change. It is best if the clinician has a good working relationship with the client at this point of the functional assessment, so that the direct focus on substance use will not be perceived by the client as threatening, and will lead to an honest, fruitful discussion. Therefore, the assessment of substance use may occur somewhat later than the other parts of the functional assessment, when the client is clearly engaged in treatment. However, the clinician is encouraged to attempt to complete the assessment within a month of initiating contact with the client, if possible.

Description of Substance Use

This section begins with obtaining a detailed description of the client's substance use. Within this part of the assessment, we suggest using the Drug/Alcohol Time-Line Follow-Back Calendar (TLFBC; Form C.5 in Appendix C)—a version of a standard approach for evaluating the pattern of substance use over the past 6 months (Fals-Stewart, O'Farrell, Freitas, McFarlin, & Rutigliano, 2000; Sobell, Maisto, Sobell, Copper, & Sanders, 1980). Many clients have difficulty accurately recalling their substance use over the past 6 months. In addition, it is common for clients to underreport their substance use over the most recent month. The clinician should be aware of these limitations in client self-reports, but not overly concerned. The most important information gathered during this assessment concerns the *pattern* of a client's substance use, including types of substances used, the approximate frequency and regularity of use, and the situations in which use most commonly occurs. The specific accuracy of the amounts of substances used is not central to understanding the client's substance use behavior. An example of a completed TLFBC is provided in Figure 4.2.

Motives

After obtaining information about the client's pattern of substance use, the clinician probes for possible reasons for using substances. At this point, the clinician may have already identified possible motives for substance use, based on the previous review of the client's psychiatric illness, psychosocial adjustment, and apparent pattern of substance use. The clinician uses this information along with additional probe questions to explore these factors in greater detail. It should be noted that clients' perceived reasons for using substances may not accurately reflect the true effects of the substances. In addition, motivational factors that clients are not aware of, or are unable to articulate, may nevertheless contribute to substance abuse. A client's perception of why he or she uses substances is only one type of information gathered by the clinician in attempting to understand motives for substance use; other sources of information include reports of significant others, reports of other treatment team members, and the clinician's own observations or hypotheses from other information obtained in the assessment. However, the client's perceptions of the reasons for using substances are often an important place to begin treatment.

Various motives are commonly associated with substance abuse in clients with mental illness (Addington & Duchak, 1997; Carey & Carey, 1995; Graham & Maslin, 2002; Mueser, Nishith, et al., 1995; Nishith, Mueser, Srsic, & Beck, 1997; Nishith, Resick, & Mueser, 2001; Noordsy et al., 1991; Test et al., 1989; Warner et al., 1994). In general, these reasons for substance use fall into four categories: self-medication; socialization; recreation; and sense of purpose, structure, or compulsion. Regarding *self-medication* motives, people with severe mental illness report using substances to alleviate troublesome symptoms (e.g., depression, anxiety, sleep disturbances, or auditory hallucinations), although substance use often worsens such symptoms in the long run. With respect to *socialization* motives, clients may have poor social skills or experience social stigma, resulting in difficulties establishing relationships with others; such difficulties may lead clients to develop relationships with more accepting and more marginalized social groups, such as persons with primary substance use disorders. Alternatively, some clients with dual disorders used substances with a peer group before they developed their mental illness, and they continue to use with these friends as a shared activ-

ity. Yet another socialization motive is that some clients report that using substances makes them feel less anxious or nervous in social settings.

Recreational motives for using substances are very common, as the effects of alcohol and drugs are usually quite rapid and predictable. The temptation to use substances simply for their pleasurable effects may be even greater in persons with severe mental illness than in the general population, as a way to combat the problem of boredom or anhedonia (lack of pleasure). Furthermore, clients often have limited money for engaging in other recreational pursuits, and the onset of their mental illness in late adolescence and early adulthood often interferes with the development of hobbies and other less harmful recreational activities. Finally, with respect to *sense of purpose, structure, or compulsion,* some clients develop severe substance dependence in which their addiction assumes a life of its own; feeding the addiction, and maintaining a routine that enables them to do so, become ends in their own right. All people have a need for meaning in their lives—a sense of purpose, something to do with their time, and a reason to live. People get meaning from their lives in a variety of ways, including family, friends, work, sports, and other recreational pursuits. For some people who lack these outlets, addiction fills the void by providing something meaningful to do.

CASE EXAMPLE

Jerome had major depressive disorder and severe cocaine dependence. He began every day with a trip to the local subway, train, or bus station at 7:30 to 8:00 A.M., where he would panhandle for money until he had enough to buy several rocks of cocaine. Then he would go to a local crack house, where he would purchase some cocaine and use it there for the next couple of hours. Although Jerome described enjoying the feeling of cocaine, it was also clear that his addiction, including his routine (or compulsion) for obtaining and using cocaine, provided him with a meaningful structure for his daily life that was as important as the "high" itself.

Insight

In the final part of the substance use section of the interview, the clinician evaluates the client's awareness of negative consequences associated with substance use, insight into having a substance use problem, and motivation to work on substance abuse. Just as the clinician avoids debate when inquiring about the client's insight into his or her psychiatric illness, the clinician also does not try to persuade the client about having a substance use disorder. Since assessment typically occurs during

Drug/Alcohol Time-Line Follow-Back Calendar (TLFBC)

Client ID: _____   Date: ____/____/____

Instructions to interviewers: The TLFBC summarizes the current month and the previous 6 months of the client's substance use. Start by asking about alcohol use, month by month, and then ask about drug use. Focus on an estimation of monthly use and the pattern of use. (More detailed instructions follow the chart below.)

Ask: For each month—(1) How many days have you used alcohol (or drugs)? (2) What kind of alcohol (or drugs) did you use? (3) How much did you use each day (on those days you drank or used drugs)? (4) What is the total number of days in _____ (month) that you drank (or used any drug at all)?

	Current month 1 (# days: 15)	Previous month 2 Aug	Previous month 3 July	Previous month 4 June	Previous month 5 May	Previous month 6 April	Previous month 7 March
Alcohol Kind	beer	beer	beer	beer	beer		↑
How much (per day)	6 pack per day						↑
How often (days/month)	10 days	20 days	20 days	20 days			↑
Total days/month alcohol used	10	20	20	20			↑
Drugs Kind (+ abused meds)	1) pot 2) cocaine	1) pot 2) cocaine	1) pot 2) cocaine 3) Klonopin	1) pot 2) cocaine			↑ ↑
How much (per day)	1) 1 joint/day 2) 1 gram/day	1) 1 joint/day 2) 1 gram/day	1) 1 joint/day 2) 1 gram/day 3) 12 extra/day	1) 1 joint/day 2) 1 gram/day			↑ ↑
How often (days/month)	1) 15 days 2) 2 days	1) 20 days 2) 3 days	1) 10 days 2) 3 days 3) 2 days	1) 20 days 2) 10 days			↑ ↑
Total days/month drugs used	15	20	12	25			↑

same pattern of use

FIGURE 4.2. Example of a completed Drug/Alcohol Time-Line Follow-Back Callendar (TLFBC).

the engagement stage, the clinician must nurture his or her relationship with the client by steering clear of debate, and focusing instead on understanding the role of substance use in the client's life.

SUMMARY

We have begun this chapter with an overview of the assessment process for clients with dual disorders, which we organize into five steps: detection, classification, functional assessment, functional analysis, and treatment planning. This is followed by a review of eight common problems with the assessment of substance use disorders in the dual-diagnosis population. These include the failure of clinicians to take a proper history of substance abuse; denial and minimization of substance use and related problems; confusion about the effects of substance use; the primary–secondary distinction; distortions related to the mental illness (cognitive, psychotic, or mood-related); the history of legal sanctions against drug use; clients' premotivational state; and different norms for substance use disorders in the severely mentally ill population compared to the general population. We have described strategies for dealing with and overcoming each of these common problems.

The reminder of the chapter has provided specific guidelines for the first three steps of assessment: detection, classification, and functional assessment. For each of these steps, we have made specific clinical recommendations and described instruments that are designed for clients with dual disorders. In the following chapter, we continue the discussion of assessment by providing recommendations and tools for conducting the last two assessment steps: functional analysis and treatment planning.

5

Assessment II: Functional Analysis and Treatment Planning

In Chapter 4, specific strategies and instruments have been discussed for accomplishing the first three steps of assessment: detection, classification, and functional assessment. This chapter addresses the last two steps: functional analysis and treatment planning. We begin the chapter by discussing principles and methods for a functional analysis aimed at identifying factors that contribute to ongoing substance abuse, or that pose a risk of relapse. We complete the chapter (and our description of the assessment process) by providing a framework for combining all of the information obtained in the previous four steps into a treatment plan that is comprehensive, can be implemented, and will serve as a basis for evaluating the success of subsequent interventions. To ensure that treatment planning is ongoing and responsive to each client's needs, we make recommendations regarding how to follow up on a treatment plan to determine whether the plan has been properly implemented, to evaluate its success, and to modify it when appropriate.

FUNCTIONAL ANALYSIS

The aim of the functional analysis is to identify the functions or roles substance use plays in the client's life. That is, what are the positive consequences of using substances for the client, and what are the negative consequences associated with developing a sober lifestyle? Put another way, *why* does the client currently abuse alcohol and drugs, and what interferes with developing more adaptive behaviors? Such an understanding can

pave the road toward developing effective treatment plans that address those mechanisms.

We begin this section by distinguishing between *functional behavior* and *adjustment*; we point out that functional behaviors do not necessarily result in good adjustment to the environment, and in fact often contribute to worse adjustment. Next, we describe why the functional analysis is a critical step of the treatment process, and identify the core characteristics of effective functional analyses. We then describe a tool for helping clinicians conduct a functional analysis of their clients' substance use behavior, the Payoff Matrix, and its utility for treatment planning.

Functional Behavior and Adjustment

People with substance use disorders typically experience a wide range of personal and social adjustment problems, yet they continue to use substances. Why do people behave in such seemingly contradictory ways? In order to address this question, we need to define *adjustment*.

Hawkins (1986) succinctly states that "the more people maximize their own and others' benefits and minimize their own and others' costs in an environment, the better adjusted they are to that environment" (p. 351). Two features of this definition deserve special attention. First, adjustment is behavior that is adaptive to the extent that it maximizes both an individual's *and others'* benefits, and minimizes their costs. Thus stealing is not adaptive because it maximizes one person's benefits at the cost of another's. Second, implicit in this definition is that adjustment is conceptualized as global and long-term, rather than immediate and short-term. Thus someone who habitually spends the past week's paycheck on weekend drug binges, and has little money left for food and bills, is not well adjusted because of the long-term effects of that behavior on his or her health and economic self-sufficiency.

The *function* of a behavior can be defined as those positive factors that the behavior serves to maximize for an individual, and those negative factors that the behavior serves to minimize for him or her. If those positive and negative consequences can be altered, the behavior should change correspondingly. Note that in contrast to the definition of adjustment, the functionality of behavior is limited to the individual (and does not include others). Furthermore, the function of a behavior is defined only in terms of the factors that influence it, not the overall benefits or costs of the behavior. Thus a behavior may be functional because it serves to produce a particular positive consequence (and the behavior would stop if that consequence could be blocked), despite the fact that it contributes to worse adjustment.

The notion that behaviors can be functional but maladaptive is an old one in clinical psychology (Mowrer, 1950). Typically, such problems result from the fact that the short-term positive consequences of a behavior have a stronger influence than the long-term negative consequences. One common example is a phobia, in which the short-term relief produced by avoiding the feared thing or situation can lead to pervasive avoidance and inability to fulfill basic role responsibilities. Another example is substance abuse, in which the short-term benefits of using substances (e.g., pleasure, social opportunities, coping with symptoms) can overshadow the negative long-term effects (e.g., poor illness control, money problems). Although anyone can get trapped in the paradox of responding to the short-term rather than the long-term consequences of behavior, clients with severe mental illnesses are especially vulnerable to it because of deficits in cognitive functioning, including the ability to anticipate and plan for future events (Green, 2001; Paulman et al., 1990; Seidman et al., 2002). People with schizophrenia may also have increased neurobiological vulnerability to the positive reinforcing effects of substances (Chambers et al., 2001). Thus understanding the functions of destructive substance use offers clues to addressing this apparently paradoxical behavior.

The Nature of Functional Analysis

To conduct a *functional analysis* is to systematically examine the positive and negative consequences of a behavior and its alternatives. As a first step in behavior change, functional analysis has a long and rich history (Bijou & Peterson, 1971; Ferster, 1965; Goldfried & Pomeranz, 1968; Goldiamond, 1974; Kanfer & Saslow, 1969; Lindsley, 1964). It has been the cornerstone of clinical efforts to change a wide range of maladaptive behaviors, ranging from anxiety to self-injurious behavior to substance abuse. At its core, the functional-analytic approach is atheoretical; the function of a behavior is defined in terms of certain factors only if changes in those factors result in a change in the behavior. From a treatment perspective, the identification of factors believed to influence substance abuse leads directly to interventions aimed at modifying those factors.

Effective functional analyses are those that readily lend themselves to treatment plans, with the accuracy of the analysis determined by its success in creating the desired behavior change. Useful functional analyses share a number of common characteristics, including their focus on behavior (rather than traits), their constructive (rather than eliminative) nature, their attention to the context in which the behavior occurs, their focus on factors maintaining the behavior (rather than etiological factors), and their ability to be empirically validated or refuted. These characteristics are described below.

Behavioral Focus

Traditional psychological assessment focuses on the evaluation of global, internal traits that are presumed to be at the root of maladaptive behavior. In contrast, functional analysis emphasizes specific behaviors and behavior patterns, and eschews intrapsychic explanations in favor of understanding the circumstances in which problems occur (Hartman, Roper, & Bradford, 1979). Thus the functional-analytic or behavioral approach is more interested in what people do, whereas the traditional approach tries to understand what people have inside them that makes them behave the way they do (i.e., their personalities) (Mischel, 1968). Focusing on behaviors rather than traits is more helpful in conducting a functional analysis, because such behavioral specificity can lead to the formation of behavioral goals that are addressed in treatment planning.

Constructive Approach

Functional analyses are most effective when they lead to treatment plans aimed at helping people develop new and more effective behavioral strategies for achieving their goals, rather than when they focus on eliminating maladaptive behaviors (Corrigan, McCracken, & Holmes, 2001; Schwartz & Goldiamond, 1975). Expanding rather than contracting clients' behavioral repertoires is more useful for two related reasons. First, there is a well-established (and ever-growing) technology for teaching new skills to individuals, ranging from social skills to coping skills to emotion regulation skills. The successful teaching of these skills to a wide range of clients with mental illness attests to their effectiveness in improving adjustment, as well as their appropriateness for clients with dual disorders. Second, maladaptive but functional behaviors can be very resistant to extinction unless another approach, less costly to the client, is identified for achieving the same desired outcomes. For example, it is often difficult or impossible to persuade a client who uses substances with a peer group to simply stop using without also helping him or her develop alternative social outlets. Similarly, the effort to limit clients' access to money to be spent on substances (e.g., payeeships; see Chapter 17) is rarely sufficient in and of itself to reduce substance abuse. As described later in this chapter, our approach to functional analysis and treatment planning is constructively oriented, rather than pathology-oriented.

Attention to Contextual Factors

Substance use and abuse do not occur in a vacuum, and examining the context in which they happen is critical to successful treatment. According to Nelson and Hayes (1986), the contextual approach to developing a functional analysis can be contrasted with a mechanistic approach. In the mechanistic approach, the clinician attempts to use internal and stable constructs to understand behavior; this is similar to the evaluation of traits in traditional assessment. From this perspective, a person who has alcohol dependence drinks because he or she has the disease of alcoholism. In the contextual approach, on the other hand, the clinician seeks to understand the situational factors in which the behavior occurs and does not occur. From this perspective, a person with alcohol dependence may drink to facilitate social interactions with others, to enjoy the "high," to relieve boredom, or to escape temporarily from depression or anxiety.

The contextual approach does not deny the possible role of biological vulnerability—as reflected, for example, by a family history of addiction—but it does not view such vulnerability as an adequate explanation for substance abuse. Instead, the contextual approach poses a different question: "Under what circumstances does a person abuse substances and what changes in those circumstances might promote a sober lifestyle?" Such a contextual approach is consistent with the facts (1) that addiction does not have a stable, predictable course and outcome in either the general population or among clients with severe mental illness, and (2) that many people with addictions successfully turn their lives around and are able to live sober and productive lives (Vaillant, 1995).

Focus on Factors Maintaining the Behavior

A functional analysis of substance use behavior is aimed at identifying those factors that *currently maintain* the behavior, and not the factors that are *etiologically responsible* for the substance use in the first place. Sometimes the same factors may be involved in both the etiology and maintenance of substance abuse, but at other times very different factors may be involved. For example, someone may initially drink and use drugs as part of a shared recreational activity with friends, but over time and with the development of mental illness, the person may shift to using substances to cope with symptoms and to maintain contacts with a shrinking peer group. Understanding which factors currently maintain substance abuse (rather than those etiologically responsible) has direct implications for treatment, which can focus on modifying those factors.

Empirical Validation

A functional analysis is a hypothesis (or a set of linked hypotheses) about the factors that maintain a client's ongoing substance abuse or that pose a risk of relapse. The utility of the functional analysis is that it leads directly to interventions aimed at modifying the factors believed to maintain substance abuse, and the success of these interventions at changing substance abuse is what provides empirical validation for the initial hypothesis (Nelson & Hayes, 1986). Alternatively, if the interventions are not successful at decreasing substance abuse, the hypotheses are not supported, and the functional analysis must be reevaluated or modified. Therefore, in order for the functional analysis to lead to fruitful treatment, it must include specific hypotheses that can be either supported or refuted by the outcome of the intervention.

It is critical that clinicians conceptualize the functional analysis of a client's substance abuse as a *hypothesis*, and that they remain open to the possibility that their hypothesis is incorrect (or *falsifiable*). Humans have a natural tendency to look for support for their hypotheses, while ignoring evidence to the contrary, and thus deluding themselves about the accuracy of their beliefs (Hayes & Nelson, 1986; Stanovich, 2001). This tendency to distort information in the service of supporting one's own convictions can have devastating effects in treatment settings, as clinicians persist in providing an intervention to clients despite overwhelming evidence pointing to its ineffectiveness.

Stating hypotheses in the functional analysis that can be supported or refuted by the success or failure of interventions that stem from them, and being willing to modify those hypotheses accordingly, enable clinicians to select and implement interventions in a systematic and scientifically valid manner (Popper, 1959). The process of conducting a functional analysis—selecting and trying interventions based on the analysis, evaluating outcome, modifying the analysis as needed, and selecting and trying other interventions until improvement occurs—is akin to conducting a series of "mini-experiments" (O'Leary & Wilson, 1975) in which the correctness of the functional analysis is determined by whether changes are produced in the desired outcomes. As multiple factors may influence substance abuse, it should be noted that a number of different functional analyses may be correct for any given client, suggesting that multiple pathways may lead to treatment success (Hawkins, 1986).

The core characteristics of a functional analysis are summarized in Table 5.1.

Conducting the Functional Analysis

Conducting the functional analysis involves tapping information about many different factors that may be involved in maintaining substance abuse (or pose obstacles to sobriety), including social (e.g., friends), affective (e.g., relief from anxiety and depression, pleasure), cognitive (e.g., the belief that "I'm normal because I use drugs"), physiological (e.g., withdrawal symptoms), and economic (e.g., money or goods obtained in exchange for drugs or a place to use substances) factors. The information incorporated into the functional analysis can be obtained from a wide range of sources, including the client, family members, friends, other clinicians, and medical records. Any and all sources of information are potentially valuable in conducting the functional analysis, and no single source of information is necessarily more

correct or more incorrect than any other. As stated in the preceding section, the accuracy of a functional analysis is determined by its success in leading to interventions that change substance abuse behavior.

The functional assessment guides the clinician in obtaining most of the information required to complete the functional analysis. Relevant information for the functional analysis can be organized with the aid of the Payoff Matrix, and summarized in the Functional Analysis Summary (both forms are provided in Appendix C, Forms C.6 and C.7). The Payoff Matrix is a tool designed to prompt the clinician to systematically identify all the possible advantages for the client of using substances (upper left quadrant), the possible disadvantages of using (bottom left quadrant), the possible advantages of not using (upper right quadrant), and the possible disadvantages of not using (bottom left quadrant). Often it is helpful to complete the Payoff Matrix in collaboration with the client (and, if possible, family members); however, no single individual's (or group of individuals') perception is necessarily accurate, and the "correctness" of the functional analysis is determined by whether it leads to fruitful changes in substance abuse. We briefly describe the types of information included in each of the four quadrants of the Payoff Matrix, followed by a discussion of its treatment implications.

Advantages of Using Substances

The positive consequences of using substances are generally easy to identify once the question has been asked. The short-term effects of substance use tend to predominate; these include pleasurable feelings, temporary reductions in negative feelings, social acceptance and affiliation, alleviation of cravings or withdrawal symptoms, and something positive and important to look forward to (Spencer et al., 2002). Although the positive ef-

TABLE 5.1. Characteristics of an Effective Functional Analysis for Substance Abuse

Characteristic	Definition
Behavioral	Focuses on specific behaviors and not on enduring personality characteristics.
Constructive	Aims primarily at developing new and more effective skills for achieving life goals, and not directly at eliminating maladaptive substance use behaviors.
Contextual	Examines how specific situations influence substance use behavior rather than assuming that substance abuse is determined by stable and unchanging forces.
Maintaining factors	Evaluates current factors that maintain substance abuse, and does not focus on etiological factors that first led to the substance abuse.
Empirical validation	Specific and testable hypotheses are formulated that are either supported or changed based on the success of treatment, rather than developing untestable theories about substance abuse that are tenaciously held regardless of treatment outcome.

fects of using substances overlap for different clients, the clinician strives to identify those specific effects that appear to be most important to each individual client, and avoids making assumptions about why the client uses substances.

Disadvantages of Using Substances

Many of the disadvantages of substance use are quite apparent, at least to clinicians and family members, and they typically play a role in identifying the client's need for dual-disorder treatment. Common disadvantages of substance abuse include relapses and rehospitalizations, financial and family problems, housing instability, loss of parenting role, risks of infectious diseases and other medical problems, suicidality and violence, and long-term increases in depression and anxiety. Clients are often aware of some disadvantages of using substances (e.g., money problems, conflict with significant others), but not others (e.g., increased relapses, risks of infectious diseases). At the same time, clients may not give the same level of importance to certain negative consequences that would be given by clinicians or family members, and they may not be motivated to reduce such consequences. For example, some clients with severe mental illness actually report an attraction to psychiatric hospitals (Drake & Wallach, 1988), and they may not be interested in reducing rehospitalizations. The clinician includes in this quadrant of the Payoff Matrix only those negative consequences that are truly experienced as negative by the individual client.

Advantages of Not Using Substances

Some of the advantages of not using substances are apparent from considering the disadvantages of substance use. Many of the negative effects of using substances are reversed when someone stops using; for instance, relapses and rehospitalizations are reduced, there is less tension in relationships, and so on (Zisook et al., 1992). In addition to identifying how negative consequences of substance abuse can be decreased, positive consequences of not using substances can be explored by helping the client evaluate how substance use may interfere with achieving personal goals, including improving the client's quality of life. Identifying advantages of not using substances may require retrospection into periods in the past when the client did not use or used less. For clients with heavy, long-term substance abuse who cannot recall when they used less, identifying possible advantages of not using substances may require some imagination and speculation. For functional-analytic purposes, the primary focus is on specifying the most prominent advantages of not using substances.

Disadvantages of Not Using Substances

A helpful way to conceptualize the disadvantages of not using substances is to ask this question: "What are the costs to the client of giving up substances?" Just as the advantages of not using substances are the opposite as the disadvantages of using, the disadvantages of not using substances are the opposite of the advantages of continuing to use. Given the many reasons clients use substances, the costs of achieving sobriety can be high. Examples of disadvantages of not using substances include problems interacting with peers who use substances; the need to establish new peer networks; lack of pleasure and enjoyment in life; problems with anxiety, depression, or sleep; and not having anything exciting to look forward to. Specifying the disadvantages of not using substances may also require retrospection or imagination for clients with heavy, long-term abuse who have had no recent periods of abstinence or reduced use.

Examples of common advantages and disadvantages of using substances, and advantages and disadvantages of not using substances, are included in Figure 5.1. Examples of completed Payoff Matrices for two clients, Jim and Sarah, are provided in Figures 5.2 and 5.3.

Clinical Utility of the Payoff Matrix

Because the purpose of the functional analysis is to understand which factors maintain the client's substance use behavior, a cursory review of the Payoff Matrix for an actively using client should reveal that the combined advantages of using substances and the disadvantages of not using outweigh the combined disadvantages of using substances and the advantages of not using. Note that the perceived short-term benefits of using substances and the short-term costs of giving up substance use often outweigh the longer-term benefits of sobriety and the costs of continued use. If the disadvantages of using substances (and the advantages of not using) appear to clearly outweigh the advantages of using (and the disadvantages of not using), then the clinician is faced with the question of why the client continues to abuse substances, and the functional analysis is incomplete.

Once a complete functional analysis has been summarized in the Payoff Matrix, there are theoretically four general ways in which substance abuse can be decreased or eliminated: (1) The positive consequences of using substances can be decreased; (2) the negative consequences of using can be increased; (3) the positive consequences of not using can be increased; and/or (4) the negative consequences of not using can be decreased. All interventions stemming from the functional analysis can be subsumed under one (or more) of these

	Using Substances	Not Using Substances
Advantages	• Feeling good • Acceptance and friendship when using with peers • Decreased social anxiety • Feeling "normal" when using with others • Escape from belief that one is a "failure" or has not lived up to expectations • Relief from depression or anxiety • Reduction or distraction from hallucinations • Help getting to sleep • Improved attention and concentration • Decreased medication side effects • Something to look forward to • Reduction in craving or withdrawal symptoms	• Better relationships with significant others • Stable and independent housing • Improved control and stability of psychiatric illness • Financial stability and control over one's money • Staying out of jail/prison • Minimized exposure to infectious diseases and better management of medical illnesses • Reduced exposure to trauma • Improved ability to pursue goals and meet major role obligations (worker, student, spouse, parent) • Better social relationships, including intimate relationships, with people who really care • No physical dependence
Disadvantages	• Conflict with significant others • Housing instability and homelessness • Relapses and rehospitalizations • Financial problems • Legal problems • Risks of infectious diseases and other medical illnesses • Increased exposure to trauma • Inability to pursue goals and meet major role obligations (worker, student, spouse, parent) • Physical dependence, leading to need for greater amounts • Sociopathic or criminal social network • Lack of an intimate relationship • Increased hallucinations or paranoia	• Lack of positive feelings • Awkwardness or peer pressure from friends who use substances • Social isolation because all friends use • Social anxiety • Feeling "abnormal" because of stigma from mental illness • Confrontation with belief that one is a failure • Persistent depression or anxiety • Distress due to hallucinations • Poor attention and concentration • Troubling medication side effects • Nothing to do or look forward to • Cravings or withdrawal symptoms

FIGURE 5.1. Examples of common advantages and disadvantages of using and not using substances, organized in the Payoff Matrix format.

	Using Substances	Not Using Substances
Advantages	• Helps get to sleep at night • Temporarily decreases auditory hallucinations • Decreased sense of social isolation	• Better relationship with family members • Psychiatric illness more controlled and fewer hospitalizations • More money to spend
Disadvantages	• Leads to conflict with other family members • Contributes to relapses and rehospitalizations • Results in money problems at end of the month	• Trouble getting to sleep • Distress due to persistent auditory hallucinations • Increased anxiety and unhappiness about lack of friends and social isolation

FIGURE 5.2. Payoff Matrix for Jim. Jim has alcohol dependence and tends to drink alone in his room on a daily basis.

	Using Substances	Not Using Substances
Advantages	• Provides temporary escape from depression and anxiety • Enjoys substance use as one of the few pleasures in life • Cocaine use provides social and sexual interaction opportunities	• More able to get and keep job • Improved severity of depression • Better management of mental illness • Decreased HIV-risky sexual behaviors
Disadvantages	• Has led to loss of several jobs • Worse depression the day after drinking or using cocaine • Avoidance of mental health treatment providers • HIV-risky sexual behaviors when intoxicated or high	• No escape for depression and anxiety • Lack of other pleasurable activities • Difficulty refusing substances from peers • Feeling more inhibited in social and sexual situations • Difficulty finding friends who don't use substances

FIGURE 5.3. Payoff Matrix for Sarah. Sarah has alcohol and marijuana abuse. Her cocaine abuse usually occurs in social situations, whereas her alcohol abuse occurs both alone and with others.

four categories. Specific interventions for each category are briefly described below.

Decreasing the Positive Effects of Substance Use. Substance use is a source of immediate, predictable, and dependable gratification. In practice, few available interventions can decrease the positive consequences of using substances; the most prominent examples of these are pharmacological treatments. One approach is the medication naltrexone, which works by blocking endogenous opiates in the brain, and has been used successfully in the treatment of alcoholism and narcotic addiction to block the "high" associated with these substances (see Chapter 19). A second example is the medication disulfiram, which blocks the pleasurable effects of alcohol by causing severe headache, nausea, and flushing (see Chapter 19). Disulfiram also increases the negative consequences of using substances, and is briefly discussed in the next section.

Increasing the Negative Effects of Substance Use. Substance abuse is naturally associated with a wide range of negative consequences, but clients persist in using despite these negative effects. There are relatively few options for increasing negative consequences, and by their very nature, these strategies tend to be coercive. Disulfiram can be included in this category (as well as in the preceding category), because it results in highly aversive physical experiences when it is combined with alcohol. Instituting financial payeeships, in which a more responsible individual controls a client's money, is another strategy for increasing negative consequences; with this method, clients are only able to regain control over their money when their substance abuse is in remission. Conditional discharges from psychiatric hospitals, or specific conditions of probation or parole from jail or prison—in all of which substance use

or abuse is explicitly prohibited—are further strategies for increasing negative consequences: Clients who use substances under these conditions risk losing their personal freedom and returning to a hospital, jail, or prison. (See Chapter 17 for more on involuntary and coerced interventions.) Although these treatment options are viable, they are limited, and represent an eliminative rather than a constructive approach to substance abuse.

Increasing the Positive Effects of Not Using Substances. There are several options for increasing the positive effects of not using substances. One strategy is contingent reinforcement, in which clients are rewarded with money, food vouchers, or other desirables for not using substances (Higgins et al., 1994; Silverman et al., 1996). Another strategy is community reinforcement (Azrin, Sissons, Meyers, & Godley, 1982; Meyers & Smith, 1995), in which clients gain natural rewards for engaging in activities that are inherently reinforcing, but incompatible with substance use and abuse (e.g., work, exercise). Yet another strategy is motivational interviewing (Miller & Rollnick, 2002), in which clients identify and begin the process of pursuing personal goals, and develop motivation to address substance abuse when they perceive it as interfering with achieving those goals (see Chapter 7).

Three more overlapping strategies that can increase the perceived advantages of not using substances include education about dual disorders, the decisional balance method, and persuasion groups. Education focuses on helping clients understand the interactions between commonly abused substances and their psychiatric illness. This can motivate clients to reduce substance use in order to manage the psychiatric illness better. The decisional balance method involves constructing a list with the client of the disadvantages of using substances and the advantages of not using substances. This method can raise client awareness and result in the decision to stop using substances (K. B. Carey, Purnine, Maisto, Carey, & Barnes, 1999; Prochaska & DiClemente, 1984; Ziedonis & Trudeau, 1997). Persuasion groups (see Chapter 9) are process-oriented groups designed to give clients opportunities to explore how substance use and mental illness have affected their lives; these opportunities can similarly lead to motivation to reduce the negative effects of substance abuse.

Decreasing the Negative Effects of Not Using Substances. Clients often cling to their substance use habits because they are naturally concerned about how they will meet basic social, coping, and recreational needs that are currently fulfilled, at least in part, by using substances. Interventions designed to decrease the costs of giving up substances are a powerful, indirect set of strategies for reducing substance abuse. They include social skills training (see Chapter 11) to improve clients' capacity to develop new relationships with people who do not use substances, or to help clients develop alternative social outlets. Clients who use substances to help them cope with symptoms can be taught a wide variety of coping skills to address such problems as depression, anxiety, sleep problems, and hallucinations. Effective pharmacological treatment (see Chapter 19) can also reduce persistent, distressing symptoms that contribute to ongoing substance abuse. Clients whose use of substances is one of their only sources of pleasure can be taught recreational skills to help them develop alternative and less destructive ways of enjoying themselves. Clients with firmly ingrained substance use habits, who might have nothing to look forward to if they stopped

using substances, can be helped to develop new meaning and sense of purpose in their lives by pursuing such goals as work, education, or resuming parental roles.

Examples of interventions based on each of the quadrants of the Payoff Matrix are provided in Figure 5.4.

TREATMENT PLANNING

Treatment planning involves combining and integrating information obtained during the first four steps of assessment into a coherent set of actions to be taken by the treatment team. The implementation of this plan is then regularly reviewed, and the plan is periodically revised and updated according to its success or failure in altering the targeted behaviors and achieving the desired outcomes. Although treatment planning for persons with dual disorders needs to address the broad range of functioning that may be impaired, our discussion here focuses on addressing clients' substance use problems, as well as the multiple interactions between these problems and psychiatric illness. Treatment plans may involve interventions that directly address substance abuse, such as helping a client develop the necessary skills to reduce or stop using substances. Treatment plans may also involve interventions that indirectly affect substance abuse by increasing compensatory skills for getting needs met in other ways, such as improving socialization skills or helping a client find competitive work in order to develop a sense of purpose in life (i.e., reducing the costs of giving up substances).

Treatment planning can be broken down into six

	Using Substances	Not Using Substances
Advantages	• Naltrexone • Disulfiram	• Contingent reinforcement • Community reinforcement • Motivational interviewing • Decisional balance method • Education about dual disorders • Persuasion groups
Disadvantages	• Disulfiram • Financial payeeship • Conditional discharge from psychiatric hospital • Probation or parole condition	• Skills training for social competence • Identifying new social outlets • Teaching skills for coping with distressful symptoms • Pharmacological treatment of distressful symptoms • Developing alternative recreational activities • Creating new and meaningful pursuits (e.g., work, school, parenting) • Teaching strategies for coping with cravings

FIGURE 5.4. Examples of interventions aimed at addressing factors that maintain substance abuse (or increase risk of relapse), based on the Payoff Matrix. Such interventions are aimed at decreasing the positive effects of using substances (upper left quadrant), increasing the negative effects of using substances (bottom left quadrant), increasing the positive effects of not using substances (upper right quadrant), and decreasing the negative effects of not using substances (bottom right quadrant).

steps: (1) evaluating pressing needs; (2) determining client motivation to address substance use problems; (3) selecting target behaviors as goals for change; (4) determining interventions for achieving desired goals; (5) choosing measurable outcomes to evaluate the effects of the interventions; and (6) selecting follow-up times to review implementation of treatment plans and their success. We discuss each of these steps below.

Evaluating Pressing Needs

In order to treat substance abuse successfully in a client with dual disorders, it is helpful to achieve as much stability as possible in the client's life. Doing so depends on a variety of factors, including the client's place of residence, the client's resourcefulness and survival skills, his or her social networks, and the extent of dual-disorder services that can be devoted to that individual. Clinicians need to balance helping their clients achieve as much stability as possible with working to treat the substance use disorder itself. In many cases, it is possible to spend all the available time trying to help clients achieve or maintain stability, while never actually beginning to work on their substance abuse. In the long run, focusing only on achieving stability is both frustrating and ineffective, because the contribution of substance abuse to instability is never directly addressed. Therefore, attention is given from the beginning not only to improving the stability of clients' lives, but also to treating their substance abuse problems.

Several different areas merit consideration when one is evaluating the pressing needs of a client with a dual disorder. Clearly, if the client presents a grave danger to his or her own safety or that of others, protective steps must be taken (as with any person with either a severe mental illness or a substance use disorder). Homelessness or housing instability is another crucial area, as it is difficult to provide effective dual-diagnosis treatment to individuals who do not have a stable residence (Drake et al., 1997). Stable housing may include living with family members, in one's own apartment, or in a supervised or supported residence. For some clients whose substance abuse is severe and has led to the loss of many housing options, temporary housing can often be found in homeless shelters until more stable housing can be found.

Sometimes a social network crisis may require attention to avert major negative consequences. For example, clients with dual disorders are often threatened with the loss of housing by family members who have become frustrated with their substance use and its attendant problems (Caton et al., 1994, 1995). In addition, a pressing problem may need to be addressed when a client is involved in a close relationship with another person that is marked by interpersonal violence on the part of either or both.

A client's psychiatric disorder may require pharmacological stabilization, in order to reduce acute symptoms that can interfere with effective dual-disorder treatment. Although such stabilization in a client who is currently abusing substances is tenuous at best, efforts to achieve it should nevertheless be made. Other areas of pressing need that may require immediate attention include providing assistance in obtaining food and clothing, and attending to medical needs for health problems.

Table 5.2 summarizes different pressing needs that may require attention in order to stabilize clients with a

---

TABLE 5.2. Common Pressing Problems in Clients with Dual Disorders, and Possible Interventions

Problem area	Possible solutions
Danger to self or others	Close monitoring; hospitalization
Housing instability/homelessness	Supported or sheltered housing
Lack of food and clothing	Providing access to food or clothing
Social network crisis	Outreach, support, and crisis resolution with family; respite care
Medical problems	Arranging and coordinating medical care
Acute psychiatric symptoms	Pharmacological evaluation and treatment
Predatory behaviors (e.g., dealing drugs, stealing, pressuring peers to give money)	Close supervision; minimizing contact with potential victims (e.g., peers)
Legal problems	Obtaining legal representation for client; coordination of integrated treatment with criminal justice authorities
Severe substance dependence	Inpatient or outpatient detoxification

dual disorder and potential interventions to address each need.

Determining Client Motivation to Address Substance Abuse

Central to the concept of the stages of treatment is the fact that dual-diagnosis treatment is always geared to the client's motivational state. Planning effective treatment requires a clinician to establish a client's stage of treatment and his or her motivation to work on the problem of substance abuse.

In order to standardize the assessment of clients' motivation to change their substance use behavior, we have developed the Substance Abuse Treatment Scale—Revised (SATS-R; McHugo et al., 1995; Mueser, Drake, et al., 1995). The SATS-R is an 8-point scale based on the four stages of treatment: engagement, persuasion, active treatment, and relapse prevention. Each stage of treatment is broken down into two substages. Behavioral anchors are used to describe the client's substance use behavior and involvement in treatment, so that reliable and objective ratings can be made. The SATS-R ranges from the low end of preengagement and engagement (characterized by no or irregular contact with a dual-disorder clinician), to the middle stages of early and late persuasion and active treatment (characterized by regular contact with the clinician and progress toward substance use reduction or abstinence), and to the final stages of relapse prevention and recovery/remission in which the client has not met criteria for a substance use disorder for at least 6 months). An outline of the SATS-R is provided in Table 5.3; the full SATS-R is given in Appendix C (see Form C.8).

Similar to the Alcohol Use Scale—Revised (AUS-R) and the Drug Use Scale—Revised (DUS-R), the SATS-R is completed on the basis of all available information, including client self-reports, observed behavior, information from treatment providers, laboratory tests, and feedback from significant others such as family members (see Chapter 4 for a discussion of the AUS-R and DUS-R, and Forms C.2 and C.3 in Appendix C for the full scales). Also similar to the AUS-R and DUS-R, ratings on the SATS-R are most accurate when they are based on a discussion involving the whole treatment team, rather than assigned by a single clinician. This discussion can be valuable because it encourages team members to reach a consensus regarding their perception of the client's motivation to change his or her substance use behavior, which is critical to identifying interventions appropriate to the client's stage of treatment. We recommend that consensus-based SATS-R ratings be completed at least every 6 months.

Ratings for the AUS-R and DUS-R are based on the *worst period* of alcohol or drug abuse over the past 6 months. In contrast, the SATS-R ratings are based on the client's *pattern of substance use* over the 6-month period, with an emphasis on the client's most recent substance abuse and involvement in treatment. This allows the treatment plan to correspond to the client's current motivational state and level of treatment participation.

CASE EXAMPLE

Frank was having significant problems with alcohol dependence 5 months ago, when he participated irregularly in dual-disorder treatment. However, over the past 3 months he has become more involved in treatment, including participation in weekly groups and meeting on a regular basis

TABLE 5.3. Summary of the Substance Abuse Treatment Scale—Revised (SATS-R)

Stage	Subscale	Behavioral description
Engagement	1. Preengagement	No contact with a counselor
	2. Engagement	No regular contact with a counselor
Persuasion	3. Early Persuasion	Regular contact with a counselor, but no reduction in substance abuse
	4. Late Persuasion	Reduction in substance abuse for less than 1 month
Active treatment	5. Early Active Treatment	Reduction in substance abuse for more than 1 month
	6. Late Active Treatment	No abuse for 1–5 months
Relapse prevention	7. Relapse Prevention	No abuse for at least 6 months
	8. In Remission or Recovery	No abuse for over 1 year

with his case manager. In addition, Frank has successfully reduced his alcohol use over the past several months and has experienced only a few problems with alcohol. Because of Frank's significant reduction in alcohol abuse and his increased involvement in treatment, he is rated on the SATS-R as being in Early Active Treatment (5).

Additional clinical vignettes illustrating ratings on the SATS-R are provided in Table 5.4.

Selecting Target Behaviors as Goals for Change

The clinician next addresses this fundamental question: "What changes are necessary in order to decrease substance abuse or to minimize the chances of a relapse into substance abuse?" This question is considered and answered within two frameworks: the stages of treatment and the functional analysis.

First, the client's stage of treatment has immediate

TABLE 5.4. Clinical Vignettes to Illustrate Ratings on the Substance Abuse Treatment Scale—Revised (SATS-R)

1. Preengagement. The person does not have contact with a dual-disorder clinician.

Jeanne lives in a single-resident-occupancy building and has high visibility in the local community because of her "strange" behaviors, which become worse when she is using substances. Police and local merchants have called the mental health center about her, and several attempts have been made by center outreach staff to get her into the center. She continues to refuse these offers.

2. Engagement. The client has had irregular contact with a clinician, but does not have regular contacts.

John, a young single man who has been diagnosed in the past as suffering from schizophrenia, occasionally shows up at the mental health center and demands to see someone. He knows he has a case manager, but cannot remember his name. He last saw his case manager 1 month ago when he wanted to get fuel assistance. His contacts with clinicians are infrequent, and usually involve wanting money, food, or cigarettes. He smokes marijuana on a daily basis, but does not speak with his case manager about it.

3. Early Persuasion. The client has regular contacts with a clinician, but has not reduced substance use.

Fred has been a client of the mental health center for many years. He was a long-time resident of the state hospital prior to his involvement at the center. Fred continues to drink at least a quart of wine daily and is not compliant with taking his antipsychotic medication. He does meet weekly with his case manager and sometimes calls when in crisis. The meetings usually deal with concrete needs and activities of daily living.

4. Late Persuasion. The client shows evidence of reducing substance use over the past several weeks.

Star binges on alcohol and cannabis, and occasionally uses hallucinogens. She lives in a supported apartment with two other clients of the mental health center. Star attends a day treatment program at the mental health center 3 days a week, attends weekly persuasion groups, and sees her case manager twice a month. In sessions, she says that she recognizes her substance abuse as a problem, and that she is considering a plan for abstinence. Her case manager reports that the number of "parties" at Star's apartment has decreased considerably, and she has not been bingeing as much.

5. Early Active Treatment. The client has reduced substance use for more than 1 month, but still experiences some substance abuse problems.

Crystal is a grandmother with years of polysubstance abuse. Her psychiatric symptoms are controlled with medication, which she receives every other week from the mental health center nurse. She sees her case manager at least monthly. Six months ago, she went on a binge of drinking and smoking crack; she went out of control, scared her daughter and her two grandchildren, and was brought to the emergency room. Since that incident, she has contracted with her clinician and her daughter not to use crack, and is trying to cut down on her drinking. She wants to be able to still drink in a controlled manner, but if this does not work, then she states that she would adopt abstinence as a goal.

6. Late Active Treatment. The client has not met criteria for substance abuse for the past 1–5 months.

Gina is a young single woman with bipolar disorder who is active in Narcotics Anonymous for her cocaine addiction. She has been abstinent for 2 months, and prior to that has had a 5-month and a 4-month period of abstinence. After her last relapse 2 months ago, she asked to be placed in a more structured living situation associated with a treatment program. She knows that cocaine is her drug problem, and uses this as a focus of her weekly meetings with her clinician. Her goals include abstinence and getting to work.

7. Relapse Prevention. The client has not met criteria for substance abuse for the past 6–12 months.

Vanessa, a middle-aged woman with major depression and a history of alcoholism, sees her clinician weekly. She has been sober for 7 months, with a brief lapse of 2 days several months ago. She became depressed over a love relationship, loss of a job, and financial problems, and slipped, but avoided falling back into regular substance abuse.

8. In Recovery or Remission. The client has not met criteria for substance abuse for over 1 year.

Jefferson is a long-term client of the mental health system. He has an excellent relationship with his clinician, where the focus is on social skills and maintaining himself in the community. For many years he had severe alcohol dependence, but he has not used any substances in over 13 months and reports no craving to do so. He takes mood-stabilizing and antipsychotic medications, and he regularly attends the local consumer-run drop-in center.

relevance to selecting target behaviors as goals (i.e., behavioral goals), because it reflects the individual's motivation to change his or her substance use behavior. In the engagement stage, clients do not have a working relationship with a clinician, and they are not motivated to change their substance use behavior. Therefore, treatment goals in the engagement stage focus primarily on establishing regular contact with clients and helping them get their basic needs met. At the persuasion stage, clients have regular contact with their clinicians, but they are minimally invested in changing their substance use behavior. In this stage of treatment, clients are often motivated to learn more and talk about their substance use, and to work on other goals that are personally relevant and that may be important later in living a substance-free, satisfying life; however, they are not motivated to work directly on their substance use problems. In the active treatment stage, clients have begun to reduce their use of substances and are motivated to achieve further reductions or abstinence. In the relapse prevention stage, when clients have not recently had problems related to substance use, there is motivation both to keep the substance abuse in remission and to work even more on improving other areas of functioning. Thus the clinician's focus of attention depends on the client's specific stage of treatment. (See Table 2.3 in Chapter 2 for a summary of stage-related goals.)

The second framework for selection of behavioral goals is the functional analysis. This analysis, as laid out in the Payoff Matrix, is used to target those factors believed either to maintain ongoing substance abuse (for clients in the engagement or persuasion stage) or to threaten a worsening of substance abuse or relapse (for clients in the active treatment or relapse prevention stage). Targeting behaviors as goals based on the functional analysis often aims at reducing substance abuse through indirect methods. Two such indirect approaches, illustrated below, include targeting behaviors that reduce the costs of not using substances (i.e., factors identified in the bottom right quadrant of the Payoff Matrix) and targeting behaviors that increase the perceived advantages of not using substances (i.e., factors identified in the upper right quadrant of the Payoff Matrix).

CASE EXAMPLES

In the case of Jim (see the bottom right quadrant of the Payoff Matrix in Figure 5.2), the hypothesized disadvantages of not using substances include increased trouble getting to sleep, distress due to persistent hallucinations, and increased anxiety and unhappiness due to lack of friends and social isolation. Potential behavioral goals for Jim to address these factors could include improved sleep hygiene, teaching coping strategies to manage hallucinations, and developing alternative social outlets with non-substance-abusing friends. Success in changing any or all of these behaviors could reduce the costs to Jim of not using substances, thereby moving him toward reduced substance use or abstinence.

In the case of Sarah (see the upper right quadrant of the Payoff Matrix in Figure 5.3), the hypothesized advantages of not using substances include improved ability to keep a job, less severe depression, and decreased risky sexual behaviors. Potential behavioral goals to address these factors could include supported employment to obtain work (Bond, Becker, et al., 2001); skills training to address problems emerging on the job (Wallace, Tauber, & Wilde, 1999); motivational interviewing to identify strategies for maintaining work (e.g., decreased substance use) (see Chapter 7); education about the longer-term effects of substance use on depression; and education and discussion about the relationship among substance use, sexual behaviors, and risk of infectious diseases, and about getting tested for infectious diseases. Success at increasing any or all of the perceived advantages of not using substances could lead to increased motivation not to use substances, and associated reductions in substance abuse.

The stages of treatment and the functional analysis represent different approaches to identifying behavioral goals for change. However, these approaches are complementary, and some common goals may emerge from both. For example, a client in the active stage of treatment who has succeeded in reducing cocaine abuse may experience difficulty achieving abstinence because of a lack of other recreational activities. From the stages-of-treatment perspective, the goal of reducing substance use and achieving abstinence (i.e., the goal of the active treatment stage) can be partly accomplished by helping the client identify and explore new leisure activities. From a functional-analytic perspective, one of the costs of giving up cocaine for this client is having to forgo the pleasures of cocaine use, and developing new leisure activities will decrease this cost of abstinence. Thus common goals can emerge from the stages-of-treatment and functional-analytic approaches to treatment planning, although other goals may be specific to one approach or the other.

When the clinician and client are selecting behavioral goals, it is best to identify several goals, to break them down into small steps and specific behaviors, and to select goals that elicit minimal resistance and have high potential for success. At least one goal should be based on the client's stage of treatment, and at least one more goal should be based on the functional analysis. In addition, the selection of behavioral goals should be determined by their relevance to changing substance use behavior and the expectation that the behaviors can in fact be altered.

The process of identifying suitable target behaviors as goals follows three steps. First, the problems that are preventing the person from progressing to the next stage of treatment need to be considered. Second, factors that maintain ongoing substance use or threaten a relapse are identified. Third, concrete behavioral goals to address these factors are specified. Examples of different problems and corresponding behavioral goals based on the stages of treatment and the functional analysis are provided in Tables 5.5 and 5.6.

Determining Interventions for Achieving Desired Goals

Once two to four behavioral goals have been selected, interventions for achieving the desired changes must be identified. In this book, we describe a broad range of different approaches for treating clients with dual disorders. When selecting treatment strategies to achieve specific goals, clinicians should bear in mind that some methods are stage-specific, whereas others are not. For example, case management, family work, and psychopharmacology are treatment modalities that can be provided at all stages of treatment. In contrast, motivational interviewing is most appropriate for the persuasion stage, and active treatment groups are most suitable for

clients in either the active treatment or relapse prevention stage. Table 5.7 provides a summary of the different stages at which different treatment modalities can be used. Sometimes a client may benefit from an intervention not usually provided at his or her stage of treatment. For example, clients in the persuasion stage occasionally benefit from attending a self-help group such as Alcoholics Anonymous or Dual Recovery Anonymous. In short, Table 5.7 provides general guidance to clinicians for matching treatment to clients' motivational states (i.e., stages of treatment), but exceptions can be made.

In addition to the fact that different treatment modalities can be used at different stages of treatment, specific treatment goals can often be achieved via different strategies and modalities. For example, the treatment goal of developing new social outlets with non-substance-abusing peers can be accomplished by engaging a client in group-based social skills training to improve conversational skills, family work to explore alternative socialization opportunities, sampling community social organizations during case management outreach, cognitive-behavioral counseling to reduce anxiety in novel social situations, or any combination thereof. Similarly, the goal of developing strategies for managing cravings in high-risk situations can be accomplished through active treatment groups, family problem solving, pharmacotherapy, or individual cognitive-

TABLE 5.5. Examples of Problems, Behavioral Goals, and Interventions Based on the Stages of Treatment

Problem	Behavioral goal(s)	Interventions
Lack of regular contact with dual-diagnosis clinician (engagement)	Regular contact with clinician	Assertive outreach; practical assistance; social network support
Lack of awareness of substance abuse–mental illness interactions (persuasion)	Knowledge of effects of substance use on mental illness	Education; persuasion groups; systematic analysis of substance use episodes
Interference of substance abuse with personally valued goals (persuasion)	Efforts to reduce substance use in order to make progress toward personal goals	Motivational interviewing; persuasion groups; vocational rehabilitation
Despite reductions in substance use, occasional "slips" in high-risk situations (active treatment)	Recognition of high-risk situations, and implementation of strategies for avoiding those situations	Active treatment groups; family problem solving; cognitive-behavioral counseling
Several months after achieving abstinence, powerful cravings to drink (active treatment)	Ability to use imagery techniques to cope with cravings	Cognitive-behavioral counseling
Relapse of substance abuse during hypomanic or manic episodes (active treatment or relapse prevention)	Development of relapse prevention plans for mania and substance abuse	Active treatment groups; cognitive-behavioral counseling; family problem solving
Desire to resume "normal" substance use after 8 months of successful abstinence (relapse prevention)	Recognition of high vulnerability to addiction when trying to use substances "normally"	Self-help groups; education; active treatment groups
Loneliness due to distance from peers who abuse substances (relapse prevention)	Improved skills for making friends and opportunities to meet new people	Social skills training; family problem solving; self-help groups

TABLE 5.6. Examples of Problems, Behavioral Goals, and Interventions Based on a Functional Analysis of Substance Abuse

Problem	Behavioral goal(s)	Interventions
Alcohol and marijuana use to relieve social anxiety	Competent skills for reducing anxiety in social situations	Cognitive-behavioral counseling for anxiety management; social skills training; pharmacotherapy
Use of substances when bored	Engaging in recreational activities regularly	Case management; community reinforcement; social skills training; family problem solving
Looking forward to getting "high" as most important part of the day	Identifying new, more personally meaningful pursuits (e.g., work, education)	Supported employment; supported education
Use of alcohol and benzodiazepines to get to sleep at night	Demonstration of good sleep hygiene skills	Cognitive-behavioral counseling
Giving in to friend's invitations to use substances	Improvement of substance refusal skills and avoidance of high-risk social situations	Social skills training; active treatment groups; family problem solving
Lack of social support for abstinence	Improvement of social support; joining alternative social group	Family education; self-help groups; case management (to identify and sample alternative social supports)
Alcohol use to cope with auditory hallucinations	Competent skills for coping with hallucinations	Cognitive-behavioral counseling; family problem solving; pharmacotherapy

TABLE 5.7. Potential Interventions at Different Stages of Treatment

Intervention	Stage of treatment			
	Engagement	Persuasion	Active treatment	Relapse prevention
Case management	X	X	X	X
Family work	X	X	X	X
Pharmacological treatment	X	X	X	X
Assertive outreach	X	X	X	
Coerced or involuntary interventions	X	X	X	
Residential programs		X	X	
Motivational interviewing		X	X	
Persuasion groups		X	X	
Cognitive-behavioral counseling		X	X	X
Social skills training		X	X	X
Vocational rehabilitation		X	X	X
Active treatment groups			X	X
Self-help groups			X	X

behavioral counseling. Selecting the optimal treatment modality depends on a combination of the clinician's skill and knowledge, the availability of different treatment modalities at the agency, the client's preference, and the client's treatment history.

A wide variety of different interventions can be used to achieve behavioral goals. Examples of specific interventions based on goals selected from the client's stage of treatment and from the functional analysis are provided in Tables 5.5 and 5.6.

Choosing Measurable Outcomes to Evaluate the Effects of the Interventions

When specific interventions have been selected to achieve behavioral goals, measurable outcomes must be identified in order to determine the interventions' success in achieving the desired changes. These outcomes should be objective, easy to observe (when possible), and clearly related to the goal in question. Whenever possible, behavioral specificity is desired. Table 5.8 provides examples of how to operationalize treatment goals in terms of measurable outcomes.

Selecting Follow-Up Times to Review Implementation of Treatment Plan

Even the best of plans is ineffective if it is not followed through. In order to maximize the success of a treatment plan, systematic efforts must be made to follow up plans and to modify them as necessary. Two types of follow-up are needed to ensure effective treatment. First,

regular monitoring needs to be conducted to determine whether the interventions have been implemented as planned. Problems with successfully delivering an intervention should be identified and resolved as soon as possible. We recommend that treatment providers monitor the implementation of their interventions for clients with a dual disorder on at least a weekly basis.

Second, the implementation of a treatment plan does not guarantee that the desired goals will be achieved. Interventions can be successful, partially successful, or unsuccessful. For example, an intervention may be successful in helping a client develop friendships with people who do not abuse alcohol, but the client's substance abuse may continue to be problematic because he or she still uses alcohol to manage sleep difficulties. Periodic reviews and modifications of the treatment plan are necessary in order to address problems that persist despite the treatment, or to move on to new problems and goals when old ones have been successfully resolved. The review and evaluation of the treatment plan also provide valuable information concerning the functional analysis, which needs to be reevaluated and often revised along with the treatment plan. We recommend that the treatment team conduct a formal review of the treatment plan and functional analysis, and modify them as necessary, every 6 months.

A treatment plan form, the Individual Dual-Disorder Treatment Plan, is presented in Appendix C (see Form C.9). Four examples of completed treatment plans, corresponding to clients at each stage of treatment, are provided in Figures 5.5 through 5.8. The Individual Treatment Review—a form for summarizing progress

---

TABLE 5.8. Examples of Measurable Outcomes for Behavioral Goals

Behavioral goal(s)	Measurable outcome(s)
Regular contact with clinician	Client participates in weekly meetings of at least 20 minutes with clinician.
Awareness of substance abuse–mental illness interactions	Client is able to identify examples of how substance use has affected mental illness in his or her life.
Recognition of high-risk situations for substance use, and development of strategies for avoiding them	Client is able to describe different high-risk situations he or she has faced, and one method for avoiding each situation.
Improved skills for making friends and opportunities to meet new people	Client initiates three new conversations per week, at least one in a novel place.
Development of alternative recreational activities	Client tries at least one new recreational activity per week and two old activities.
Improved sleep hygiene skills	Client uses three new sleep hygiene skills and maintains record of sleep.
Ability to refuse offers to use substances	Client can skillfully refuse offers to use substances during practice role plays, *and* reports using skills in real-life situations.
Improved skills for coping with auditory hallucinations	Client uses three different coping strategies for dealing with hallucinations that result in decreased distress.

Individual Dual-Disorder Treatment Plan

Client: <u>Duane</u>   Date: <u>XXX</u>

Primary clinician: <u>Bob</u>

Psychiatric disorder (Axis I): <u>Major depressive disorder (with psychotic features)</u>

Alcohol Use Scale—Revised: <u>3 (alcohol abuse)</u>

Drug Use Scale—Revised: <u>5 (severe cocaine dependence), 3 (marijuana abuse)</u>

Substance Abuse Treatment Scale—Revised: <u>2 (Engagement)</u>

Stage-Wise Goals

Problem	Goal	Intervention	Treatment modality	Responsible clinician(s)
1. Lack of contact with treatment providers	Meet weekly w/client for at least 20 minutes	Assertive outreach to meet w/client in community	Case management	Bob, Karen
2. Family stress poses threat to client's housing stability	Reduction of stress and resolution of immed. crises	Connect w/family members in home to assess needs	Family intervention	Karen
3.		and resolve severest problems		

Goals Based on Functional Analysis

Problem	Goal	Intervention	Treatment modality	Responsible clinician(s)
1. Client reports using in response to depression	Improved stabilization of depresson	Pharmacological treatment; assertive	Pharmacological; case management	Bertha, Bob
2.		outreach to ensure med. adherence		
3.				

Date of treatment plan meeting with client: <u>XXX</u>

Date of treatment plan meeting with family: <u>XXX</u>

Date of next review of treatment plan: <u>XXX</u>

FIGURE 5.5. Example of a completed Individual Dual-Disorder Treatment Plan for client in the engagement stage.

made in implementing planned interventions, obstacles and problems encountered, and goals achieved since the last treatment plan—is also included in Appendix C (see Form C.10). Specific forms for summarizing family interventions are described in Chapter 14 and also included in Appendix C (see Forms C.17, C.18, C.19).

SUMMARY

This chapter has discussed the last two of the five steps of assessment (detection, classification, functional assessment, functional analysis, and treatment planning). We have begun the chapter with a discussion of the aim of a functional analysis of substance use behavior, which is to develop an understanding of the factors (e.g., so-

cial, coping, recreation) that maintain substance abuse or pose a risk of relapse. The identification of factors that maintain substance use and abuse has important implications for treatment, as interventions may need to address them in order for treatment to be successful. We have introduced the Payoff Matrix (see Appendix C, Form C.6) as a tool for conducting the functional analysis, in which the major advantages and disadvantages of using substances are identified, as well as the advantages and disadvantages of *not* using substances. Treatment can be aimed at modifying any of the "payoffs" of using or not using substances in order to decrease substance abuse.

We have concluded the chapter with an explanation of how to plan dual-disorder treatment. Treatment planning is conducted according to the following se-

Individual Dual-Disorder Treatment Plan

Client: <u>Maria</u>   Date: <u>XXX</u>

Primary clinician: <u>Betty</u>

Psychiatric disorder (Axis I): <u>Schizophrenia</u>

Alcohol Use Scale—Revised: <u>5 (severe alcohol dependence)</u>

Drug Use Scale—Revised: <u>3 (marijuana abuse)</u>

Substance Abuse Treatment Scale—Revised: <u>3 (Early Persuasion)</u>

Stage-Wise Goals

Problem	Goal	Intervention	Treatment modality	Responsible clinician(s)
1. Not aware of substance effects on mental illness	Awareness of three sub. effects on mental illness	Psychoeducation about dual disorders	Cog.-beh. couns., persuasion groups	Betty, Clarence
2. Does not view sub. abuse as interfering w/personal goals	Seeing sub. abuse as inconsistent w/goals	Exploring goals and interactions w/sub. abuse	Mot. interviewing, persuasion groups	Betty, Clarence
3.				

Goals Based on Functional Analysis

Problem	Goal	Intervention	Treatment modality	Responsible clinician(s)
1. Uses alcohol to cope w/hallucinations	Acquire three new coping skills	Teaching strategies for coping w/hallucinations	Cog.-beh. couns.	Betty
2. Uses marijuana for recreation	Identify/try four new rec. activities	Prob. solving to identify new act., arranging/	Cog.-beh. couns., case mgmt.	Betty
3.		accomp. client to act.		

Date of treatment plan meeting with client: <u>XXX</u>

Date of treatment plan meeting with family: <u>XXX</u>

Date of next review of treatment plan: <u>XXX</u>

FIGURE 5.6. Example of a completed Individual Dual-Disorder Treatment Plan for client in the persuasion stage.

quence: (1) evaluating pressing needs; (2) determining client motivation for change; (3) selecting behavioral goals for change, based on both the functional analysis (i.e., the Payoff Matrix) and the client's motivational state (i.e., stage of treatment); (4) determining interventions for achieving desired goals; (5) choosing measurable outcomes to evaluate the effects of the interventions, and (6) selecting follow-up times to review implementation of treatment plans and their success. In order for treatment to be effective, formal reviews of the functional analysis and treatment plans need to be conducted at least every 6 months.

Individual Dual-Disorder Treatment Plan

Client: _Eddie_   Date: _XXX_

Primary clinician: _Victor_

Psychiatric disorder (Axis I): _Schizoaffective disorder_

Alcohol Use Scale—Revised: _4 (alcohol dependence)_

Drug Use Scale—Revised: _4 (amphetamine/marijuana dependence), 3 (cocaine abuse)_

Substance Abuse Treatment Scale—Revised: _6 (Late Active Treatment)_

Stage-Wise Goals

Problem	Goal	Intervention	Treatment modality	Responsible clinician(s)
1. Difficulty resisting offers to use substances	Competence in skills for refusing offers	Improve soc. skills for sub. use situations	Soc. skills training	Victor, Rose
2. Occasionally uses in high-risk situations	Avoidance of high-risk situations	Identify and avoid high-risk situations	Active tx. groups; family prob. solving	Victor, Rose
3.				

Goals Based on Functional Analysis

Problem	Goal	Intervention	Treatment modality	Responsible clinician(s)
1. Feels lonely avoiding soc. situations w/friends who use	Make new friends who don't use	Improve social skills; identify ways to meet people	Soc. skills tr., active tx. groups	Victor, Rose
2. Boredom/desire to use when nothing to do, but interest in working	Find work in areas of interest	Assist in finding and keeping job	Fam. prob. solv., vocational rehab.	Victor, Rose, Bill
3.				

Date of treatment plan meeting with client: _XXX_

Date of treatment plan meeting with family: _XXX_

Date of next review of treatment plan: _XXX_

FIGURE 5.7. Example of a completed Individual Dual-Disorder Treatment Plan for client in the active treatment stage.

Individual Dual-Disorder Treatment Plan

Client: <u>Tara</u>   Date: <u>XXX</u>
Primary clinician: <u>Samantha</u>
Psychiatric disorder (Axis I): <u>Bipolar I disorder</u>
Alcohol Use Scale—Revised: <u>1 (alcohol abstinence)</u>
Drug Use Scale—Revised: <u>1 (cocaine abstinence; dependence in remission)</u>
Substance Abuse Treatment Scale—Revised: <u>7 (Relapse Prevention)</u>

Stage-Wise Goals

Problem	Goal	Intervention	Treatment modality	Responsible clinician(s)
1. Tempted to try "controlled" cocaine use	Awareness of vulnerability to relapse	Peer support	Active tx. groups; self-help groups	Samantha
2.				
3.				

Goals Based on Functional Analysis

Problem	Goal	Intervention	Treatment modality	Responsible clinician(s)
1. Frustration over low-paying job w/no future	Improve job qualifications	Supported education	Case mgmt.	Samantha
2. Intermittent depression	Improve depression	Teach depr. self-mgmt. skills	Cog.-beh. couns.	Samantha
3. Conflict w/spouse	Improve conflict res. skills	Teach communication/ prob.-solv. skills	Fam. prob. solv.	Jeremy

Date of treatment plan meeting with client: <u>XXX</u>
Date of treatment plan meeting with family: <u>XXX</u>
Date of next review of treatment plan: <u>XXX</u>

FIGURE 5.8. Example of a completed Individual Dual-Disorder Treatment Plan for client in the relapse prevention stage.

III

Individual Approaches

6

Stage-Wise Case Management

Case management is the central clinical intervention for the community treatment of clients with dual disorders. We begin this chapter with a description of the role of case management in providing integrated treatment for clients with dual disorders. We then provide background by discussing the clinical case management model (see Chapter 3 for a description of the organization of treatment teams that provide case management). The remainder of the chapter is devoted to describing specific activities within each of the three general functions of case management: psychotherapeutic work; advocacy and clinical coordination; and promoting rehabilitation and recovery. As the specific goals and activities used by case managers differ at each of the four stages of dual-disorder treatment (engagement, persuasion, active treatment, and relapse prevention), these goals and activities are discussed separately for each stage.

THE ROLE OF STAGE-WISE CASE MANAGEMENT IN DUAL-DISORDER TREATMENT

Dual disorders are complex, influencing all spheres of clients' lives, and affecting the lives of others around them (including family and friends). As outlined in this book, integrated treatment of dual disorders requires a comprehensive array of services. These include psychotherapeutic treatments that directly target substance abuse, whether delivered to individuals (Part III), in groups (Part IV), or to families (Part V). They also include ancillary interventions, such as approaches to housing (Chapter 16), coerced or involuntary interventions (Chapter 17), vocational rehabilitation (Chapter

18), and psychopharmacological treatment (Chapter 19). Considering the range of potential treatment options, the complexity of identifying and prioritizing treatment goals, and the limited cognitive capacity of many clients with dual disorders (due to the effects of mental illness, the effects of substances, or their combination), one clinician needs to take responsibility for ensuring that such a client's needs are assessed, that systematic treatment planning takes place, that interventions are delivered in a coordinated fashion as intended, and that treatment has its desired effects (or, if not, that treatment is suitably altered). The case manager works with the client to fulfill this vital function, and therefore serves as the "glue" that holds together and ensures the integration of the various components of treatment.

In order to integrate these various components into a coherent treatment delivery package, the case manager must always be aware of the client's stage of dual-disorder treatment and focus on delivering services that meet the treatment goals for that stage. Without this coordination, it is very easy for a clinician to slip into providing services that are well intended but inappropriate to a client's stage of treatment. This can cause confusion, disruption, and rebellion. Case managers also have to monitor their own interventions and to be careful that their goals and eagerness to help do not outpace clients' progress through stages of treatment.

The goal of case management in the *engagement stage* of treatment is to establish a relationship that gives the case manager access to the client on a regular basis. This relationship also needs to allow for regular discussion of the client's psychiatric symptoms and substance use in an open and honest fashion. Therefore, all interventions in the engagement stage are focused on building connections between the client and the treatment team, and on having the client experience these connections as welcoming, helpful, and nonthreatening. At a minimum, the client needs to experience a lack of adverse responses from team members; ideally, he or she should experience positive reinforcement associated with sharing information with the team. Client information sharing is critical to all future treatment efforts. Therefore, either suggesting that the client change his or her behavior or disapproving of the client's current coping strategies is incompatible with the goals of the engagement stage. Once case managers grasp the importance of focusing all behavioral change efforts on reinforcing honest dialogue, it becomes much easier for them not to jump ahead with active treatment interventions.

In the *persuasion stage*, the goal of treatment shifts to helping clients develop motivation to change their substance use and mental illness management behaviors. The critical emphasis is on development of motivation at this stage, not on behavioral change. Even the best active treatment interventions are doomed to failure without motivation; this is why it is critical to focus on the development of motivation before moving on to active treatment. Therefore, interventions at this stage focus on supporting clients in carefully examining all available information about their psychiatric illness and substance use, as well as determining their goals and developing hope for achieving them. Clearly, a poorly timed active treatment intervention provided during the persuasion stage can result in failure that undermines the development of hope and motivation for a positive change.

In the *active treatment stage*, the goal is to provide the client with the skills and tools necessary to succeed in changing illness management, substance use, or both. Therefore, the interventions at this stage focus on helping clients decrease substance use, achieve and sustain sobriety, and/or improve medication adherence and participation in rehabilitation programs. At this stage, the behavioral and rehabilitation technologies are tapped that have been proven effective in managing specific aspects of addictions in severe mental illness. These techniques maximize the client's chances of succeeding in meeting newly developed goals and sustaining that success over time. The case manager's task in this stage of treatment is to coordinate the different aspects of care, so that they will work in harmony to uniformly reinforce active treatment goals.

In the *relapse prevention stage*, the goal of treatment shifts from maximizing success in a narrowly defined objective for the short term to maintaining that success for a sustained duration. Treatment goals are expanded to include a wider range of lifestyle changes that will enhance and support the client's overall outcomes.

The key to success at this stage is shifting primary responsibility from extensive professional supports to the client, and facilitating the client's further growth in self-reliance and self-efficacy. The case manager also encourages the client to become further integrated into the community, and to seek opportunities to serve as a role model for other clients who are struggling in the early stages of treatment (e.g., in persuasion groups; see Chapter 9).

THE CLINICAL CASE MANAGEMENT MODEL

Clinical case management has been the dominant model for coordinating and delivering psychiatric treatment for persons with severe mental illness since the 1980s (Harris & Bergman, 1987; Kanter, 1989). Clinical case management includes both the brokerage and advocacy functions found in the *brokerage model of case management*, as well as the delivery of direct clinical care. The overall goals of clinical case management are to assess client needs, to identify and provide necessary services to meet those needs, and to monitor outcomes to determine the success of treatment or need for other services.

Clinical case management is most effective when it is provided in the context of a multidisciplinary treatment team that includes a case manager, a psychiatrist, and a variety of other professionals (such as a nurse, master's-level clinicians, and a vocational specialist). In recent years and across multiple treatment settings, the clinical case management model has evolved to incorporate aspects of the *assertive community treatment (ACT) model* (Allness & Knoedler, 1998; Stein & Santos, 1998) and the *strengths model* (Rapp, 1993). These features, which are described below, are important enhancements to clinical case management for clients with dual disorders.

In the original brokerage case management model, most services were provided by other clinicians, with the case manager serving mainly in the role of broker (Intagliata, 1982). The clinical case management model modified the brokerage model by specifying that case managers are more than brokers; they are also clinicians, who through their close working relationships with clients are in a unique position to provide clinical services (Kanter, 1989). Because more clinical services are provided directly, the chances of clients' not receiving critical services because of poor follow-through on referrals can be minimized—an especially important concern for clients with dual disorders.

The ACT model was first developed to meet the needs of a subgroup of clients with severe mental illness who were prone to frequent relapses and rehospitalizations, due to their inability or unwillingness to go to local mental health centers for treatment (Stein & Test, 1980; Test & Stein, 1980). This model differs from clinical case management in several ways (Allness & Knoedler, 1998; Stein & Santos, 1998). First, most services are provided to clients in their natural settings in the community, rather than in the clinic, to ensure that necessary services are delivered. Second, a multidisciplinary treatment team is established that is responsible for providing most services to clients, continuing the clinical case management trend away from brokering services to direct service provision. Third, in order to decrease staff burnout and improve coordination of care across different clinicians, cases are formally shared across members of the treatment team. Fourth, because of the outreach necessary to engage clients, and the emphasis on direct provision of services, smaller caseloads are used—typically approximately 1 clinician per 10 clients, rather than 1 clinician per 30 or more clients. Although many mental health centers have established ACT teams to address the needs of a subgroup of clients with severe mental illness who heavily utilize emergency and inpatient treatment services (Bond, Drake, et al., 2001), the ACT model has influenced routine clinical case management as well. Specifically, outreach is a common component of clinical case management, as are shared caseloads on multidisciplinary treatment teams.

Finally, the strengths model of case management emerged in response to concerns that approaches to case management (and treatment in general) for persons with severe mental illness have tended to overemphasize the limits and impairments associated with psychiatric illnesses, at the cost of overlooking the strengths that clients can harness toward achieving their personal goals (Sullivan, 1992). In contrast to being primarily oriented toward the elimination of psychopathology, the strengths approach focuses on identifying clients' aspirations and competencies; niches in the community that facilitate adaptive functioning; and resources and opportunities in the community, including social supports, that can be harnessed to help them pursue those goals (Rapp, 1993, 1998b). The key propositions of the strengths model are summarized in Table 6.1. This positive focus is reflected in the constructive approach to dual-disorder work that is described throughout this book. It begins with an assessment process that emphasizes building new competencies rather than simply attempting to suppress substance abuse (Chapters 4 and 5). It continues with helping clients understand and become empowered by setting their own recovery goals (described later in this chapter); stimulating clients' motivation to better their lot in life (Chapters 7 and 9); and improving social support and relationships with friends (Chapter 11), family members (Part V), and other poten-

---

TABLE 6.1. Key Propositions of the Strengths Model of Case Management

1. The quality of niches people inhabit determines their achievement, quality of life, and success in living.
2. People who are successful in living have goals and dreams.
3. People who are successful in living use their strengths to attain their aspirations.
4. People who are successful in living have the confidence to take the next step toward their goal.
5. At any point in time, people who are successful in living have at least one goal, one relevant talent, and confidence to take the next step.
6. People who are successful in living have access to the resources needed to achieve their goals.
7. People who are successful in living have a meaningful relationship with at least one person.
8. People who are successful in living have access to opportunities relevant to their goals.
9. People who are successful in living have access to resources and opportunities for meaningful relationships.

Note. From Rapp (1998b). Copyright 1998 by Oxford University Press. Reprinted by permission.

---

tial supporters in the community, including residential (Chapter 16) and employment (Chapter 18) supports.

FUNCTIONS AND ACTIVITIES OF CASE MANAGEMENT

The specific activities of stage-wise case management can be divided into categories reflecting these three general functions: psychotherapeutic work; advocacy and clinical coordination; and promoting rehabilitation and recovery. The activities in each of these categories are described below.

Psychotherapeutic Work

Activities falling within the case management function of psychotherapeutic work include developing a working alliance with the client, individual counseling, psychoeducation about dual disorders, and family work. These activities are discussed below for each stage of treatment.

Shaping an Effective Working Alliance

The *working alliance* is the therapeutic relationship between the case manager and client. As the goals of case management for clients with dual diagnoses are somewhat different from the goals of other therapeutic relationships, the alliance that will support the therapeutic work necessary to achieve those goals may also be somewhat different. Focusing on the working alliance as a practical therapeutic tool can also help with the management of clinicians' personal reactions to difficult clients.

The working alliance developed between case manager and client throughout dual-disorder treatment involves a consistently supportive stance that respects the client's ability to make decisions about his or her substance use, given complete information about consequences of use and hope for change. The working alliance evolves from reinforcing the client's contact with the clinician and establishing a trusting relationship, to the clinician's and client's becoming partners in exploring the specific effects of substance use in the client's life. In later stages, some clients appear to prefer to have their clinicians become somewhat confrontational in pointing out slippage toward pitfalls, while other clients require a more supportive stance throughout.

Engagement Stage. At the engagement stage, the therapeutic alliance is initiated, and a foundation is built to support the work ahead. As the goal of this stage of treatment is to establish open, honest communication, it is critical for the case manager to model these behaviors. Therefore, if coerced or involuntary intervention is being contemplated or if communications are received from collateral resources, this information is shared with the client openly. The case manager is also more likely to provide practical help and support without concern about enabling substance use in this stage, because he or she is focused on fostering hope and ensuring that the client experiences involvement with the treatment system as helpful and worthwhile.

Persuasion Stage. The case manager has established a therapeutic alliance with the client by the persuasion stage. He or she now has the delicate task of maintaining unconditional positive respect for the client, while at the same time increasing his or her awareness of the adverse consequences of substance abuse and/or poor mental illness management. The risk at this stage is that the case manager becomes associated with the adverse consequences, and the therapeutic relationship is threatened by the client's desire to avoid thinking about those consequences. Therefore, it is very important for the case manager to take a stance of allying with the client against the disease. This places the focus clearly on the illness (mental illness and/or substance abuse) as the source of aversive stimuli. The client clearly experiences the case manager as allied with him or her by virtue of the manager's nonjudgmental, supportive stance.

Many case managers make the mistake of communicating disapproval or confronting self-destructive behaviors in this stage. This often causes a rift between a case manager and client in their working alliance. It creates a focus on the case manager's values and may induce feelings of shame and guilt in the client. It is helpful for the case manager to divert feelings of disapproval toward the illness rather than the client. Keeping the focus on the illness, and conceptualizing it as an external factor that causes harm to the client, preserves the therapeutic alliance while also permitting an open exchange concerning substance use and its consequences.

The psychodynamic concept of the therapist as a mirror can be useful in the persuasion stage, with some modification. The case manager's role is not to judge the client's behaviors, but rather to help him or her see consequences of the illness that the client may not be aware of. Therefore, the case manager merely focuses the client's attention on the illness's natural consequences for his or her life, rather than trying to convince the person that substance use or medication noncompliance is problematic on principle. Clearly, dual-disorder work requires greater therapeutic openness than the traditional psychodynamic concept of the reflective mirror implies.

Active Treatment Stage. The full force of the nonjudgmental, compassionate working alliance is put to work toward the goal of achieving sustained sobriety in the active treatment stage. The case manager may deliver individual cognitive-behavioral therapy and may also be the client's group therapist during this stage. Therefore, the case manager is actively involved in coaching and supporting the client, as well as reminding him or her of goals set during the persuasion stage. The working alliance in this stage is an extension of the alliance developed during the two previous stages: The case manager carefully avoids endorsing sobriety or alterations in illness management skills on principle, but rather uses the evidence from the individual's life experiences and decisions made during the persuasion stage to support continued progress.

Slips into substance use/abuse or into treatment nonadherence during this stage are viewed as learning opportunities rather than failures. The clinician helps the client do a careful behavioral analysis of events and feelings before, during, and after each slip. The goal of this analysis is to identify where the active treatment plan may have broken down, and then to use this information to fine-tune the plan, in order to increase the client's chance of preventing future slips or relapses. Clients are reminded that slips are a common part of the process of recovery and are not signs of failure or causes for hopelessness. A client is encouraged to celebrate the period of success that he or she had leading up to the slip, and to recognize that those periods of success may be growing incrementally. If a slip becomes a sustained relapse, the clinician should carefully reassess the client's stage of treatment and shift treatment interventions accordingly.

Relapse Prevention Stage. The working alliance in the relapse prevention stage combines elements of the alliance developed in the persuasion and active treatment stages. The clinician continues to use the supportive stance in fine-tuning the cognitive-behavioral interventions that are maintaining the client's success, while gently directing his or her attention toward the risks to which the person is exposed in other areas of his or her life. Discrepancies between current progress and life goals are identified to develop motivation for expanded lifestyle improvement. The clinician focuses the client's attention on becoming fully aware of improvements in his or her life and attributing them to the active treatment stage, in order to boost self-efficacy. The clinician may start to be able to use the client's commitment to maintaining an active treatment gain, such as sobriety, to justify the importance of examining further therapeutic steps. It is important to be careful not to take commitment to sobriety or treatment adherence for granted, however, and to continue checking in with the client to acknowledge that these remain desired goals.

Individual Counseling

In the clinical case management model, as previously discussed, case managers both help clients negotiate the treatment system and serve as clinicians directly providing services themselves. Case managers are involved in providing individual counseling for clients with dual disorders throughout all four stages of treatment. The focus of counseling shifts from being primarily supportive during the earliest stage of treatment, to exploring the effects of substance abuse and poor control of mental illness and developing strategies to address these issues in the intermediate stages, to the prevention of relapses in the last stage of treatment.

Engagement Stage. In the engagement stage, individual counseling consists primarily of supportive therapy. Therapy sessions may be quite informal and take place in whatever setting the client may be found, including homeless shelters, hospitals, or the streets. Therapy may be brief and woven into other activities, such as transportation to receive benefits, doctors' appointments, or housing options. The focus of supportive counseling in this stage is on practical life issues, helping clients recognize the limitations or suffering created by their current lifestyle, and instilling the belief that they deserve better.

Persuasion Stage. Motivational interviewing (Chapter 7) is the individual counseling technique predominantly employed in the persuasion stage. Miller and Rollnick (2002) have described this technique in detail. Motivational interviewing may need to be applied for extended periods of time in addressing multiple adverse consequences before some clients with a dual disorder develop motivation for change. Cognitive-behavioral counseling focused on psychosocial rehabilitation—including social skills training, teaching coping strategies for managing persistent symptoms, and identifying alternative leisure and recreational activities— can also be useful at the persuasion stage. As clients develop better skills for getting their social, coping, and leisure needs met, their reliance on substances for achieving these needs often decreases.

Active Treatment Stage. At the active treatment stage, when clients are motivated to address their substance use problems, cognitive-behavioral substance abuse counseling (Chapter 8) is most useful. Many clients experience difficulties attaining sustained reductions in their substance use, or maintaining abstinence for prolonged periods, because of vulnerability to triggers and exposure to high-risk situations for substance abuse (e.g., social situations, persistent symptoms, boredom). Therefore, as a client moves from persuasion to active treatment, cognitive-behavioral counseling intensifies and becomes more focused on developing skills that will support sobriety.

Relapse Prevention Stage. As the client achieves a sustained remission of substance abuse, cognitive-behavioral counseling is extended to other areas of the client's life, such as work, social relationships, spirituality, and parenting. Relapse prevention principles as described by Marlatt and Gordon (1985) are also employed. If the client uses a self-help group as part of the recovery process (i.e., a Twelve-Step program), principles of that program may be woven into the active treatment and relapse prevention stage individual counseling as well (see Chapter 12).

Individual Psychoeducation

The term *psychoeducation* refers to the provision of information about psychiatric and substance use disorders, using didactic and interactive methods to ensure comprehension of relevant material (Anderson, Reiss, & Hogarty, 1986; Goldman & Quinn, 1988). Psychoeducation is a critical and long-term function for clients with dual disorders and their families, because there is so much to learn. An educational approach is consistent with the motivational development process, which assumes that a client equipped with adequate knowledge, self-awareness, and decision-making skills can make better choices. Educating clients communicates respect both for their need to know about their disorders and for their decision-making capacity. Educating family members or other significant supports is the first step to engaging them as members of the treatment team. Educational handouts for clients and family members are provided in Appendix B. These handouts can be used in individual, group, or family sessions.

Engagement Stage. In the engagement stage the case manager should assess the client's knowledge about mental illness and substance use disorders. Basic information may be provided about the biological basis and chronic nature of both types of disorders, as well as the rationale for currently prescribed treatments. The goal of this stage is to provide information that clients want, while not overwhelming them with excess and unrequested information, or prematurely trying to persuade them that they have substance use problems.

Persuasion Stage. As a working alliance develops and the client enters the persuasion stage, psychoeducation is continued and expanded, and the topic of substance abuse can be addressed more directly. An understanding of the distinctions among abstinence, nonproblematic substance use, abuse, and dependence is valuable to helping clients assess their own problems related to substance use. Learning to distinguish psychiatric symptoms from emotions and medication side effects is likewise important. A client should also be educated about all available treatment options, in order to consider active treatment interventions and match his or her needs to available options.

Active Treatment Stage. Psychoeducation about treatment options continues at the active treatment stage, with a shift in focus to helping the client further reduce substance use or attain abstinence. Education may directly address substance use or abuse; aspects of the mental illness that may interfere with achieving or maintaining sobriety; or personal choices that may support a sober lifestyle. For example, a client who identifies nonproblematic use of marijuana as his or her goal could benefit from information about the subtle long-term effects of marijuana on energy and motivation, the increased risk of relapse, and the recognition of withdrawal symptoms. The client could also benefit from information about techniques for managing insomnia or stress through diet, exercise, relaxation techniques, or meditation (see Table 10.2 in Chapter 10), or information about strategies for coping with symptoms or social situations related to marijuana use.

Relapse Prevention Stage. Psychoeducational efforts shift to a broader focus on holistic health and well-being once a client's substance abuse is in sustained remission. Information about the effects of smoking, poor diet, or a sedentary lifestyle on both psychological and physical health, as well as methods for successfully establishing lifestyle changes, are all relevant topics during this stage. Many clients become actively involved in researching health information for themselves in this stage and can be taught how to obtain this information from their health care providers. Clients in the relapse prevention stage can also serve as important role models to their peers. They can provide information about what worked for them in their recovery process or journey in a way that other clients find helpful. The process of helping to educate others enables clients in the relapse prevention stage to take perspective on what has contributed to their success, which can further solidify their gains.

Strategies for conducting psychoeducation are summarized in Table 6.2.

Family Work

Family intervention is a core ingredient of integrated dual-disorder treatment (see Part V), and working with family members is a key component of clinical case management. A case manager may be directly involved in providing family intervention, such as conducting behavioral family therapy (Chapter 14) or leading a multiple-family group (Chapter 15); alternatively, another clinician on the team may provide family services. Regardless of whether the case manager or another clinician provides family intervention, at least some family work is involved in effective case management, and these functions are described below (see Chapter 13 for more general guidance on family work). For clients with little or no ongoing contact with family members, the

---

TABLE 6.2. Strategies for Conducting Psychoeducation

- Present didactic information.
- Review educational handouts on different topics.
- Ask questions to assess clients' understanding of presented information.
- Prompt clients to explore how pertinent information is related to their personal experiences.
- Adopt clients' language to ensure good communication and avoid misunderstandings and conflict.
- Assign homework to read or review written materials on educational topics (e.g., educational handouts; Appendix B).
- Probe to identify gaps in knowledge and desire for additional information.
- Review previously covered topics by asking questions.

same principles of family work can be applied to other people who have caring relationships with the client.

Families are highly involved in the lives of their loved ones with dual diagnoses, but clinicians are often unaware of the extent of their involvement (Clark & Drake, 1994). Family members may inadvertently reinforce inappropriate behaviors when attempting to help a relative. Usually the goals of family members are quite similar to those of the treatment team, even though their actions may appear to be at odds initially. Therefore, it is critical to develop a strong working alliance with the family members, to invite them to participate on the treatment team, and to coordinate therapeutic efforts with them. Over time, family work leads to a productive alliance between the treatment team and the family, and to the utilization of family support and resources to help a client progress toward recovery goals.

Engagement Stage. In the engagement stage, case managers often need to explore with clients the potential benefits of involving family members in their treatment. Such benefits may include decreasing the stress on all family members, preventing future crises, and helping clients make progress toward their personal goals. Through helping clients see that involving their relatives in treatment is in their best interest, and through providing support and addressing clients' concerns, case managers can be effective in gaining clients' consent to this involvement.

Relatives can be engaged in treatment in a variety of settings, but conducting outreach to families in their homes is an especially effective strategy. Meeting with families "on their own turf" is more convenient for relatives, and enables case managers to engage some reluctant family members. Outreach can also provide invaluable information about current sources of stress, ongoing substance use and abuse among relatives, and potential crisis situations.

Clients who have engaged in treatment themselves may be resistant to having the treatment team contact their families early in the course of treatment, even after reviewing the potential benefits of involving relatives. When this happens, a case manager should respect a client's wishes in this stage and focus on forming a trusting therapeutic relationship. If the client has given consent to sharing information with the family, trust is enhanced by keeping the client informed of any information shared between the case manager and relatives.

When a client has not given consent for the clinical team to share privileged information with the family, the clinical team can legally receive whatever information is offered. Again, this receipt of information should be fully disclosed to the client, so that the honesty of the relationship with the case manager is not compromised.

When family members wish to provide information to the clinical team without the client's knowledge, the case manager should attempt to avoid this by helping the family members address the reasons why they wish to do so. The most common reason is the fear that the client will be upset by the sharing of information; this fear typically reflects the belief that the client is in denial about the illness. If so, that denial will only be enabled by continuing to keep secrets about others' assessment of the client's behavior.

Some clients who are reluctant to participate in treatment come referred by family members. Engagement may start by developing an alliance with the family members and educating them about the client's illnesses. The family may be able to arrange early contacts with a client who is resistant to or afraid of meeting with a professional. Sometimes even relatives living across the country can be valuable in providing background information, encouraging the client to accept contacts, and using their resources to reinforce initiation of treatment.

Persuasion Stage. In the persuasion stage, the case manager makes a more concerted effort to initiate contact with relatives whom it was not appropriate to contact in the engagement stage, due to the focus on developing a therapeutic alliance with the client and the client's resistance to involving family members. In many cases, clients who resist family contact can be assisted to examine the sources of their reluctance and trace them back to the consequences of mental illness and substance abuse. When family members are involved in treatment, the persuasion stage is ideal for providing education to them about dual disorders. Psychoeducation provides useful opportunities to explore the effects of substance abuse and poor management of the psychiatric illness on both the client and the family members (see the previous discussion of psychoeducation). Because focusing on addressing the client's psychosocial needs is an important activity in this stage, garnering family support and identifying strategies for addressing these needs are other goals of family work.

As the case manager assesses the family situation, he or she may find that some family members are abusive, predatory, or caught in addictions themselves. It may be appropriate to help the client gain distance from and set appropriate boundaries with family members who are not supportive of the client's attempts to move toward recovery. On the other hand, not all clients want more distance from possibly destructive family members, and it is important for clinicians to respect these preferences. In such a situation, it is generally preferable for the case manager to attempt to engage these family members, to provide psychoeducation about the client's dual disorders, and to strive to reach a consensus about what treatments are in the client's best interest.

Active Treatment Stage. In the active treatment stage, all resources, including the family, are put to work to support the client in attempting to achieve behavioral change of substance use or illness management. The family may specifically provide reinforcement for success in the form of financial and material rewards (e.g., assistance in purchasing a vehicle, additional time spent with the client, permission to reenter family functions). It is usually best for relatives not to make current levels of support contingent on success, as that would mean depriving the client of this support if he or she failed to succeed. This could lead to a downward spiral of discouragement. Rather, family members are encouraged to give "bonus supports" to mark successes in the active treatment stage. Typically, trying to bribe a client into sobriety who is not motivated for it is of little success. However, small mementos to mark milestones of success, such as dinner with the family to celebrate a week's sobriety, can be very useful in making the family's pride in the client's success overt.

Some clients who are estranged from their families are reluctant to involve relatives before they have achieved some sobriety. Family members may also not want to invest their energies into reestablishing a relationship with a client before sobriety has been achieved. In the active treatment stage, after the client has achieved several months of sobriety, the case manager can reach out to these family members to explore engaging them in treatment.

Relapse Prevention Stage. During relapse prevention, the focus of family intervention may extend to repairing burned bridges with family members, including children whose custody may have been lost during active stages of illness. As clients expand their positive lifestyle, changes in interpersonal relationships and developing positive social relations with families are common goals. Some clients return to live with family members who have evicted them in the past because of inappropriate behaviors. Family members are encouraged to recognize the importance of minimizing a client's exposure to substance use and abuse, celebrating small gains, managing stress, and avoiding viewing slips as failures. In this way, they can become extensions of the treatment team who are accessible for more of the day, expanding the client's support system and facilitating his or her work toward recovery goals.

Table 6.3 summarizes the different activities included within the function of psychotherapeutic work in stage-wise case management.

Advocacy and Clinical Coordination

Together, advocacy and clinical coordination constitute the most long-standing and critical element of case management. Advocacy is important because cognitive impairments and psychiatric symptoms characteristic of severe mental illness often make clients unable to advocate for themselves. Clinical coordination is required because clients typically have multiple needs and must interact with multiple treatment providers; in order to ensure efficiency, a case manager must take responsibility for ensuring that the appropriate services are delivered and that they achieve their desired effects. The specific activities within this general function of stage-wise case management include advocacy, promoting follow-through, providing practical help and benefits, obtaining and maintaining housing, coordinating medication treatment, using close monitoring and legal constraints (when necessary), and responding to crises.

Advocacy

Advocacy involves taking steps to ensure that clients' rights to basic services, entitlements, and treatment are observed. Advocacy efforts may be applied to a specific client's situation (e.g., obtaining access to an appropriate treatment program) or to that of clients with a dual disorder as a group (e.g., advocating with an employer to begin hiring clients). The Americans with Disabilities Act of 1990 (and its subsequent updates and revisions; see Equal Employment Opportunity Commission, 1997) represents a powerful advocacy tool: It requires that employers and institutions treat all individuals equally, regardless of their disability status. Since clients with dual disorders may be discriminated against by landlords, employers, and even the legal system, it is important for case managers to educate themselves about the Americans with Disabilities Act and to refer to it when advocating for their clients' needs.

Engagement Stage. Advocacy efforts can be critical to establishing a connection with the client. Helping the client gain access to services or negotiate the legal system can be a powerful step toward establishing a trusting relationship. Because the goals of treatment in the engagement stage are not to create change, but rather to establish hope and a working alliance, the case manager does not worry about advocacy efforts' enabling substance use at this stage. After the client has been engaged in treatment, the case manager can modify his or her advocacy efforts to reduce or eliminate possible enabling of substance use behavior.

TABLE 6.3. Activities within the Function of Psychotherapeutic Work in Stage-Wise Case Management

Work	Engagement	Persuasion	Active treatment	Relapse prevention
Shaping an effective working alliance	• Conduct outreach to establish regular contact. • Keep communication open, honest. • Provide practical help and support.	• Maintain unconditional positive regard. • Explore effects of substance abuse and mental illness. • Ally with client against illnesses.	• Support progress in sobriety and illness management by using evidence from client's life. • View slips in substance abuse as learning opportunities and part of recovery process.	• Boost self-efficacy by focusing attention on gains made in substance abuse. • Redirect attention to other areas for change.
Individual counseling	• Provide supportive counseling. • Weave informal discussion into other activities (e.g., transportation to doctor's appointments).	• Use motivational interviewing to establish discrepancy between substance abuse and goals. • Initiate psychosocial rehabilitation to address social, coping, and recreational needs.	• Provide cognitive-behaviorial counseling to reduce substance use or maintain abstinence. • Continue with psychosocial rehabilitation. • Encourage client to explore self-help groups.	• Help client develop relapse prevention plans. • Continue with psychosocial rehabilitation. • Support continued involvement in self-help groups for clients who choose this.
Psychoeducation	• Assess knowledge of mental illness and substance abuse. • Provide information that clients want. • Avoid overwhelming clients with information.	• Provide information about mental illness, substance abuse, and their treatment. • Use interactive teaching methods.	• Give focused information related to client's specific goals pertaining to substance abuse. • Use interactive teaching methods.	• Provide information related to health, well-being, and lifestyle change. • Help clients learn how to obtain information themselves. • Explore a client's becoming a peer educator for others.
Family work	• Explore benefits of family work with client. • Conduct outreach to connect with family members. • Offer support and help to address pressing crises in families.	• Make more effort to engage relatives of clients previously unwilling to include their families. • Educate family members about dual disorders, and explore consequences of substance abuse. • Enlist family support to address client's psychosocial needs related to substance abuse.	• Conduct outreach and engage reluctant relatives. • Facilitate family support of client's reduction in substance abuse. • Involve relatives in addressing psychosocial needs.	• Help client repair burned bridges to reestablish relationships with estranged relatives. • Enlist family support for sustained lifestyle changes.

Persuasion Stage. As the therapeutic relationship develops, advocacy efforts are coupled with the process of helping the client to identify the consequences of substance use. For instance, when advocating for a client who has lost his or her driver's license for driving while intoxicated, the case manager draws attention to the impact of current behaviors on the client's chances of success. The clinical treatment team is often asked to write a letter to the court in these situations. The treatment team makes it clear to the client that it will always report honestly. This report can be very helpful to a client who is willing to work with the team by providing some verification of substance use. A plan may be developed for the client to submit a series of random urine drug screens, so the results can be reported to the court to document abstinence. The case manager carefully positions him- or herself as an advocate for the client in this process, rather than as an agent of the legal system. At the same time, the case manager may help the client achieve a period of abstinence.

Active Treatment Stage. As gains are made in substance abuse, advocacy efforts shift toward helping the client obtain access to services or social settings that now have become appropriate, despite problems in the past. For example, advocating with a landlord in a good neighborhood to accept a client with a history of multiple evictions during times of poor control may allow the person to change environmental cues and increase chances of success. The case manager may be able to offer the support of the treatment team and the availability of regular in-home monitoring to the landlord as a form of "collateral." Advocacy efforts may also shift to helping the client obtain access to formal education, jobs, peer counselor roles, and membership on committees (of the community mental health center or the local Alliance for the Mentally Ill chapter). Establishing life roles and responsibilities will further the client's commitment to the recovery process and provide him or her with opportunities to help others.

Relapse Prevention Stage. As sustained sobriety is attained, advocacy efforts shift toward helping clients develop the skills and knowledge to advocate for themselves. Teaching self-advocacy involves helping clients (1) understand applicable labor, eviction, and antidiscrimination laws; (2) learn how to obtain more information about their rights; and (3) develop better assertiveness skills. Case managers may still be involved in advocacy efforts, especially when the mental illness is severe, but efforts are aimed at helping the client develop as strong self-advocacy skills as possible.

Promoting Follow-Through

For many clients with dual disorders, a case manager's work has just begun when he or she advocates for access to housing, jobs, or clinical programs. The case manager then has the daunting task of promoting follow-through with clients who traditionally have high rates of nonadherence to treatment plans. The case manager has to maintain a delicate balance: keeping responsibility for follow-through squarely in a client's corner, while trying to maintain credibility with those people on the receiving end of the advocacy efforts. Following the stages of treatment helps reduce the failure of clients to follow through on referrals to stage-inappropriate interventions. Educating employers, landlords, and program managers about the likelihood of a referral's success, anticipated problems, and available supports can avoid surprises, maintain the case manager's credibility, and facilitate the relationship with referral sources.

Engagement Stage. Promoting follow-through early in the treatment process must be approached quite delicately, to avoid creating a psychological rift between the client and case manager. Promoting follow-though may involve reminding a homeless client of the reasons he or she previously cited for wanting to have an individual apartment, and to encourage the client to stick with housing that is consistent with this goal. Case managers may provide behavioral incentives such as increased supportive contacts to reinforce appropriate follow-through. If there is a financial payee in place, appointments to pick up spending money can be coordinated with treatment appointments to increase the likelihood of showing up. A careful functional analysis may be required to identify the reinforcers for the client's current behavior (i.e., lack of follow-through) and ways they might be modified to maximize the client's chances of follow-through (see Chapter 5). Family members and significant others can reinforce a client's follow-through as well, if this is not perceived as manipulative by the client.

Persuasion Stage. The behavioral reinforcement of follow-through may be expanded in the persuasion stage to participation in persuasion groups, vocational services, and individual counseling sessions. When a client repeatedly fails to follow through, the case manager should try to put him- or herself in the client's shoes to understand why the client did not show up. Is the person afraid that he or she will be judged for being intoxicated? Are appointments at inconvenient times of day, when the client would normally be sleeping or engaged in another important activity? Is the client being taken advantage of by predatory individuals who may be present in the waiting room or outside the treatment center? This analysis may lead to an obvious solution to increase follow-through, such as meeting in a safer or more convenient location (e.g., the client's home or a community setting), or meeting at a time when the client is unlikely to have been using substances.

At this stage, a family member may offer additional supportive contacts or resources to the client as a reinforcement for following through with treatment on a regular basis. For example, a client's parents might offer to take him or her to the movies each weekend, in addition to their usual social contacts, if the client demonstrates medication adherence during the previous week. The case manager should also involve the client in analyzing difficulties with follow-through, to examine whether they may represent consequences of substance use or poorly controlled mental illness. Getting clients involved in the analysis process and the development of expectations of success for themselves can ensure that the clinical team is not working harder than the clients at achieving good follow-through.

Active Treatment Stage. In the active treatment stage, clients assume greater responsibility for following through, although they still may require support as they make commitments to lifestyle changes and support programs that may be threatened when their motivation wanes. Clients commonly experience decreases in motivation when they get beyond the anticipation of success in early action and move into the hard work and monotony of carrying out their plan over time. Case managers are careful to repeat the motivational interviewing steps (Chapter 7), helping clients to refocus on goals that spurred their interest in making change in the first place. Clients may need to recall the pain and consequences they experienced when using substances. Even in the active treatment stage, it is important not to assume that a client will be motivated to follow through because it is the "right thing to do," as this implies an external judgment about the client's life and can quickly breed defensiveness and rebellion. Therefore, the case manager invests effort in supporting the client's decision-making and recovery process, trusting that decisions made by the client will have a more powerful effect on long-term behavior than will decisions made by others.

Relapse Prevention Stage. In the relapse prevention stage, clients set goals to expand their recovery to other areas of lifestyle change, and follow-through on those plans becomes a natural part of the recovery process. The case manager can now step back from promoting follow-through, as it is much more valuable to guide the client at developing skills in monitoring and promoting his or her own follow-through. In the relapse prevention stage, the consequences of failing to follow through are also less devastating. The case manager may make room for clients to learn from their mistakes. Clients are trained to use logs or maintain journals to monitor their motivation levels and behavioral follow-through. They are also taught to examine goals carefully before they set them, to ensure that they are prepared to take on the work of behavioral change. The case manager helps the client to observe patterns of follow-through with commitments over time, and to gain insight into internal and external barriers to follow-through and strategies for overcoming them.

Providing Practical Help and Benefits

A core case management duty is assisting clients in obtaining such basic needs such as food and clothing, as well as financial support and health insurance benefits. (Shelter, another basic need, is discussed separately below.) This work is particularly necessary in managing the client with a dual disorder as substance abuse is associated with financial instability and poor self-care

among these persons. Assistance with basic needs is also important to developing clients' sense of hopefulness for positive change, and serves as the foundation to building a recovery process.

Engagement Stage. Practical help and assistance shows the client that the clinician has something to offer him or her. This is key to establishing a trusting relationship with a client who may fear the consequences of entering into treatment. Practical help and assistance are not used as bribery to change behavior. Rather, they are used to build a relationship, which is the goal of the engagement stage. Therefore, practical help and assistance with obtaining benefits are provided without demands on or expectations for clients in this stage, other than that they will do their part to follow through with commitments.

Persuasion Stage. The process of providing practical help and assistance begun in the engagement stage continues in the persuasion stage with addressing any unmet needs; the client may only now be willing to accept help with some of these. Some such needs may come up as a consequence of substance abuse, such as inability to buy food because money has been spent on drugs. During the persuasion stage, the case manager is careful to weave providing practical help in with the process of developing motivation to heighten the client's awareness of the consequences of substance use. The case manager also sets clear limits on the number of times he or she will provide assistance with a behavior directly related to substance use, in order to increase the client's responsibility for maintaining basic needs. On the other hand, it is not reasonable to expect clients to be able to manage the consequences of their disorders on their own before active treatment begins. The process of addressing basic needs (including obtaining benefits) assists in developing motivation by instilling hope in clients that things can be better, while directing attention to barriers to meeting their needs that are consequences of their dual disorders.

Active Treatment Stage. Most basic needs have been met by the active treatment stage. It is useful to help clients who have recently achieved sobriety realize that they will thus experience an increase in standard of living, such as being able to use money previously spent on substances to purchase adequate clothing, nutritious foods, or meet other basic needs. Clients who still have basic unmet needs are provided with assistance to address these needs; however, there is an increased focus on helping clients learn how to get their own needs met, including how to use natural supports (e.g., family members) to this end.

Relapse Prevention Stage. With sustained sobriety, case managers increase the efforts they have begun making in the active treatment stage to expand clients' ability to provide for their own basic needs. A client who begins working at any point during the stages of treatment may need particular assistance with coordinating employment income and benefits (see Chapter 18). Clients can "get ahead of themselves" by earning an income that results in termination of benefits before they are able to sustain that level of employment. Therefore, the case manager has a vital role in educating clients carefully about the limits of employment income allowed for each benefit that they are receiving, and assisting them in identifying employment they can sustain in the long run.

Obtaining and Maintaining Housing

Clients with dual disorders are vulnerable to housing instability and homelessness, as their illnesses often lead to erratic, agitated behaviors that result in eviction (Drake, Osher, & Wallach, 1989). They may spend all of their money obtaining substances and fail to pay rent. By the time many clients enter treatment, obtaining housing is a major problem. Clients may be at the point of discharge from the hospital with no place to go. They may be homeless and either living on the streets or staying with various friends and relatives. Case managers often find that landlords refuse to rent to clients who have previously been evicted with large unpaid bills or damage done to apartments. The housing that is available may be substandard or expose clients to high-risk, substance-using environments. Helping clients find and maintain safe housing appropriate to their stage in treatment can be instrumental in promoting their progress into recovery (see Chapter 16).

Engagement Stage. At the engagement stage, the case manager helps homeless clients obtain housing, or helps clients living in independent but substandard housing to improve their standard of living. As a case manager focuses primarily on developing a working alliance with a client and instilling hope, there is no attempt to move toward "dry" (substance-free) housing in this stage. Instead, the case manager focuses on helping the client recognize that he or she deserves better living conditions, and that such conditions exist. The case manager can assist the client in locating and moving into housing if needed, and will not interfere with the client's choice of "wet" housing (where he or she may use substances freely). Despite the lack of prohibitions against substance use, the goal is to establish a safer living arrangement than the client's current residence. If the case manager is considering referring the client to a group home or similar professionally run residence, the limits on substance use and consequences for violating them must be clearly explained prior to moving in, so that the client can make an informed choice. This enables the case manager to maintain a trusting alliance with the client and avoid being placed in the position of having to enforce limits in a punitive fashion later.

Persuasion Stage. Once a therapeutic relationship develops, the case manager works to help the client make a connection between housing consequences (e.g., eviction or unsatisfactory living conditions) and substance-using behaviors, as part of the motivational development process. If the client begins to experiment with making reductions in substance use, movement toward "damp" housing may be appropriate. This is housing in which the client may return home after substance use, but may not use in the home. A move to safer living conditions with less exposure to drug dealers or persons using substances may also facilitate reductions in use during the persuasion stage. If the client lives with his or her family, the case manager can engage the family members in determining limits on substance use and associated behaviors at home during this stage. If family members themselves are actively using substances and unable to support the treatment process, the client may need to obtain more stable and supportive housing elsewhere.

Active Treatment Stage. As a client achieves sobriety, "dry" housing is appropriate where such housing options exist and the client desires them. These options may include a residential treatment facility (Brunette et al., 2001) or an apartment where strict limits on substance use and associated behaviors are set by the landlord. If the client is living with family members, the case manager can work with them to manage the psychiatric illness and keep the home free of substances. Some clients may return home to live with their families as part of an active treatment sobriety plan.

Relapse Prevention Stage. With sustained sobriety, the case manager works with the client to improve his or her quality of life through achieving higher-quality housing in safe settings, at a higher level of independence than may have been acquired during the active treatment stage. As in the active treatment stage, "dry" housing remains appropriate, although clients in the relapse prevention stage should become able to set their own limits on using substances in their homes. As clients increase their social and occupational functioning, they may also now have the resources to support a higher standard of housing. Such a move can make the gains of the clients' recovery concrete and motivate sustained abstinence.

Clients who attain sobriety though a residential treatment program may have limited skills in maintaining sobriety in independent housing. A return to situations and social networks associated with past substance use can have a powerful effect on stimulating craving. Substantially increased supports and skills training interventions are usually necessary at the point of transition out of a residential dual-diagnosis program, even when a client has achieved prolonged sobriety.

Coordinating Medication Treatment

Any multidisciplinary treatment team for clients with dual disorders should include a psychiatrist or other prescriber as a core member. As such, the prescriber should establish his or her own therapeutic working alliance with each client. However, the case manager usually has greater contact with the client than the prescriber does and can serve a vital role in observing signs and symptoms of illness, as well as medication responses. It is vital that the team have an integrated approach to pharmacology, so that each client gets a consistent and well-reinforced message about recommended medication treatments. Experienced case managers often advocate with the team psychiatrist for medication interventions when they see opportunities to enhance their clients' control of the illness (see Chapter 19).

Engagement Stage. In the beginning, case managers focus primarily on educating clients about their current medications or proposed medication treatments. They often help their clients obtain access to medications. The case managers also monitor the timeliness of prescriptions and refills as an indicator of medication adherence.

Persuasion Stage. In the persuasion stage, case managers become more active in monitoring medication adherence. Stabilizing mental illness facilitates clients' capacity to address substance use. Clients are strongly encouraged to report their medication usage pattern honestly, and to describe any adverse effects they may be experiencing. They are strongly encouraged to present requests for medication changes to their prescriber, rather than altering their regimen on their own. It is important that a case manager be able to obtain an appointment with the prescriber within a reasonable time frame. Otherwise, the client will disregard the medication regimen rather than put up with perceived adverse effects.

When clients do not take their medication as pre-

scribed, a careful behavioral analysis is performed, as with substance use. Contributors to medication nonadherence are addressed, and behavioral interventions are considered for a client who wants to achieve better control over symptoms through medications. Cognitive impairments can interfere with clients' ability to take medication regularly, and *behavioral tailoring* can be used to overcome the effects of these deficits (Mueser, Corrigan, et al., 2002). Behavioral tailoring includes helping clients develop strategies for incorporating taking medication into their personal routines—such as simplifying their medication regimen (e.g., taking medications as few times as possible per day); combining taking medication with their daily activities (e.g., brushing teeth, eating breakfast, getting ready for bed); and building prompts to take medication into their routines (e.g., using Post-it Notes to remember to take medication, strapping a toothbrush to a medication bottle with a rubber band so that the client is reminded to take medication when he or she brushes teeth).

For clients who are not motivated to use medications to manage symptoms, an awareness of the consequences of nonadherence to the medication regimen is developed. Clients who understand medications and who make an active, informed choice for the treatment they desire will be most likely to adhere to the regimen. The principles of motivational interviewing (as described in Chapter 7) can be applied to medication nonadherence to help clients understand how taking medication may help them in achieving their personal goals (Kemp, Hayward, Applewhaite, Everitt, & David, 1996). Strategies for increasing medication adherence are summarized in Table 6.4.

TABLE 6.4. Techniques for Increasing Adherence to a Medication Regimen

- Simplify medication regimen (e.g., reduce total number of medications taken).
- Reduce number of times per day medication must be taken (e.g., once per day).
- Review and discuss benefits of taking medication.
- Dispel inaccurate beliefs about medication (e.g., that medications are addictive).
- Review side effects of medication and options for managing them.
- Identify the client's personal goals, and explore how taking medication may help achieve them (i.e., motivational interviewing).
- Evaluate support or lack of support for taking medication among significant others.
- Develop strategies for incorporating taking medication into the client's daily routine, such as morning hygiene or eating meals (i.e., behavioral tailoring).
- Consider depot antipsychotic medications when poor adherence to oral antipsychotic medications persists.

Active Treatment Stage. Continued behavioral tailoring and motivational interviewing approaches are often required in the active treatment stage to develop motivation and skills for taking medication as prescribed. As efforts to help clients evaluate the benefits of taking prescribed medications and learn skills for taking them regularly achieve success in the persuasion stage, supports for prompting medication adherence can be decreased, while case managers continue to monitor clients' use of medication. Pharmacological interventions to reduce craving for substance use are appropriate in this stage (e.g., naltrexone; see Chapter 19). It may also be appropriate to use medications to support abstinence from substances (e.g., disulfuram for alcohol). Detoxification may be another part of the active treatment stage and require medication intervention. Since detoxification often involves the use of potentially addictive medications and is more commonly performed on an outpatient than an inpatient basis, the case manager has a vital role in close monitoring the use of medication during this stage. Monitoring may be required from several times a week to several times a day.

Relapse Prevention Stage. In the relapse prevention stage, clients take even more responsibility for coordinating their own medication treatment. A case manager teaches a client skills in negotiating effectively with his or her prescriber. Clients are trained to monitor and log symptoms, to report them effectively, and to advocate for changes. If medication monitoring is in place, the frequency is gradually tapered as clients take increasing responsibility for adherence to their chosen medication regimen. Even clients who must have a guardian's consent to medication can take greater responsibility for monitoring their own medication adherence as they become stabilized. Many clients can learn to recognize the early warning signs of illness exacerbation, and develop relapse prevention plans for averting full-blown relapses (Herz et al., 2000). Such plans may include using doses of medication "as needed" to prevent a further escalation. Clients in this stage can gradually take responsibility for requesting refills directly from their prescriber when due, picking up medications from the pharmacy, filling a weekly Mediplanner if needed, and monitoring medication effects and side effects.

Using Close Monitoring and Legal Constraints (When Necessary)

Many clients with severe mental illness are resistant to treatment and present potential danger of harm to themselves or others if not treated. Coercive treatments are used even more often for clients with dual disorders, due to the consequences of substance abuse. Even when treatment is voluntary, clients with dual disorders have a high rate of nonadherence to treatment plans (Miner et al., 1997). Therefore case managers treating such clients must have a clear understanding of the legal constraints available in their state and be comfortable using them when necessary (see Chapter 17).

Engagement Stage. Some clients may come to treatment with involuntary conditions already in place. For example, a client coming from a state hospital may have either a guardian or a conditional discharge with extended commitment to community treatment. The case manager is then faced with the challenge of establishing a trusting working alliance with the client, for whom he or she is also acquiring the responsibility of monitoring and enforcing a coercive intervention. Other clients may present at intake with such dangerous behaviors that an immediate coercive intervention is called for at the start of the engagement stage. Some clients may never engage in treatment until forced to by a legal constraint.

The dilemma that case managers face is that the goals of the engagement stage are not to change behavior, yet most coercive interventions take place in premotivated clients who are unable to engage in treatment voluntarily. Therefore, case managers must approach legal constraints with great care. The best strategy that we have found is to objectify the criteria for a legal constraint and attribute them to society and the legal system. In this way, the behaviors that a client must demonstrate in order to avoid involuntary consequences are made clear, and are not experienced as coming from a case manager. Complying with the legal constraints becomes the client's responsibility. The case manager's role becomes defined as having the responsibility to report honestly to the legal system, and to assist the client in acquiring the skills needed to avoid involuntary consequences (e.g., adherence to prescribed medication).

Persuasion Stage. In the persuasion stage, clients are assisted in making connections between legal constraints and their substance-using or treatment-nonadherent behaviors. This allows blame for the legal constraint to be projected outward from the relationship between client and case manager and onto the illness (addiction or mental illness), which can be vilified. Close monitoring of voluntary clients becomes appropriate at this stage, as well as gathering the data necessary for making connections among treatment nonadherence, substance use, and subsequent adverse consequences.

Case managers working with clients in the persuasion stage are often faced with the dilemma of whether or not to invoke a constraint to limit the clients' adverse behaviors, which may also limit their experience of consequences related to their substance use or medication nonadherence. Such decisions must be individualized and involve weighing the risks and benefits of each approach, choosing one, and trying it consistently for a predetermined period of time. Outcomes are improved by periodically reevaluating the risk and shifting strategies if the approach has not been successful. These decision points must include clients and their family members, so that the parameters of the treatment program are clear. When clients make active decisions about their treatment, they feel more invested in the outcome. Close monitoring in this stage includes regular screening for alcohol and drug use, as well as observation of clients taking their medication.

Active Treatment Stage. At the active treatment stage, close monitoring continues and may intensify to support clients in meeting their goals and keeping slips into substance use from becoming full relapses. However, the team tends to back off from legal constraints in this stage, letting clients use their increased motivation to take greater responsibility for freedom from harm to self or others. Clients who previously might have required involuntary hospitalization may request voluntary intensive interventions for detoxification or stabilization of psychotic symptoms in this stage. Family members or other significant people in a client's life (e.g., employers or self-help group sponsors) may participate in close monitoring for the client during the active treatment stage.

Relapse Prevention Stage. The process of close monitoring continues in the relapse prevention stage, but responsibility for it is gradually shifted to the client. The client learns the importance of keeping very close track of his or her emotional responses to stressful situations, experiences of cravings, and thoughts of no longer needing treatment. The roles of case managers in the relapse prevention stage are training clients to recognize the importance of continued monitoring to reduce the risk of relapse, and training them in the skills of monitoring and logging their emotions and behaviors.

Legal constraints can often be dropped or allowed to expire in this stage. There can be an important sense of gratification and recognition for a client who is able to graduate from the need for coerced or involuntary treatments into self-motivated and self-guided treatment. These transition points should be celebrated to increase the client's sense of pride and accomplishment.

Responding to Crises

Crisis is opportunity. Case managers who approach crises in this fashion discover that being available to serve their clients during crises offers enormous opportunities for the work of dual-disorder treatment. During times of crisis, clients tend to be most acutely aware of the painful consequences of their substance use or poor illness management, and they are most willing to consider behavioral changes. Clients may also reveal the depth of their psychiatric symptoms, which they might otherwise hide from their treatment team. Some clients become overly dependent upon crisis services or use emergency services in place of regular treatment. This may require a case manager to discuss the pattern with such a client and discover what factors contribute to it, in order to identify a mutually acceptable response that can better meet the client's needs.

Engagement Stage. For some clients, the experience of an acute crisis represents a valuable opportunity for case managers to engage them actively in treatment. It is critical at this stage that the team be available for crisis response, in order to establish a relationship with clients who have been resistant to treatment and who have rejected previous efforts to engage them. Giving clients support and defining treatment plans can help involve them in treatment. Identifying social issues, such as housing instability or lack of funds, may clarify an underlying cause of some presenting crises and lead to solutions. For example, clients who consistently pursue hospitalization a week or two after receiving their monthly benefits check, and then pursue discharge shortly before the next check should arrive, may be assisted by having a payee appointed to help them spread their money out though the month.

Persuasion Stage. In the persuasion stage, crisis response gives the case manager an awareness of acute and painful consequences of substance use that can be used in the motivational development process. The consistency of the case management team across the spectrum of clinical activity allows a knowledge base to be built that can be used to increase a client's awareness of the need for change. Clients in this stage may also go to emergency rooms or primary care physicians seeking opiates, benzodiazapines, or other commonly abused substances. The availability of the dual-disorders team to consult and provide guidance in treatment response will both ensure a consistent treatment approach and be greatly valued by the medical care team.

Active Treatment Stage. During the active treatment stage, crisis response often centers around relapses. The case manager approaches slips or relapses as opportunities for learning about the behavioral sequence that led up to substance abuse, and then for fine-tuning the sobriety plan. The client is encouraged to engage in a full behavioral analysis, once he or she is sober enough to participate in one constructively, and to reassess treatment goals (see Chapter 8). Slips should always lead the case manager to reassess whether the client remains in the active treatment stage or has moved back into persuasion; this reassessment guides the treatment response. The case manager must also be careful not to reinforce the substance-using behavior by giving excessive attention or treatment resources to the client selectively during periods of relapse. It is usually most helpful to provide a terse assessment at the point of intoxication and advise the client to go home and "sleep it off." The person can return the next day when sober to process the slip, regroup, and redefine the treatment.

Relapse Prevention Stage. Crises tend to diminish further as longer-term sobriety is attained and clients become more able to rely on their own resources or those of their social network for responding to emotional crises. If slips or episodes of illness occur, the team responds as it does in the active treatment stage. Immediate assessment and stabilization are provided, followed by reassessment once sobriety or symptom stabilization has been regained. Clients can usually take more responsibility for managing their treatment in the relapse prevention stage. They may use a medication "as needed" to manage their symptoms from home, rather than being hospitalized, in order to maintain their social and work schedule. Case managers work with clients during periods of stability to anticipate further crises and to assist them in writing their own response plans for how they would like to see future episodes of illness managed (Copeland, 1997).

Stage-wise activities within the advocacy and clinical coordination function of case management are summarized in Table 6.5.

Promoting Rehabilitation and Recovery

Stage-wise case management involves actively helping clients achieve rehabilitation goals, and inspiring them to develop and pursue their own personal recovery goals. Whereas much of the psychotherapeutic work of case management is oriented toward addressing substance abuse and illness management skills either directly or indirectly, the rehabilitation- and recovery-promoting function of case management is aimed mainly at improving overall psychosocial functioning and developing a sense of positive self-esteem and self-worth. Such a focus is critical to helping clients develop the belief that they are capable of changing their lives, and creating positive lives worth living without substances. Three specific activities of stage-wise case man-

agement are included within this general function, including increasing structured activity, developing social/leisure skills and lifestyle change, and facilitating recovery.

Increasing Structured Activity

All people have a need for some meaningful activity during their lives. Unstructured time is commonly described by clients with dual disorders as a cue for using substances. Furthermore, unstructured time tends to aggravate hallucinations and delusions in clients with psychotic disorders (Corrigan, Liberman, & Wong, 1993; Rosen, Sussman, Mueser, Lyons, & Davis, 1981; Wong et al., 1987). Therefore, helping their clients to find constructive activities to fill their daily lives is an important role of case managers. In order to avoid long-term dependence on mental health services and to maximize community integration, it is optimal to strive to involve clients in naturally structured activities in the community, such as volunteer or paid work and affiliation with religious or social groups. These connections can also strengthen and broaden clients' social networks and supports.

Engagement Stage. In the engagement stage, the case manager's primary role is to assess the client's level of involvement in structured activity in a nonthreatening and nonjudgmental way. The case manager may help the client evaluate the degree of structure in his or her life, and explore from the client's perspective possible disadvantages of a lack of meaningful structure. The case manager can offer hope that engagement in treatment will result in opportunities for desired structured activities, which the client may presently perceive as beyond reach. However, little attempt is made to change the client's behavior at this point unless the client strongly desires it. At times it may facilitate the engagement process to connect in terms of an activity-related goal, such as helping a client find a job.

Persuasion Stage. As the therapeutic relationship develops, the case manager works actively to help the client establish regular, constructive activities in his or her life. Such involvement in structured activities can foster hope for positive change and highlight areas in which substance use or nonadherence to psychiatric treatment creates barriers to successfully maintaining desired structured activities. Work is the most common structured activity that clients are motivated to engage in. Loss of income from work after being fired for showing up intoxicated or missing too many days of work can be a powerful natural consequence. Alternatively, having a better income, feeling better, and taking pride in

TABLE 6.5. Activities within the Function of Advocacy and Clinical Coordination in Stage-Wise Case Management

Activity	Engagement	Persuasion	Active treatment	Relapse prevention
Advocacy	• Help clients gain access to housing, medical care, or legal representation.	• Explore consequences of substance abuse in the context of advocating for client needs.	• Help clients obtain services, housing, or privileges that their substance abuse formerly prevented access to. • Expand advocacy to other areas and roles (e.g., work, formal education).	• Help clients learn how to advocate for themselves.
Promoting follow-through	• Reinforce follow-through on basic services. • Coordinate treatment appointments with other activities (e.g., money management).	• Use motivational interviewing to ease lack of follow-through. • Conduct a functional analysis to troubleshoot poor follow-through. • Involve family in promoting follow-through.	• Support client decision making by shifting responsibility for follow-through to client. • Use motivational interviewing when follow-through wanes. • Enlist family support for appropriate follow-through.	• Step back from promoting follow-through. • Allow clients to learn from own mistakes. • Encourage logs or journals to develop follow-through skills.
Providing practical help and benefits	• Furnish practical help and benefits without expectations or demands.	• Address needs for which client previously rejected help. • Develop motivation by exploring effects of substance abuse while providing practical help. • Set limits on help addressing consequences of current substance abuse.	• Help clients experience increase in standard of living (e.g., more control over money soon after achieving sobriety).	• Expand clients' ability to get own basic needs met.
Obtaining and maintaining housing	• Help clients find housing. • Help client improve quality of housing. • Explore "wet" (tolerant of substance abuse) housing.	• Help client make connection between housing problems and substance abuse. • Explore "damp" housing (substance use permitted outside residence). • Help client change housing to setting with less substance abuse.	• Help client improve quality of housing after achieving sobriety. • Explore "dry" (substance use not permitted) housing.	• Help client find more independent, higher-quality housing. • Provide skills training and supports to foster living in independent housing.
Coordinating medication treatment	• Provide access to doctor and medication. • Educate client about medication effects. • Help client fill prescriptions.	• Monitor medication adherence. • Use behavioral tailoring to help clients take medication as prescribed. • Use motivational interviewing to address nonadherence.	• Facilitate evaluation of medications to reduce cravings or substance abuse relapses. • Coordinate detoxification. • Decrease prompts to take medications.	• Teach skills to negotiate medication issues with prescriber. • Train recognition of early warning signs of symptom relapses. • Decrease frequency of medication monitoring.
Using close monitoring and legal constraints (when necessary)	• Objectify criteria for legal constraints. • Attribute legal constraints to society and legal system. • Clarify role of case manager.	• Assist client in making connection between legal constraint and substance abuse or treatment nonadherence. • Closely monitor voluntary clients. • Screen substance use and observe medication adherence.	• Reduce legal constraints. • Maintain close monitoring.	• Drop legal constraints or allow to expire. • Shift monitoring to client. • Train self-monitoring skills.
Responding to crises	• Use crisis situation to establish relationship with disengaged clients. • Identify social factors that may contribute to crisis.	• Help clients make connection between crisis and substance abuse. • Ensure consistency of crisis response across treatment providers.	• Conduct an analysis of factors contributing to substance abuse relapses. • Avoid giving excessive attention to brief lapses of substance abuse.	• Facilitate skills for self-management of crises. • Work to improve prediction and prevention of future crises.

one's accomplishments are powerful natural reinforcers associated with work; they can gradually build a client's willingness to increase investment in constructive activities and reduce investment in substance use or illness symptoms (see Chapter 18).

Active Treatment Stage. As clients make progress toward reducing substance use or achieving abstinence, issues of boredom, lack of social contact, and not knowing what to do with oneself often arise; addressing these issues is critical to avoiding relapse. Therefore, the focus on structured activity continues. A client is assisted in filling up his or her day with therapeutic and vocational activities, as well as constructive social activities with family members, self-help groups, or religious organizations.

Clients whose active treatment goals include improved management of psychiatric symptoms also benefit from increased structured activity to keep their minds focused on external stimuli and to reduce preoccupation with internal stimuli. The more a client develops patterns of focus on external stimuli (e.g., pursuing educational goals, involvement in work), the more natural and comfortable it becomes to let go of preoccupation with internal stimuli. This process may lead to stable decreases in symptoms over extended periods of time.

Relapse Prevention Stage. Clients in the relapse prevention stage are assisted in expanding their structured activities to new areas, such as increased time devoted to recreation and social relationships, which may have been neglected through years of mental illness and substance abuse. Clients may need a great deal of basic coaching to achieve regular involvement in exercise or social organizations. They may need help with acquisition of basic conversational or other social skills (see Chapter 11).

Clients with negative symptoms (e.g., anhedonia, apathy) may have particular difficulty following through on plans to increase structured activity. Negative symptoms should be carefully assessed and aggressively treated through medication whenever possible (see Chapter 19). In addition, clients with negative symptoms may require extensive support, prompting, and encouragement from their case managers (and significant others) to follow through on plans for structured activity. Both clients and their significant others may benefit from developing specific coping strategies aimed at combating negative symptoms that interfere with follow-through, such as positive self-statements for small steps taken, frequent positive feedback for daily accomplishments, and helping the clients be mindful of their long-term goals (Mueser & Gingerich, 1994; Mueser,

Valentiner, & Agresta, 1997). Over time, the more a client participates in an activity that may feel unnatural at first, the more natural it becomes. Furthermore, clients' stamina for engaging in structured activity tends to increase gradually as their experience and familiarity with the routine increase.

Developing Social/Leisure Skills and Lifestyle Change

Most clients with dual disorders have extremely limited recreation and leisure skills, as well as highly impaired social skills. They often live a self-destructive lifestyle and have suffered many physical consequences of their mental illness and substance abuse (e.g., poor nutrition, dental decay, head traumas, broken bones, hepatitis, HIV, sexually transmitted diseases, and emphysema). Most clients approach the process of recovery with a focus on what they are giving up in the early stages. They fear the loss of the drug or alcohol they may have relied on as a coping mechanism or as their only experience of pleasure from a very early age. Most clients with dual disorders have little idea how to experience pleasure or relaxation without drug use. Without substances, they are like fish out of water. One job of case managers through the stages of treatment is to help clients shift from a focus on what they are losing to a focus on what they are gaining. Helping clients experience the joys and pleasures that can be gained from vigorous exercise, meaningful interpersonal relationships, or appreciation of nature's beauty can help them to find new meaning in life and to experience the process of recovery as rewarding and positive. Facilitating lifestyle changes in clients overlaps with increasing meaningful structure in their lives, but it includes other changes as well, such as improved relationships.

Engagement Stage. In the engagement stage, the case manager focuses primarily on assisting the client in assessing his or her current level of social, leisure, and recreational activity. The client may be guided to recognize things that he or she enjoyed at a previous point in life but is currently missing out on, or positive relationships that have turned sour or have ended. The case manager does not attempt to change the client's behavior at this point, but rather focuses on creating a recognition that things could be different with treatment and instilling hope for positive change in the future.

Persuasion Stage. As the relationship between the case manager and client evolves, the client is helped to begin sampling pleasurable recreational activities. It usually works best to start with activities the client has already had some interest or involvement in, or has previously engaged in but has since ceased. These experiences may rekindle fond memories and past pride in athletic accomplishments or other abilities, which can serve as a contrast to the client's present state. Some clients may feel demoralized by their loss, but many can be helped to find motivation for pursuing an age-appropriate level of competence and involvement in sports or other recreational activities. Walking is the simplest and most accessible activity for most clients. In either rural locations or urban parks, clients may have access to a natural area. A walk in the woods can help the client relax, and can often facilitate a therapeutic engagement and an honest exchange with someone who might feel too threatened or paranoid in an office setting.

Clients who want to increase their contacts with others can benefit from exploring options for social contacts (e.g., community organizations, self-help groups) or from reestablishing relationships with family members or friends. Some clients with social skill deficits may benefit from systematic skills training (Bellack et al., 1997) to improve their competence in relating to others (Chapter 11). Social skills training can also be helpful in addressing problems in existing relationships that clients want to improve (e.g., frequent conflict, lack of intimacy, aggression or exploitation). Some of these relationships may be with other people who have active substance use problems—which can be problematic, as clients have limited motivation to reduce their substance use in the persuasion stage. In such situations, case managers focus on helping the clients develop better skills for addressing relationship problems with significant others, regardless of whether those individuals are abusing substances. At the same time, the case managers look for opportunities to help clients see the problematic nature of their relationships with people who abuse substances, and to instill motivation for healthier relationships with people who do not use (i.e., motivational interviewing; Chapter 7).

Active Treatment Stage. As the client develops experience with different social and recreational activities, and substance abuse decreases, the case manager assists him or her in establishing a routine of new activities to replace the role of substance use. These activities can also provide new avenues of reinforcement to replace the void left by reduced substance use or abstinence. Particular attention is given to activities and relationships that are associated with a sober lifestyle and perhaps inconsistent with substance use. For example, vigorous athletic activity may help increase clients' awareness of the adverse effects of their previous lifestyle on their physical health, and thus may increase motivation for sobriety. As improving social skills typically requires extended periods of time, skills training

(Chapter 11) often continues into the active treatment and relapse prevention stages.

Some clients prefer to focus on a single change during the active treatment stage (e.g., sustaining abstinence from alcohol or a drug that they were using heavily), and may experience other lifestyle changes as overwhelming or distracting. Other clients, however, find that either spending time with certain social networks or remaining sedentary and isolated is so associated with their substance abuse that it is hard for them to maintain abstinence without developing a broader lifestyle change. Virtually all clients find it difficult to change substance-using behaviors without a substantial change in their social network, and they commonly report that establishing a new social network, is difficult (Drake, Brunette, & Mueser, 1998). In the active treatment stage, case managers focus strongly on helping clients identify and sample constructive social options where substance use is less likely to occur.

Relapse Prevention Stage. In the relapse prevention stage, case managers assist clients in expanding their recovery process to include a wider array of social and recreational options. Clients are helped to make change toward a healthy lifestyle that is free from substance misuse of all kinds. Case managers use the focus on achieving pleasure, relaxation, and increased interest in social and leisure activities to compete with these old behaviors. Clients are extensively educated about the benefits of regular exercise, good nutrition, giving up smoking, and stress management for both physical and mental health.

Facilitating Recovery

Recovery is a concept emanating from the self-help and consumer movements; it refers to a process of redefining one's life not through illness and disability, but through relationships and abilities (Anthony, 1993; Deegan, 1988; Fisher, 1992; Leete, 1989). In other words, clients who are able to make the transition from negative self-images of hopelessness, severe mental illness, and addiction to identities defined by work, social relationships, and recreational pursuits will be able to find motivation for the hard work of managing their dual disorders. Learning how to manage such disorders becomes worthwhile when the efforts serve the larger purpose of allowing a person to explore and expand his or her horizons. Although recovery is described by clients as a personal inner journey that cannot be taken for them by anyone else, professionals may be able to play a role in facilitating the recovery process (Noordsy et al., 2000; Torrey & Wyzik, 2000). Recovery should not be confused with rehabilitation. *Rehabilitation* is a process of facilitating increased involvement in functional activities, often with the use of behavioral techniques such as social skills training. *Recovery* is the change in identity and self-esteem associated with the belief that one is a productive contributor to society and has a meaningful life, despite the presence of chronic illness (Deegan, 1988).

Engagement Stage. The case manager's primary role early in treatment is to portray the recovery process to the client as a source of hope. The case manager describes the experiences of other clients who have been able to make the transition from a life ravaged by mental illness and addiction to a life filled with gratification and purpose. The client is not pressured to change, but rather is educated about the possibilities that exist.

Persuasion Stage. In the persuasion stage, clients are encouraged to actively envision their lives as they would like to see them in the state of recovery. This process of brainstorming hope and dreams for the future is allowed to become as grandiose and unrealistic as a client desires. The case manager's goal is to better understand the client and help the client better understand him- or herself. Personal strengths are identified and highlighted, as these qualities are critical to helping clients perceive themselves as worthwhile and capable individuals who can make progress toward desired changes. These goals and dreams then allow a contrast to the client's present state, as well as the definition of small steps that may be involved in getting from one place to the other. This is where realism is introduced (e.g., "What can you do today to get one step closer to where you'd like to be 5 years from now?"). Additional strategies for helping clients understand how their substance abuse interferes with their ability to achieve personal goals, and supporting clients as they begin to work on their substance abuse problems, are described in Chapter 7.

Active Treatment Stage. As the client begins to attain sobriety, he or she can make a commitment to taking a significant step toward future goals by making a substantial behavioral life change. During the active treatment stage, clients frequently become discouraged, demoralized, and overwhelmed by the hard work of obtaining sobriety; they may long for the easy "fix" of drugs or alcohol. The case manager works to keep the recovery goal alive and to maintain motivation through recognition and building on personal strengths. The recovery process also makes the motivation for behavioral change very personal. Clients are not giving up substance use to help the treatment team or to manage an abstract diagnosis. Rather, they are taking themselves one step closer to important goals—such as regaining the right to parent their children; taking pride in themselves as athletes or employees; or making meaningful, creative contributions in the arts.

Relapse Prevention Stage. In the relapse prevention stage, case managers assist clients in actualizing their recovery goals and expanding their recovery to other areas. This is the "payoff" stage, in which the hard work of the active treatment stage now allows a client to accomplish things that were previously out of the question. The client may seek a better job, obtain a driver's license, or resume pursuing an educational goal. The case manager assists the client in continuing to explore his or her possibilities and potentials, to create more and more distance between the past and the person's current self-definition while remaining mindful of the risk of relapse. Again, it is critical to keep the ownership for the recovery process and its direction with the client. The case manager's role is to encourage reflection, perspective, and open-minded exploration of potential.

The stage-wise case management activities within the function of promoting rehabilitation and recovery are summarized in Table 6.6.

SUMMARY

Case management is the core service delivery intervention for clients with dual disorders. The dominant model employed is the clinical case management model, in which the case manager both coordinates treatment and works as a clinician with the client. This approach is informed by the ACT model, which emphasizes outreach, teamwork, and direct (rather than brokered) service delivery; and by the strengths model which focuses on clients' assets (rather than pathology) and building on natural supports to helping clients achieve personal goals. Paramount to all effective case management is establishing a good therapeutic relationship with the client.

Case management is conducted in accordance with the stages of treatment to ensure that interventions are properly matched to each client's motivational state. The functions of stage-wise case management can be divided into three general categories: psychotherapeutic work; advocacy and clinical coordination; and promotion of rehabilitation and recovery. The specific stage-wise case management activities within each of these functions are described in the chapter (and summarized in Tables 6.3, 6.5, and 6.6).

TABLE 6.6. Activities within the Function of Promoting Rehabilitation and Recovery in Stage-Wise Case Management

Activity	Engagement	Persuasion	Active treatment	Relapse prevention
Increasing structured activity	• Assess client's level of involvement in structured activity. • Avoid concerted efforts to change client's behavior.	• Help establish regular constructive activities in client's life (e.g., work). • Identify positive changes in new activities as they are explored. • Develop positive expectations.	• Identify activities to fill void left by reduced substance abuse (e.g., boredom, lack of social contact). • Encourage focus on external rather than internal stimuli, to reduce psychiatric symptoms.	• Expand structured activities to new areas (e.g., recreation, social relationships). • Provide encouragement and coaching to maintain regular exercise or involvement in social organizations.
Developing social/leisure and lifestyle change	• Assist clients in assessing current social leisure and recreational activities. • Create recognition that things could be different, and instill hope for improvement.	• Facilitate sampling recreational activities. • Explore resumption of previous social and recreational activities.	• Establish route of recreational activities. • Focus on lifestyle changes incompatible with substance abuse (e.g., exercise). • Facilitate development of new social outlets.	• Expand range of social/leisure activities and of lifestyle changes. • Provide education about health benefits of regular exercise, nutrition, and stress management.
Facilitating recovery	• Portray recovery process as source of hope. • Describe experiences of others who have recovered from dual disorders.	• Envision future state of recovery. • Explore how substances interfere with steps toward recovery. • Identify client strengths to use in making progress toward recovery goals.	• Keep recovery goal alive through encouragement and focus on client's strengths. • Celebrate small successes as steps toward recovery goals.	• Actualize and expand recovery goals. • Keep ownership for recovery and its direction with clients.

7

Motivational Interviewing

One of the most common challenges for clinicians treating dual disorders is working with clients who are engaged in treatment, but who do not view their substance abuse as a problem, who express little or no desire to change their substance use behavior, or who profess an interest in changing but nevertheless continue to use. Clients in the persuasion stage of treatment frequently deemphasize or altogether deny the negative consequences associated with their substance use (see Chapter 2 for a review of the stages of treatment and their relationship with the stages of change). Clinicians' efforts to confront them about their substance abuse frequently meet with resistance and can even result in their disengaging from treatment. With direct confrontation, some clients admit to the negative consequences of their substance use, and may even endorse a goal of reducing or stopping substance use. However, clients who give in to this type of pressure often lack the personal resolve to work on their substance abuse problems, and their verbal agreement to begin reducing or stopping substance use is rarely accompanied by actual behavior change. The net results of repeated efforts to persuade such a client of the negative consequences of substance use are often frustration for both the clinician and the client, and a strain on their working alliance.

Motivational interviewing is a set of therapeutic strategies designed to help clients understand the impact of substance abuse on their lives in their own terms. Motivational interviewing is typically provided in the context of the individual relationship between the clinician and the client (hence its inclusion in the "Individual Approaches" part of this book). However, the principles of motivational interviewing can also be applied in group and family treatment approaches, as briefly described at the end of this chapter and elaborated in Chapters 9 and 14. In this chapter, we describe how to use motivational interviewing strategies for clients with dual disorders—strategies based on the model developed for facilitating change by Miller and Rollnick (2002).

Although motivational interviewing has been conceptualized as an intervention for addressing substance abuse in ambivalent people, the intervention can be applied to a wide variety of clinical problems. For example, Swanson and colleagues (1999) provided inpatients with dual disorders with a brief motivational interviewing intervention to increase attendance at outpatient treatment appointments following hospital discharge. Kemp and colleagues (Healey et al., 1998; Kemp et al., 1996, 1998) used motivational interviewing to increase medication adherence in clients with psychosis. Corrigan, McCracken, and Holmes (2001) have described the use of motivational interviewing in assessment and the setting of rehabilitation goals for persons with severe mental illness. Thus the principles of motivational interviewing have broad applicability for addressing problematic behaviors (including substance abuse and nonadherence to treatment recommendations) that interfere with clients with dual disorders in achieving their personal goals.

THE ROLE OF MOTIVATIONAL INTERVIEWING IN DUAL-DISORDER TREATMENT

Lack of motivation is one of the most common and pervasive problems clinicians cite among clients with dual disorders. The purpose of motivational interviewing is to help clients recognize how their substance abuse interferes with their ability to achieve personally valued goals—rather than the goals of clinicians or of society at large—and become motivated to work on their substance abuse in order to pursue these goals. Some personal goals may be identified in the assessment process, but additional or more important goals may be targeted as the process of motivational interviewing unfolds. Helping clients articulate personal goals and explore how substance use interferes with achieving these goals—which is the core of motivational interviewing—requires a strong working alliance between the client and clinician. Therefore, the core of motivational interviewing is most appropriate for clients who are in the persuasion and active treatment stages (see Table 5.7).

As we explain in the next section, the first step of motivational interviewing is to express empathy, and it typically begins in the engagement stage of treatment and overlaps with the five-step assessment process (see Chapters 4 and 5). However, empathic listening is a general clinical skill useful in engaging clients in treatment, and it is not unique to motivational interviewing. In addition, motivational interviewing strategies may occasionally be incorporated into the relapse prevention stage, but it is usually not a primary focus of treatment at this stage. For these reasons, motivational interviewing is not listed as an intervention for the engagement or relapse prevention stages in Table 5.7.

All clients who are actively using substances and currently experiencing negative consequences of this use are appropriate for motivational interviewing, as well as clients who have recently experienced such problems. The assessment process can be useful in identifying goals that are the focus of motivational interviewing work with clients. Specifically, the functional analysis of substance use behavior involves pinpointing the potential benefits of not using substances for the client (Chapter 5). Examples of such benefits include improved stabilization of the psychiatric disorder, ability to obtain and maintain independent housing, better chances of getting a job or resuming parental responsibilities, better health, and more money to spend. However, these advantages have often been insufficient to motivate clients to give up their use of alcohol and drugs. There are many reasons why this may be so. For example, clients may not be invested in working toward "advantages" of sobriety identified by clinicians or relatives, or they may believe that they are incapable of making significant changes in their lives. Motivational interviewing is a critical treatment strategy that can help clients (1) to focus on and take steps toward positive goals identified in the functional analysis (or to refine those goals through further discussion); (2) to develop insight into how their substance use interferes with achieving their goals; and (3) to make early efforts to address their substance abuse, in order to continue

their pursuit of personal goals. Becoming adept at helping clients develop internal motivation for change is one of the most valuable skills a clinician can develop.

WHAT IS MOTIVATION?

Motivation is a commonly used word, but each person attaches his or her own meaning to it. To some people, it refers to what a person wants or says he or she wants, regardless of what the person actually does. Others use the term *motivation* more restrictively, to refer both to articulated desires and to actual effort toward achieving those goals. Considering the centrality of the concept of motivation to this chapter, it is important to be as specific as possible in defining our use of this term.

We use the same definition of *motivation* as that proposed by Miller and Rollnick (2002): Motivation can be understood not as something that someone *has*, but as something that someone *does*, involving recognizing a problem, finding a way to change, and then starting and sticking with that change strategy.

Individuals say they want to change their substance use for a variety of different reasons—many unrelated to personal motivation, such as the desire to please others and fear about the loss of benefits or support. However, these verbal reports are often unrelated to behavior observed by others (Addington, el-Guebaly, Duchak, & Hodgins, 1999). For this reason, an emphasis is placed on defining motivation based on the client's behavior, not just his or her verbal statements.

Thus a client who states a wish to reduce drinking, but shows no actual efforts or success at decreasing alcohol use, is not considered motivated (or sufficiently motivated) to reduce alcohol use, despite his or her verbal statements. In contrast, an individual who not only expresses a desire to reduce alcohol use, but has either made efforts to cut down or has succeeded in reducing consumption, is considered motivated to reduce alcohol use. Note that the emphasis on using behavioral change to define motivation is consistent with the behavioral anchors used to define different stages of treatment on the Substance Abuse Treatment Scale—Revised (SATS-R; for discussion, see Chapter 5; see Appendix C, Form C.8, for the SATS-R itself). That is, before an individual progresses to the active stage of treatment (where the focus of treatment is on substance use reduction itself), he or she must demonstrate some success or repeated efforts at reducing substance use. Therefore, the primary goal of motivational interviewing is to motivate clients to address their substance abuse (i.e., persuasion work) and to support them in their early efforts to cut down substance use or achieve abstinence (i.e., active treatment work).

STEPS, AIMS, AND STRATEGIES
OF MOTIVATIONAL INTERVIEWING

Overview

Traditional confrontational approaches to treating people with substance use disorders fail with clients with dual disorders for several reasons. Sometimes a clinician's pressure to change actually pushes a client to be more aware of the other parts of his or her ambivalence toward change, increasing resistance to change. Another problem is that clinicians often focus on the consequences that *they themselves* believe are most important, rather than appealing to *clients'* own values and perceptions. Motivational interviewing differs from direct confrontational approaches by shifting the focus away from the consequences of substance abuse most apparent to a clinician, and exploring the possible consequences from a client's own perspective. To the extent that confrontation occurs, it is between the client's personal goals and preferences, not the clinician's goals and the client's substance use behavior.

Motivational interviewing begins with the process of listening, exploring, and trying to understand the client's experiences in a dialogue free of judgment and agenda. Next, the goals and personal values of the client are explored, in order to determine life changes that the client can be engaged to work toward. When such changes have been identified, the client and clinician begin to explore the steps necessary for achieving them. In the process of determining how to achieve a goal, the clinician looks for opportunities to consider the possible role of the client's substance use in interfering with that desired goal. When clients begin to see that their substance use is an obstacle to achieving their own goals, cognitive dissonance develops between their beliefs and values on the one hand, and their continued substance abuse on the other. A client can reduce this dissonance between achieving personal goals and substance use behavior by making efforts to cut down using substances or to stop altogether. The process of creating dissonance, exploring the implications of changing substance use behavior, and developing the confidence that change is possible can be slow but rewarding. The conclusion of successful motivational interviewing is a client's taking personal responsibility for working on substance abuse, with the help of the clinician, because the client has come to understand that this is in his or her own best interests.

We break the clinical skills involved in motivational interviewing down into five steps: expressing empathy, establishing personal goals, developing discrepancy, rolling with resistance, and supporting self-efficacy. These steps are almost identical to the steps described by Miller and Rollnick (2002). The one difference is that we have added the step of establishing personal goals, because this requires considerable time, effort, and clinical skill in clients with dual disorders, but is distinct from either expressing empathy or developing discrepancy.

Expressing Empathy

The Aim of Expressing Empathy

The ultimate aim of motivational interviewing is to help clients view their substance use as a problem for their own reasons. In order to accomplish this, it is imperative that a clinician establish a trusting, therapeutic relationship with a client that can withstand the cognitive dissonance the client subsequently develops. Thus the aim of the first step of motivational interviewing is to understand the client's world from his or her own perspective. Many of the skills for accomplishing this are basic psychotherapeutic skills, as described below.

Strategies for Empathic Listening

Good *active listening behaviors* are important for demonstrating understanding and empathy to clients. Examples of such behaviors include good eye contact; facial expressiveness that is responsive to the content of what the client is saying; body oriented toward the client; and other "encouraging" behaviors, such as head nods and small verbal interjections (e.g., "I see," "Uh-huh," "I understand"). These verbal and nonverbal behaviors convey the clinician's interest in the client and attention to what is being said.

Reflective listening is a powerful method for checking out what is heard and demonstrating understanding. In reflective listening, the clinician paraphrases his or her understanding of the client's message. The closer the clinician sticks to the client's language, the easier it is to verify that the message has been heard correctly. Reflective listening serves two main functions. First, repeating back to the client what the clinician has heard concretely demonstrates to the client that his or her communication has been understood. Second, hearing one's own statements reflected back with a minimum of interpretation can lead to further elaboration, refinement, and exploration. In this way, reflective listening can help clients develop a better understanding of their own thoughts, feelings, and experiences.

Reflective listening is useful when the clinician understands what the client has said, and wishes to demonstrate this to him or her. At other times, the communication may be less clear, and the clinician needs to ask *clarifying questions* to ensure that he or she has understood the client properly. Asking clarifying questions can be especially useful in work with clients whose communication skills are limited by cognitive impairment, psychotic distortions, severe depression, or agitation. Clarifying questions can be asked in a simple yes–no format as a check on the clinician's understanding of the client—for example,

> "It sounds like you were pretty upset when your sister called your doctor and case manager in order to have you hospitalized. Is this correct?"

Alternatively, open-ended clarifying questions can be asked that request the client to elaborate on a specific point, as in this example:

> "It sounds like when you began drinking again 3 months ago, there were a lot of different things going on in your life. Could you tell me a little bit more about what was happening to you around the time you resumed drinking?"

There is a difference between asking clarifying questions and questioning or challenging what a client says. Asking clarifying questions helps the clinician determine whether he or she has understood the client correctly. Questioning or challenging the client, on the other hand, is aimed at directly changing the client's behavior, which is incompatible with the aim of understanding the person's world. Similarly, judging the client, expressing doubt about his or her statements, and providing unsolicited advice are not part of empathic listening and do not help to express empathy.

The aim of expressing empathy, and clinical strategies for achieving this aim, are summarized in Table 7.1.

TABLE 7.1. Aim and Strategies for Expressing Empathy in Motivational Interviewing

Aim: To understand the client's world.

Clinical Strategies:
- Practice active listening behaviors:
  - Good eye contact.
  - Responsive facial expression.
  - Body oriented toward the client.
  - Verbal and nonverbal "encouragers" (e.g., head nods, saying "I see").
- Use reflective listening (i.e., paraphrasing the client).
- Ask clarifying questions.
- Avoid:
  - Challenging the client.
  - Expressing doubt.
  - Passing judgment.
  - Giving unsolicited advice.

Establishing Personal Goals

The Aim of Establishing Personal Goals

Expressing empathy to the client builds the necessary foundation upon which the exploration of goals is based. In order to develop a dissonance between the client's goals and substance use, personal and meaningful goals must be established. The aim of this step is to identify goals that are important to the *client*, not simply goals that the clinician or others think the person should have. If the client's true desire for a personal goal is tenuous, then the likely result when dissonance is created between substance use and achieving that goal will be devaluing or discarding the goal, rather than addressing the problem of substance use. The time and effort expended during empathic listening will result in an understanding of the client that will help the clinician determine when the client has articulated personally meaningful goals.

Establishing goals can be especially difficult in work with severely ill individuals whose lives have been fraught with disappointment and despair. Many clients with dual disorders appear to have given up on their hopes and desires, and seem passively to accept their dismal lot in life. For these individuals, not having goals has its advantages; if they have no goals, they cannot be disappointed by the failure to achieve a goal.

Clinicians need to understand clients' passive acceptance of the status quo, and appreciate that such acceptance may serve as a protective shield against disappointment. In this respect, helping clients believe that change is possible and searching for goals with personal meaning involve a certain amount of risk taking on the parts of both clients and clinicians. Clients need to be supported in breaking out of their self-protective shells of resigned acceptance into contemplating the possibility that change is in fact possible, while believing at the same time that failure is not inevitable. Clinicians need to be willing to risk instilling hope in clients who have given up, and to work actively with clients to ensure that some progress is made toward goals. Furthermore, clinicians need to take steps to minimize the chances of failure, and to help clients deal with disappointment on the rocky road to achieving personally meaningful goals.

Strategies for Establishing Personal Goals

When a clinician is trying to begin a dialogue with a client about goals, it is often best to avoid using the term *goal*. Many clients regularly participate in treatment-planning meetings in which they are expected to identify short-term goals to work on for the next 3–6 months. The emphasis in these meetings is often on goals that are of limited interest to the clients. In addition, the routine of goal setting and attainment as a part of treatment planning may seem mechanistic to many clients, who reluctantly participate in the process because it is a requirement of receiving services from the treatment center. Rather than using the term *goal* when talking about desired life changes, clinicians may simply explore with clients how they would like things to be different, their aspirations, and even their fantasies.

Clients' truest desires have often become submerged following many years of frustration, and they themselves may not be able to readily identify goals to work toward. Rather than focusing on current goals, a useful alternative in such cases is to explore what clients were like when they were younger, the activities they engaged in, the people they admired, and the things they hoped to do as they grew older. It is often much easier to get a client to talk about the past then the present, and by finding out more about the client's life at an earlier age, the clinician gathers valuable information in a comfortable, nonthreatening, and low-expectation manner.

When the conversation focuses on the here-and-now, clients often become stymied because of the multiple problems they see posed by their present circumstances. Such clients need help thinking of their present circumstances differently, in order to come up with goals toward which they may be motivated to work. One useful strategy for eliciting possible goals is to ask questions such as these: "If you didn't have these kinds of difficulties, how would things be different? What would you be doing right now? What would you have that you don't currently have?" By asking questions in this manner, a clinician encourages a client to imagine what life would be like if some of its difficulties were removed (e.g., psychiatric illness, poverty, loneliness, etc.). Facilitating clients' ability to think about how they would like their lives to be different naturally leads to the identification of goals related to those desires.

In the process of identifying goals to work on, a clinician is faced with the question of which goals are most suitable to work on with a client and how ambitious the goals should be. This question can best be restated as follows: "Which types of goals are *not* appropriate for collaborative work?" The clinician should avoid agreeing to work with the client on only two types of goals: (1) goals that are clearly delusional in nature, and (2) goals that are potentially harmful to the client and/or others.

As an example of the first type of unsuitable goal, a client with a fixed delusional belief that she had invented the Boeing 747 stated that her goal was to obtain the money she believed she was owed by the Boeing Corporation for her invention, and she requested the clinician's assistance in achieving this goal. The clinician acknowledged the client's belief that she had invented the 747 (without agreeing or disagreeing with it), but declined to work with her toward getting compensation, and steered the conversation to goals not based on delusions.

As an example of the second type of unsuitable goal, one client defiantly told his clinician that his only goal was to drink himself to death. The clinician responded with some humor by saying,

"I understand that you said that you would like to drink yourself to death. I'd say you've been doing a pretty good job of that by yourself, and that you don't need any help from me on that! How about if we talk about some other ways that I might be helpful to you?"

For the most part, clients with dual disorders have the same goals and ambitions as people in the general population. They want to love and be loved by someone else; to have a family; to live in clean, comfortable, and safe housing; to eat good food; to do something meaningful with their time; to own various possessions; and to engage in fun activities. Although each individual's goals are unique, the general nature of these clients' goals and desires is no different from anyone else's. Examples of the kinds of goals clients have worked toward are provided in Table 7.2.

Clinicians (and even clients) may have mixed feelings about working toward very ambitious goals, such as having a family or owning a car. However, there are several reasons for working in earnest toward any goal that a client genuinely wants, no matter how ambitious that

---

TABLE 7.2. Examples of Goals Identified by Clients in Motivational Interviewing

Finding a job	Getting one's own apartment
Completing high school	Resuming parenting responsibilities for one's offspring
Finding a girlfriend	Reestablishing relationships with one's siblings
Getting a driver's license back	Handling one's own money
Getting married	Buying a car
Losing weight	Playing in a band
Rekindling a relationship with an old boyfriend	Enrolling in an aerobics program
Going fishing with one's father	Becoming a professional writer

goal may be. First, neither a clinician nor a client can accurately forecast the future for the client, and the recovery movement has emphasized that it is the client, not the professional, who has the right to define desired outcomes (Carling, 1995; Deegan, 1992; Madera, 1988). We have seen individuals with dual disorders make dramatic changes in their lives and accomplish remarkable goals. For example, one of us (Lindy Fox) experienced the breakup of her first marriage and loss of custody of her children, amidst a severe case of bipolar disorder and alcoholism that involved over 20 hospitalizations. Over the following 10 years, Lindy became abstinent from alcohol, remarried, rekindled her relationships with her children, resumed her schooling, and became a dual-diagnosis clinician and research interviewer. Who could have predicted that such improvements would take place? No one has the right to tell a client that he or she cannot attain an ambitious, but not delusional, goal.

A second reason for working toward ambitious goals is that the success of the effort is not determined so much by whether or not the final goal was achieved as by the progress made toward that goal. As we discuss in the next section, once a goal has been established, steps are identified that are necessary in order to achieve that goal. Even when the final goal is not achieved, substantial and meaningful improvements may occur in the client's life. Furthermore, based on the earlier successful steps toward achieving a stated goal, and the accompanying change in perspective, the client's goal may shift and become the focus of new efforts.

CASE EXAMPLE

An unemployed woman with polysubstance abuse expressed a long-latent desire to become an actress in TV commercials. In discussions with her clinician, it was agreed that she would need some work experience and employment history before she began exploring how to get into TV commercials. The client's substance abuse had interfered with her previous efforts to keep jobs, and she began the process of decreasing (and eventually stopping) her use of alcohol, cocaine, and marijuana. Several months after successfully working as an assistant to a florist, the client announced that she had decided she no longer wanted to pursue becoming a TV actress, and was interested instead in going to cosmetology school and becoming a cosmetologist. This new goal was more realistic, and she was eventually successful in achieving it.

A third reason for working with clients toward personally meaningful, long-term goals is that people are willing to work the most and endure the greatest hardship to achieve goals that they care the most about. Clients are not willing to stop using alcohol and drugs in order to achieve goals that lack meaning and personal importance. By their very nature, meaningful goals also tend to be ambitious; thus such goals have the potential for harnessing client motivation to change, whereas less ambitious and more rudimentary goals do not.

The aim of establishing personal goals, and clinical strategies for doing this, are summarized in Table 7.3.

Developing Discrepancy

The Aim of Developing Discrepancy

After a personally meaningful goal has been identified, the clinician and client explore it, develop steps for achieving it, and determine barriers that must be overcome to achieve it. Once the clinician has created a safe, neutral, and supportive environment in discussing how the client can make progress toward a goal, the client can identify his or her substance use disorder as a barrier, and thus can develop motivation to work on substance abuse. The aim of this step is to help the client see his or her own substance abuse as inconsistent with achieving an important personal goal, so that the client will become motivated in this way.

It should be stressed, however, that the process of identifying goals and helping clients take steps toward achieving these goals is not pursued only for the purpose of developing a discrepancy between the client's substance abuse and those goals. Indeed, it would be disingenuous for a clinician to explore and pursue goals with a client solely for the purpose of addressing substance abuse, without concern for achieving the goals themselves. Rather, identifying goals and developing concrete steps for achieving them are important parts of the shared decision making that characterizes the client–clinician relationship in an integrated treatment

---

TABLE 7.3. Aim and Strategies for Establishing Personal Goals in Motivational Interviewing

Aim: To establish goals that are genuinely personal and meaningful for the *client*, in order to increase the client's willingness to work toward them.

Clinical Strategies:
- Talk with the client about his or her:
  - Aspirations.
  - Desires for how things could be different.
  - Fantasies about how things should be.
- Get to know what the client was like in the past, such as finding out about his or her:
  - Preferred activities.
  - Admired people.
  - Personal ambitions.
- Don't discourage the client from expressing ambitious goals.

program. From this vantage point, motivational interviewing elegantly capitalizes on the fact that substance abuse often interferes with individuals' personal goals.

Strategies for Developing Discrepancy

Critical to the development of discrepancy is the recognition that people tend to value insights they arrive at on their own more than ones that are supplied to them by others. Indeed, experimental evidence indicates that direct confrontation about delusional beliefs tends to *increase* conviction in those beliefs, rather than to *decrease* it (Milton, Patwa, & Hafner, 1978). The negative effects of direct confrontation may be partly due to *psychological reactance* (Brehm, 1966; Fogarty, 1997), or the tendency for people to reject options if they view them as limiting their range of choices (Corrigan, River, Lundin, Penn, & Kubiak, 2001). This means that the clinician must avoid directly confronting or even pointing out the contradictions between the client's substance use behavior and his or her personal goals. Rather, the clinician structures the discussion in a way that is conducive to the client's seeing this discrepancy on his or her own.

A useful strategy for accomplishing this is the *Socratic method*. The Socratic method is named after the teaching style used by Socrates with his students, as exemplified in Plato's *Republic* and other writings. The Socratic method involves asking the student (client) a series of questions that eventually leads to a conclusion. Each question builds on the answers to previous questions, so that conclusions are reached through a natural and logical progression. Rather than being told the answer to any particular question, the client reaches a conclusion based on his or her answers to the different questions. The principal advantage of using the Socratic method over lecturing or directly confronting clients is that people are more likely to accept their own answers to specific questions than answers someone else tells them.

In order to develop discrepancy, most personal goals need to be broken down into a series of smaller goals. Through use of the Socratic method, the clinician can help the client break down a large, seemingly unattainable goal into a series of smaller, more manageable steps. We provide an illustration below of how this can be done.

CLINICIAN: Joe, we've been talking together about some of the things that are really important to you. You've told me that someday you would like to have your own family, meaning a wife and kids.

JOE: Yeah, I'd really like that.

CLINICIAN: Well, that's a really great long-term goal to work toward. Would you like to do some thinking together about how you might achieve that goal?

JOE: Okay.

CLINICIAN: Having a family is a pretty big goal. I've found that it's sometimes helpful to take a big goal like this and break it down into a bunch of smaller goals. Then you can work on these smaller goals, one at a time. What do you think about that, Joe? Should we work on just the big goal, or should we try to break it down into some smaller goals?

JOE: Let's work on the smaller goals.

CLINICIAN: Okay. Let's do some brainstorming together and figure out some of the possible steps you might need to take toward your goal. I'll keep track of the different possible goals on this blackboard. Joe, if you're going to get married, what is something you need before you get married?

JOE: A marriage license?

CLINICIAN: That's true, you'll need a marriage license. What do you need to have before a marriage license? Who are you going to marry?

JOE: A girlfriend?

CLINICIAN: Right. It helps to have a girlfriend before you get married. Do you have a girlfriend right now?

JOE: No. But I'd like one.

CLINICIAN: Okay, so that's another goal on the way to your bigger goal—having a girlfriend. Let's talk about what you need in order to have a girlfriend. What would be a possible step toward getting a girlfriend?

JOE: I don't know. I don't know very many people.

CLINICIAN: All right, that's a good point, Joe. It's helpful to have some friends and to be able to meet new people in order to get a girlfriend.

JOE: Yes, but I don't know where to meet new people, and I don't know what to say when I meet them.

CLINICIAN: Those are some really good points, Joe, and maybe we could look at this as one of the first goals to start working on. What do you think about the goal of working on what to say in order to help you meet new people?

JOE: Sounds good to me.

When the critical steps toward achieving a goal have been identified, the clinician begins the delicate work of exploring the possible interactions between the client's substance abuse and achieving those steps. There are several ways of accomplishing this. First, the clinician can avoid direct reference to substance use, and instead employ the Socratic method to prompt the client to evaluate possible difficulties with achieving his or her goal. Through selective questioning and reinforcement, the client can be brought closer to understanding how substance abuse interferes with achieving a desired goal. The advantage of this strategy is that the client assumes the primary responsibility for appreciating the role of the substance abuse as an obstacle to achieving a personal goal. Second, the clinician can ask the client whether his or her substance use interferes with accomplishing a step toward the goal. This strategy can be effective, although a disadvantage is that such direct questioning can be too "leading" and may backfire. Third, the clinician may assume the opposite position, and ask the client how his or her substance use *helps* achieve a particular goal. We continue with the example of Joe:

CLINICIAN: We've agreed to work together on how to meet new people and what to say when you meet them.

JOE: Right.

CLINICIAN: We can work on improving your ability to start and have interesting conversations with others by doing some role plays together. You also might be interested to know that there is a social skills training group offered at this center, for helping people develop better skills for getting to know other people. How's that sound?

JOE: Okay.

CLINICIAN: How about the goal of finding places to meet new people?

JOE: I don't really know where to meet people. I don't go out very much.

CLINICIAN: So what do you do with most of your spare time at home?

JOE: Drink, I guess.

CLINICIAN: I see. How do you think staying at home and drinking at night helps you meet new people?

JOE: Meet new people? (*Puzzled*) Probably it's not very helpful.

CLINICIAN: Well, what do you think? Does your drinking help you meet new people?

JOE: I don't think it helps very much.

CLINICIAN: It doesn't? If we can identify some new places for you to meet people, what are you going to need to do in order to get out? What about your drinking?

JOE: I guess I'd better not drink on the night that I go out. If I got sloshed, I don't think I'd go out.

CLINICIAN: That's a good point, Joe. Maybe you could pick some nights to go out and meet some people, and on those nights you could avoid drinking. What do you think of that idea?

JOE: I'll give it a try.

As exemplified in the use of the Socratic method to help clients break down large goals into smaller ones, and to evaluate the role of substance abuse in interfering with the attainment of personal goals, the clinician strives to avoid arguing with the client at all costs. Arguments invariably undermine the success of motivational interviewing, and tend to strengthen rather than weaken a client's beliefs. In order to develop discrepancy successfully, the clinician needs to work collaboratively with the client, rather than in opposition. Such collaborative work is necessary in order to create a situation in which the client argues with him- or herself, allowing dissonance to emerge.

The aim of developing discrepancy, and strategies for achieving this aim, are summarized in Table 7.4.

Rolling with Resistance

The Aim of Rolling with Resistance

Developing discrepancy between substance use and desired goals naturally leads to contemplating the implications of behavior change. Even when clients identify important goals and demonstrate an awareness that their substance use interferes with achieving those goals, they often resist change. In order to maintain a dialogue with a client that addresses problems related to substance abuse, the clinician must be able to "roll with" the client's resistance—that is, to acknowledge and deal with it, while at the same time avoiding direct confrontation. Only in this manner can the resistance be effectively overcome, which is the aim of this step. Although some degree of resistance is natural to all

---

TABLE 7.4. Aim and Strategies for Developing Discrepancy in Motivational Interviewing

Aim: To help the client see that his or her personal goals are inconsistent with current substance abuse behavior, and thus to motivate the client to work on the substance abuse.

Clinical Strategies:
- Use the Socratic method to help the client reach his or her own conclusions.
- Break large, long-term goals into smaller, more manageable steps.
- Use questions to explore with the client how substance abuse may interfere with achieving personal goals.
- Avoid direct argumentation.

change, Miller and Rollnick (2002) point out that significant resistance is an important signal that the client is not yet ready for change, and that more groundwork is needed before true change can be undertaken. Some of the same skills involved in developing discrepancy and avoiding argumentation are employed in dealing with resistance to change in substance abuse, such as the Socratic method. Additional strategies for rolling with resistance are described below.

Strategies for Rolling with Resistance

It is important for clinicians to recognize that resistance to change is a normal and natural part of the change process, and should not be overpathologized. Any individual contemplating a significant change in his or her life wavers back and forth in the process of deciding whether to act. Part of the indecision is due to the fact that changes, by their very nature, involve entering into unfamiliar territory and giving up what is known and predictable. People often cling to what they know largely because it is familiar, despite tremendous costs of maintaining the status quo. This is often the case with clients with dual disorders, who experience a multitude of negative consequences related to their substance abuse, but are afraid of what life will be like without the comforts and routine of their alcohol and drug use habits.

Rather than directly opposing or confronting a client's normal resistance to change, it is preferable to explore it in order to fully understand the basis for the client's concerns. Exploring resistance involves asking the client about how he or she views the change process, and eliciting concerns about potential consequences. Clients may want to change their own substance use behavior, but resist actual change because of concerns about achieving sobriety. In order to address these concerns, the clinician needs to evaluate with the client the possible changes associated with achieving sobriety, especially the perceived costs. The functional analysis of substance use behavior (Chapter 5), in which the possible disadvantages of sobriety are identified, may provide clues to the costs of giving up substances—and thus to possible sources of resistance. This discussion can then lead to the identification of strategies for minimizing or managing these costs.

Clients may be concerned that if they stop using substances they will have no outlets for leisure and recreation; that they will not be able to handle social situations involving substance use; that they will have trouble sleeping, dealing with anxiety, or handling depression; or that they will not be able to handle the stress and strain associated with assuming new responsibilities, such as work, a closer relationship with someone, or more independent living. In order to overcome

resistance to change, a clinician needs to identify a client's specific concerns and to problem-solve how these concerns may be addressed. This approach acknowledges that making significant changes is a difficult process, but that it can be facilitated by an open, matter-of-fact discussion.

Ambivalence is a fundamental part of change. Clients become attached to their substance use habits (Miller & Rollnick, 2002), and despite awareness of the high costs of these habits, they may be afraid to give them up. Although clients have some awareness of both sides of change, they may veer away from change, especially if clinicians adopt the role of advocating for change. A useful alternative is for a clinician to discuss some of the advantages of a client's *not* changing, which can lead the client to assume the other position and own the side that represents change. Consider this example:

CLIENT: I'm all mixed up. Sometimes I think I want to change, and then again I don't.

CLINICIAN: It seems like there are some pretty strong reasons for not changing your drinking right now. It's a good way of getting together with your friends, and it's something to do. And it's dependable.

CLIENT: Yes, that's right.

CLINICIAN: Drinking is actually a pretty positive force in your life.

CLIENT: Well, it is, but there are the problems too!

CLINICIAN: Problems? Like what?

CLIENT: I get into fights with my family. I miss appointments. I run out of money at the end of the month. . . .

Several other approaches to overcoming or sidestepping resistance are identified by Miller and Rollnick (2002). With *simple reflective listening*, the clinician demonstrates that he or she is listening by paraphrasing back to the client what has been said, as in establishing empathy. With *amplified reflection*, the clinician reflects back what the client said, but exaggerates part of the communication. This amplification, if not grossly overdone, can help the client see the other side of what he or she is saying—as in this example:

CLIENT: I really enjoy the feeling of getting high. I don't know if I could give it up. But it's interfering with my trying to go back to school.

CLINICIAN: Getting high is very important to you, and you don't think you could give it up.

CLIENT: I do like the feeling. I've given up smoking pot a few times before, but I kept coming back to it.

CLINICIAN: You've tried to quit before, and you're pretty sure you won't be able to quit, even if you want to.

CLIENT: I do want to stop.

CLINICIAN: But you know you can't.

CLIENT: Maybe I can. Maybe this time will be different.

CLINICIAN: Should we see if there's a way of making this effort even more successful?

CLIENT: Sure.

The aim of rolling with resistance, and strategies for achieving that aim, are summarized in Table 7.5.

Supporting Self-Efficacy

The Aim of Supporting Self-Efficacy

Once clients have begun to understand that their substance abuse interferes with their goals, and their concerns about change have been addressed, they still need to muster the energy required to set the change process in motion. This requires the fostering of hope, which is the aim of this last step in motivational interviewing. When clients are on the brink of making substantial changes in their lives, the belief that such changes are possible and attainable can be the most critical factor. Because hope provides the psychic fuel that makes change possible, instilling hope is a vital part of the therapeutic process at all stages of treatment.

Strategies for Supporting Self-Efficacy

When contemplating with the client the possibility of change, the clinician should model a confident, upbeat, optimistic attitude. The clinician needs to acknowledge the client's doubts and prior frustrations, while remaining positive about the fact that change is possible and is within the client's reach. Recognizing past difficulties,

---

TABLE 7.5. Aim and Strategies for Rolling with Resistance in Motivational Interviewing

Goal: To overcome the client's resistance to change in substance abuse behavior, by acknowledging and dealing with it but avoiding direct confrontation.

Clinical Strategies:
- Don't overpathologize resistance—it's normal.
- Rather than opposing resistance, explore it.
- Identify and problem-solve the client's specific concerns about attaining sobriety.
- Express the disadvantages of change to get the client to own the side of change.
- Use simple reflective listening or amplified reflection.

---

while simultaneously looking toward the future, demonstrates to the client that it is possible to be both optimistic and realistic about the prospects of change.

Self-efficacy for change can be supported by exploring past accomplishments with the client. These accomplishments may predate the onset of the dual disorders, may have occurred more recently, or both. Raising a child, attaining abstinence for a 1-year period, working a job, assuming household responsibilities, getting a general equivalency diploma (GED), maintaining an apartment, adhering to a medication regimen, attending dual-disorder services regularly, or quitting smoking are examples of accomplishments clients may have experienced that clinicians can draw attention to. Helping clients identify their own personal strengths and success stories encourages them to take pride in their accomplishments, and to realize that they are capable of achieving personal goals—even ambitious ones, such as decreasing or stopping substance use. This recognition is key to supporting clients' self-efficacy and instilling the belief that they are capable of successfully changing their behavior.

Some clients with dual disorders have experienced a seemingly endless stream of setbacks, obstacles, and apparent failures. With such an individual, identifying plausible accomplishments can be a daunting task; however, the failure to identify successes is tantamount to conceding to the client's self-perception that he or she is a failure. In work with clients who have experienced such a multitude of hardships, it can be useful to *reframe* the clients' endurance of such hardships as testimony to their personal strength and determination. Reframing provides clients with an alternative way of reconceptualizing their past experiences by transforming them from examples of failure to examples of their personal assets. We provide several examples of reframing common hardships experienced by clients with dual disorders as evidence of their ability to succeed in the face of dire circumstances.

Homelessness is a common consequence of dual disorders (Drake, Wallach, & Hoffman, 1989), and from society's point of view, the inability to keep stable housing for oneself is a sign of dismal failure in one of life's most basic areas. In line with this, clients often view their bouts of homelessness as examples of personal failure. To counter these negative self-perceptions, the experience of coping with homelessness can be reframed as an example of a client's resourcefulness in surviving under harsh circumstances. Being homeless requires basic survival skills, including the ability to find shelter and food, to safeguard one's possessions, and to protect oneself from others. Homelessness also requires certain social skills, such as the ability to negotiate for temporary shelter, to barter, and to deal with numerous strangers. Rather than being viewed as an example of personal failure, homelessness can instead be reframed as a challenging life experience that the client has met, successfully managed, and at times overcome.

Suicidal thinking and suicide attempts are unfortunately common in clients with dual disorders (Bartels et al., 1992). The struggle with the meaning of life, the temptation to end it all, and unsuccessful suicide attempts are often viewed by clients as potent examples of their personal failures. However, like homelessness, clients' struggles with significant suicidality can be reframed as evidence for their personal strength and fortitude. Individuals with suicidal thoughts and attempts frequently cope with these urges on a day-to-day basis, resisting the impulse to hurt themselves on repeated occasions. When a suicide attempt does occur, it is often only after strenuous efforts to resist ideas of self-injury. Rather than looking at such struggles as signs of their failures, clients can reframe these experiences as successful battles they have waged against their own self-destructive impulses. Even clients who have made serious attempts to end their own lives can be helped to reconceptualize these experiences as examples of a drive to live that is stronger than any conscious attempts to end life. Such personal strength is an example of an ability to overcome great odds. This ability can be harnessed to work in earnest on the problem of substance abuse.

There are many other examples of difficult circumstances that clients with dual disorders manage or overcome. Dealing with persistent psychotic symptoms, such as chronic auditory hallucinations; surviving childhood and adult traumas, such as sexual and physical abuse; experiencing severe poverty or deprivation; and spending time in jail are all common challenges in clients' lives that can be reframed as examples of the clients' personal strengths and resourcefulness. Reframing is extremely useful, because it can help a client view any difficult life circumstance in a positive light, and thus can create hope that change is possible. To put it another way, reframing can help clients by instilling the belief that "that which doesn't kill me makes me stronger."

The aim and strategies for supporting self-efficacy are summarized in Table 7.6.

MOTIVATIONAL INTERVIEWING IN GROUP AND FAMILY WORK

The focus of this chapter has been on motivational interviewing in individual counseling. However, the same principles of motivational interviewing described above can also be applied in group- and family-based interven-

---

TABLE 7.6. Aim and Strategies for Supporting Self-Efficacy in Motivational Interviewing

Aim: To foster hope in the client that he or she can achieve desired changes.

Clinical Strategies:
- Express optimism that change is possible.
- Review examples of the client's achievements in other areas.
- Reframe prior "failures" as examples of the client's personal strengths in coping with such problems as:
  - Homelessness
  - Suicidality
  - Persistent psychotic symptoms
  - Time in jail
- Use reflective listening.
- Acknowledge past frustrations, while remaining positive about the prospects of change.

---

tions. We briefly highlight the relevance of motivational interviewing to group and family interventions for dual disorders, which are described later in this book.

Group Intervention

Motivational interviewing techniques play a prominent role in persuasion groups (Chapter 9). These groups are aimed at helping clients understand the impact of substance abuse on their lives by creating an environment conducive to the sharing of personal experiences related to substance use, including both positive and negative experiences. As clients discuss their experiences, the group leaders strive to foster an open, honest exchange of stories and viewpoints; encourage group members to validate each other's experiences; and step in when necessary to block criticism, judgment, and strong confrontation. These strategies parallel the expression of empathy in motivational interviewing.

During the course of persuasion groups, the leaders are alert to clients' expression of personal goals. Although eliciting personal ambitions in persuasion groups is not an explicit goal, it frequently happens. When goals are identified, it provides an opportunity for the leaders to explore the possible interactions between the clients' substance use and the steps necessary to achieve those goals. This exploration can result in the clients' beginning to perceive a discrepancy between attaining their goals and continuing to use substances, leading to motivation to address the problem of substance abuse. In line with the principles of motivational interviewing, the leaders avoid direct confrontation when developing discrepancy, and use a combination of the Socratic method and involvement of other group members to help clients evaluate whether their substance use interferes with their personal goals or values.

Finally, persuasion groups provide valuable role-modeling opportunities for clients who express interest in changing their substance abuse, but who nevertheless resist change or feel hopeless that change is possible. Persuasion groups typically include clients who are in either the persuasion stage or the active treatment stage, and occasionally clients who are in the relapse prevention stage. The participation of clients who have succeeded in reducing their substance use and achieving abstinence (i.e., clients in the active treatment and relapse prevention stages) provides clients in the persuasion stage, who are struggling with the prospect of change, with positive role models showing that change is possible. Clients who still believe that change is not possible can be confronted by clients in later stages of treatment, who can convincingly argue that because they succeeded in changing, others can too. Ultimately, such confrontation works to support clients' self-efficacy in regard to reducing their substance abuse, should they desire to do so.

Active treatment groups are aimed at helping clients who are motivated to work on their substance abuse reduce use and/or achieve stable abstinence (Chapter 10). As clients in the active stage of treatment are by definition motivated to work on substance abuse, there is no need to develop discrepancy between their goals and substance abuse. However, relapses of substance abuse occur in active treatment, and clients often become frustrated with their progress toward personal goals, leading to ambivalence about change and threats to self-efficacy. As in persuasion groups, the presence in active treatment groups of other clients who have made improvements in substance abuse and progress toward personal goals provides positive role models to struggling clients, resulting in hope and improved self-efficacy concerning their ability to continue making important life changes.

Motivational interviewing techniques can also be employed in social skills training groups (Chapter 11), although the focus of these groups is not directly on developing client motivation to work on substance abuse. Social skills training groups are aimed at improving interpersonal competence, in order to help clients develop rewarding relationships with non-substance-abusing peers and handle common social situations in which substances are abused. For clients in the persuasion stage, skills training is primarily focused on helping them achieve goals related to improving their relationships. In the process of learning skills related to achieving these goals, opportunities spontaneously arise in which a discrepancy can emerge between a client's substance abuse and his or her personal goals or relationships. In addition, the emphasis in social skills training on frequent social reinforcement, gradual shaping of

behavior toward desired goals, and programmed generalization of skills into the community ensures that clients experience numerous successes over the course of training; these further strengthen their belief that change is possible.

Thus motivational interviewing strategies can be used in a group format. Persuasion groups provide numerous opportunities for exploring personal goals, developing discrepancy between goals and substance abuse, overcoming resistance to change, and supporting self-efficacy. Active treatment groups are also appropriate for motivational interviewing, especially for dealing with resistance to change and problems with self-efficacy for clients who have become frustrated with the slow rate of change or frequent setbacks. Social skills training groups provide other opportunities to use motivational interviewing techniques, including developing discrepancy and supporting self-efficacy about clients' ability to achieve important goals as they improve their social competence.

Family Intervention

Similar to group intervention, motivational interviewing techniques can also be applied in family intervention. The most straightforward application of motivational interviewing is in work with families in behavioral family therapy (BFT) as described in Chapter 14. However, motivational interviewing techniques also have applications in multiple-family groups, described in Chapter 15.

In work with families of clients with dual disorders, early contacts focus on providing support and expressing empathy, in order to understand the experiences and perspectives of family members living with or in close contact with the clients. Substance abuse is not given priority during most early contacts with family members, unless they spontaneously express concern and a desire to address substance abuse. With most families, discussions of substance abuse occur after the clinician has developed a thorough understanding of family members' perceived needs.

Psychoeducation is a core ingredient of BFT, and many families are prepared to begin working on the problem of substance abuse after they have been educated about the nature of clients' mental illness, the principles of treatment, and interactions with substance abuse. Clients in these families may progress to the active treatment stage with relatively little time spent in persuasion, and no need to develop discrepancy between goals and substance abuse. However, clients in other families (and sometimes their relatives as well) continue to be unconvinced about the importance of addressing substance abuse even after educational sessions have addressed the interactions between substance abuse and severe mental illness. With these families, a motivational interviewing approach is taken to develop discrepancy, using the method of family problem solving. Individual or family goals are identified as the focus of shared family work. In line with the principles of motivational interviewing, the steps toward achieving the goals are identified, with the clinician prompting family members to explore the possible interference by substance abuse to achieving the goal. When developing discrepancy in a client or relatives, the clinician assumes the role of a facilitator and teacher of the problem-solving method, thereby avoiding argumentation and allowing family members to take responsibility for recognizing the problems posed by substance abuse to achieving valued goals. This application of motivational interviewing is identical to that provided in the individual format, except that it involves family members (including the client).

Finally, family work, in both the persuasion and the active treatment stages, involves helping families overcome their ambivalence about change, and instilling the hope that change can be achieved even after many years of frustration. Just as an individual client needs help in overcoming resistance to change and developing self-efficacy that they are capable of change, so do family members—who have experienced many defeats and frustrations in maintaining a close relationship with a relative with a dual disorder.

Thus motivational interviewing techniques have broad applicability in working with families. The strategies are useful for understanding the concerns of family members, motivating them to examine and address the role of substance abuse in a client's life, and encourag-

ing them that they are capable of change, despite the frustrations they may have experienced.

SUMMARY

This chapter has elucidated the principles of motivational interviewing for clients with dual disorders. Motivational interviewing is a set of strategies designed to help clients understand the impact of substance abuse on their lives, to deal with ambivalence about changing their substance use habits, and to become motivated to address their substance use problems. Because motivational interviewing is primarily aimed at clients with whom clinicians have a working relationship, but who have limited motivation to work on their substance abuse, it is most appropriate for clients in the persuasion or active treatment stages.

The primary aim of motivational interviewing is to help clients understand that their use of substances interferes with their own personal values and goals. Clients' recognizing the impact of substance abuse on their own goals, rather than the goals of others, leads to motivation to change substance abuse behavior because it is seen by the clients as in their own best interest. The motivational interviewing process can be broken down into five steps: expressing empathy, establishing personal goals, developing discrepancy (between substance abuse behavior and achieving desired goals), rolling with resistance, and supporting self-efficacy. Motivational interviewing is often used as an individual intervention. However, the same techniques can also be used in a group format (especially in persuasion groups; see Chapter 9) and in family intervention (especially BFT; see Chapter 14).

8

Cognitive-Behavioral Counseling

Individual substance abuse counseling is a mainstay of treatment for dual disorders, and most clients benefit from a combination of motivational interviewing (Chapter 7) and cognitive-behavioral treatment. This chapter describes how to provide individual *cognitive-behavioral counseling* for clients with dual disorders. We begin with a discussion of the role of such counseling in the stage-wise treatment of dual disorders, with an emphasis on its importance in the later stages of treatment (active treatment and relapse prevention). The remainder of the chapter addresses the specific goals and techniques of cognitive-behavioral counseling at each of the four stages of treatment (engagement, persuasion, active treatment, relapse prevention), and provides clinical examples to illustrate these methods.

THE ROLE OF COGNITIVE-BEHAVIORAL COUNSELING IN DUAL-DISORDER TREATMENT

Cognitive-behavioral counseling is a general approach to helping people overcome problems and make progress toward personal goals. Based on the principles of learning, it is aimed at teaching clients new and more effective skills for improving health, self-care, and self-regulation; anticipating, preparing for, and managing stress; behaving more effectively in social situations; and minimizing or coping with unpleasant thoughts and feelings. Cognitive and behavioral skills are taught with a combination of methods. These include teaching clients how to systematically identify and modify the antecedents and consequences of problematic thoughts, feelings, and behaviors; teaching new skills through demonstration (modeling); having clients rehearse new behaviors

in sessions; assigning homework to practice skills; and providing frequent positive reinforcement (e.g., verbal praise) to strengthen skill acquisition. In short, the focus of cognitive-behavioral counseling is on learning skills for managing problems and achieving goals, not on fostering insight into the nature of one's problems.

Broadly speaking, motivational interviewing can be considered a type of cognitive-behavioral counseling, because it often involves the systematic application of learning principles to help clients develop motivation to change self-destructive behaviors. However, in this book we separate motivational interviewing from other approaches to cognitive-behavioral counseling. The emphasis in motivational interviewing is on helping clients understand how their substance use keeps them from achieving their goals (i.e., insight); it places relatively little emphasis on teaching skills for achieving goals. In actual practice, counseling clients may shift back and forth between motivational interviewing techniques and the cognitive-behavioral strategies discussed in this chapter, resulting in a blend between the two approaches.

Cognitive-behavioral counseling can be incorporated into individual, group (see Chapters 10 and 11), or family (see Chapter 14) formats. We focus in this chapter on individual cognitive-behavioral counseling. Clients with dual disorders frequently complain of difficulty tolerating group settings, particularly in the early stages of treatment. Although individual counseling may not be helpful for all clients, it provides an important alternative (or complement) to group- or family-based interventions for dual disorders. Therefore, the treatment team should be prepared to provide individual cognitive-behavioral counseling alone for some clients or during some phases of treatment, while combining it with such interventions as group intervention, self-help, or family work for other clients. Occasionally, a client may receive only individual counseling throughout the course of treatment if he or she has particular difficulty tolerating other interventions.

Cognitive-behavioral counseling has the great advantage of being highly portable and easily blended with other interventions. In other words, a client who has difficulty making scheduled appointments or committing to regular group attendance may be able to receive individual counseling during a spontaneous drop-in at the treatment center, a home visit, or an emergency contact. Clinicians often combine cognitive-behavioral counseling with case management activities designed to address practical life needs, such as assistance with shopping or activities of daily living (see Chapter 6). Indeed, it blends well with practical life interventions: It often yields data related to the consequences of substance abuse or poor mental illness management in a client's life, and the counseling in these contexts is less threatening because it is less direct.

Cognitive-behavioral counseling can be used with clients with dual disorders to address problems related to either their substance abuse or their psychiatric disorder (Beck, Wright, Newman, & Liese, 1993; Miller & Rollnick, 2002; Monti et al., 2002). There is an enormous clinical and research literature on the cognitive-behavioral treatment of mental illness, with interventions focused on a wide range of different problems (e.g., depression, anxiety disorders, anger, sleep problems, hallucinations, and delusions). Cognitive-behavioral therapy is one of the most effective forms of psychotherapy known. In this chapter, we focus more narrowly on the application of cognitive-behavioral counseling to help clients with dual disorders progress through the stages of substance abuse treatment; we address more briefly its application in treating the symptoms and impairments of psychiatric disorders.

COGNITIVE-BEHAVIORAL COUNSELING AT THE FOUR STAGES OF TREATMENT

As in all treatment approaches for clients with a dual disorder, the aims and specific strategies of cognitive-behavioral counseling depend on clients' motivation to work on their substance abuse and their progress in reducing their use. At the earlier stages of treatment, before clients have developed strong motivation to address substance abuse issues (i.e., the engagement and early persuasion stages), clinicians focus mainly on expressing empathy and using the other steps of motivational interviewing to connect with clients and motivate them to work on their substance abuse; they reserve the use of cognitive-behavioral counseling for helping clients cope more effectively with their psychiatric problems. Changing substance use behaviors is not a major focus of cognitive-behavioral counseling at these stages, because clients are presumed to lack the basic motivation to modify these behaviors.

Cognitive-behavioral counseling has an important role to play later in the persuasion, active treatment, and relapse prevention stages of treatment. At the persuasion stage, when a therapeutic relationship has been established but clients lack strong motivation to work on their substance use problems, cognitive-behavioral counseling can help clients develop more effective skills for getting their coping, social, and recreational needs met, especially in areas related to their motives for using substances (see "Functional Analysis" section in Chapter 5). As clients become more proficient at getting their needs met in ways other than using substances, their reliance on substances decreases, their awareness of the negative effects of substances increases, and along with it their desire to work on these problems.

As the motivation to work on substance abuse develops, and the client progresses into the active treatment stage, cognitive-behavioral counseling focuses directly on substance abuse, including developing and following through on plans for reducing substance use, attaining sobriety, and dealing with cravings and other high-risk situations for using substances. When sustained sobriety has been attained, in the relapse prevention stage, cognitive-behavioral counseling is aimed at bolstering skills for responding to slips in substance use, preventing relapses, and developing a healthier lifestyle.

Information obtained during the five-step assessment process (see Chapters 4 and 5) has direct implications for selecting the targets of cognitive-behavioral counseling, which are informed by a client's stage of treatment. For clients in the engagement and persuasion stages, the functional assessment and functional analysis are useful for specifying the costs of reducing substance use (e.g., increased distress due to symptoms, lack of recreational activities), and cognitive-behavioral counseling can be used to decrease these costs (e.g., teaching strategies for coping with symptoms or developing new recreational activities). For clients in active treatment or relapse prevention, the functional assessment and functional analysis are useful for identifying potential risk factors for substance use or relapse (e.g., increased symptoms, cravings), and cognitive-behavioral counseling can directly address those risk factors. Generally, risk factors for substance use or abuse in the active treatment and relapse prevention stages can be addressed by reducing clients' exposure to such situations (e.g., avoiding situations where substances are used) or increasing clients' ability to resist using substances in those situations (e.g., increasing ability to refuse offers to use, improving ability to cope with symptoms or cravings to use). We describe below the aims and strategies of cognitive-behavioral counseling at each of the four stages of treatment, which are summarized in Table 8.1.

Engagement Stage

In the engagement stage, the clinician focuses on establishing a working alliance built on an open, honest discussion of substance use. Therefore, individual counseling focuses on establishing and reinforcing this behavior. Clinicians create openings for clients to discuss their substance use, and respond with careful reflective listening without judgment or criticism. The goal of cognitive-behavioral counseling in this stage is to alter verbal behavior, not substance use behavior. In other words, the clinician focuses all of his or her efforts on reinforcing clear communication about substance use, without attempting to alter the use itself.

From their past treatment experiences, some clients may expect clinicians to attempt to change their substance use behavior, and they may be defensive initially about discussing their substance use. When a client inquires about the clinician's opinion or expresses his or her own judgment about substance use, the clinician must be careful to emphasize empathy (i.e., "I'm concerned for you") over judgment. Restraint at this stage will pay off in establishing a pattern of honest communication and the client's sense of responsibility and self-direction of treatment down the line.

Environmental cues (e.g., empty beer bottles, drug paraphernalia, or signs of financial distress) may create opportunities to begin discussion of substance use with reluctant clients. A clinician should be careful not to make a client feel as though he or she has been "caught" when these cues are present. On the other hand, the clinician does not want to set the stage for ignoring glaring signs of substance use and abuse. The clinician should leave plenty of room for the client to bring up the subject of substance use. If obvious cues are ignored by the client, the clinician may calmly observe the signs of substance use that are present and give the client the opportunity to go into as much detail as he or she feels comfortable with. This can take several sessions for very resistant clients. When clients are willing to divulge information about their use of substances, the clinician praises their courage in sharing these details to reinforce further discussion. This results in clients' feeling increasingly comfortable talking about their use of substances and about the factors appearing to contribute to it. Consider this example:

CLIENT: You don't understand how difficult it is to cope with all of this.

CLINICIAN: It sounds like it's very difficult.

CLIENT: Sometimes you've got to get high just to get away from it all when things get real bad. It helps me cope. It's better than killing myself or somebody else.

CLINICIAN: It's better than hurting somebody.

CLIENT: I've got a lot to deal with. You just don't understand how bad it gets.

CLINICIAN: I really respect your honesty and courage in sharing that with me. I hope that I can help you to cope as I understand more about what you go through.

TABLE 8.1. Aims and Strategies of Cognitive-Behavioral Counseling for Clients with Dual Disorders

Stage of treatment	Focus	Aim	Strategies
Engagement	Verbal behavior	To increase communication about substance use (or mental illness management)	Express empathy; create openings; selectively reinforce honest communication about substance use (or mental illness management)
Persuasion	Perceptions and motivation	To increase motivation for change in substance use and/or mental illness management	Use motivational interviewing techniques; develop a detailed behavioral analysis; use functional assessment and analysis
Active treatment	Physical behaviors	To reduce substance use and improve mental illness management	Create a behavioral action plan; develop alternative responses to craving; use slips productively by learning from them
Relapse prevention	Risk factors	To reduce risk of relapse	Refine action plan; expand recovery; develop a healthy lifestyle that is inherently reinforcing

The engagement stage may last just a few weeks or many months. Cognitive-behavioral counseling sessions should follow the client's lead during the engagement stage—reinforcing honest discussion about mental illness and substance use, but not directly initiating discussion about these topics. Premature use of persuasion techniques may disrupt the process of developing the trust necessary for open and nonjudgmental communication to occur.

Persuasion Stage

Once the client is comfortable talking with the clinician more openly about substance use, he or she is ready to move on to persuasion-stage counseling. The goal of cognitive-behavioral counseling in this stage is to help the client develop an understanding of the pattern of events surrounding substance use, especially its consequences, and to develop motivation to change substance use behaviors (see Chapter 7). Therefore, counseling sessions focus on an exploration of behavioral, cognitive, and emotional events before, during, and after substance use, along the lines described for conducting the functional assessment and functional analysis (Chapter 5). These discussions also focus on rekindling interests in life goals, identifying barriers to change, and developing hope.

Exploring and understanding the events that lead up to each instance of using substances, and the results of this behavior, aids the clinician in overcoming the temporal reinforcement of substance use by increasing the clients' awareness of the full range of its antecedents and consequences. This helps clients become more comfortable with letting go of substance use. Exploring the potential benefits of reduced substance use increases clients' awareness that changes in substance use lifestyle may result in personally relevant positive outcomes. This process increases the client's motivation for moving toward a healthier lifestyle and developing more effective coping strategies (Prochaska, Norcross, & DiClemente, 1994).

Facilitating Recognition of Substance Abuse's Consequences

The exploration of substance use behavior must be approached with skill. The client may perceive substance use as his or her only solace in a lonely and terrifying existence. Directly challenging the person's use may threaten the working alliance and can lead to dishonesty and deception. It is critical to avoid slipping into attempts to alter behavior before motivation is developed.

By definition, clients with substance use disorders frequently experience adverse consequences of their use. However, a clinician should not rush into trying to convince a client that these adverse events prove the existence of a problem. Instead, more lasting insights are developed by allowing the effects to speak for themselves to the client, and by facilitating an open-ended discussion. Clinicians can increase their credibility with their clients by accepting that some episodes of use may not result in adverse consequences, or that positive consequences as well as negative ones may occur. If an environment of honesty is created, a client is less likely to adopt a superficial bias toward substance use to balance a perceived bias against use by the clinician.

The eventual aim is not only to assist in-session examination of substance use, but also to get clients into the habit of more closely examining the process involved in their use. As clients are encouraged to evaluate such factors as what they think and how they feel before and after using, they are able to continue the work of therapy on their own between regularly scheduled sessions. This extra work may enable the clients to arrive at a better understanding of both the motivating factors and the costs of substance use (i.e., the functional analysis). These insights are all the more valued because they originate with the clients themselves, rather than with their clinicians.

Although direct questioning may be used at times, a clinician needs to get a client to ask the important questions whenever possible. The technique of reflective listening, described in Chapter 7, is very useful in directing the client's attention to certain questions without asking him or her directly. As a client describes the details of a substance use episode, the clinician responds by reflecting on something the client said. For example, even when a client appears disheveled at a counseling session, the clinician lets the client take the lead in beginning the discussion:

CLIENT: I was over at a friend's house, and before I knew it, a party was going on.

CLINICIAN: It sounds like you were having a good time at your friend's house.

CLIENT: Yes, I was. And then somebody broke out some beer. So I had a few beers with my friends.

CLINICIAN: You decided to join your friends for a few beers.

CLIENT: Right. The only trouble was, things got a little out of hand, and I had a few too many.

CLINICIAN: Too many beers?

CLIENT: Yes. I didn't have any trouble going to sleep,

but it was really hard getting up this morning, and I still feel a little groggy.

This technique has several advantages. First, it clearly communicates attentive listening and understanding. Second, it encourages the client to go into further detail by keeping attention on the story. When clinicians prematurely extract some meaning or draw a conclusion, clients are often distracted into responding to the interpretation rather than fleshing out their understanding in further detail. Third, keeping the focus on the client's story and away from the clinician's interpretations reduces the chances that the client will feel judged by the clinician. This facilitates the continued maintenance of an environment of open and honest communication, in which the clinician is genuinely interested in understanding the client's life experience. This often leads to greater trust and makes it possible for the client to reveal ambivalence about using substances, as well as more superficial attitudes toward it. Finally, as the motivational process proceeds, the clinician can use reflective listening to direct attention toward important themes, in line with motivational interviewing (again, see Chapter 7). As the client presents his or her story, the clinician carefully selects specific details and reflects these back in order to increase the client's attention to certain key areas for recovery, including the person's understanding of the effects of substance use on his or her life.

As the exploration of events before and after substance use continues, the client's attention is drawn to events further and further from the actual episodes of use. Most clients are primarily aware of the euphoric and reinforcing aspects of substance use, since these occur closest in time to the use. Clinicians can help clients get a more complete perspective by increasing their awareness of withdrawal symptoms (if any) and cravings prior to substance use, as well as hangovers, insomnia, anxiety, dysphoric moods, and exacerbations of psychiatric symptoms that may occur many hours or days after use of the substance has ceased. Many clients confuse withdrawal symptoms with symptoms of their mental illness, and believe that their substance of choice quiets their mental illness by relieving this withdrawal. Clients may also believe that the exacerbation of their symptoms caused by substance use actually represents their baseline level of symptoms, because their deterioration to this level may have been gradual. If, for example, a client can be helped to discover that his or her psychiatric medication dosage has been increased in order to compensate for substance-induced symptom exacerbations, this may represent an important, tangible adverse consequence of substance use.

Exploring Potential Benefits of Not Using Substances

During the persuasion stage of treatment, a counselor also tries to reduce a client's ambivalence about a substance-free lifestyle as part of the motivational development process (Prochaska et al., 1994). This is achieved through helping the client focus on life goals that may be incompatible with substance use (see Chapter 7). As a desire to achieve successful work, improved relationships, heightened athletic performance, or better health is developed, it becomes clear that the client's success in achieving these goals will hinge on investment in self-care and independence. Negotiating life with a severe mental illness is hard enough without substance use to complicate matters. A clinician can highlight these advantages of sobriety when opportunities present themselves—for instance, transporting a client to a local food bank to pick up food:

CLIENT: I need $15 for a haircut.

CLINICIAN: Have you run out of the money your payee gave you on Monday?

CLIENT: Yeah. I had to pay back some money I borrowed and buy cigarettes, so I'm all out. I'm sick of having a payee. I wish you people would let me have my own money.

CLINICIAN: I wish you could have your own money, because it's a hassle for me, too. I think you could manage it responsibly if it weren't for using substances. The Social Security Administration requires that disability payments go to meet your basic needs. I look forward to the day when we can tell them that you don't need a payee any more.

CLIENT: You can tell them that now, as far as I'm concerned.

CLINICIAN: Well, actually, it *is* under your control. All we do is report the truth; when your behaviors show that you can use your disability payments to support your basic needs, we are obligated to let Social Security know. Besides, that's exactly what we want to see happen. It will be a sign of success when you can manage your own money, and a whole lot less work for us, too.

A critical step in exploring the benefits of not using is the identification of previous interests, skills, and accomplishments. A survey of the client's activities in childhood and young adulthood prior to the onset of dual disorders may reveal athletic or artistic interests, as well as educational or work achievements. Assisting the client to sample these activities again can be very helpful in rekindling interest. Clients may also find that their performance or concentration is limited by substance use, and they may thus gain motivation to improve their physical and mental health. Clients who do not have a history of engaging in currently accessible recreational or academic activities can be assisted in sampling alternatives. Developing specific and detailed plans—including time lines and follow-up review dates, rehearsal of any difficult parts, and tracking of clients' involvement and enjoyment—can help.

Hopelessness is a major contributor to lack of motivation for change. When clients feel no hope for the future, it is logical to engage in behaviors that give them short-term pleasure or relief, even when they result in long-term deterioration. During the process of exploring abilities, hopes, and dreams, it is critical to focus on the development of hope for a better life. This can be done by describing treatment successes, introducing the client to peers who have achieved successful recovery, and helping the client to achieve small successes (e.g., decent housing or paid part-time employment).

As described in more detail in Chapter 7, it is important never to denigrate even the most grandiose goals that clients present. Clients are developing dreams and aspirations here. A portrait of each client emerges in the personal goals he or she sets—a portrait that may differ substantially from the client's present circumstances. The clinician assists the client in exploring this fully and identifying the steps toward achieving his or her goals. The latter process introduces realism and allows the clinician the opportunity to guide the client in identifying barriers to achieving goals.

A "can do" attitude toward life goals is important in the clinician during this work. Clients can be energized by their clinicians' belief in them and an attitude that all problems can be solved if broken down into small enough parts. When a clinician is also a client's case manager (as is often the case), he or she can directly link progress in individual cognitive-behavioral counseling to practical life interventions that help the client to achieve a series of successful steps toward personal goals over time. This process builds hope and motivation further.

Some clients overtly identify their substance use or poor management of their mental illness as a barrier to progress, and set goals to change these behaviors as part of the steps toward achieving their life goals. The development of motivation is more subtle in many other clients, however. They may feel too ashamed or defeated to make a specific statement of motivation for change. Instead, as they become progressively energized about work, relationships, and recreational activities, they may start to let go of their attachment to substance use. They may start to develop a pattern of reduced substance use

as its consequences interfere with their developing recovery process. The clinician should not force such a client to "say uncle," but rather should help him or her to appreciate the gradual progress made toward goals and to celebrate these successes. This process will reinforce the client's developing self-esteem and self-efficacy, as well as the developing belief in his or her own potential to achieve a life defined though roles and relationships rather than through illness and disability.

CASE EXAMPLE

Greg was a 36-year-old man with schizophrenia and alcohol abuse. For 6 months he had been working with his case manager, Tom, whom he had been seeing regularly. At Greg's request Tom had helped him obtain a 6-hour-per-week job at a local recycling center. On Mondays, Wednesdays, and Fridays from 10:00 A.M. to 12 noon, Greg worked at the center. He was having trouble making it to work on time, and his boss was considering firing him. Tom and Greg discussed the problem, and Tom asked Greg what his drinking had been like since he started work. Greg said he was drinking three to four beers nightly to relax. Tom suggested that on nights before Greg was to work, he try cutting down to one beer and see whether that made it easier to get up on time. Greg agreed to give it a try; he found that cutting down did make it easier to get up, and he was able to maintain his job.

Active Treatment Stage

Once clients have developed sustained motivation for a lifestyle change, they are ready to move into active treatment counseling. In the active treatment stage, the goal of cognitive-behavioral counseling is to teach a client the skills necessary for reducing substance use and achieving abstinence (if desired), combined with better illness management. The clinician (and the case manager, if this is someone else) review the information generated from the detailed behavioral analysis conducted during the assessment process (functional assessment and functional analysis; see Chapter 5), which is refined in the persuasion stage of cognitive-behavioral counseling (see the preceding section). This information is then used to create a *behavioral action plan* with the client. (Similar plans may be constructed to increase illness management, but we do not emphasize them here.) Individual targets in the biological, psychological, cognitive, interpersonal, and environmental arenas are all addressed in this plan. The clinician works collaboratively with the client to identify reinforcers of substance use, to develop a specific plan for change, and to practice aspects of the plan that would benefit from behavioral rehearsal.

Clients may set goals in active treatment that do not fully address all of their needs. For example, a client may choose to continue using one substance (e.g., alcohol) while becoming abstinent from others (e.g., cannabis), or attempt to control use of a substance that he or she is currently dependent upon (e.g., to limit drinking to one or two drinks per day, or to use cannabis only on weekends). Clinicians should avoid criticizing clients for setting goals of "controlled use," despite the relatively small chances of such goal's being fully realized.

In our experience of treating dual disorders, we have observed that recovery from substance use disorders is often a gradual process, with reduction in substance use often preceding abstinence, and some clients succeeding in continuing to use substances without apparent untoward effects. Making any steps in the right direction helps a client to build motivation for developing a broader recovery over time. Therefore, the clinician helps the client identify the risks and benefits of a particular behavioral action plan, and fully supports the client in pursuing the goals established in the plan, even when they represent only partial steps in the right direction. Once a client has achieved a partial success and reaped some personally relevant benefits, it usually becomes easier to take further steps. This is consistent with the process of breaking down goals into smaller, more manageable steps.

Once the client has set goals, the behavioral action plan can be created. Such a plan has three components: *attaining the action goal* (sobriety, reduced use, or medication compliance), *managing craving*, and *managing slips*.

Attaining the Action Goal

In order to establish a behavioral action plan, the clinician helps the client identify the range of reinforcers of substance use behavior and works collaboratively to develop strategies to address each one. Specific reinforcers are identified in the process of conducting the functional assessment and functional analysis, as described in Chapter 5 and summarized in the client's Payoff Matrix. For example, a client with substance dependence whose active treatment goal is to achieve sobriety may need to address withdrawal symptoms, anxiety, insomnia, low self-esteem, and a substance-using social network, all of which have contributed to the pattern of substance use. The clinician can assist the client in identifying alternative strategies for managing each of these issues and choosing the level of change he or she is prepared to commit to at this time. Table 8.2 identifies typical strategies for addressing common problems that interfere with reducing substance use. Additional strategies can be identified by consulting the vast clinical

and research literature on cognitive-behavioral treatment of psychiatric disorders and symptoms.

Writing a behavioral action plan with the client helps diminish ambiguity, increase confidence, and clarify responsibilities. At a minimum, such a plan should include a start date; a clear action goal; a detoxification plan (if necessary); specific steps to be taken by the client, clinician, and collateral supporters; and a review date. The start date should give the client enough time to get prepared for the work ahead and to inform peers, family members, and other supportive persons of his or her plans. The review date specifies when the plan will be reviewed and revised. If problems arise or a slip occurs, the plan may be reviewed sooner.

It is important to strike a balance between encouraging the client to follow through with his or her plan and viewing the plan as a work in progress that requires continual updating and improvement in order to remain relevant. The client and significant other participants should all have their own copies of the plan. A typical behavioral action plan might include a detoxification period, medication adjustments, increased structured activities, increased family and social support, and enrolling in an active treatment group (Chapter 10). A sample behavioral action plan is provided in Figure 8.1.

Initially, clients may not be prepared to commit to changes that would be most likely to support their sobriety, such as altering their environment or their social network. For clients to retain ownership of their behavioral action plans, it is important for them to make the final choice of steps they are committed to follow through on, after a careful appraisal of the probability of success. A plan is continually refined over time as weak links are identified. It is generally more productive for clients to learn from experience that they need to take further steps in disengaging from a social network in order to achieve success, rather than to be coerced into agreeing to plans that they are not prepared to carry out. If a clinician keeps a client focused on maintaining motivation for his or her action goal, the steps to success will flow naturally from roadblocks as these are identified.

The following case example illustrates how developing and following through on a behavioral action plan is an ongoing process, in which the clinician collaborates with the client in formulating and implementing the plan, and then evaluates and troubleshoots the plan after the client has made some attempts to implement it.

CASE EXAMPLE

When José and his clinician, Peter, developed a behavioral action plan for José's decision to stop smoking crack, they identified hopelessness, depression, a desire to fit in, and having money as reinforcers or triggers of cocaine use for

TABLE 8.2. Typical Strategies for Addressing Common Problems That Interfere with Reducing Substance Use

Problem	Strategies
Withdrawal symptoms	• Inpatient detoxification • Outpatient detoxification • Social support • Improved hydration and nutrition
Insomnia	• Sleep hygiene techniques • Adequate housing • Adequate bedding • Medication adjustment • Sleep cycle adjustment
Anxiety	• Behavioral relaxation techniques (e.g., breathing retraining) • Gradual exposure to feared thoughts/situations • Training in basic yoga techniques, or referral to a class • Medication adjustment • Adequate treatment for underlying psychosis • Cognitive restructuring • Cognitive-behavioral therapy for social anxiety
Depression	• Medication adjustment • Scheduling pleasant activities • Cognitive-behavioral therapy for depression • Interpersonal psychotherapy • Self-help books about depression • Family/couple treatment to address relationship problems
Poor social skills	• Social skills training • Social network development
Limited social network	• Joining a YMCA or health club • Joining a hobby-based group (e.g., reading group at library) • Joining a social organization (e.g., Lions' Club, Rotary Club) • Joining a church • Joining a self-help group (e.g., Alcoholics Anonymous, Dual Recovery Anonymous) • Integrated competitive employment • Getting involved in a consumer advocacy organization
Boredom	• Getting a job • Starting a hobby (e.g., stamp collecting, reading) • Exercising daily (e.g., walking) • Taking a class • Learning to use a computer • Surfing the Internet • Volunteering • Establishing a schedule
Hallucinations	• Medication adjustment • Coping strategies (distraction, relaxation, self-talk) • Cognitive-behavioral therapy for psychosis

Action plan for: <u>John Doe</u>   Clinician: <u>Stacey</u>
Start date: <u>9/15/02</u>   Review date: <u>11/15/02</u>

Action goal: To stop smoking marijuana   Responsible Person(s):
Detox plan: • 3–5 days in respite bed
                          • 28 days at home   John
                          • Log of withdrawal symptoms   Dr. Smith
                          • Medication for insomnia/anxiety if needed

Reinforcers: Anxiety, boredom, "everyone I know smokes marijuana"

Sobriety Plan:
1. John will not purchase marijuana.
   • John will avoid drug dealers.   John
   • John's mother will hold his money and take him shopping for groceries. Mrs. Doe

2. John will decline offers to smoke marijuana.
   • John will practice drug refusal skills.   John and Stacey
   • He will avoid peers who smoke marijuana.   John
   • He will say "no" and leave if offered marijuana.   John
   • He will find a new apartment away from drug users and dealers.   John and Stacey

3. John will manage anxiety better.
   • John will get relaxation skills training.   John and Stacey
   • Medication will be adjusted as needed.   Dr. Smith
   • John will register for yoga class at YMCA and attend weekly with his mother. John and Mrs. Doe
   • He will take a walk every day and enjoy the outdoors.   John (Stacey will go with John
                                                                          for the first week)

4. John will get support for staying sober.
   • John will attend active treatment dual-disorder group weekly.   John and group leader (Stacey
                                                                          will provide ride first 4 weeks)
   • He will go to a movie and dinner with his mother every Saturday if sober the week before. John and Mrs. Doe
   • He will attend NA once a week with Stacey to see if he likes it.   John and Stacey

5. John will fill his time with constructive things to do.
   • John will increase his work hours.   John and his boss
   • He will meet with Stacey on Monday, Wednesday, and Friday at 10 A.M. John and Stacey
   • He will keep a schedule.   John
   • He will go to the library with his mother and pick out things to read every 2 weeks. John and Mrs. Doe

6. John will develop friends who don't use marijuana.
   • John will learn social skills in social skills training group.   John and group leader
   • He will practice starting a conversation.   John and Stacey
   • He will attend the chess club at the community center.   John

FIGURE 8.1. Sample behavioral action plan.

José. José's initial behavioral action plan included a brief hospitalization to detoxify himself and stabilize his suicidality; participation in a dual-disorders active treatment group (Chapter 10); medication adjustment to treat depressive symptoms (Chapter 19); and a payeeship to manage his disability payments (Chapter 17). José also found a job and began to work part-time (Chapter 18). José did not want to give up his social network, however, feeling that he could say "no" to offers to use even if his friends were using. Peter helped José to think carefully through the risks associated with being around people who are using substances, and to recall how hard it had been for José to say "no" in the past.

José reduced contact with his peers for a few weeks, but began to spend more time with them thereafter. He proudly reported his ability to say "no" to offers to use, and reluctantly participated in role-playing refusal skills with Peter (Chapter 11), feeling that he did not need to practice. Then José had a relapse during which he used cocaine with friends at a party, and then engaged in high-risk sexual behaviors in order to obtain more cocaine. As they reviewed the events leading up to his relapse, José recognized that when he was feeling hopeless and depressed, his exposure to friends who used cocaine served as a powerful trigger for him to use cocaine. The problem wasn't that José couldn't say "no" to his friends' offers to smoke crack when he was feeling down; the problem was that José didn't want to say "no" when he felt bad about himself, and was looking for solace and approval from others. José now decided that he had to avoid his cocaine-using peers, because he did not want to jeopardize his new job, and he was also worried about acquiring HIV infection. José and Peter modified his behavioral action plan to include development of new friendships with coworkers, including improved social skills for making friends with people who did not use substances.

Managing Cravings

The second step in active treatment is establishing a plan for managing cravings for substances. Cravings tend to come in waves that peak and then diminish within 5–10 minutes if substances are not used. Cravings diminish with the duration of abstinence, but strengthen after using.

One helpful strategy for managing cravings is to encourage clients to create a written list of behaviors that they can engage in to soothe themselves and pass time until the cravings subside. Clients with severe substance dependence have difficulty identifying and selecting alternative behaviors in the midst of cravings. Identifying suitable alternative behaviors in advance, and making a list of them that can be carried wherever a client goes, can help the client remain focused on his or her sobriety goal and avoid giving in to cravings when they occur. Actual role playing of the experience of having a craving, followed by consulting the list of alternative behaviors and selecting and engaging in a behavior, can further increase the client's resolve and ability to follow through on the behavioral action plan. Involving significant others in the plan for managing cravings can further increase the likelihood that this component will be implemented successfully. Common alternative behaviors for the management of cravings are included in Table 8.3.

The clinician should collaborate closely with the client to evaluate the effectiveness of the managing-cravings component of the behavioral action plan, and to help and support the client in using the list of alternative behaviors. New alternatives can be added to the list if needed, as the client discovers what does and does not work. With time, experience, and support, the client will be able to identify and develop expertise in using an effective set of alternative behaviors for managing his or her cravings.

Managing Slips

Finally, the client and clinician should anticipate slips of substance use. A *slip* refers to substance use by a client who has been abstinent. The slip may be very brief (even as little as a single drink or puff of marijuana), and may be associated with few or no negative consequences. We distinguish a *slip* from a *relapse:* A slip is a minor return to substance use or abuse, whereas a relapse is a more substantial setback involving more prolonged substance abuse and more severe negative consequences. It is more difficult to define a slip in a client who chooses to continue using small amounts of substances, and who is able to avoid negative consequences due to minimal use. For such individuals, a slip can be conceptualized as an increase in the amount of a substance used, or the experience of negative consequences related to use.

Slips are common in active treatment. In dealing with a slip, the clinician wants to strike a balance between preventing discouragement by normalizing slips on the one hand, and maintaining high expectations for success in sobriety on the other. Slips into substance use are never viewed as "failures," but rather as opportunities to learn how to improve the behavioral action plan.

When the clinician is developing a plan for managing slips, highest priority is given to maintaining an open, honest relationship by encouraging the client to describe any slips as soon as possible. The clinician conducts a careful evaluation with the client of the events before, during, and after substance use, gathering all the available information about what may have contributed to the slip and what might reinforce ongoing use. The clinician and client then return to the behavioral action plan and refine it based on the information gained.

Slips often occur soon after a client has achieved a brief period of abstinence, and modifying the behavioral action plan as soon as possible is important for maintaining the client's motivation and prolonging the period of abstinence. Significant others can play an important role in helping clients follow though on their behavioral action plans (see Chapters 13–15). In the following case example, the clinician and client responded to a slip by deciding to involve the client's husband more in her sobriety plan.

CASE EXAMPLE

Mary had cut down significantly on her use of alcohol and drugs, and had achieved abstinence for the past 10 days.

TABLE 8.3. Examples of Alternative Behaviors for Coping with Cravings

Taking a walk	Seeking verbal support
Deep breathing	Using coping self-statements
Listening to music	Praying
Eating a healthy snack	Watching a movie or video

When meeting with her clinician, she described a situation where she began having severe cravings for alcohol. Mary had a pattern of going to the grocery store and buying scratch lottery tickets instead of food; along with this behavior, she would begin to crave beer and marijuana. Mary and her clinician talked about ways she could handle her cravings. One suggestion was that she not go shopping alone. Her husband was supportive of her not drinking and agreed to shop with Mary. If Mary continued to have cravings even when shopping with her husband, he agreed to do the grocery shopping alone.

As this case illustrates, harnessing positive social relationships can be important in modifying a behavioral action plan in response to a slip. However, relationships can also contribute to slips, and these social contacts need to be addressed in modifying the sobriety plan. For example, if a client has slipped into substance use at the encouragement of old friends, counseling may focus on the social network. Does the client consider these individuals true friends, even though they apparently do not respect the integrity of the client's decisions? Does the client have a problem with his or her self-image as an abstinent individual? Does the client lack the confidence to be proud of attaining abstinence without having to feel strange or different? Does the client lack a well-rehearsed response to offers to use substances? As clients identify the factors that contributed to a slip, they feel less like "failures" and build personal motivation for taking more effective steps to ensure the future success of their action goals. The process of responding to and examining social factors that contribute to a slip, while providing encouragement for progress made, are illustrated in the following dialogue.

The client has been abstinent from marijuana for the past 2 months when he reports a recent slip to his clinician:

CLIENT: I got high last night.

CLINICIAN: You got high?

CLIENT: Yeah. I was with a bunch of my old friends, and they were passing a joint around. I told them I wasn't using, but after a while I got feeling like such a jerk, just sitting there while everyone else was having fun.

CLINICIAN: You felt like a jerk?

CLIENT: Yeah. They must have all thought I was stuck up or trying to prove something by not using.

CLINICIAN: How did you know they were thinking that?

CLIENT: Well, I guess I don't really know what they were thinking, but it seemed kind of strange just sitting there while everyone else was using.

CLINICIAN: Would it be correct, then, to say that you have learned that when you're around other people who are using, it makes you feel awkward and uncomfortable, and that can be a trigger for using?

CLIENT: Yes, I guess that's right.

CLINICIAN: What happened next? How did you get from feeling uncomfortable about not using to actually picking up the joint?

CLIENT: I just kept thinking about how good it feels to get high. At first, I told myself I wasn't going to use, but then I started craving it so bad I could feel it. Then, next thing I knew I was picking it up, not even knowing what I was doing.

CLINICIAN: You felt a craving.

CLIENT: Yeah, my body ached for it. There was no resisting that craving when it got that bad.

CLINICIAN: So, are you saying that when physical craving gets to a certain point, you find yourself unable to resist using?

CLIENT: Yeah.

CLINICIAN: And the craving started after you felt awkward about being the only one who wasn't using.

CLIENT: Yeah.

CLINICIAN: Where do you want to go from here?

CLIENT: I don't want to go back to using. It was awful. I couldn't stop, and I blew all my money.

CLINICIAN: How could we refine your behavioral action plan for keeping sober from what we've learned today?

CLIENT: I can't hang around with those guys any more, and if somebody I'm with starts using, I've just got to get out of there. I thought I'd be okay because they weren't pushing me to use it, and they knew I was trying to get clean. But it didn't work. I just can't be around it.

CLINICIAN: Let's not forget that you put together 2 months of clean time before this slip. Isn't that the longest you've been clean since you started using?

CLIENT: Yes.

CLINICIAN: And you didn't fall back into a full-blown relapse. You were able to recognize where you were headed and get back on target with your goal.

CLIENT: Yes.

CLINICIAN: Do you think you could have done that 6 months ago?

CLIENT: Nope, I guess not.

CLINICIAN: Let's keep focused on building your success and putting together longer and longer periods of sobriety, starting with today. You have done amazing work in getting this far and in learning so much from your slip. Now you have even better tools to work with from here. Let's revise your sobriety plan, and then think about something positive you can do for yourself today to remind you that you've made a lot of progress.

During the active treatment stage, the client and clinician remain narrowly focused on the action goal, as this in itself is usually a substantial challenge. Any factors that interfere with succeeding at the goal are brought into the behavioral action plan to support its success. However, maintaining the focus on achieving the action goal by minimizing other changes helps to avoid distraction; it thus maximizes the chances of success, which will build hope. It is often helpful in this stage to reframe the goal as gaining health rather than decreasing or quitting use of a desired substance. This helps the client make the cognitive shift from viewing the action step as a loss (losing something fun) to viewing it as a gain (gaining better health). The clinician frequently helps the client to recognize the gains he or she has made during progress through the active treatment stage. However, the focus stays on attaining the action goal until the client and the clinician agree that it has been solidly achieved.

Relapse Prevention Stage

In the relapse prevention stage, the work of continually refining the behavioral action plan continues. Slips occur less frequently, and information is gleaned from them if they occur to improve the plan further. In addition, the focus on gaining health, eliminating self-destructive behaviors, and improving illness self-management is expanded. Clients are helped to examine aspects of their lifestyle that may increase their chances of relapses into substance abuse or their psychiatric disorder. Examples of lifestyle problems that can lead to relapse include social isolation, poor physical health, use of other substances (e.g., caffeine and nicotine), medication nonadherence, interpersonal dependency, lack of structured activity, or living in a high-risk environment. Gradually, the client and clinician develop motivation for tackling those issues that leave the client most vulnerable to a relapse. A behavioral action plan is developed around each risky behavior, and the client is assisted in achieving a series of successful lifestyle alterations.

Movement toward recovery guides work in the relapse prevention stage. As described in previous chapters (see especially the "Facilitating Recovery" section of Chapter 6), recovery is the process of movement from a self-concept defined by sick roles and disability to one defined by relationships, life roles, and responsibilities (Deegan, 1988; Fisher, 1992; Frese & Davis, 1997). Recovery also involves a shift in behavior, with illness mastery and community integration replacing dependency and institutionalization (Anthony, 1993; Chamberlin & Rogers, 1990). Recovery is distinct from remission: Remission is defined as relief from symptoms, whereas recovery involves making the most of one's life despite having one or more chronic illnesses.

Clinicians can be helpful in promoting recovery (Noordsy et al., 2000; Torrey & Wyzik, 2000). The principles of facilitating recovery are woven into the clinical approach outlined throughout this book, and cognitive-behavioral counseling can play a vital role in promoting clients' development of the skills necessary to pursue personal life goals. During dual-disorder treatment, there is a focus on hope from the engagement stage onward. Training in life skills begins in the persuasion stage. Encouraging movement beyond excessive dependency on treatment into natural community supports and social networks becomes the focus of the relapse prevention stage.

Therefore, in addition to expanding the breadth of lifestyle interventions, the client and clinician shift the balance of responsibility and authority in their work during the relapse prevention stage. The clinician increasingly refers to the client's experience, rather than his or her own, in resolving issues. Clients are taught to use their increasing experience and developing self-knowledge to answer questions, as well as to use strategies for solving problems. Clients who have not previously been taught the steps of problem solving (defining the problem, brainstorming solutions, evaluating solutions, selecting the best solution, planning for implementation, review, and troubleshooting; see Chapter 14 for more on problem solving) can benefit from training in these steps, which they can use to progress toward recovery goals and deal with obstacles they encounter along the way (D'Zurilla & Nezu, 1999; Nezu & Nezu, 1989).

Now, rather than relying primarily on the team's supports for maintaining sobriety and developing motivation for a new behavioral change, clients look to their family members, friends, and coworkers for some of this support. They increase their reliance on self-help organizations, new social networks, and community-based structured activities (e.g., work). Therefore, the clinician uses cognitive-behavioral counseling in this stage with an eye toward a gentle transition that will eventually make him or her obsolete. As clients move into sustained recovery, they may also find that providing support to others is a powerful way of strengthening their own commitment to a healthier lifestyle (Campbell, 1997; Gartner & Riessman, 1977; Madera, 1988).

Clients with dual disorders may have particularly good long-term outcomes once they achieve recovery from their substance use disorders. Their mental illness symptoms may become much more readily manageable once substance use ceases and lifestyle improvements are made. Many clients with dual disorders have relatively intact cognitive and affective abilities, which are necessary to negotiate the substance-using world. Once they achieve sustained recovery and learned requisite skills, clients in relapse prevention may be able to terminate intensive services and continue maintenance medication treatment with little or no need for cognitive-behavioral or other rehabilitative services.

CASE EXAMPLE

John's father had expressed concern about John's sleeping to the clinician. According to his father, "John has been taking his medications and he hasn't had problems with drugs or alcohol for almost a year, but all he ever does is sleep. Yesterday he got up to take his medications, and then went back to bed and slept until afternoon." The clinician raised this issue with John, after informing him of his discussion with his father.

CLINICIAN: Tell me about your sleep.

CLIENT: Oh, I sleep pretty well.

CLINICIAN: What time do you generally go to sleep?

CLIENT: Usually around 8:00 or 9:00.

CLINICIAN: And when do you get up for the day?

CLIENT: Oh, it depends on if I have anything to do or not. If I've got to be somewhere, I get up around 8:00 or 9:00.

CLINICIAN: And if not?

CLIENT: Oh, well, sometimes I sleep in until 10:00 or 11:00.

CLINICIAN: Do you have any concerns about sleeping so much?

CLIENT: There's nothing to do. Sleeping is better than getting into trouble.

CLINICIAN: What have you learned about having time on your hands?

CLIENT: I guess sitting around with nothing to do can be a trigger for me. That's why I had that slip last year. But sleeping keeps me away from people and keeps me out of trouble.

CLINICIAN: True. What else contributes to your sleeping so much?

CLIENT: I fall asleep right after I take my medication. It makes me tired.

CLINICIAN: Anything else?

CLIENT: I haven't been using my BiPAP machine [for sleep apnea] for a couple of months.

CLINICIAN: And what happens when you don't use it?

CLIENT: I don't know. I guess I don't breathe as good when I sleep.

CLINICIAN: And that may contribute to feeling tired most of the time?

CLIENT: Yeah, I guess so.

CLINICIAN: What are some solutions to feeling sleepy all the time?

CLIENT: I guess I could start wearing the BiPAP machine again.

CLINICIAN: What about your medications?

CLIENT: There's nothing I can do about my medications—I need to take them.

CLINICIAN: If you're having side effects from your medication, what can you do about that?

CLIENT: I guess we could go back in and see the doctor and tell him about it.

CLINICIAN: Exactly. You're the authority on the effects your medication has on you. Dr. Smith can only improve your medication with your input.

CLIENT: Yes, and we should get in to see him.

CLINICIAN: Perhaps later on in this session we could do a role play of what you can say to Dr. Smith?

CLIENT: Okay.

CLINICIAN: I get the sense that this problem is more a concern of your father's and mine than it is your own. What do you stand to gain by sleeping so much?

CLIENT: I don't know. Sleeping keeps me out of trouble.

CLINICIAN: Would it make sense, then, that if you had something else to do to help you stay out of trouble, you wouldn't have to sleep so much?

CLIENT: I think so. I can get up and get going when there is something to do.

CLINICIAN: Yes. We have been working on finding some structured activity that is meaningful for you for a while.

CLIENT: That would be good.

CLINICIAN: I don't think our plans will succeed for very long until you have something to do with your time.

CLIENT: Yes, I guess you're right.

CLINICIAN: Working on structured activities would

help you with reducing your vulnerability to relapses, too.

CLIENT: Yes.

CLINICIAN: Remember that vocational counselor you
met with last year?

CLIENT: Yes, but I only saw him once.

CLINICIAN: Would you be willing to meet with him
again, to get a sense of how he might help you?

CLIENT: Yes, I should probably do that. Things are a lot
different now, and I think I might be ready to work
on that.

CLINICIAN: How about if we practice what you could
say when you meet with him again?

CLIENT: Okay.

SUMMARY

This chapter has outlined the use of cognitive-behavioral substance abuse counseling for people with dual disorders. Cognitive-behavioral counseling is a general approach to psychotherapy that is based on the systematic
application of theories about learning to human problems, with an emphasis on developing new skills and
competencies for overcoming problems and achieving
life goals. Although such counseling has numerous applications in addressing the mental health concerns of
clients with dual disorders, and there is a large clinical
and research literature attesting to its effectiveness for
numerous problems (e.g., reducing depression, anxiety,
anger, psychotic symptoms, improving sleep), the primary focus of this chapter has been on the use of cognitive-behavioral counseling to address substance abuse.

Many of the skills employed in cognitive-behavioral counseling overlap with those used in motivational interviewing (Chapter 7), and counseling often involves
shifting back and forth between or blending the two approaches. In general, however, motivational interviewing is most useful in the earlier stages of dual-disorder
treatment, and cognitive-behavioral substance abuse
counseling is most useful in the later stages. In the engagement and persuasion stages of treatment, cognitive-
behavioral counseling focuses mainly on creating a supportive and reinforcing environment in which substance
use can be discussed, and on conducting an exploration
of the circumstances in which substance use and abuse
occur. Such exploration often leads to motivation to
change substance use behavior.

The most valuable applications of cognitive-behavioral substance abuse counseling are in the active treatment and relapse prevention stages, when clients have
developed a clear motivation to address their substance
use problems, and they have a desire to learn new skills
for accomplishing this. In the active treatment stage,
cognitive-behavioral counseling focuses on helping clients developing behavioral action plans, based on a
careful behavioral analysis of the antecedents and consequences of substance use. These plans are designed to
enable clients to reduce (or stop) using substances; to
identify and avoid "high-risk" situations for relapse; to
respond rapidly to slips, in order to prevent them from
developing into full-blown relapses; to learn from relapses; and to promote a healthier lifestyle. In the relapse prevention stage, behavioral action plans are refined as necessary, with increased attention given to
helping clients develop the skills necessary to pursue
recovery goals, to decrease reliance on treatment, and to
increase self-sufficiency.

IV

Group Interventions

9

Persuasion Groups

Stage-wise treatment groups, including *persuasion groups* (described in this chapter) and *active treatment groups* (described in Chapter 10), are group interventions specifically designed to meet the needs of clients with a dual disorder at these respective stages of treatment. Persuasion groups are aimed at helping clients develop an understanding of how substance use has affected their lives, to become motivated to work on reducing their use of substances, and (if desired) to achieve abstinence. These goals are accomplished by creating an accepting group environment in which clients are free to discuss their experiences with alcohol and drugs without fear of judgment, social censure, or confrontation. Providing a safe haven for clients to talk about some of the positive aspects of their substance use opens the door for an honest exploration of the negative consequences—an exploration that often leads to the emergence or rekindling of interest in working on substance abuse.

In this chapter, we provide the necessary information for clinicians to establish and lead persuasion groups for clients with dual disorders. We begin with a discussion of the role of persuasion groups in integrated dual-disorder treatment, followed by logistical considerations for setting up and conducting these groups. We next discuss therapeutic principles of persuasion group work, guidelines for leading groups, and the structure of group sessions. We end with a discussion of group process, topics for persuasion groups, and curricula-based persuasion groups. A number of educational handouts useful in persuasion groups are included in Appendix B.

THE ROLE OF PERSUASION GROUPS IN DUAL-DISORDER TREATMENT

Substance use and abuse frequently occur in social settings, both in the general population and among persons with severe mental illness. As a consequence, clients receive substantial encouragement and approval from others for continuing to use (Alverson, Alverson, & Drake, 2001). This reinforcement is often a barrier to perceiving the negative effects of substance use and developing a desire to address it. A group psychotherapeutic approach can create an awareness of the effects of substance use on clients' lives, while it also harnesses the potential benefits of social support from peers. As a result, clients can be motivated to reduce substance use. But an awareness of negative effects can only emerge in a group context (i.e., a persuasion group) in which there is total freedom for clients to express their thoughts and feelings about substance use, which can then be facilitated and processed by group leaders.

During treatment planning (Chapter 5), strong consideration should be given to referring all clients who are in the persuasion stage of treatment to persuasion groups, whether or not they are also receiving individual (Part III) and/or family (Part V) psychotherapeutic treatment modalities. Clients in this stage who are participating in social skills training groups (Chapter 11) may also benefit from participation in persuasion groups. Once a clinician has established regular contact with a client, though substance abuse continues to be problematic, the client is in the persuasion stage and can be involved in a persuasion group. In our experience, between 50% and 75% of clients with dual disorders who are in this stage of treatment can eventually be engaged in persuasion groups. Prior to the persuasion stage, a clinician typically lacks the rapport and strength of the therapeutic relationship to encourage a client to participate in a group with a major focus on substance use.

Clients who participate in persuasion groups can benefit from continued participation in such groups even after they move from the persuasion into the active treatment stage—and, for some clients, the relapse prevention stage as well. As clients progress into the later stages of treatment, the benefits they derive from participation in persuasion groups changes. At first, clients benefit most from exploration of their own experiences with substance use, the gradual connection of substance use and long-term adverse outcomes, and the ensuing motivation to change. These clients also receive social support from other clients in the group and from the leaders for examining their own experiences and reconsidering their conclusions about alcohol and drugs. In the later stages of treatment, clients benefit most from being positive role models who are respected by the leader(s) and other members for the progress they have made. They receive social support for maintaining the healthier, substance-free lifestyle they have achieved.

As clients progress beyond the persuasion stage of treatment, they sometimes become frustrated with the focus of a persuasion group on the open-ended exploration of substance use, and begin to feel that it no longer meets their needs. Those clients who are interested in working directly on strategies for reducing their own use or maintaining abstinence, rather than talking about experiences with substance use, should graduate from the persuasion group. These clients may benefit from joining an active treatment group (Chapter 10) or a self-help group (Chapter 12), if either is available.

LOGISTICAL CONSIDERATIONS

In this section, we describe logistical factors related to the setting up and running persuasion groups. For the sake of simplicity, we assume that the typical persuasion group is conducted with outpatients receiving services at a local community mental health center. However, other settings for persuasion groups are possible, such as Department of Veterans Affairs, county, or private mental health clinics; inpatient units (for intermediate or long-stay clients), forensic settings (e.g., jails or prisons); or day treatment programs.

Leadership

Persuasion groups work best with two leaders. It is preferable if one leader has expertise in treating severe mental illness, and the other has expertise in the addictive disorders. Both leaders should be familiar with dual diagnosis, including the major symptoms of mental illnesses and the psychology of addiction. In addition, at least one of the two leaders should be part of a team that provides other treatment services to the agency's clients with dual disorders, or should have close linkages to these teams.

Integration of Group Treatment with Other Interventions

If one or both of the group leaders also belong to the treatment team, they will develop considerable knowledge of the clients, their lives, and their treatment outside the group. Such a linkage ensures that group principles will be reinforced in the community through any other psychotherapeutic treatment being provided, including case management (Chapter 6), motivational interviewing (Chapter 7), cognitive-behavioral counseling (Chapter 8), and family interventions (Chapters 13–15). This coordination of treatment also makes it possible for the group leaders to suggest to other team members specific interventions that may benefit a particular client, based on the client's progress during the persuasion group. For example, to help a client who expresses in the group a strong desire to quit using alcohol, but is frustrated by numerous unsuccessful attempts, a leader might facilitate a discussion between the client and his or her doctor about the possible benefits of a pharmacological treatment for alcoholism (e.g., disulfiram, naltrexone, or clozapine; see Chapter 19).

The integration of persuasion groups with other services at the direct provider level also helps ensure that clients do not receive contradictory messages from different clinicians about their dual disorders. This coordination forces clinicians to maintain an open dialogue about each client's current stage of treatment, and to select interventions appropriate to the client's motivational state. Close contact between the persuasion group leaders and other treatment providers also enables the treatment team to remain abreast of the clients' progress in substance abuse treatment, including setbacks, and to modify their interventions accordingly.

Setting

Persuasion groups can be conducted in any setting that is convenient to the clients and leaders. For clients receiving outpatient mental health services, the mental health center, day treatment program, or clinic is usually most convenient. In some circumstances, an alternative setting in the community—such as a YMCA, a local church, a community recreational center, or a group home—may be preferable if it is more accessible to the group participants. Community settings may also be perceived by some clients as less stigmatizing than treatment centers, and thus may be more acceptable. As noted earlier, persuasion groups can also be conducted in psychiatric inpatient settings or in forensic settings. However, as discussed in more detail in Chapter 17, there are natural limitations to persuasion groups conducted in relatively long-term institutional settings, because of the difficulty of establishing a milieu in which clients can talk openly and without fear of recrimination about their ongoing use of substances.

Size

Groups should be large enough to provide a variety of active peers and role models in different stages of recovery. Generally, the group should have at least 4 to 6 active members, and not more than 12. When a small agency is starting to identify clients for stagewise dual-disorder treatment groups, it may be desirable to combine persuasion and active treatment groups into a single group, and to split them later when sufficient numbers of clients have reached the active treatment and relapse prevention stages. Groups larger than 12 clients become unwieldy and reduce reluctant clients' opportunities to participate. When groups become too large, they can be split into several groups meeting at different times to maximize the convenience and frequency of offerings. This can be an opportunity to develop specialized offerings, such as gender-specific, diagnosis-specific, or language-specific groups.

Timing and Frequency of Meetings

Persuasion groups meet weekly, often shortly before or after the weekend, when periods of heavy drug and alcohol use are likely to be fresh in clients' minds. Groups can be scheduled more frequently for special circumstances. For example, conducting persuasion groups two or three times a week can be useful during a stressful period when clients may be at increased vulnerability to heavier substance abuse (e.g., the holiday season), or in settings where more intensive treatment is provided, such as inpatient, forensic, or partial hospital (day treatment) programs.

Duration of Meetings

Short, focused group meetings are most successful. When groups meet for a brief duration, it reduces intensity and enables clients who have limited attention spans to attend. Some groups run 45 to 60 minutes, while others have two 20- to 25-minute sessions separated by a short break. Leaders can meet during the break or after the group session to review the process, plan strategy, and log the group members' progress.

Admission and Attendance

Acknowledging a problem with alcohol or drug use is not a prerequisite for joining the group, as many clients in the persuasion stage lack such insight. Reluctant clients should be encouraged to attend in order to learn more about their mental illness, substance use, and their interactions. Regular attendance should be encouraged and made part of the treatment plan, although clients who attend irregularly may also benefit and should not be turned away. Groups are usually open to clients who only attend on an occasional, drop-in basis, where their future participation is continually encouraged and reinforced.

Motivating Clients

Establishing a persuasion group at a mental health center can take time. Many groups have trouble attracting members at first. It is important to choose a name for the group that will reflect the educational nature of the group (such as "Good Health," "Health Education," or "Feeling Better"), so that members will not get the impression that going to the group represents admitting to a problem with substance use. Often members of the initial persuasion group can be involved in identifying a name for the group after several sessions have been conducted.

In order to facilitate attendance at groups, it can be helpful to serve refreshments, such as coffee, juices, fruit, or other snacks. Scheduling a group field trip or recreational activity can attract new members. Ensuring that the group is extremely supportive to participants during the early sessions also encourages attendance.

Clients can be motivated to participate in persuasion groups by explaining to them that these groups offer people the opportunity to discuss their personal experiences with others—including experiences with alcohol and drugs—in a nonjudgmental, supportive social milieu. Clients are informed that the desire to change substance use behavior is not a requirement to participate in such a group, although if they are interested in reducing use, they may find the group helpful. For a client who is either ambivalent or anxious about participating in the group, a clinician can facilitate his or her attendance by arranging transportation to the group, meeting with the client immediately before or after the group, attending some of the group sessions with the client, or having the client meet with the group leader(s) or other clients to learn more about the group and to get questions and concerns addressed. For some clients, it can be helpful if the clinician schedules events important to them (e.g., receiving medications or a weekly benefit allotment) to coincide with the group. Occasionally, compulsory attendance is arranged as a condition of probation, parole, or hospital discharge.

THERAPEUTIC PRINCIPLES

The stated goal of persuasion groups is to help members learn more about the role that alcohol and drugs play in their lives. As such, persuasion groups are psychoeducational, interactive, and supportive. These flexible groups take a nonjudgmental approach, and capitalize on the members' tendencies to be more open to and influenced by feedback and support from their peers than from treatment providers. Clients expect treatment providers to view their substance use as a problem and not to understand what it is like to manage a mental illness. Peers' assessments are often viewed as more valid and unbiased. Leaders adhere to several therapeutic principles in developing a group process conducive to helping clients understand, and develop the motivation to address, the effects of substance abuse.

Avoidance of Confrontation

Persuasion groups are significantly less confrontational than traditional substance abuse groups. They assume that genuine acceptance of a substance abuse problem occurs over time in the context of peer group support, education, and the experience of ongoing negative consequences from substance use. Since dual-disorder treatment frequently begins before clients become aware of substance abuse problems and before they actively seek help, the early treatment process occurs in a different context from traditional addiction treatment.

Group leaders attempt to facilitate peer interactions and feedback exchange about the members' experiences with alcohol and drug use. The leaders must be fairly active, though, to maintain the group's focus on substance abuse and its interactions with psychiatric illness. An example of avoiding confrontation while facilitating peer interaction on the topic of substance abuse is provided below.

JOE: I haven't been drinking as much as I used to.

LEADER: That's great, Joe. How about smoking pot?

JOE: Yeah, I smoke a few times a week, when it comes around. It doesn't hurt, so I figure, "Why not?"

LEADER: What do you think, Sarah?

SARAH: I stopped drinking a year ago, and I was still smoking pot. That was okay for a while, but then I was doing speed and coke with it, and I ended up in the hospital, so I don't do it any more. They put me on lithium there, and it makes me shake. Do you think that's the right medication for me?

LEADER: Are things better for you now that you're not using drugs?

SARAH: Yes, I'm not so scared.

Facilitation of Peer Interaction

Whenever possible throughout the group, the leaders strive to facilitate peer interaction. Feedback and suggestions from peers seem more legitimate to clients than the "biased" viewpoints of leaders during discussions of substance use, including its benefits and consequences. Group leaders should delay their own comments until other members have had a chance to contribute. An example of facilitating such peer interaction is given below.

LEADER: How was your weekend, Fred?

FRED: Okay. I had a six-pack last night to put me to sleep.

LEADER: How did you sleep?

FRED: Well, I fell asleep—no problem.

LEADER: Okay.

FRED: I woke up around 3:30 with "cotton mouth" and had a few cigarettes. I couldn't get back to sleep, so I just walked around in my apartment and smoked until it was light. (*Pause*)

JUDY: That used to happen to me sometimes when I was drinking. I always felt worse the next day. I don't know why I kept doing it. (*Pause*)

LEADER: How do you feel today, Fred?

FRED: Nerved up.

Low Expectations, but Support for Attendance

Group leaders strive to create an atmosphere of tolerance for individual differences; they have low expectations for active participation in the group, but provide continued support for attendance at the groups. Members who have difficulty tolerating the stimulation of the group may leave early if they feel uncomfortable, making it easier for them to come into the group in the future. Other members may have difficulty talking at all. Leaders occasionally invite them to contribute during the sessions. In general, though, maintaining members' comfort in the group is more important than prompting active participation.

CASE EXAMPLE

One client, Justin, participated regularly in a persuasion group for an extended period of time while almost never actively contributing to the group discussion. After a year in the group, Justin indicated to the members that he had decided he wanted to go on disulfiram to manage his alcoholism, which had continued unabated. One of the group leaders relayed Justin's interest to his treatment team, and he was subsequently given a trial of disulfiram. The trial was successful, and Justin soon progressed to the active treatment stage.

Psychoeducation

Lengthy didactic presentations are avoided, since they almost invariably exceed members' capacity for attention. To stimulate interest and discussion, leaders may occasionally provide relevant brief presentations, films, readings, and exercises. Group leaders are always on the lookout to provide education about substance abuse, mental illness, and their interactions. Psychoeducation may take the form of leading a discussion about a specific topic, or seizing an opportunity to help clients understand their own experiences in terms of their dual disorders. Relevant topics for presentations include the educational handouts in Appendix B and other topics of potential interest to the group participants (see the later section on specific discussion topics and activities).

Leaders may point out that the perceived benefits of substance use are often short-term, while the actual harms are delayed and long-lasting. Clients are usually able to enumerate the short-lasting benefits, since many know that drugs and alcohol can help them fall asleep, put them in a good mood, relieve anxiety, and make them feel good. They readily connect these effects—not the longer-lasting effects—with substance use, because the time elapsed between use and effect is short.

The group members need time, and experience with feedback from the group, to recognize the long-lasting corollaries: Falling asleep right away corresponds with the delayed effects of insomnia and early awakening; the immediate good mood corresponds with the depressive aftereffects; and the relief from anxiety corresponds with the increased anxiety following the episode. Feeling good when using substances has the

longer-term results of poor health and feeling bad. Furthermore, the biological vulnerability that characterizes clients' psychiatric disorders makes them even more susceptible to the effects of substances at much lower amounts than in persons without mental illness (Mueser, Drake, & Wallach, 1998). Members are often able to grasp that they have "sensitive brains" requiring special care.

CASE EXAMPLE

Nate abused alcohol regularly and also suffered from severe anxiety. During a group session, Nate explained that he used alcohol to calm his nerves, and that he found it moderately effective for controlling his anxiety. Upon further questioning, Nate acknowledged that his anxiety was often worse the day after heavy drinking. The leader used this opportunity to elicit other members' experiences, who verified the association between alcohol abuse and worse anxiety the next day. The leader explained to Nate that the temporary improvement in anxiety, followed by a worsening, was the effect of *rebound anxiety*. In other words, substances that tend to relieve anxiety temporarily by slowing activity of the nerve cells often make the anxiety even worse, making the nerve cells hyperactive when they wear off and are no longer in a person's body. Through this education and peer input, Nate realized that alcohol was actually making his anxiety worse in the long run, and he developed motivation to stop drinking.

Use of Motivational Approaches

One important way that clients in persuasion groups develop an interest in decreasing their use of substances is by realizing how it interferes with their goals and values. Leaders always need to be on the lookout for opportunities to use motivational strategies to stimulate clients' awareness of substances' effects on their lives, and to develop hope that change is possible. Motivational interviewing techniques, described in detail in Chapter 7, involve developing in clients a sense of discrepancy between their ongoing use of substances and their achievement of personal goals. When clients perceive this discrepancy as personally relevant, they often become motivated to begin working on their substance abuse. In the context of persuasion groups, the discrepancy can emerge out of either discussions with peers, the leaders, or a combination of both.

Persuasion groups can assist their members in developing their personal goals and hope for achieving them, as well as in recognizing ways that substance use may interfere with achieving these goals. Sessions can focus on life goal development when acute client needs for support after episodes of use are low. Leaders can weave prompts about goal development into weekly discussions. They can also encourage members to consider the effects of substance use on members' goals by posing questions at opportune times. An example of using motivational strategies is provided below.

CARMEN: One of the things that cocaine and alcohol do for me is to help me forget about what a mess my life is. It make me feel good, even if it's only for a short period of time.

BOB: I know what you mean. It's such an escape.

LEADER: Carmen, I'd be interested in knowing what you mean when you talked about making a mess with your life. Could you give us an example of something you're not happy about?

CARMEM: Sure, that's easy. My daughter. She lives with my mother. I wish I could be a real mother for her. I really miss her.

JULIE: That sounds tough, Carmen.

BOB: Yes. My parents were always drinking and fighting, and I missed out on my childhood. It seems like I was raised to drink, and here I am.

LEADER: I agree, Carmen. It sounds like this is something real important to you.

CARMEM: It is. But I feel so stuck sometimes.

LEADER: When you talked about being a "real" mother for your daughter, what did you mean? Could you give us some examples of what would make you a "real" mother for her?

CARMEM: For one thing, I'd be seeing her more often, and really become a part of her life. I miss that now.

BOB: So why don't you see her? Can't you just stop in and see her?

CARMEM: I don't want her to see me when I'm smashed or high. And my mother doesn't like it.

LEADER: So using helps you forget the pain of not being there for your daughter, but it also gets in the way of going to see her when you can?

CARMEM: I guess I need to cut down. Or see her on days I haven't used.

JULIE: You can do it, Carmen. I've started to cut down myself, and I know it can be done.

Patience and Optimism

Leaders sometime find themselves becoming impatient with members who continually use substances week after week, despite clearly negative consequences. The nonjudgmental style of a persuasion group rarely leads members to rapid acceptance of a need for change. Consequently, leaders should be prepared for a process that takes place gradually over time, as members share many episodes of substance use. The experience of participating in groups and watching some members successfully address their substance use eventually gives both clients and leaders a greater sense of hope.

CASE EXAMPLE

Bruce was 24 years old when he came to the community mental health center for treatment, following several years of hospitalization for unremitting psychosis. He was referred to the persuasion group after his case manager became aware of his regular marijuana and alcohol use, and a careful assessment revealed that he met criteria for alcohol dependence and marijuana abuse. In the group, Bruce reported his belief that he had damaged his brain with LSD in adolescence and caused himself to hear voices. He said that drugs were bad for his brain. Bruce regularly stated his intention to stop using marijuana, alcohol, and cigarettes, but always reported using again by the next meeting. He stated that alcohol helped him to fall asleep, and the he used marijuana because it helped him feel more connected with God. His speech was often disorganized and tangential. He usually rocked in his seat during the group, and often asked to leave early when he was unable to dominate the group discussion by talking about his delusions.

The group leaders helped Bruce to communicate more effectively by summarizing his comments for others. Group members explained to him that his marijuana and alcohol use were probably worsening his symptoms, counteracting the beneficial effects of his medication, and leading to the need for higher doses of the medication. Bruce discovered a familial component to his substance abuse when he completed a genogram of relatives with mental illness or addictive disorders as part of a group exercise (discussed later in this chapter).

Over 2 years, Bruce became more comfortable in the group and stayed for longer periods of time, sometimes for an entire session. As he gradually discontinued using marijuana and decreased his alcohol use, group members gave him positive feedback on his improved appearance and social skills. Bruce appreciated the feedback from other members, which further encouraged him to seek a sober lifestyle.

GROUP GUIDELINES

Persuasion group leaders can establish several guidelines (or ground rules) for the group by facilitating discussion among the participants. These guidelines are discussed below.

Confidentiality

Honesty and an open sharing of experiences among group members are essential in order for clients to develop genuine insights into their substance abuse. However, to encourage free discussion, it is important that group members feel secure in disclosing private information about themselves without fear of this disclosure spreading to nonmembers. Therefore, it is helpful to establish in the group the expectation that the sharing of experiences between members is confidential, should be kept within the confines of the group, and should not be discussed with others outside the group.

Leaders should bear in mind that their ability to enforce this rule of confidentiality is limited. Leaders cannot control what group members say to others outside the group, and excluding members for breaking confidentiality would disrupt the group, which would do more harm than good. Rather, discussing confidentiality among group members sensitizes the participants to the importance of respecting the privacy of others by not divulging information about them to nonmembers. Violations of confidentiality should be discussed in the group, and peer pressure should be developed to reduce the likelihood of further breeches.

Alcohol and Drug Use

In contrast to the policies of most groups for substance abuse, clients who present to a persuasion group session under the influence of alcohol or drugs are usually *not* automatically excluded from participating in the session. Clients who show up at a session inebriated or high may be permitted to participate as long as their behavior is not disruptive. Either during or after the group session (either immediately after the session, or when the client is sober again but before the next group meeting), the leader can elicit the inebriated client's perceptions of the group session in order to explore whether the client thought the group session was useful, and to determine whether he or she felt uncomfortable or awkward during the session. Clients who use alcohol or drugs before a group session are often ambivalent about their use and may be concerned about how the leaders and other group members will react to them. The leaders can use this situation to avoid criticizing such a client openly, while at the same time evaluating with the client whether using substances before a group session is beneficial to him or her and to other group members. A common outcome of this discussion is for the client to commit to not using substances before attending group meetings in the future.

The primary rationale for not excluding clients who use substances before a persuasion group session is that such exclusion goes counter to the core philosophy of these groups, which is *inclusion*, not exclusion. Most clients who are participants in persuasion groups have been excluded from a wide range of both therapeutic interventions and social situations. Prohibiting such clients from participating in persuasion groups runs the risk of disengaging them from treatment and increasing their social marginalization. By contrast, a no-exclusion policy makes it more difficult for these clients to drop out of treatment—and preventing dropout is an important goal of persuasion groups.

The presence of an inebriated peer typically elicits powerful responses from other group members. This energy often strengthens group resolve and peer support for abstinence, and may lead to substantial movement of the group culture into motivational development. At the same time, the leaders should try to prevent tension and confrontation from becoming so strong that the inebriated client drops out of the group.

Disruptive Behavior

Disruptive behaviors—including angry outbursts, monopolizing the discussion, extreme argumentativeness, repeated tangentiality, or severe preoccupation with psychotic symptoms that interferes with group intervention (e.g., responding to hallucinations, accusing others based on delusions)—need to be curtailed by the leaders to maintain the integrity and safety of the group. At first, when such a behavior occurs, the leaders can respond by either redirecting the disruptive client or ignoring the behavior. If the problematic behavior persists, the leaders can directly address the problem by speaking to the client about it, explaining how it interferes with the group, asking other members to say how it makes them feel, and requesting that the client desist from the behavior. Depending on the nature of the problem, one of the leaders can offer to meet individually with the client after the group to discuss his or her concerns. If these tactics are unsuccessful at stopping the disruptive behavior, the client can be asked to leave the session (or escorted out by one of the leaders) and invited to come back to the next group meeting. By responding to disruptive behavior in this way, the leaders demonstrate their concern over the welfare of the whole group, while showing respect, flexibility and a desire to respond to the needs of individual clients.

Clients with active psychotic symptoms can benefit from participating in persuasion groups just as nonpsychotic clients can, but their tenuous contact with reality requires that special allowances be made. Although redirection may occasionally be necessary, paying selective attention to on-topic contributions and ignoring irrelevant statements are often sufficient to keep clients with persistent psychotic symptoms actively involved in the group. We provide an example below of how a leader managed a client with psychotic symptoms (Bruce, the client described earlier).

LEADER: Has anyone else had problems with symptoms getting worse when they used drugs?

BRUCE: When I was 14 or 15 years old, I used to take acid. I think it damaged my brain cells and made me hear voices. Ever since I took acid, I can feel this rushing and pressure in my head. These kids would give it to me and laugh at me. The damaged cells ooze out toxins out of the neurolimbic cell endings and shoot protoplasm down my spine in electronic pulses that send pain to my back and legs and my feet, and—and they feel like they are rotting into—

LEADER: —Bruce, it sounds like you had a lot of problems with symptoms after you used acid. Thank you for sharing that with us.

Some clients with severe psychotic symptoms or marked cognitive impairment have great difficulty following the unstructured process of a persuasion group. Although their problems may or may not be actively disruptive to the group, their ability to benefit may be limited by their poor attention. Such clients may benefit more from participating in social skills training groups (Chapter 11) than in persuasion groups, because skills training groups are more structured and predictable, and less oriented toward group process and establishing insight.

Respect for Others

Persuasion groups derive their clinical effectiveness from providing a safe social environment for clients to explore and share their experiences with alcohol and drugs. Fundamental to creating such a group atmosphere is engendering a sense of mutual respect among the group members. This respect includes an understanding that each person has the right to make decisions concerning his or her own life without being criticized, judged, or devalued by other group members.

Disrespect between group participants can take many forms, but the most common form occurs when a client in one of the later stages of treatment (either active treatment or relapse prevention) is harshly critical of a client in the persuasion stage for his or her continued substance use. The leaders can employ several strategies to ensure that group members demonstrate respect for each other. Leaders can directly address the issue by introducing a discussion of the topic and elicit-

ing feedback from members about what it means to be respected, instances where they have felt either respected or disrespected, and ways members within the group can show respect to one another. When one member appears to be judging another, the leaders can remind the member that all people have the right to live their lives in their own unique ways; that there are multiple pathways to recovery; and that genuine change must come from within, not in response to pressure from others. Critical group members who have achieved more control over their substance abuse can also be encouraged to examine their own experiences and to reflect with the group about their own pathways to recovery, including the times when they experienced the greatest despair.

CONDUCTING THE FIRST PERSUASION GROUP SESSION

It is helpful for the leaders to structure the first meeting of a persuasion group in order to allay clients' concerns and to stimulate discussion. This helps to avoid uncomfortable silences, while specifying to participants the focus of discussion at each point of the meeting. Over time group sessions will become less structured than the first session, while adhering to a basic structure described in the next section.

The primary topics that should be covered during the first persuasion group meeting are a brief explanation of the rationale for the group, introductions and brief sharing among participants, and a discussion of rules for the group. These topics are described below, with approximate time allotments summarized in Table 9.1.

Presenting the Rationale for the Group

Group participants are informed that the purpose of the persuasion group is to provide an opportunity for people who have experienced difficulties in life because of mental illness and substance use to share their experiences and viewpoints with each other. It is

TABLE 9.1. Outline of First Persuasion Group Session

Topic	Time allotment
Rationale for group	5–10 minutes
Introductions	15–20 minutes
Discussion of guidelines for the group	15–20 minutes
Wrap-up	5–10 minutes

usually best if leaders avoid reference to specific terms for substance use disorders (e.g., *addiction, substance abuse, substance dependence*) and specific terms for mental illnesses (e.g., *schizophrenia, bipolar disorder*) at this point, since the participants may find these labels objectionable or believe that they do not apply to them. The focus of the rationale is on getting people with similar experiences together to talk about their lives and to explore whether they want to make changes. A brief explanation is usually sufficient, such as the following:

"I'd like to welcome everybody to this meeting today, and tell you what a pleasure it is to see you. My name is Jamal, and this is my coleader, Samantha. We'd like to spend a few minutes talking with you about this group, and then to spend a few minutes getting to know each other.

"This group is for people who have had a mental illness and some problems related to using alcohol or drugs. The goal of the group is to provide a safe place for people to talk about their experiences with their mental illness and coping with it, and about the effects of alcohol or drugs on their lives, including either positive or negative effects. You might not think you've had one of these problems, and that's okay. You were invited to participate in this group because your case manager, or someone else on your treatment team, thought it would be helpful to you. We're not going to judge you, and we want you to have the freedom to truly speak your mind and to use this group to your own best advantages. Any comments or thoughts about the ideas behind this group?"

Introductions by Members

When any questions have been answered, and the leaders have facilitated a brief discussion about the group (there may be none), introductions by the different participants are done. These introductions serve to "break the ice" by letting each person tell the others a little about him- or herself. Participants should not be pressed to give specific details about their lives or circumstances if they prefer not to. Leaders can ask a few follow-up questions if these seem needed to clarify a client's introduction. Leaders should strive to make the group atmosphere as tolerant and accepting as possible. A leader can initiate the round of introductions as follows:

"Let's introduce ourselves. I'm Jamal, and I work as a case manager on the C team. Let's go around in a circle. I'd like each person to introduce himself or herself, and to give a brief explanation about

how you came to this group. (*Turns to the client on the left.*) Shelby, do you mind starting this off?"

Discussing Group Rules

When the introductions have been completed, the leaders next begin a discussion about guidelines or rules for the group (e.g., Table 9.2). The purposes of this discussion are to clarify expectations for participation in the group, and to emphasize the importance of mutual respect and tolerance for different members' beliefs and perceptions. The leaders can put forth some guidelines, but at least some suggestions should be elicited from the participants. All suggested rules should be acknowledged, though not every possible one needs to be included; nor should too many rules be identified (e.g., over six or seven). Rules may be modified based on group discussion. For example, the suggested rule that "No one can attend the group if he or she has used alcohol or drugs that day" might be altered to "Try not to use alcohol or drugs before attending the group." Reasons for including rules (or not including them) should be briefly discussed. Rules that have been agreed upon should be written down and posted. This discussion can be initiated as follows:

"We'd like to spend a little time talking about guidelines for participating in this group. Guidelines can be helpful because they let everyone know what is expected of them, and what they can expect from other people. One guideline that I like is that one person speaks at a time—no interrupting. That way, each person gets to say what's important to him or her, without worrying that someone else is going to cut them off. Does anyone have any ideas of guidelines for the group that they would like to suggest?"

Wrap-Up

After the guidelines for the group have been discussed, the leaders close with some observations about the group, and remind participants of the date and time of the next group session. Final questions and comments are handled, and the session ends.

TABLE 9.2. Examples of Persuasion Group Rules

- One person speaks at a time.
- No interrupting.
- Come to the group on time.
- No name calling or put-downs.
- Respect personal differences.
- Everybody who wants to speak gets a chance.

THE STRUCTURE OF FURTHER PERSUASION GROUP SESSIONS

After the initial group session, subsequent sessions follow a general internal structure that consists of the members' check-in, the discussion topic or activity, and closing remarks. We describe these structural components of further sessions below, and summarize the time allotted to each component in Table 9.3.

Members' Check-In

Persuasion group sessions often begin with a *check-in*. That is, each member reports about his or her use of alcohol and drugs since the last meeting. This discussion must be kept nonjudgmental, so that members will feel safe in giving honest accounts of their substance use. The check-in among group members can be initiated several weeks after the group has begun, when members have begun to feel comfortable with each other, and substance use has already become a topic of conversation. Clients who prefer not to talk about their use, or who deny use in the face of evidence to the contrary, are not challenged.

When members discuss their recent use of substances, the leaders help them explore what led up to each episode; to identify internal emotional states before, during, and after the substance use; and to explore the consequences of use. Beneficial and adverse consequences of substance use are evaluated and weighed against each other. All members are encouraged to contribute to the discussion, perhaps by offering advice or relating a similar experience.

The weekly review of substance use can become such an expected routine that members initiate it on their own. Regular members often find this exercise helpful in supporting their attempts to achieve periods of relative sobriety or abstinence. When clients face opportunities to use substances between group meetings, they know they will be reporting their use in the next group. This continuity may remind clients of things they discussed in the group, which may support their ability to say "no."

A member may share a substantial adverse conse-

quence of substance use or poor illness management, such as an arrest, jailing, eviction, hospitalization, or major fight with a friend or family member. A member who has struggled with substance use may have achieved a period of abstinence. A member may have promised him- or herself never to use again after a particularly distressing episode of drug use or bad hangover. A member who has begun to moderate his or her use of substances may have relapsed back into heavy use.

Typically, a leader will point out that such an issue is important to come back to if the member does not make the request him- or herself. The group then continues the check-in until all members have had a chance to share. If several issues come up during the check-in, the leaders assist the group in prioritizing the follow-up discussion and managing the group time to ensure that all issues are addressed. The flexibility of the focus maximizes relevance of persuasion groups by ensuring that topics of discussion are immediately helpful and usable in the members' lives. This approach also establishes a norm of group problem solving and mutual support, as well as an investment in the outcome of each other's struggles.

Discussion Topics and Activities

Persuasion groups may have a topic or activity selected by the leaders intended to stimulate discussion among members. In a mature persuasion group, the weekly check-in will often uncover material that will become the topic of the main part of the session. In contrast to learning-oriented group interventions for dual disorders, such as social skills training (Chapter 11), the primary purpose of introducing specific topics is not to teach critical information or skills. Instead, such topics serve as vehicles for initiating group discussions of issues related to substance use and abuse. Fostering lively interaction among group participants is the main goal; the leaders are not especially concerned that a topic be adequately covered, that members actually learn the relevant information, or that participants stick to the topic at hand. As long as the discussion concerns substance use, mental illness, or their interactions, the leaders allow the group discussion to evolve spontaneously, without trying to confine it to the preselected topic. As group members become more familiar with each other and the relatively unstructured format of the group, topics for groups often become unnecessary, and group sessions "take off" on their own after the initial members' check-in. Specific topics and activities for persuasion groups are discussed in a later section of this chapter.

A variety of different materials can be used in persuasion groups. Information can be presented on a

TABLE 9.3. Outline of Subsequent Persuasion Group Sessions

Topic	Time allotment
Members' check-in	10–15 minutes
Discussion topic or activity	30–45 minutes
Closing remarks	5–10 minutes

blackboard, flipchart, or posters, or in written handouts, such as those provided in Appendix B. Self-help materials from organizations such as Alcoholics Anonymous and Narcotics Anonymous are usually not helpful in persuasion groups. Most participants in these groups are still having difficulties with substance abuse, and introducing them to self-help concepts directly aimed at achieving and maintaining abstinence is premature for their stage of treatment (see Chapter 12).

Closing the Session

Toward the end of the session, the leaders begin to wrap up and do closing remarks. At a minimum, this wrap-up should include a statement that the session is about to end; praise or specific observations about the discussion; an invitation to group members to make any final comments; and a reminder to the members about when the next group meeting will take place. Members may be asked to participate in selecting a topic for the next meeting.

Depending upon the content of the group discussion, the leaders may also prompt a brief discussion at the end of the session to check on members who may be under unusually high levels of stress, suicidal, very symptomatic or otherwise distressed, or vulnerable to a relapse of either severe (and harmful) substance abuse or their psychiatric disorder. In the event that the leaders or members are concerned about one of these issues in a member, time can be set aside at the end of the session to review the situation (and others' concerns) with this member, and to determine a plan of action that is both agreeable to the member and has the likelihood of reducing his or her risk of harmful consequences. In some cases, the leaders may arrange to meet with the member after the session to help resolve the situation. When one member has experienced an especially difficult time, and he or she has shared this with the group, it is important that this be followed up at the next session—so that other members are reinforced for their concern, and, if the problem was successfully managed, they can receive some credit for helping resolve the difficulty.

GROUP PROCESS

A good persuasion group often runs itself, with the leaders' involvement limited primarily to keeping the group on the topic of substance abuse and mental illness, facilitating peer interaction, and asking occasional questions to promote personal exploration among members. *Group process* refers to the interactions among the members, which, if successful, lead to new insights or renewed motivation to work on the problem of sub-

stance abuse. Leaders have several ways of facilitating group process and helping members in the persuasion stage progress to the active treatment and relapse prevention stages.

First, group leaders should focus on eliciting the experiences of members whenever possible. Negative experiences are common among persons with dual disorders. Encouraging group members to share their experiences conveys to them that they are not alone and validates them, which in and of itself can be a source of relief. In addition, talking about personal experiences can lead to the sharing of coping strategies between members, as some members may have successfully managed these problems in the past and are eager to help others do the same.

Second, the leader can encourage discussion among members by asking questions that prompt them to reconsider their beliefs about substance abuse. Questions can be framed in an open-ended manner that invites contributions from all members, but is intended to have its main impact on one member. Used in this way, the group process can sometimes persuade a client that substance abuse is problematic (or that it can be addressed) when the leaders alone would be unsuccessful. An example of using group process to help a member reevaluate his substance abuse is provided below.

CHARLIE: I know smoking weed and drinking has been a problem for some people, but I've never had that problem. It makes me feel fine.

LEADER: How about the rest of you? Does anyone have any thoughts about what Charlie just said?

DARLENE: I like the feeling of alcohol, too. It makes me feel relaxed. But pot and cocaine make me paranoid, so I've stopped using them.

RONALD: The problem isn't with the symptoms; it's other stuff.

LEADER: Could you tell us a little more about that, Ronald?

RONALD: I used to use up all my money on booze, and then I'd run short by the end of the month and have to hit my mother up for some extra.

LEADER: What was that like?

RONALD: Bad. Once she called the police on me. I was drunk, and I said I was going to bust down the door.

DARLENE: I knew you when you were a drinking man, and you were *bad*. And mean.

RONALD: Yes, I guess so.

CHARLIE: I don't drink *that* much.

LEADER: Darlene, has your drinking been a problem

for any of your relationships, like with family or friends?

DARLENE: I don't see my family much. My boyfriend sometimes complains when I pass out on him.

LEADER: That bothers him?

DARLENE: Yes. I sometimes get carried away and drink more than I should, and then I black out or something. He doesn't think I'm much fun when that happens.

LEADER: What do you think, Charlie?

CHARLIE: Maybe she shouldn't drink so much.

LEADER: Maybe. How about yourself? Have there been any down sides to your drinking and smoking pot, even though they make you feel good?

CHARLIE: I don't know. No one complains.

DARLENE: That's because you're alone at home most of the time when you are drinking!

CHARLIE: I guess so—there's no one to complain.

LEADER: Is that okay with you, that there's no one to complain?

CHARLIE: Not really. I get kind of lonely.

RONALD: Does drinking make you feel less lonely?

CHARLIE: Maybe a little, but I still feel lonely when I'm drinking.

LEADER: It sounds to me like you're not happy about that—spending a lot of time drinking alone.

CHARLIE: Yes. Drinking makes me feel good, but then I get isolated and feel very alone.

DARLENE: You don't have to be alone, Charlie.

LEADER: That's something we could work on together.

A third strategy leaders can use to facilitate group process is to be willing to hold back and "go with the flow" when the group is engaged in a discussion about substance abuse. Simply providing brief, validating comments, but not trying to influence the direction of the conversation, is often sufficient for a therapeutic group process to develop. When this happens, the leaders more closely resemble the other group members; free exchange is maximized; and sharing of personal experiences and perspectives is enhanced.

SPECIFIC TOPICS AND ACTIVITIES FOR PERSUASION GROUPS

As noted earlier, discussion topics and activities provide a focus to the persuasion group by encouraging the participants to consider their use of substances from a par-

ticular angle. An entire group may revolve around one topic introduced by the leaders at the beginning of the group, or the group may shift from the discussion topic to another on its own. During the first several weeks of starting a persuasion group, the leaders should be prepared at each group session to introduce a new topic. However, as members get to know each other, as the ground rules of the group become familiar, and as the members' check-in at the beginning of the group becomes standard, leaders must be prepared to abandon the selection of discussion topics and allow the natural group process to take over. Once a group has reached a level of maturity, the leaders can occasionally select discussion topics to vary the group format.

We briefly describe examples of topics and activities for persuasion groups below. Leaders and clients can identify additional ones that may be suitable.

Genogram Exercise

A *genogram* is a picture that is used to summarize family relationships across several generations (Marlin, 1989). Genograms are used for a variety of purposes by either professionals or laypeople: to describe and learn patterns from family history about medical problems, difficulties in family or personal functioning, or other areas of interest (Carter & McGoldrick, 1988). In persuasion groups, a genogram exercise can help group members see that substance use disorders and psychiatric illnesses often run in families. This can be helpful in reducing members' shame and guilt about having dual disorders, and helping them understand that there may be a hereditary basis for the disorders.

The leader begins the discussion by inviting group members to consider the possible role of family history in psychiatric and substance use disorders. This is followed by the genogram exercise itself. The leaders illustrate how to complete a genogram on a blackboard or flipchart; each member then completes his or her genogram, with the leaders providing assistance as necessary. When all members have completed their genograms, the leaders facilitate a sharing discussion among the members on the topic. This topic can be extended to cover several persuasion group sessions if time requires it.

In a genogram, it is most common to depict three generations of family members, with the person completing the genogram and his or her siblings at the bottom level, the parents (and their siblings) on the next level above, and the grandparents (and their siblings) at the top level. Some basic rules for completing a genogram include the following: Males are drawn with rectangles or squares, females with circles or triangles; enough space should be left under each person's symbol to designate whether the person has a psychiatric disorder, a substance use disorder, or both; siblings are arranged in descending order of age from left to right; marriages can be depicted with an "=" sign, and divorces by drawing a dash through the "=" sign; an "✕" is drawn through a person who is dead; children can be connected to their parents by drawing a line down from the "=" sign to them. Figure 9.1 illustrates a family genogram (note that the "=" sign was not used in this case).

Not all clients can identify relatives with either a substance use problem or a mental illness. When this occurs, clients should be informed that many different sets of factors are involved in determining a person's vulnerability to substance-related problems and mental illness, of which family factors (including genetic factors) are only one set. Genograms help clients understand the biological roots of at least some of their problems, while appreciating that not all family members are affected in the same way.

Educational Topics

A variety of different educational topics can be used to stimulate conversations about substance abuse. Table 9.4 provides examples of educational topics, and many others are possible. Educational topics are presented with a combination of informed didactic teaching and an interactive exchange of experiences among the group members. Specific curricula about psychiatric disorders, medication, the stress–vulnerability model, and substance abuse are contained in Appendix B in the form of handouts. Key points from these handouts can be summarized in the persuasion group and used as a springboard for discussion. Topics involving substance

TABLE 9.4. Examples of Educational Topics for Persuasion Groups

- Physiological and psychological effects of alcohol and specific drugs (book handouts)
- Symptoms of mental illness (book handouts)
- The stress–vulnerability model of psychiatric illness (book handout)
- Medications (book handouts)
- Dealing with stress
- Coping with symptoms
- Communication
- Solving problems
- Orientation to self-help organizations
- Activities for relaxation and pleasure
- Cues associated with craving
- Work: Finding and keeping a job
- Effects of substance use on relationships and family

abuse can include the names of commonly used psychoactive substances, their effects (both positive and negative), and common reasons for using them. Discussions of psychiatric disorders can address the names and symptoms of major mental illnesses, their biological basis, their treatment, and the course of each illness. Group discussion of the stress–vulnerability model can facilitate an understanding of how the biological vulnerability underlying psychiatric illness can make clients more susceptible to the biological stress of the effects of moderate or even small amounts of alcohol or drugs. Discussion of this model can also give members hope that the long-term course of their psychiatric illness can be successfully managed by minimizing stress, improving coping skills, adhering to prescribed medications, and reducing (or preferably avoiding) use of alcohol and drugs.

Other educational topics, such as dealing with

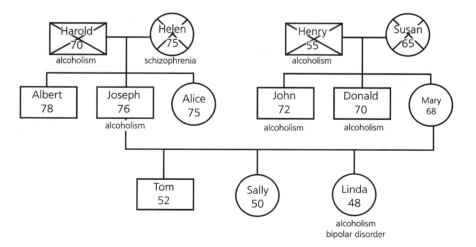

FIGURE 9.1. Example of a genogram completed by a member of a persuasion group.

stress, identifying alternative recreational activities, and solving problems, serve to review common coping strategies for handling many of the day-to-day problems experienced by clients with a dual disorder. Curricula for these topics can be drawn from a variety of sources, including self-help books, professional books, and the leaders' own clinical and personal experiences. Ideas for educational topics can be the focus of group discussions, so that members have input into the topics selected.

Social Skills Training

Although persuasion groups are different from social skills training groups (described in Chapter 11), training of specific skills can be a useful topic on occasion, and can lead to fruitful discussion in a persuasion group. It can also be used to help a member acquire a specific skill that he or she discovers a deficiency in during the persuasion group, the acquisition of which would be helpful to the motivational development process (e.g., drink refusal skills). In social skills training groups, the primary goal is to systematically teach new skills through extensive practice, including both role playing in the group and homework assignments for clients to practice the skill on their own. In contrast, when social skills training is used in persuasion groups, less emphasis is placed on extensive practice with new skills, and more attention is turned to facilitating group discussion about the relevance and need for the skills. The use of active role playing in the group often helps to "break the ice" in the first few sessions of a persuasion group, through the active, experiential learning involved in role playing and sharing feedback.

Social skills training is conducted following the standard sequence of steps described in Chapter 11 and expanded in greater detail in other books (Bellack et al., 1997; Liberman, DeRisi, & Mueser, 1989; Monti et al., 2002). As indicated above, however, when a skill is introduced in a persuasion group, the leaders need not follow each step of skills training in a rigorous fashion. When introducing skills, the leaders should work to elicit a rationale from the members about the relevance of the skills to both substance abuse and day-to-day situations. For example, conversational skills can be useful in helping members establish connections and friendships with people who do not abuse substances. Learning how to express angry feelings and how to compromise and negotiate with others can help members whose substance use is associated with (or exacerbated by) strong levels of interpersonal conflict.

Modeling of each skill by the leaders is an important step that should not be skipped. Modeling shows to the group members that the leaders are willing to be just as actively involved as the members, and the role-play demonstration often provokes much discussion. It is preferable if each client has the opportunity to practice the skill in a role play at least once, but extensive practice in multiple role plays is not required. The primary focus of feedback is on what each client did well in his or her role play, with the leaders prompting members to give feedback directly to this client. Negative feedback is cut off at first, and later (after positive feedback) it is rephrased in the form of encouraging suggestions. The net result of participating in the role plays, receiving feedback, and giving feedback to others is to help members think about the specific skills they can use to achieve interpersonal goals, and to validate their own ability to use these skills in appropriate situations.

Like other topics in persuasion groups, social skills training can be done ad hoc, in response to a group member's need emerging during the course of the group, as well as in preplanned sessions. Examples of useful social skill topics for persuasion groups include starting and maintaining conversations, expressing positive feelings, expressing negative feelings, compromising/negotiating, making requests, and refusing requests or offers. The curricula for teaching these and other skills are summarized in Chapter 11.

Guest Speakers

After cohesion has developed in the group, an occasional invited guest speaker can provide a useful springboard for lively discussion. Guest speakers can address a number of different topics selected by the group leaders, the members, or both. Examples of guest speakers include another client from a later stage of treatment who can discuss his or her experiences of recovery from substance abuse (i.e., someone in the relapse prevention stage); a psychiatrist who can talk about new medications; a psychiatric consumer who can talk about self-help and recovery from mental illness; a supported employment specialist who can talk about the benefits of work and how to get jobs; a benefits expert who can talk about Supplemental Security Income, Social Security Disability Insurance, and substance abuse; and an addiction expert who can discuss the psychology and physiology of addiction. Leaders should be familiar with invited speakers and their general message before they meet with the group, and should also prepare speakers for the needs and norms of the group.

"War Stories"

Most persons with past or recent histories of substance abuse enjoy sharing their experiences with others. Clients often become especially animated when swapping what many call "war stories" about their exploits involving alcohol and drugs, and these discussions can even develop a competitive edge as each person tries to top the other with an even wilder account. These exploits typically involve extended benders, the consumption of huge quantities of alcohol and/or drugs, and narrow escapes from the law or other authority figures. Devoting a group to telling these stories can be a useful persuasion group exercise.

Many group members may have participated in other groups in which accounts of their experiences with alcohol and drugs, especially positive accounts, are frowned upon or are prohibited outright. The censorship of such topics often breeds resentment in clients who have at least some positive feelings about their use of substances (such as feeling intensely "alive," uninhibited, or temporarily free of anxiety when under the influence of substances). These clients often feel that discussing only the negative aspects of substance abuse is one-sided and does not validate their true experiences with substances. Obtaining and using substances, especially illegal ones, may be one of the few things a client has been competent at in his or her life. Preventing clients from talking about their true experiences with substances often makes them less honest about the costs of their substance abuse, and can result in their harking back to a romantic (and usually distorted) vision of the "good old days."

Allowing clients to swap war stories is a group topic that energizes members, while providing social validation for their experiences. Of equal or greater importance, allowing these stories opens up the door for the leaders to explore with members the dangers they found and the consequences or aftermath of these events. Though going down this road may be painful for many clients, especially those who have suffered the worst losses, most are willing to do so when their positive experiences have been acknowledged.

Fun Sessions

Although the major work in persuasion groups is on exploring the effects of substances on members' lives, devoting a session simply to having fun can build cohesion and good will among all members. Fun sessions can involve a recreational activity or outing where there is no expectation that issues related to substance abuse will be raised. Examples of activities for a fun session include going on a picnic, going bowling, going to the beach, visiting a park, or going to a fair. Activities that are unlikely to promote interaction between members, such as going to the movies, should be avoided.

Art Projects

Art projects can provide persuasion group members with opportunities to express themselves nonverbally and to share their perceptions through discussion. Either each member can do something that expresses his or her unique perspective, or each member can contribute to a shared work of art. An example of an art project that can be done either by individual members or as a group is making a collage of what life is like on versus off alcohol and drugs. When the art has been completed, members discuss the images, share their perspectives, and explore their meanings.

CURRICULA-BASED PERSUASION GROUPS

Persuasion groups are usually conceptualized as process oriented rather than aimed at teaching specific information and skills based on a preplanned curriculum. However, the basic format of a persuasion group can be adapted to make it curricula based while still providing ample opportunities for members to process the effects of substance abuse or poorly managed mental illness on their lives, and to develop motivation to address those problems. Curricula-based persuasion groups employ the same therapeutic principles as in more process-oriented groups while incorporating more formal interactive teaching methods.

There are several advantages to conducting curricula-based persuasion groups over purely process-oriented groups. First, curricula-based groups may decrease anxiety among less experienced clinicians who have not led process-oriented groups, and who may be concerned about successfully stimulating group process. Second, some clients may prefer curricula-based groups because they may be attracted to specific topics that will be covered in the group. Third, it may be easier to train new clinicians to conduct curricula-based persuasion groups over process-oriented groups, since the format and focus of sessions are more structured.

The primary disadvantage to curricula-based persuasion groups is that they are time limited rather than time unlimited, as in more process-oriented persuasion groups. Despite the focus of a persuasion group on helping clients progress from the persuasion stage to the active treatment stage, some clients may remain in the persuasion stage after completing a time-limited curricula-based persuasion group. In such circumstances, clients can be invited to participate in another round of the group, likely benefiting from additional exposure to the material on a second (or even third) round of the group. Table 9.5 provides an outline of a 21-week curricula-based persuasion group.

SUMMARY

A *persuasion group* is a process-oriented, stage-wise group intervention designed to help clients with a dual

TABLE 9.5. Curriculum Outline for Persuasion Group

Session #1: Introduction of facilitators and group participants
- Purpose of group
- Overview of group rules
- What is mental illness?
- How are mental illnesses diagnosed? (diagnostic interviews after ruling out medical causes)

Session #2: Introduction to the concept of recovery
- Recovery from mental illness (see Mueser, Corrigan, et al., 2002)
- Recovery from substance use problems
- What does recovery mean to each person?
- Recovery as the process of setting personal goals and getting on with one's life
- How the management of mental illness and substance use problems can facilitate the recovery process
- Encourage clients to begin setting personal recovery goals

Session #3: Schizophrenia and Related Disorders (book handouts)
- Characteristic symptoms
- Epidemiology, onset, course, biological theories
- Treatment
- Participants encouraged to discuss symptoms, diagnoses

Session #4: Mood Disorders (major depression, bipolar disorder: book handouts)
- Same format as Session #3

Session #5: Anxiety Disorders (posttraumatic stress disorder, panic disorder, agoraphobia, phobias, obsessive–compulsive disorder: book handout on PTSD, supplemented with information from DSM-IV on other anxiety disorders)
- Same format as Session #3

Session #6: Stress–Vulnerability Model (book handout)
- Description of Stress–Vulnerability Model
- Nature and origins of biological vulnerability
- Stress and its potential effect on the course of mental illness
- Coping more effectively with stress
- Beneficial effects of social support
- Positive effects of medication
- Negative effects of alcohol and drugs
- Treatment principles: stress reduction, building coping strategies, medication, reduction of alcohol and drug use

Session #7: Medications for Psychiatric Disorders (book handouts)
- Antipsychotics, antidepressants, mood stabilizers
- Effects of medications on symptoms and prevention of relapses
- Side effects
- Strategies for enhancing adherence to medications
  - Evaluating pros and cons of taking medication
  - Behavioral tailoring: fitting taking medication into person's daily routine, including natural prompts to take medication (e.g., medication stored next to toothbrush)
  - Simplifying medication regimen (e.g., talk with doctor about taking fewer medications fewer times per day)
  - Involving significant others in reminding person to take medication
  - Use of "Mediplanners" to organize medications each week
- Consider inviting team psychiatrist(s) or nurse(s) as guest speaker(s)

Session #8: Substance Use, Part I: Introduction (book handout)
- Background on history of substance use
- Different types of drugs and their effects, including positive and negative effects
- Encourage participants to talk about their experiences with different types of substances

Session #9: Substance Use, Part II: Motives and Consequences (book handout)
- In-depth discussion of common motives for using substances, including:
  - Social motives
  - Recreational motives
  - Coping with symptoms and negative moods
  - Alleviation of substance withdrawal symptoms
  - Providing structure and something to look forward to
- Consequences of substance use
  - Understanding high vulnerability to negative consequences of substance use
  - Substance abuse (defined)
  - Substance dependence (defined)
    - Psychological dependence
    - Physical dependence

(continued)

TABLE 9.5. *(continued)*

Session #10: Substance Use, Part III: Treatment (book handout, Payoff Matrix)
- Stages of treatment concept
- Review of different treatment approaches
- Group members evaluate their own stage of treatment
- Payoff Matrix exercise (pros and cons of continued substance use and pros and cons of sobriety)
- Exploration of ambivalence
- Identification of obstacles to sobriety

Session #11: Coping with Negative Feelings I: Anxiety/Fear
- Discussion of how people use substances to cope with anxiety and its drawbacks
- Brainstorm strategies for coping with anxiety
- Encourage participants with anxiety to select at least one strategy for coping with anxiety
- Plan on how to implement and monitor the effects of strategies for coping with anxiety for each participant
- Examples of coping strategies:
  - Use relaxation strategies (e.g., breathing retraining)
  - Gradually approach/expose oneself to feared but safe situations
  - Challenge beliefs that feared situations/stimuli are in fact threatening
  - Acknowledge fearful feelings but do not let them control your behavior
  - Write about personal experiences that contributed to feelings of fear and anxiety

Session #12: Coping with Negative Feelings II: Depression/Sadness
- Same format as Session #11
- Examples of coping strategies:
  - Schedule pleasant events to engage in on a regular basis
  - Exercise (especially vigorous exercise)
  - Challenge self-defeating thoughts/beliefs about hopelessness, helplessness, worthlessness, and other negative thoughts
  - Problem-solve about conflict in social relationships that may be contributing to sad feelings
  - Identify positive self-statements about strengths to counter negative thoughts

Session #13: Coping with Negative Feelings III: Anger
- Same format as Session #11
- Examples of coping strategies:
  - Forgive the other person(s)
  - Problem-solve to address current problems contributing to angry feelings
  - Practice verbally expressing feelings in a constructive, nonhostile manner
  - Challenge beliefs about others' responsibility, overly idealistic notions about how the world "ought" to be (rather than how the world is)
  - Identify anxious/fearful feelings that anger may be "protecting" the person from

Session #14: Coping with Negative Feelings IV: Guilt/Shame
- Same format as Session #11
- Examples of coping strategies:
  - Challenge beliefs about one's own responsibility and awareness about the behaviors in question
  - Reevaluate unrealistic expectations of perfection and remind oneself that "to err is human"
  - Attempt to redress the situation, make amends, or seek forgiveness from the person who was wronged
  - Do something else that is good for others in order to compensate for past behavior

Session #15: Dealing with Social Situations I: Alternatives to Social Use
- Discuss how substance use is used to facilitate social interactions, such as:
  - Use with friends to maintain social relationships
  - Use of substances to fit in socially with people who may have substance use problems
  - Use of substances to decrease social anxiety, including sexual/intimate situations
- Discussion of advantages/disadvantages of common social motives
- Group identification of alternatives to social use
- Encourage participants to select at least one alternative to social use and plan on how to implement it

Session #16: Dealing with Social Situations II: Managing Substance Use Situations
- Identification of common social situations involving substance use, such as:
  - Running into friends who are using substances
  - Encountering a former drug connection/dealer
  - Being pressured to use substances
  - Being enticed to use substances (e.g., free substances, in connection with sex)
- Role play substance refusal skills (see Chapter 11)

Session #17: Leisure and Recreation
- Discuss how using substances feels and consider recreational motives
- Consider how substance use patterns often develop early in life and inhibit formation of other recreational interests
- Use group discussion as a springboard to identifying "healthy pleasures" or alternative recreational interests
- Encourage participants to select at least one alternative recreational activity and plan on how to implement it

(continued)

TABLE 9.5. *(continued)*

Session #18: Health and Wellness (book handout on Infectious Diseases)
- Provide information and discuss issues related to substance abuse and health, such as:
  - Infectious diseases (e.g., hepatitis, HIV)
  - Nutrition
  - Exercise
  - Sleep hygiene
  - Nicotine
- Consider strategies for making positive health-related changes and removing obstacles to change
- Encourage participants to select at least one health-related change and plan on how to implement it

Session #19: Goal Setting and Recovery, Part I: Building Self-Confidence to Change
- Return to discussion of recovery, what it means to each person
- Open discussion of goals, including reduced substance use or abstinence, or improved psychiatric illness management, for participants who did not establish these as goals in Session #2
- Consideration of individual situational factors that maintain or increase substance use and/or exacerbate mental illness
- Exploration of roadblocks to making personal changes

Session #20: Goal Setting and Recovery, Part II: Establishing a Personal Recovery Plan
- Next steps: help group members identify individual goals in their recovery process, focusing on strategies for reducing risk and decreasing ambivalence, using lots of examples of small, feasible life changes
- Develop a personal recovery plan for achieving goals, considering:
  - What is the precise goal? (be as specific as possible!)
  - What steps need to be taken to achieve the goal?
  - What is the timetable for taking different steps?
  - What personal resources does the person have that will help in achieving the goal?
  - What resources are needed to achieve the goal (such as money, people, information, skills)?
  - Who can be helpful in achieving the goal?
- Sharing between participants' personal recovery plans

Session #21: Termination
- Highlights of curriculum, from participants' varying perspectives
- Discussion of gains, insights acquired through group process
- Sharing of next personal steps in recovery

Note. This curriculum outline was developed by Kim Mueser, Peggy Sherrer, and Lindy Fox.

disorder understand the impact of substance abuse on their lives. These groups are most appropriate for clients who are in the persuasion stage of treatment, although the groups benefit from having some participants who have progressed to the active treatment or relapse prevention stages. Persuasion groups are nonconfrontational, are highly tolerant of members' individual differences, and are oriented primarily toward fostering peer interactions on the topics of substance abuse and management of mental illness. Leaders look for opportunities to use the group process as a vehicle for educating members about the interactions between mental illness and substance abuse, encouraging them to examine their experiences

with alcohol and drugs closely, and providing mutual support to meet the challenges of their lives. Special topics for groups can be selected to stimulate group discussion, such as family programs, education, special speakers, and social skills training. As an alternative to purely process-oriented persuasion groups, curricula-based persuasion groups can be conducted that focus on teaching information about dual disorders, skills for addressing basic needs and problematic social situations, and developing hope and motivation to work on substance abuse and improved management of mental illness. In the next chapter, we discuss the second type of stage-wise treatment group: active treatment groups.

10

Active Treatment Groups

Active treatment groups are the second type of stage-wise treatment groups. When members of persuasion groups (Chapter 9) move into the active treatment stage, they may find it helpful to move into active treatment groups. The focus of persuasion groups is on helping clients understand the impact of substance abuse on their lives and become motivated to work on their substance-use-related problems. Because persuasion groups need to maintain this focus, they cannot invest much time in teaching skills for decreasing substance abuse itself. In active treatment groups, on the other hand, all members have already developed an awareness of substances' negative effects on their lives, and the focus of group work shifts explicitly to helping participants reduce substance use further or successfully maintain abstinence.

In this chapter, we describe how to initiate and conduct active treatment groups. We begin by considering the overall role of active treatment groups in dual-disorder treatment, and the question of which clients are appropriate to participate in these groups. This is followed by discussion of the logistical details of organizing and conducting active treatment groups. We next discuss core therapeutic principles of facilitating these groups, followed by a review of the structure of group sessions, and the use of group process to support the goals of substance use reduction and abstinence. Different topics and activities for active treatment group sessions are then reviewed. Finally, we compare the relative advantages of separate persuasion and active treatment groups to those of combined groups.

THE ROLE OF ACTIVE TREATMENT GROUPS IN DUAL-DISORDER TREATMENT

Active treatment groups, like their precursor persuasion groups, can be an effective treatment component for dual disorders because they can harness social support from peers. In most treatment settings that develop active treatment groups, the formation of a separate active treatment group takes place several months or even longer after a successful persuasion group has been in place, when the need for a group that directly supports substance use reduction and abstinence becomes more apparent. The identification of clients who are appropriate for and most likely to benefit from active treatment groups flows naturally from those who have made the most progress in developing motivation to address their substance abuse during persuasion groups, although some clients who have not participated in persuasion groups may also benefit.

Based on information obtained and updated during assessment and treatment planning, referral to active treatment groups should be considered for all clients who are in the active treatment or relapse prevention stages. Because the explicit aim of these groups is to help clients further reduce substance abuse or maintain abstinence, clients whose substance abuse continues to be active and severe are not suitable candidates for such groups. Although referral of clients to active treatment groups is usually most effective when they have reached the active treatment stage, clients who have begun to decrease their substance abuse significantly and have succeeded in using substances less or achieving abstinence for a period of several weeks (i.e., clients who are in late persuasion) may also benefit from active treatment groups.

The duration of participation in an active treatment group varies from one client to the next. Some clients choose to participate in such groups for relatively brief periods of time (ranging between 3 and 9 months), and are able to progress into the relapse prevention stage with no setbacks. These individuals benefit from the focus of active treatment groups on practical relapse prevention strategies, and from group members' support for the progress they have made. Ceasing participation in active treatment groups for these clients is often associated with involvement in self-help organizations for addictive disorders available in the community, such as Alcoholics Anonymous (AA), Narcotics Anonymous (NA), or Dual Recovery Anonymous. For other clients, participation in active treatment groups may continue for up to several years. For these individuals, such groups serve as an important source of social support. Clients with poor social skills have the most difficulty affiliating with community self-help groups (Noordsy et al., 1996). Furthermore, the emphasis on skills for avoiding relapses and coping with urges to use is critical for maintaining their sobriety and minimizing the severity of relapses. For clients who decide they want to stop participating in an active treatment group, it is important for the leaders to consider with them other potential sources of social support for maintaining the gains they have made in managing their substance use disorders.

Clients in active treatment groups sometimes experience partial or full relapses into substance abuse. Although one goal of active treatment groups is the prevention of relapses, another goal is to minimize the severity of relapses that do occur. Clients who experience a partial relapse (or a full relapse that is brief in duration) often receive needed abstinence skills, social support for coping with and recovering from the relapse, and benefit from continued participation in the active treatment group. If a relapse is sustained over a significant period of time (i.e., several weeks), the group is unlikely to be helpful to these clients, and their continued presence in the group may harm group morale. In such a case, the leader should discuss with the client a temporary return to the persuasion group until the person's substance abuse is once again under control.

LOGISTICAL CONSIDERATIONS

Most of the logistical elements of running active treatment groups are the same as those reviewed in Chapter 9 for persuasion groups. However, some aspects differ between the two types of groups. In this section we briefly review the logistics of conducting active treatment groups, and highlight differences (where they exist) between these groups and persuasion groups.

Like persuasion groups, active treatment groups benefit from having two leaders, and it is best if each leader comes from a different professional background (i.e., a mental health professional and a substance abuse professional). And like leaders of persuasion groups, leaders of active treatment groups need to have direct contact with the clients' treatment teams, in order to ensure the fullest integration of mental health and substance abuse treatments. In addition, the setting of active treatment groups (usually at a mental health center), the size of groups (6–12 participants), and the timing (one session per week) are similar to those of persuasion groups.

One difference between active treatment and persuasion groups can be the duration of treatment sessions. Whereas sessions rarely last longer than 75 minutes in persuasion groups, sessions in active treatment groups—because of the focus on learning specific skills and shared group support—can last up to 90 minutes, in addition to a scheduled break midway through the group. Active treatment groups need not last as long as 90 minutes; however, most clients are able to sustain attention over longer periods of time when they have reached the active treatment and relapse prevention stages.

In persuasion groups, attendance is left open; clients are encouraged to attend, but there is a high tolerance for irregular and even occasional attendance. In active treatment groups, on the other hand, regular attendance is more strongly encouraged, and an informal expectation is established that clients will attend the group unless they have an important reason for not attending. As in persuasion groups, clients in active treatment groups can have their participation included as part of their treatment plan. However, when a client's attendance is irregular, the leaders can directly confront the client about his or her commitment to the group, in an effort to achieve appropriate follow-through.

One final distinction between persuasion and active treatment groups concerns the issue of motivating clients to participate. In persuasion groups, when substance abuse is active, many clients have limited motivation to participate; special steps must be taken to harness their motivation to attend groups (e.g., offering refreshments, providing transportation, arranging to meet with a client immediately after the persuasion group). When clients have successfully decreased their substance use or have attained abstinence, the motivation to participate in active treatment groups is much stronger, due to their desire to avoid relapses. Because of this high level of motivation, less effort is needed to motivate clients' involvement in active treatment groups through external rewards. For example, refreshments do not need to be served at active treatment groups (although they are still an option group members might enjoy), and special meetings need not be arranged around the times of group meetings. Although less inducement is usually necessary to motivate clients to participate in active treatment groups, motivational strategies may be useful on an occasional basis, such as during the early stages of a relapse into substance abuse.

THERAPEUTIC PRINCIPLES

The therapeutic principles that guide active treatment groups differ to some extent from those of persuasion groups. In persuasion groups, clients are at a relatively fragile point during the process of recovery from a substance use disorders. They have often been only recently engaged in treatment; their tolerance for discussing substance-use-related topics may be limited; and they are often highly sensitive to criticism or perceived social challenges. Clients in active treatment groups are less vulnerable, with higher tolerance for conflict and less susceptibility to spontaneously dropping out of treatment. Consequently, in comparison to persuasion groups, the therapeutic principles of active treatment groups involve addressing substance abuse and related problems more directly, and focusing specifically on strategies to promote further reduction of substance use or to maintain abstinence. To illustrate the role of active treatment groups in facilitating recovery from substance use disorders, we provide a clinical vignette describing the progress of one group member.

CASE EXAMPLE

After 2 years in a persuasion group, April came to recognize that her regular marijuana use increased her paranoia and her auditory hallucinations. She decided to stop smoking marijuana following a hospitalization for an exacerbation of psychotic symptoms, because she did not want to return to the hospital. Early withdrawal had taken place in the hospital, but she used the active treatment group to discuss her cravings for marijuana and to develop skills for resisting the impulse to return to smoking marijuana. Other members related similar experiences during their first 6 months of abstinence, supported her decision to quit, and pointed out that she would have to go through craving all over again if she smoked again.

April attended a few NA meetings at the encouragement of the group leaders, but she was too anxious to continue. She discovered in the active treatment group that her concern about her boyfriend's drinking also increased her craving for marijuana, and she learned to let go of her attempts to control his drinking. After two brief episodes of marijuana use led to immediate paranoia, she was able to sustain abstinence. Three months later, her psychiatrist reduced her dosage of antipsychotic medication, because her psychotic symptoms were markedly diminished. She continued to attend the persuasion group as a role model for others, and the active treatment group to support her abstinence.

We discuss the therapeutic principles guiding active treatment groups in greater detail below.

Permissible Confrontation

Whereas confrontation is almost always avoided in persuasion groups, clients in active treatment groups have sufficient commitment to working on their substance abuse problems, and a strong enough relationship with their treatment providers, to withstand interpersonal confrontation. More often than not, confrontation takes place in the form of one peer's confronting another about the other's minimization or denial of problems related to substance use, or his or her perceived invulnerability to relapse. Such confrontation is especially helpful early in a relapse, when the relapsing client may be receptive to feedback from others, and before the substance use behavior has become reentrenched.

Although confrontation is acceptable in active treatment groups, the leaders must nevertheless strive to maintain a calm, respectful, and supportive group atmosphere that is conducive to the participation of all members. Avoiding emotionally charged interactions is important, because many persons with severe mental illness are exquisitely sensitive to interpersonal stress (Butzlaff & Hooley, 1998), and such stress in the group increases their risk of withdrawal from the group, disillusionment, and/or increased psychiatric symptoms. Therefore, a leader should intervene if a confrontation involves raised voices, significant anger, accusations, or put-downs.

If emotionally charged confrontation does occur, a leader can intercede to request that the confronting client restate his or her comments in a less critical and more helpful manner. This feedback can be facilitated if the leader provides specific information about the client's behavior during the interaction. For example, the leader could say,

"Jeremy, I noticed that you sounded pretty angry with John when you confronted him about starting to drink at parties again, and you raised your voice quite a bit. I think you have some very important feedback to give to John, but your anger may get in the way of the message. It would be helpful if you could tell John specifically what you are concerned about and why you feel that way, without raising your voice so loudly."

Facilitation of Peer-to-Peer Interaction

Leaders are always on the lookout for opportunities to facilitate direct peer-to-peer interaction during active treatment groups. Whereas in persuasion groups these interactions take the form of sharing experiences and giving feedback about substance abuse, in active treatment peer interactions are focused more directly on providing suggestions for dealing with high-risk situations, cravings, and early signs of a relapse. As the clients in an active treatment group have extensive experience (both individually and collectively) in working toward the goal of overcoming substance abuse, their feedback to one another is often highly valued; indeed, it is frequently viewed as more credible than feedback provided by the leaders. The fact that participants in an active treatment group share a common goal often makes facilitating peer interactions a straightforward task.

Psychoeducation

As described in Chapter 9, psychoeducation has an important role to play in facilitating discussion and understanding of the nature of dual disorders. In active treatment groups, psychoeducation continues to have an important role. Clients' motivation can make them even more receptive to information that may help in achieving their recovery goals. Common psychoeducational topics in active treatment groups overlap with those in persuasion groups; they include the nature and symptoms of specific psychiatric disorders, the principles of their treatment, interactions between substance abuse and mental illness, biological and psychological aspects of addiction, management of cravings and high-risk situations, and self-help principles and groups. Written materials and handouts, such as those contained in Appendix B and in other formal curricula, can be freely utilized in active treatment groups.

In addition to formal psychoeducation, the leaders are alert to informal opportunities to educate clients about dual disorders and strategies for handling common problems. These opportunities may occur when a client encounters difficulty managing a problematic symptom that contributes to the desire to use substances (e.g., overwhelming anxiety); when a client anticipates encountering a high-risk situation; or when a client discusses the belief that a return to controlled

substance use is a feasible alternative to abstinence. Given the substantial difficulties clients with severe mental illness often have in generalizing didactic training, it is desirable to tie psychoeducation to specific dilemmas that they are currently experiencing whenever possible.

Teaching Skills and Behaviors

Leaders help group members develop specific skills and behaviors to facilitate their goals of reducing substance use and maintaining abstinence. Groups focus on the skills of being appropriately assertive, giving and receiving criticism, refusing drinks and drugs, and managing thoughts about alcohol or drug use. Members learn to recognize situations that increase their risks for using substances, and to use relapse prevention techniques for the management of these situations.

The behavioral principles used in addiction treatment can effectively guide active treatment groups for clients with dual disorders (see Chapter 8). The behavioral approach involves developing intra- and interpersonal skills that clients frequently lack, especially basic social skills. Employing behavioral principles as they are used in addiction treatment doubly benefits clients with a dual disorder since the clients learn skills both for coping with mental illness and for coping with substance abuse recovery. In active treatment groups, behavioral skills training is often provided in a spontaneous fashion in response to members' immediate needs, and is intermingled with equal attention to group process and social support among the members. Active treatment group leaders are always on the lookout for examples of skills deficits that emerge in members' narratives and can be responded to with specifically targeted skills training. Providing such training to address an immediate need can increase its effectiveness. Dual-diagnosis groups that are focused more specifically on the development of social and coping skills, and that are oriented toward teaching specific curricula of skills, are described in Chapter 11.

Supporting Abstinence and Self-Help Concepts

Although exploring and attending self-help groups such as AA are actively encouraged as an adjunct to obtaining sobriety, attendance at such groups is not a requirement of active treatment. Work in active treatment groups will sometimes focus on developing skills for participation in the self-help groups. For clients who cannot use self-help programs (and there are many such clients), active treatment groups attempt to provide comprehensive treatment and support for reduction of substance use and abstinence. Further details on the role of self-help groups in recovery from dual disorders are provided in Chapter 12.

In addition to supporting the use of self-help groups, the leaders and members may bring in materials from self-help programs to increase members' familiarity and comfort with these programs. They may also quote useful principles and slogans from such organizations, making the content available to members who do not attend self-help meetings. Examples of useful self-help slogans from Twelve-Step programs that can be referred to in active treatment groups include "One day at a time," "Keep it simple," "First things first," and "Easy does it." However, the more overtly religious aspects of many traditional self-help programs are downplayed in active treatment groups, as some clients find these concepts difficult to accept, and it may spark delusional preoccupation about religious themes for others.

We provide an example of the positive use of concepts emanating from self-help programs in a group discussion below.

JASON: I can see that my drinking got me into trouble and I need to stop, but it's not fair that I can't ever drink again.

ANN: I think you should take one day at a time.

LEADER: Could you give Jason help with that, Ann? Why is taking one day at a time helpful?

ANN: Well, Jason, you're getting way ahead of yourself worrying about whether you can have a beer when you're 50. You're more likely to drink today if you're worrying about that. What you need to do is decide each day that you're not going to drink that day, and leave tomorrow to tomorrow.

GUIDELINES FOR ACTIVE TREATMENT GROUPS

Most of the guidelines for running active treatment groups are similar to those for persuasion groups discussed in Chapter 9. The issue of confidentiality is discussed with group members, in order to encourage clients not to discuss information revealed by other clients outside the group. Not interrupting or being disruptive in the group is another important guideline to discuss with members, as is showing respect for other group members. These guidelines can be discussed with group members at the introductory session, and can be reviewed by old members as new ones join the group.

One guideline that is different in active treatment groups from persuasion groups concerns the use of alcohol or drugs prior to participation in a group session. In Chapter 9, we have recommended that persuasion group leaders show tolerance by allowing members who have used substances before a group session to participate in the session, provided that their behavior is not disruptive. In contrast, we recommend that active treatment group leaders establish this clear expectation: Use of substances before a group session is not allowed, and if a member shows up for a session clearly inebriated or high, he or she will be asked to skip that session and to come to the next one sober. Substance use prior to meeting with an active treatment group is clearly inconsistent with the focus of such a group on reducing substance use and maintaining abstinence. Furthermore, the use of substances before a group session may impede clients' ability to learn important skills for managing urges to use substances in the future.

THE STRUCTURE OF ACTIVE TREATMENT GROUP SESSIONS

The structure of active treatment group sessions (after the initial one) is similar to that in persuasion groups, with a members' check-in, discussion (including addressing specific topics relevant to one or more members), and closing. However, the emphasis in each of these sections is more practical and less oriented toward group process than that in persuasion groups. With the check-in, each member reviews high-risk substance abuse situations he or she encountered in the past week, and describes how these situations were managed. As different clients' experiences are discussed, the leaders are alert to special difficulties encountered by one or more clients in managing their desire to use substances or actual use. When each member has had an opportunity to relate his or her experiences over the past week, leaders may return to one or two group members who experienced particular problems, and facilitate a group discussion on the management of those situations or their aftermath. Once group cohesion has developed and members are familiar with this routine, the check-in and subsequent focus on individual clients occur naturally and requires little direct prompting by the leaders.

When the focus of attention shifts to individual clients, the group can provide help to these clients in several different ways. Simply giving emotional support to clients who have been experiencing urges to use, or who may be in the early stages of a relapse, can be a powerful way of letting them know that they are not alone in their struggle to recover from substance abuse, and that others understand what they are going through.

In addition to providing emotional support, other clients can give practical advice. Such advice can be based on the clients' own personal experiences in dealing with similar situations, common sense, or knowledge of how others have handled similar situations. The leaders can facilitate sharing advice by prompting group members, or by leading a problem-solving discussion focused on addressing a client's specific situation. An example of facilitating a problem-oriented discussion among clients in response to the difficulties experienced by one client is provided below.

JANE: I've been having a lot of trouble with craving lately. I just can't stop thinking about having a drink.

LEADER: Maybe we could look at what's going on for you. What's been happening in your life?

JANE: Well . . . my grandmother died a couple of weeks ago. I really miss her. Now that I think of it, that's when it started. Now the craving is even worse.

LEADER: Her dying must have stirred up some really strong emotions for you, and it's hard to cope with feelings like that. Maybe your natural response is to want to drink, to calm down. If we could think of other ways of dealing with those feelings, you might not have the cravings. Does anyone have any other ways we can deal with these strong feelings? (*Goes to the blackboard.*)

JOHN: I'd call my case manager.

SALLY: Call someone . . . that's a good idea. If it were me, I'd call my brother, or probably my sister.

SUSAN: You could call me when you're feeling that way.

TIM: How about going for a walk, maybe with a friend?

ROGER: Maybe you'd like to treat yourself to something you'd really enjoy, like a long bath or a good meal.

LEADER: I'd probably go for a good workout in the gym. But what about you, Jane? Are there any ideas that you could use, starting today?

JANE: Yeah, I think I could take a walk . . . I could walk over to my sister's house and visit with her.

LEADER: That sounds like a good idea. You know, there's something else to think about here. It's a good idea when you are haunted by a loss like this to actually schedule time for grieving. Promise yourself you'll spend an hour, or a few hours each day, allowing yourself to grieve. At the same time, then, promise yourself freedom from those thoughts for the rest of the time.

Active treatment groups often focus on a topic raised by one or two clients during the check-in at the beginning of the group, and the leaders work spontaneously with group members to develop practical solutions to the problems raised by the clients. Sometimes a topic raised by one client at the beginning of the group

has immediate importance to several other group members, and more than one session can be devoted to exploring and working on that topic. As an alternative to working on topics spontaneously raised at the beginning of the group, the leaders may introduce new topics or activities as the focus of group work, following the check-in by the members. Examples of specific topics and activities for active treatment groups are described in a later section of this chapter.

GROUP PROCESS

Group process in active treatment groups is primarily based on peer-to-peer interactions; often only limited input by leaders is required. The primary role of the leaders in attending to process issues is to help members share practical advice for dealing with the problems they encounter. An additional role is to ensure that all members contribute to the group discussion—that the more talkative members do not dominate the group, and that the quieter ones do not fall by the wayside.

Group process is also facilitated when the leaders use modeling to demonstrate how certain substance abuse situations might be handled, and to share their personal experiences in coping with similar problems. Such experiences may relate to substance abuse (e.g., the road to recovery for leaders who are recovering from addiction themselves, or the reductions in use that commonly occur with age for others as work, family, and physical health become priorities); however, leaders may also address how they have handled unpleasant feelings, interpersonal conflicts, and other stressful experiences. A leader can serve as a role model and offer his or her experiences to clients as an example of one way of handling the situation. That can be followed up by encouraging others to share their opinions and experiences. Thus the group leaders stimulate group process by first modeling the sharing of perspectives, and then encouraging other members to do the same.

SPECIFIC TOPICS AND ACTIVITIES FOR ACTIVE TREATMENT GROUPS

Topics and activities for teaching and facilitating group discussion may spontaneously develop over the course of a group session in response to the specific needs of one or more members, or can be planned in advance of a group. The general theme of these topics/activities is teaching specific skills or techniques for managing common problems or achieving common goals related to recovery from substance abuse. The level of formal instruction can vary from relatively didactic (but interactive) instruction to facilitating a discussion with no formal teaching. In this section, we describe several topics and activities for active treatment groups; many others are possible.

Teaching Social Skills

Social skills training in active treatment groups usually occurs on an ad hoc basis, when the need arises; it is not usually based on formal, preplanned curricula as described in Chapter 11. Also in contrast to formal social skills training, the specific component steps of a skill are often not articulated in advance, and skills are usually not modeled in advance by the leaders. However, similar strategies are used to improve social skills, albeit in a somewhat less structured manner. These strategies include modeling, role playing, and positive and corrective feedback. More information about conducting social skills training is provided in Chapter 11 and in books by Bellack and colleagues (1997) and Monti and colleagues (2002).

Participants in active treatment groups often need help with specific social situations, such as learning how to set limits on substance-abusing friends who attempt to take advantage of them. They learn social skills for handling such situations through group interaction, and help each other with support outside the group. Discussing and practicing social skills can help group members learn how to manage relationships with significant others, including parents, friends, or partners. Clients often feel that they are being criticized, and at the same time that they are unable to ask for what they want.

These clients are also especially challenged by the stresses of social situations. Coaching can help them develop skills for meeting new people and starting conversations. An example of helping a client improve his conversational skills is provided below.

BILL: Boy, I almost had a drink on Friday night.

KEN: What happened?

BILL: Well, I was at the nightclub listening to music, and I felt really uncomfortable. It was like I was the only one there who wasn't drinking. I wanted to ask someone to dance, but I can't talk to women when I'm not drinking. I just can't say anything when I'm not drinking.

LEADER: Has anyone else had this experience?

JOE: Yes.

JIM: It happens to me all the time.

STEVE: I don't have any trouble. Women are always friendly to me.

KEN: Well, what do you say to them?

LEADER: Let's make a list of what you can say to introduce yourself. Something that reveals a little about yourself is a good opener. (*Goes to the blackboard.*)

STEVE: I sometimes say, "I really like this music, don't you?" (*Leader records as group makes a list of introductions.*)

LEADER: Okay, Susan, would you be the woman Bill wants to dance with? Bill, pick something from the list that feels like your words, look at Susan, and try it out.

BILL: I really like this music. How about you? I'm Bill; what's your name?

Clients can learn specific words for saying "no" to offers for drugs or alcohol, and they can then practice refusing an offer in role plays. One member of the group role-plays making an offer, while another member (usually the one who has brought up the difficulty of refusing) role-plays saying "no." We provide an example below.

JOE: My friends asked me to buy beer for them the other night. I didn't want to buy it for them; I just didn't want to be a part of it. I wasn't going to drink.

ANN: Did you?

JOE: Well, I bought the beer, but I didn't have any. I didn't know what to say.

LEADER: How do you feel about it now?

JOE: I wish I hadn't, but I wanted to hang around with them.

ANN: They aren't much for friends if you can't hang around them unless you buy beer.

JOE: Well, I used to drink with them. They don't understand.

LEADER: We could role-play this situation, and you could practice telling them you don't want to buy beer for them. You may also want to think about how safe it is to be around people who are drinking.

JOE: But they're my friends.

PETER: You can come over to my place if you want to talk to someone who isn't drinking. We can go to an AA meeting sometime, too.

LEADER: You can meet a lot of sober people there. Okay, Joe, how about practicing how you might handle this type of situation if it comes up again?

JOE: Okay.

LEADER: Ann, would you play the role of someone trying to convince Joe to buy the beer?

ANN: Right now?

LEADER: Sure. You two can sit where everyone can see you well. (*The role play is set up.*)

ANN: Hey Joe, we need some beer. Be a good guy and get us a six-pack at the store.

JOE: No, I don't want to.

ANN: Come on, we really need you to.

JOE: (*Speaking to the leader*) I don't know what else to say.

LEADER: Let's make a list of suggestions for Joe on the board. Then I'd like all of you guys to coach him on how to say it like he means business. Let's cheer him on. (*Group makes a list of ways to say "no."*)

LEADER: Okay, let's try that again. Joe, Ann, are you ready?

ANN: Hey, Joe, how about a six-pack, old buddy?

JOE: Sorry, Ann, not tonight.

PETER: Firmer and louder.

STEVE: Be definite.

JOE: Sorry, Ann, I'm not going to buy beer for you any more. (*Group congratulates Joe.*)

Sleep Hygiene Instruction

Problems with sleep—including sleeping too much, sleeping too little, and sleeping at the wrong times—are common in clients with a dual diagnosis. Psychiatric illnesses are often associated with significant sleep disturbances. Individuals with depression may experience problems getting to sleep, staying asleep, or early morning awakenings (or, alternatively, a need for inordinate amounts of sleep). Clients in a manic or hypomanic phase of bipolar disorder often experience a decreased need for sleep. Individuals with schizophrenia commonly reverse the usual sleep cycle by sleeping in the day and being awake all night.

Clients often use substances in an effort to normalize their sleep cycles. The substance use may then become part of the clients' daily routine, such as heavy drinking or marijuana use before going to bed at night. When clients attempt to change their substance use habits, problems with sleep often become even more apparent or emerge for the first time. Focusing a group discussion on direct instruction about sleep hygiene can be a fruitful topic for an active treatment group. Examples of good sleep hygiene habits are provided in Table 10.1, and others can be identified by consulting self-help books on the topic (Catalano, 1990; Hauri & Linde, 1996).

We provide an example below of addressing problematic sleep hygiene in a client. Such discussion can be

TABLE 10.1. Good Sleep Hygiene Habits

- Don't do any work at least 1 hour before going to bed.
- Avoid drinking beverages with caffeine (coffee, some teas, some sodas) at least 5 hours before going to bed.
- Develop a relaxing routine to do for at least 30 minutes before going to bed (reading, listening to music, relaxation exercises, warm bath).
- Don't stay in bed more than 15 minutes if you can't get to sleep; get up and do something relaxing for at least 15 minutes before going back to bed.
- If problems or stressful thoughts bother you, write them down so you can put them aside.
- Go to bed and get up at about the same time each night, even if you got less sleep than you desired the previous night.
- Avoid napping the day after you get a poor night's sleep.
- Exercise regularly, especially in the afternoon.

easily expanded to address similar problems in other group members.

JOE: I just can't get to sleep. I wish I had something to help me get to sleep.

LEADER: Joe, could you share with the group what happens when you try to get to sleep at night?

JOE: Well, I get into bed. I know I'm going to have trouble sleeping, and I just lie there tossing and turning, and I get more and more angry because I can't sleep.

LEADER: What happens when you get angry?

JOE: Then I really can't fall asleep, and that's when I think about having a beer to put me out.

LEADER: Actually, sleep experts recommend that you not stay in bed more than 15 minutes if you can't fall asleep. You can avoid getting angry by getting up and doing something pleasant, like reading or watching TV until you feel tired. Then it will be easier to fall asleep.

JOE: I see.

LEADER: You may find you feel better the next day with a half hour less sleep than if you drink a beer. Alcohol suppresses sleep function, so that one feels less rested the next day.

SUSAN: Sometimes when I can't sleep, I use a relaxation exercise. It really makes me feel sleepy.

Teaching Skills for Coping with Unpleasant Feelings

Persons with dual disorders often experience a range of unpleasant feelings that contribute to their vulnerability to substance use. Teaching members specific skills for coping with feelings of anger, anxiety, restlessness, boredom, and hopelessness can enable them to resist strong temptations to use substances. Clients learn to express anger appropriately, to say what they need to say, and to release anger through exercise. For anxiety and restlessness, group members learn to get relief from social contacts and exercise, and they practice relaxation skills. They can also learn to use positive imagery and to let negative feelings pass, knowing that the feelings are short-lived.

When a group session focuses on coping with unpleasant feelings, leaders help members learn to label and manage the emotional experiences they have been obliterating through drug and alcohol use. They come to appreciate the gradual improvements in their mental health and life stability that come with sobriety. Helping group members develop more effective coping strategies involves both sharing different ideas and teaching specific skills, such as relaxation and imagery exercises. Leaders can further assist clients in managing unpleasant feelings by employing strategies based on the concept of *mindfulness*—that is, helping clients develop the ability to recognize, accept, and tolerate negative feelings, without allowing them to dictate their behavior or dominate their consciousness (Hayes, Strosahl, & Wilson, 1999; Langer, 1989; Linehan, 1993; Segal, Williams, & Teasdale, 2002).

Managing Cravings

Clients in active treatment and relapse prevention often experience strong cravings for alcohol and drugs. When these cravings are related to the experience of negative emotions, the strategies described in the preceding section may be employed. However, cravings can also present a challenge to clients even when they are not directly associated with strong negative feelings. A discussion focused on each member's experience of cravings, and successful strategies members have employed to manage these cravings, can be a useful activity for the group.

One helpful strategy for dealing with cravings is the use of imagery. Members can learn to use imagery to get beyond cravings for substances, and to change positive images of alcohol or drug effects into images of hangovers, withdrawal, psychotic symptom exacerbations, and other negative consequences of substance use. The leaders may actively guide individual clients in developing images to focus on to combat cravings, or may suggest images in the course of the group discussion. We provide an example below of how a leader introduced the use of imagery to a client who reported experiencing difficulties with cravings for alcohol.

JANE: Most of the time I feel fine, but sometimes I'm sitting alone in my apartment and I start thinking about drinking again, and all the good times. I end up craving it. Sometimes it's so strong I could taste it. That's really tough.

LEADER: Do you ever think about the other things that happen when you drink, like getting sick or having a blackout?

JANE: Or fighting with my boyfriend and getting thrown out. That's what happened the last time I drank—I ended up in jail.

LEADER: You might think about those things at home when you're craving for a drink.

JANE: Okay.

LEADER: Let's do a little imagery exercise to help you practice how you can deal with the next time you have a craving to drink. When you think about the different negative experiences you've had related to your drinking, which one jumps to your mind as the worst?

JANE: That time I ended up in jail. Definitely.

LEADER: Okay. Now when you remember that experience—winding up in jail—which part of it stands out most in your mind?

JANE: I remember when they closed the cell door, and the guard walked away, I thought, "Shit, I've really done it this time. What if no one bails me out? What's going to happen to me here?"

LEADER: Good. That's a very clear memory to work with. Now what I'd like you to do, Jane, is to close your eyes and relax a little.

JANE: (*Settles herself in her chair and closes her eyes.*) Okay.

LEADER: Now I'd like you to remember exactly what it was like at the moment when the guard closed the door of your cell in the jail, and you thought those thoughts to yourself. Let me know when you have a good image of that moment.

JANE: Okay. The guard just shut the door.

LEADER: How do you feel?

JANE: Scared. Guilty. Upset.

LEADER: Good. You can open your eyes now. You've just created a very powerful image, Jane, and you can use that image the next time you have a craving to drink. That image will counteract all the positive images you may have about having a drink.

JANE: I think I could do that.

LEADER: Great. Let's talk a little about situations in which you've experienced cravings, so that you can be prepared to use your imagery strategy to combat the craving.

Examining Self-Help Programs

All clients in active treatment groups should be encouraged to consider using available self-help programs in their community as resources for maintaining sobriety, and as sources of social support from other sober people. Many clients use these programs successfully (Noordsy et al., 1996). In active treatment groups, one or more sessions can be devoted to reviewing self-help concepts and discussing the nature of self-help groups in the community, such as AA or NA. Group members benefit from learning more about both the philosophy of self-help programs, and the structure and expectations of a typical self-help meeting.

To familiarize members with the nature of self-help groups, leaders can discuss with group members how meetings are run, conduct a role play of a typical meeting, or invite a member of a self-help program to attend a group session and describe it to the members. In selecting self-help programs as possible options for active treatment group members, leaders should be familiar with the groups, including their attitudes toward people who are taking psychiatric medications. Leaders often stay abreast of the nature of various meetings through the reports of their clients who attend them. This familiarity should prevent a leader from referring a client to a self-help group whose members disapprove of psychopharmacology.

When discussing self-help groups, leaders should bear in mind that many clients either do not participate in these groups or participate only marginally, and leaders must respect their preferences. Active treatment groups can provide their members with an opportunity to learn more about self-help groups, without making attendance at such groups an expectation. More information about the role of self-help groups for clients with dual disorders is provided in Chapter 12.

Developing a Relapse Prevention Plan

Clients in active treatment benefit from anticipating the possibility of a relapse into substance abuse in the future, and developing plans for minimizing such a relapse or its severity. During a group session focused on helping members develop their own relapse prevention plans, leaders can encourage members to share with one another strategies that have and have not been effective in staving off relapses. This sharing of experiences can be combined with providing a basic structure that will enable each member to come up with a personal relapse prevention plan.

Before group members begin working on relapse prevention plans, the leaders can elicit from them reasons why developing such a plan may be helpful. This can be achieved by asking open-ended questions about the benefits of doing this. Next, the leaders can facilitate a brief discussion about each client's most recent potential or actual relapse, including important events that appeared to lead up to the possibility of relapse, and how the client responded to these. Discussion of the most recent relapse (or the successful avoidance of a relapse) is followed by consideration of specific triggers for relapse (negative emotions, substance-using environments, craving) and high-risk situations (e.g., interpersonal conflicts, social situations involving substance use, being alone, getting a paycheck). Each client identifies those triggers and high-risk situations that have been related to his or her substance abuse and relapses in the past.

Following discussion of situations that increase clients' risk of relapse, the leader encourages members to share their thoughts about strategies they can use as alternatives to alcohol or drug use in those situations. It is important that group members determine their own plans for avoiding or dealing with high-risk situations, although they may receive feedback in formulating these plans from other group members and the leaders. These plans can be role-played, to increase clients' resolve to follow through on them and to give them feedback from others on their skills.

Finally, it can be helpful if members consider how they might respond to the early part of a relapse, including a *slip* (i.e., an abstinent client's drinking or using drugs on one occasion, or beginning to use again before experiencing negative consequences), in order to avert a full-blown relapse. The *abstinence violation effect* refers to the tendency of persons with substance use disorders who have achieved abstinence to have rapid, full-blown relapses once a minor amount of alcohol or drug use is resumed (Sobell & Sobell, 1993). Prompting clients to consider how they might respond to the situation of consuming some alcohol or drugs before substance abuse has become severe can avert a major relapse. For example, clients may find it helpful to call another group member, a group leader, a family member, a self-help sponsor, or their case manager in the early stages of a relapse, to request help in preventing a full-blown relapse.

Relapse prevention plans can be developed informally with group members, and each member's plan can be recorded on a standard form provided in Appendix C (see Form C.12). Individuals who have completed relapse prevention plans in their individual work may be invited to bring their plans to the group and to share them with other group members. Clients should also be encouraged to consider sharing their relapse prevention plans with significant others (such as family members), because these individuals can support them and may play a helpful role in averting a relapse. The steps in developing a relapse prevention plan are summarized in Table 10.2.

Dealing with Relapses

Although a major goal of active treatment groups is the prevention of relapses into substance abuse, relapses are nevertheless bound to happen in some clients. Helping members focus on dealing with recent relapses is an important group topic. Members can be encouraged to write down their internal or interpersonal struggles during the week, so that they can work on them in the group. Through this, they often gain a greater sense of responsibility for managing both their psychiatric and their substance use disorders.

The use of the recovery model also helps clients with a dual diagnosis to manage both of their disorders simultaneously. The recovery model involves getting on with life despite chronic illness (Anthony, 1993; Deegan, 1988). Clients with severe mental illness may be caught up in hopelessness about their lives. Years have passed, and the illness remains. When a client with dual disorders begins to see recovery from the substance abuse, some hope develops. The person sees the change and feels a sense of control. Recovering from substance abuse, and the benefits that this brings, are

concrete reminders that one's quality of life can improve despite chronic mental illness.

Clients can learn that they do not have to be cured to continue recovering; that small gains are important; and that strength comes from appreciating both their own and others' progress, no matter how small the gains. Clients come to appreciate that quality of life is measured in life roles and responsibilities, not in diagnostic terms. Focusing on regaining meaningful life roles takes the place of focusing on substance abuse. Slips and relapses are not failures, but opportunities for new learning. Clients see that recovery is not an "all-or-nothing" phenomenon. As the days or weeks of abstinence (or of nonproblematic use) increase, their continuity is bound to improve. Recognizing this "big picture" is crucial for self-efficacy and recovery. Clients must be able to look forward to gradual progress despite temporary setbacks. Acceptance, balanced with hopeful expectations, helps keep the recovery process on course.

The concept of recovery as a journey, rather than a discrete goal, can be expressed through an illustration depicting *Recovery Mountain* (Roberts et al., 1999; Sobell & Sobell, 1993). This illustration shows the process of recovery from substance abuse as similar to climbing a mountain, in which the trip is punctuated by a variety of changes in terrain; these symbolize the various processes of coping skills, warning signs, relapses, and increasing periods of sustained remission. The group leaders can facilitate a discussion of the recovery process by using the Recovery Mountain Worksheet (see Appendix C, Form C.14), in which each member identifies personal warning signs of relapse and coping skills for warding off or minimizing such relapses.

Practicing Relaxation Skills

Helping clients develop skills for relaxation can help them regain control over anxiety and cravings. A variety of different strategies can be taught, such as combining progressive muscle relaxation with pleasant imagery. Members can also use relaxation strategies to manage problems with insomnia.

One of the reasons why clients with dual disorders sometimes have difficulties incorporating new skills into their lives is that they forget to practice these skills. To help clients get into the practice of using relaxation, relaxation exercises combined with either deep breathing or pleasant imagery may be used routinely as a means of closure for active treatment group sessions. In addition to frequent practice of relaxation skills in the group, clients can be encouraged to share with each other personal relaxation strategies they have used successfully, and to develop plans for practicing relaxation skills on

---

TABLE 10.2. Steps in Developing a Relapse Prevention Plan

- Review past experiences with either relapses or near-relapses.
- What situations were associated with relapses?
- What triggers signaled a possible relapse?
- How were major relapses avoided?
- What didn't work in preventing relapses?
- Identify personal "high-risk" situations for a relapse into substance abuse
- Formulate a plan for:
  - Avoiding high-risk situations,
  - Dealing with unexpected or unavoidable high-risk situations.
- Identify specific triggers for possible relapse, such as moods, images, self-statements, or environments.
- Develop a plan for how to respond to triggers for relapse.
- Consider what skills or alternative options you will need to avoid returning to alcohol or drug use:
  - Social skills.
  - Skills for dealing with anxiety, depression, anger.
  - Recreation and leisure activities.
  - Something meaningful to do with your time.
- Identify someone you can contact if you begin to have a relapse (including use of alcohol and drugs), before a full-scale relapse has occurred.
- Share your relapse prevention plan with someone (or more than one) who cares about you.

TABLE 10.3. Resources for Relaxation

Benson, H. (1975). *The Relaxation Response*. New York: Avon.

Charlesworth, E. A., & Nathan, R. G. (1984). *Stress Management: A Comprehensive Guide to Wellness*. New York: Ballantine Books.

Davis, M., Eshelman, E. R., & McKay, M. (1995). *The Relaxation and Stress Reduction Workbook* (4th ed.). Oakland, CA: New Harbinger.

Elkin, A. (2001). *Stress Management for Dummies*. Foster City, CA: IDG Books.

Goudey, P. (2000). *The Unofficial Guide to Beating Stress*. Foster City, CA: IDG Books.

Lehrer, P. M., & Woolfolk, R. L. (Eds.). (1993). *Principles and Practice of Stress Management* (2nd ed.). New York: Guilford Press.

McKay, M. (1997). *The Daily Relaxer*. Oakland, CA: New Harbinger.

O'Hara, V. (1996). *Five Weeks to Healing Stress: The Wellness Option*. Oakland, CA: New Harbinger.

their own. There are many different books and guides for helping people develop relaxation skills. Some recommended resources are listed in Table 10.3.

Increasing Pleasant Activities

Making the transition from a substance-abusing lifestyle to one free of substance use can be difficult as clients reluctantly forgo the immediate pleasures of alcohol and drugs. For some clients, substance use is their primary source of pleasure, and in its absence they may be troubled by boredom, depression, anhedonia, and anxiety. Helping active treatment group members identify and schedule pleasant activities can enable them to meet their basic leisure and recreational needs, and develop habits that will become reinforcing through producing more lasting and genuine pleasure.

A group discussion about increasing pleasant activities can be initiated by exploring with group members the importance of enjoyable activities in their lives, and the need to fill the gap left behind by drug and alcohol

use. This can be followed by a brainstorming activity in which members are encouraged to describe pleasant activities—either ones that they have previously engaged in or ones they might be interested in engaging in. During the discussion, the leaders can emphasize that *positive addictions* are activities that are noncompetitive, do not depend on others, and have some value (physical, mental, or spiritual) for a person. Such positive addictions are valuable substitutes for substance use; individuals can improve their performance with practice, while at the same time accepting their level of performance without self-criticism. Examples of pleasurable activities are provided in Table 10.4.

When members have generated a list of possible pleasant activities, the leader then discusses the importance of scheduling these activities. A major advantage of scheduling pleasant activities is that it increases clients' likelihood of engaging in them, and eventually of making them into routines. Clients are encouraged to set aside a certain amount of personal time each day (e.g., 30–60 minutes) in which they may engage in pleasant activities. The goal of setting aside this time is to achieve a balance between the things the clients should do and those things that they want to do, so that they can feel satisfied with their daily lives. During the group discussion, the leaders can elicit from group members or emphasize that the more fun things people do, the less they will miss alcohol or drugs, and the less vulnerable they will be to a relapse into substance use. An exercise sheet for recording and scheduling different pleasant activities is contained in Appendix C (see Form C.13).

SEPARATE OR COMBINED PERSUASION AND ACTIVE TREATMENT GROUPS?

The persuasion and active treatment approaches described in this and the preceding chapter can be provided within one group or in two separate, sequential

TABLE 10.4. Examples of Pleasurable Activities

Taking a walk	Yoga or meditation
Cooking	Writing (journal, short stories, poetry, a book)
Reading a book	Going to a museum
Learning a sport (golf, tennis, bowling, martial arts, Ping-Pong, skiing)	Joining a club or organization
Going to the gym	Going on the Internet
Running, swimming, or cycling	Listening to music
Sewing, knitting, or crocheting	Playing games (cards, chess, bridge)
Art—painting, sculpture, photography, collage	Home repair
Playing a musical instrument	Woodwork
Singing	Taking a trip to the beach, woods, mountains
Involvement in local theater	Participating in team sports—baseball, basketball, touch football

TABLE 10.5. Advantages of Separate Groups versus Combined Groups for Persuasion and Active Treatment

Advantages of separate groups
- Clients have a better opportunity to be with true peers (those who are in the persuasion stage with others in the persuasion stage, and likewise for clients in active treatment).
- Active treatment functions are kept from overwhelming persuasion functions (and vice versa).
- Clients in the persuasion group can aspire to step up to the active treatment group.
- More frequent meetings are available to individuals who need more.
- Individuals can return to an appropriate group when relapse or relapse prevention indicates.

Advantages of combined groups
- Clients in the persuasion stage have role models in several different stages of recovery.
- Clients in the active treatment stage have a chance to reinforce their progress by serving as role models for people in earlier stages of treatment.
- More clients are available for an effective group process (6 or more are needed).
- Specialty group programming can occur even when an agency has a small number of clients with dual disorders or is just beginning groups.

groups. Even when separate groups are operating, they have considerable overlap in functions. Active treatment usually begins in the persuasion group. On the other hand, the active treatment group may need to return to persuasion functions when a member is in or near relapse. In fact, relapse prevention is a part of ongoing active treatment.

The major differences between the groups are in the members and the activities tailored to their needs. For clients in the active treatment stage of recovery, meeting with others who share the goal of cutting down substance use or maintaining abstinence is supportive. Such clients may find it valuable to meet apart from people who are still actively abusing substances and are working on persuasion. Similarly, persuasion group members may find the lower level of expectation in a persuasion group more tolerable, and this may facilitate their further engagement in treatment.

When an agency is first starting specialty treatment for clients with dual disorders, one group may suffice until several members are prepared to move on to the active treatment phase. Separate groups help to prevent active treatment functions from overwhelming new members, and to prevent persuasion functions from holding back members who are starting to develop healthier lifestyles without substance abuse. On the other hand, separating members into two groups may reduce the size of each group to an ineffective number (less than six members); it may also siphon off the more successful members, who are able to serve as role models to persons who are still in early persuasion.

Members who join the active treatment group may continue to come to the persuasion group as role models, helping to move the group norm in the direction of substance use reduction and abstinence. Clients at this level often benefit from the opportunity to attend both persuasion and active treatment groups. The advantages and disadvantages of conducting combined or separate persuasion and active treatment groups are summarized in Table 10.5.

SUMMARY

Active treatment groups are stage-wise dual-disorder treatments that follow *persuasion groups*. In contrast to persuasion groups, where the focus is on helping members understand the effects of substance abuse on their lives, the focus of active treatment groups is on helping members to reduce their use of substances further, to achieve abstinence (when clients desire this), and to prevent relapses into substance abuse. Reduction of substance abuse and relapse prevention are achieved through a combination of engendering group support for shared goals, developing new skills for dealing with high-risk substance abuse situations, and improving other aspects of members' day-to-day lives. The emphasis on developing more effective skills for dealing with vulnerability to substance abuse and improving one's life leads to a strong focus on cognitive-behavioral strategies in active treatment groups. We have discussed several specific topics and activities for active treatment groups, including social skills training, sleep hygiene instruction, teaching coping skills, managing cravings, examining self-help programs, developing relapse prevention plans, dealing with relapses, practicing relaxation skills, and increasing pleasant activities. We have concluded with a consideration of the relative merits of combining persuasion and active treatment groups into a single group versus conducting separate groups.

11

Social Skills Training Groups

Social skills training groups are aimed at teaching clients specific skills for getting their interpersonal needs met and for handling common situations involving alcohol and drug use. Such groups are focused primarily on teaching particular skills that are important for functioning effectively without alcohol or drugs. In their strong emphasis on skills development, these groups differ from the stage-wise treatment groups discussed in Chapters 9 and 10, which use therapeutic group process as the primary vehicle for change. Social skills training has applicability to a broad range of clients with dual disorders.

In this chapter, we provide clinicians with the necessary ingredients to initiate and conduct social skills training groups for clients with dual disorders. Although we focus on the group format for conducting social skills training in this chapter, the training steps and the curricula are applicable to individual work with clients (such as individual cognitive-behavioral counseling; see Chapter 8). We begin with a discussion of the role of social skills training in integrated treatment for dual disorders, and address which clients are most appropriate for such training. We next review the conceptual foundations of social skills training, and then address logistical aspects and specific procedures for conducting skills training groups. We next discuss strategies for ensuring that skills taught in a group will generalize to clients' natural settings. Then we consider social skills training curricula for clients with dual disorders, and provide guidance concerning strategies for enhancing skill generalization. We conclude with a case example, describing (in somewhat greater detail than in the case examples given to this point in the book) how a client with a dual disorder benefited from participating in a skills training group. More detailed information on organizing

and conducting social skills training groups for clients with psychiatric disorders can be found in Bellack and colleagues (1997), and similar information for clients with addictions can be found in Monti and colleagues (2002).

THE ROLE OF SOCIAL SKILLS TRAINING IN DUAL-DISORDER TREATMENT

Social skills training has a critical role to play in the recovery of many clients from dual disorders, and the application of such training on an individual basis or in stage-wise treatment groups has been alluded to in several earlier chapters (Chapters 6, 8–10). Social skills training groups allow clinicians to focus more extensively on skills development in the context of a supportive milieu, thereby increasing clients' opportunities to practice and acquire the skills required to establish a satisfying and sober lifestyle. Improving social skills is an especially critical goal in the persuasion stage of treatment (when clients lack the motivation to change their substance abuse, and may use substances in order to get their social needs met or to cope with moods and symptoms) and during active treatment (when clients show a desire to work on their substance use problems, but may not have the skills to deal with common social situations involving substances).

The functional assessment (Chapter 4) and functional analysis (Chapter 5) of substance use behavior provide a framework for understanding the potential role of social factors in maintaining substance use for clients in the persuasion and active treatment stages, or in threatening relapses for clients in the active treatment and relapse prevention stages. Social skills training can be used to address those factors. Individuals with dual disorders often use substances in order to gain affiliation and acceptance by others. Several specific social motives are commonly implicated as reinforcing substance use in these clients (Alverson et al., 2001). For some, substance use is a long-standing shared activity among peers, and ongoing use is a natural continuation of those relationships. Others may be socially rejected because of their mental illness, and find acceptance in the social networks of people who abuse substances. Such social networks are often receptive to individuals with dual disorders, who may contribute valuable resources such as money and housing. Still others may use substances to lower their anxiety in social situations, or to deal with other unpleasant feelings that interfere with their relationships with others, such as anger or depression. These costs of reducing substance use (summarized in the bottom right quadrant of the Payoff Matrix, as described in Chapter 5; the Payoff Matrix form itself is provided in Appendix C, Form C.6) may present a barrier to motivating clients to forgo their use of substances in order to develop a healthier lifestyle. Based on the functional analysis, social skills training should be considered as an intervention for clients in the persuasion, active treatment, or relapse prevention stage, to help them develop the necessary skills to satisfy their basic social, mood, and recreational needs without using substances.

In addition to skills for getting their basic needs met, clients in the active treatment or relapse prevention stages benefit from improved skills for handling common social situations in which substance use takes place. Clients who have many substance-using individuals in their social networks have greater difficulty in decreasing their substance abuse over time (Trumbetta et al., 1999). Various social situations may make it difficult for them to resist offers to use substances. For example, friends with whom a client has used substances may resist the notion that he or she has decided to cut down or stop using substances, leading to peer pressure. A client may encounter a drug dealer with whom he or she has done business in the past, who implicitly or explicitly threatens the person to buy drugs. Dealers may even give drugs away at first in an attempt to entice clients and get them hooked again. These types of situations require effective social skills if clients are to be successful in resisting offers or pressure to use substances, and skills training groups can be used to help clients acquire these skills.

The vast majority of clients with a dual disorder can improve their interpersonal skills through participation in social skills training groups. Because almost all clients can benefit from the focus of skills training on improving social relationships, there is no need to con-

duct separate groups for clients at different stages of treatment. The highly structured approach of skills training, the emphasis on mastering specific skills, and the deemphasis on group process as a therapeutic agent results in few conflicts between clients at different stages of treatment. In addition, because the focus of skills training groups is on the development of new skills for a range of different social situations, rather than on group process as in persuasion groups (Chapter 9) and active treatment groups (Chapter 10), clients can benefit from participating in both stage-wise and social skills training groups.

The decision about whether to involve clients in stage-wise treatment groups, social skills training groups, or both should be based on a combination of factors. Many clients with severe mental illness have impaired social skills, especially those with schizophrenia (Bellack et al., 1990; Bellack, Mueser, Wade, Sayers, & Morrison, 1992; Bellack, Sayers, Mueser, & Bennett, 1994), and poor social skills are strongly correlated with poor social functioning (Mueser & Bellack, 1998). Clients with impaired social skills clearly benefit from social skills training, which has been shown to improve social functioning (Dilk & Bond, 1996; Heinssen et al., 2000). Thus the quality of a client's interpersonal functioning, as determined in the functional assessment (Chapter 4), should be the primary determinant of whether the client is engaged in a skills training group.

CONCEPTUAL FOUNDATIONS OF SOCIAL SKILLS TRAINING

Social skills training is based on the assumption that effective social functioning requires the smooth integration of specific component skills. To the extent that individuals have deficits in such skills, their social competence will be diminished. The aim of social skills training is thus to improve clients' social functioning through improving component skills. It is helpful to begin by considering the different types of social skills, as well as non-skill-related factors that can affect social performance.

Types of Social Skills

Effective interpersonal communication and behavior require three broad types of skills: *perceptual*, *cognitive* (or *problem-solving*), and *behavioral* skills (see Figure 11.1). First, in order to be socially effective, an individual must accurately perceive relevant social information in the situation, such as other persons' feelings, their probable motives, and the public or private nature of the situation. Without these necessary perceptual skills,

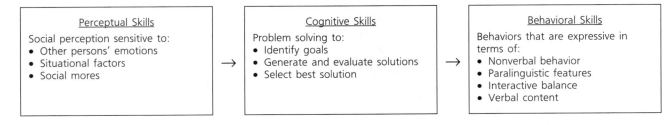

FIGURE 11.1. Three types of skills necessary for effective interpersonal communication and behavior: perceptual, cognitive (problem-solving), and behavioral skills.

inappropriate or insensitive behaviors are more likely to occur. Second, when an individual has accurately "sized up" a social situation, he or she needs cognitive (or problem-solving) skills to decide what to do. These skills involve formulating a goal, identifying possible options for achieving that goal, evaluating the options, and selecting the best option. Effective problem-solving skills set the stage for the behavioral skills that follow.

Third, once a response has been selected, behavioral skills are needed to implement it. Behavioral skills can be divided into several types, including *nonverbal behaviors, paralinguistic features, interactive balance,* and *verbal content.* Nonverbal behaviors include the person's facial expression, posture, eye contact, use of gestures, and interpersonal distance. Paralinguistic features are the vocal qualities of speech, including voice tone (pitch and inflection), loudness, fluency, and affect. The combination of nonverbal behaviors and paralinguistic features is critical to determining the "meaning" and overall effectiveness of communication. For example, an individual who responds to an offer to use alcohol by avoiding eye contact and answering in a meek tone of voice, "No, thank you, I'd rather not have a drink," is more likely to be pressured to drink than is someone who responds with the same words but in a loud, confident, assertive tone of voice, while looking the other person in the eye.

Interactive balance, the natural "give-and-take" of a conversation, is determined by how long it takes to respond to the other person (latency of response) and the amount of total time each person talks. Individuals who take longer to respond verbally to another person often make that person feel uncomfortable or awkward, because the spontaneous ebb and flow of the conversation is constrained. People who interrupt others may also interfere with the conversation by making it feel rushed or clipped. Similarly, the relative amount of time each person spends talking can affect the overall quality and ease of the conversation. If one person dominates the conversation, the lack of reciprocity may make the other person feel left out. Or if one person says very little in response to the other, this passivity may leave the other person feeling that he or she is bearing all the weight of

the conversation, and again lack of reciprocity becomes a problem. For clients with cognitive deficits, especially many clients with schizophrenia, achieving a satisfactory interactive balance can be quite challenging: Their slower speed of information processing increases their latency of response, resulting in an unnaturally slow conversational flow (Mueser, Bellack, Douglas, & Morrison, 1991). Despite these difficulties, extensive practice of conversational skills can help these clients overcome many of their deficits (Matousek, Edwards, Jackson, Rudd, & McMurry, 1992).

The final component of behavioral skill is verbal content, which includes the specific words and phrases that are communicated, independent of how they are said. Verbal content is important, because it conveys the central message the person wants to communicate. The appropriateness of verbal content can be a problem when a client is actively psychotic, or has difficulties judging relevant social features of the situation (e.g., his or her level of familiarity with the other person). For example, disclosing intimate personal information to someone who is not well known can be awkward for the other person, and can lead to social rejection of the discloser. The verbal content of communication is also critical to identifying good topics for conversation. In addition, responding assertively, such as making a request, refusing an offer to use substances, or asking someone to change his or her behavior, requires careful attention to the verbal content of the communication. For example, appropriate use of feeling statements and specificity in referring to another person's behavior, while avoiding a hostile or angry tone of voice, can avoid putting the other person on the defense when one is making a difficult request (e.g., "I would appreciate it if you wouldn't ask me to get high with you"). In social skills training, the verbal content of different communication skills is broken down into component steps, and training focuses on systematically teaching those steps.

The different components of behavioral skills, including nonverbal behaviors, paralinguistic features, interactive balance, and verbal content, are summarized in Table 11.1.

TABLE 11.1. Behavioral Social Skill Components

Nonverbal skills	Interactive balance
Eye contact	Latency of response
Facial expression	Amount of time talked
Interpersonal distance	Responsiveness
Body orientation	
Posture	Verbal content
Gestures	
	Specific verbal message
Paralinguistic features	Use of phrases and choice
	of words
Loudness	
Voice tone	
Affect	
Fluency	
Clarity	

Non-Skill-Related Factors That Can Affect Social Functioning

Although social skills are important for effective communication, not all problems in social functioning are the result of poor social skills. Non-skill-related factors can also influence social performance. If an individual lives in an unsupportive social environment or has access to few resources, poor social functioning may naturally occur. In addition, if the person's environment is not receptive to new social skills, training may not successfully transfer from the group to the natural environment.

Various client characteristics can also influence social functioning, independent of social skill level. Clients with severe depression or anxiety may feel too negative about themselves or be too fearful to initiate or work on improving social relationships. Other problems with motivation, such as anhedonia, may similarly interfere with social adjustment, regardless of a person's actual social skills (Blanchard, Bellack, & Mueser, 1994; Blanchard, Mueser, & Bellack, 1998). Finally, medication side effects, such as drowsiness, can interfere with social adjustment. In particular, *akinesia* (a mask-like appearance lacking facial expressiveness) and *akathisia* (an inner feeling of restlessness associated with nervous behaviors, such as fidgeting and pacing)—both side effects of antipsychotic medications—can make clients with schizophrenia less effective communicators.

Clinicians need to be aware of these non-skill-related factors that can influence social functioning, and (when appropriate) to take steps to minimize or eliminate them. Sometimes those factors interact with social skills training over time. For example, skills training may encourage a depressed individual to try to resolve a conflict with another person, which results in an improvement in mood. Similarly, an unreinforcing social environment may partly reflect a client's own difficulties in obtaining reinforcement from others; as he or she becomes more responsive and enjoyable to interact with, others may reciprocate and become more socially reinforcing.

LOGISTICAL CONSIDERATIONS

Duration and Frequency of Sessions

Social skills training group sessions usually last between 40 and 60 minutes, although longer sessions can be conducted if a break is scheduled in the middle. It is preferable if sessions can be conducted at least twice a week, although once per week is also feasible. Skills training procedures focus on teaching new skills and engaging clients in extensive practice of these skills, resulting in the *overlearning* of skills to the point where they become automatic. Conducting multiple skills training sessions per week provides more opportunity for clients to acquire the rudimentary steps of each skill, with homework assignments outside the session serving to reinforce gains. The focused, positive, and highly structured nature of social skills training makes it possible for clients with a dual disorder to participate in multiple training sessions per week without any negative effects.

Program Length

There is no simple answer to the question to the question of how long a skills training group should be conducted. Bellack and DiClemente (1999) have described a social skills training program for clients with schizophrenia and substance use disorders that is provided over a 6-month period. Roberts and colleagues (1999) have developed a skills training program for helping clients manage substance abuse situations that requires 3–4 months to complete. Jerrell and Ridgely (1995a, 1995b) reported positive effects of a skills training program provided to clients with dual disorders over an 18-month period.

One factor that influences the optimal duration of a skills training group is whether the group focuses on a narrow range of social skills (e.g., skills for managing substance abuse situations) or a broader range of skills (e.g., conversational, friendship, and assertiveness skills, as well as substance abuse situations). (See "Curricula for Social Skills Training," below.) The fewer the skills taught, the shorter the necessary duration of the group. Improved social functioning through skills training (e.g., quality of interpersonal relationships) requires that training be conducted over an extended period of time. For example, the strongest research supporting the effects of skills training for improving social functioning in schizophrenia has involved at least 1 year of intensive training (Liberman et al., 1998; Marder et al., 1996).

Although longer-term skills training is needed to produce lasting benefits, briefer social skills training groups for clients with dual disorders who are hospitalized is feasible and may help them become more aware of the importance of substance abuse in their lives. For example, Mueser, Fox, Kenison, and Geltz (1995) developed a 6-week skills training group for inpatients with dual disorders that included such skills as starting and maintaining conversations, expressing negative feelings, refusing offers to use substances, and problem solving about alternative recreational activities. The inpatient setting offers unique advantages in working with such clients. For example, substance abuse often precipitates hospitalization, increasing the motivation of some clients to address their addictions. In addition, hospitalized clients are readily available to participate in groups, and they tend to have a minimum of programming aimed at psychosocial rehabilitation.

Number of Participants

The optimal number of participants for a social skills training group is between 6 and 8. As few as 2 or 3 clients can participate in a skills training group, and as many as 10. It is critical that each member of the group be given enough time to participate in two to four role plays per session. When the group size exceeds 10 members, it becomes difficult or impossible for all participants to be engaged in role plays in each group session.

Setting

Social skills training groups can be conducted in a wide range of settings, including a mental health center, an inpatient treatment program, a partial hospital or intensive outpatient treatment program, a residential program, or another location in the community. Clients who live together in a group home can participate in skills training sessions provided at their residence. The meeting space should be large enough that the chairs can be arranged in a circle, with enough space in the middle for conducting role plays. The room should also be equipped with a blackboard, easel, flipchart, or other accessories for recording information from the group.

Reinforcement for Participation

Although social skills training groups are often stimulating and fun, they also require clients to make significant efforts to practice the skills and use them on their own. Providing refreshments is one way of reinforcing clients' participation in these groups. Refreshments can be served either during each group session or, if consuming the refreshments interferes with focusing on the skills training, after the session. Participants often enjoy socializing informally with other group members and the leaders over refreshments after a group session has ended. These socialization opportunities also provide leaders with valuable information about members' conversational skills, as well as a more natural setting to practice skills learned in the group.

Leadership

It is best if skills training groups can be conducted by two leaders, although one leader is feasible. Having two leaders makes it easier to ensure that all clients are actively engaged in the group; one leader can assume major responsibility for presenting the skills training curriculum, while the other makes sure that all participants are actively involved in the group and are receiving instructions and feedback tailored to their individual levels of skill.

There are several important qualities involved in good leadership of a social skills training group. Leaders need to be enthusiastic in their work with clients, and able to recognize and reinforce small steps toward desired goals. Leaders also need to be able to take a behavioral approach to skills training, focusing their feedback on the specific skill components that are necessary for effective social interactions. In addition to focusing on behaviors rather than the development of insight, leaders need to be able to engage clients in frequent active role playing, and to avoid lengthy discussions in the group. Finally, because social skills training leaders themselves are important role models for group members, they need to have good social skills.

Orientation of Clients

In order to engage clients in a social skills training group, it is desirable to have at least one individual orientation meeting with each client. This orientation meeting should be conducted by one or both of the leaders. If there is concern that a client will be hesitant about participating in the skills group, and if he or she has a good relationship with another clinician, it can also be helpful if this other clinician also participates in the orientation meeting.

The purpose of the orientation meeting is to explain the rationale for social skills training, to help clients identify personal goals for participating in the group, to describe the nature of skills training (including role playing), and to set positive expectations for participation in the group. The rationale for social skills training can be described as helping people develop skills for making friends, improving relationships with others, dealing with conflict and other problems, and standing up for oneself.

Following a general description of the purpose of skills training, the leader explores with the client specific goals he or she may have for which such training would be helpful. Specific goals vary from one client to the next, and may also depend on a person's stage of treatment. Clients in the persuasion stage are most likely to identify goals related to developing new or better friendships, establishing intimate relationships, or dealing with conflict. Although these goals may also be identified by clients in the active treatment stage, these clients are also more likely to identify substance-abuse-related interpersonal goals, such as dealing with substance abuse situations or developing relationships with non-substance-abusing peers. These goals can be articulated, and the leader can explain how social skills training can help clients achieve them.

When the personal relevance of improved social skills has been established, the leader explains how the social skills training group works, including the meeting times, the focus on learning specific skills (as opposed to engaging in a general discussion), the positive nature of the group (i.e., the emphasis on positive feedback among group members and the avoidance of criticism or negative feedback), and the active use of role playing in all groups. Clients' experiences with role playing are elicited and any remaining questions are answered.

CURRICULA FOR SOCIAL SKILLS TRAINING

Clients with dual disorders can benefit from learning a wide range of interpersonal skills. The types of social skills that can be taught are divided into four broad categories: skills for dealing with substance use situations; conversational and friendship skills; assertiveness and conflict management skills; and problem-solving skills. These skills have a long history of being successfully taught both to clients with severe mental illness (Bellack et al., 1997) and to those with substance use disorders (Monti et al., 2002). We provide a brief synopsis of each of these general skill areas, with more detail about skills for handling substance use situations. For further information about specific curricula for social skills training groups, see Bellack and colleagues (1997), Monti and colleagues (2002), and Roberts and colleagues (1999).

Drink and Drug Refusal Skills

As clients progress from the late persuasion stage though active treatment and relapse prevention, they are invariably confronted with social situations in which

they are offered or pressured to use substances by friends, acquaintances, or drug dealers. Indeed, the number of abstinence supporters in the social networks of clients with a dual disorder is predictive of the likelihood that they will reduce or eliminate substance abuse (Trumbetta et al., 1999). Although many such social situations may be avoided, the ability of clients to resist offers to use substances is key to their success in cutting down on use or achieving abstinence.

Table 11.2 summarizes five different skills, including their component steps, for dealing with offers or pressure to use substances. Clients often have multiple occasions to use these skills, and many situations require a combination of skills. Not all of the skills (and not all steps of each skill) are appropriate for every situation involving substance abuse. For example, when a client encounters a drug dealer who offers or pressures the client to use, repeated refusal and leaving the situation are effective, but suggesting an alternative activity is not. Clients are encouraged to practice the different skills in role plays, and to discuss the situations in which each skill might be useful.

Skills training groups may include clients in the persuasion stage who are not yet motivated to reduce their substance use. With these clients, the leader

---

TABLE 11.2. Skills for Refusing Alcohol or Drugs, and Their Component Steps

Direct refusal
- Say "no" first.
- Suggest an alternative.
- Request the person to stop asking if he or she persists.
- Avoid making excuses.

Repeated refusal ("broken record").
- Say "no" first.
- Keep saying "no" each time the person offers.
- Point out that you have already said "no" to the offer.

Providing an explanation (leveling)
- Say "no" to the offer.
- Explain why you are choosing not to use any more.
- Refer to problems with health, mental health, or other consequences of substance use.

Expressing a negative feeling (for persistent offers)
- Tell the person how you feel when you are pressured to use substances.
- Explain your intention not to use substances.
- Request that the other person stop.
- Suggest an alternative (optional).

Leaving the situation
- Explain that you find the situation stressful.
- Tell the person you need to leave.
- Tell the person you would be happy to see the person later, in a different situation (optional).

should invite them to participate in the role plays, but should not pressure them to participate. Clients in the persuasion stage are often willing to practice substance refusal skills in role plays, despite their ambivalence about cutting down. Clients who resist practicing these skills can be involved in role plays in which they play the role of the other person inviting someone to use substances. These clients can then be asked to critique the role-play performance of other clients at resisting offers to use substances, and asked for suggestions about how they can be more effective. Positively engaging clients in the persuasion stage on the topic of dealing with substance use situations, without putting pressure on them to adopt an abstinence stance, sometimes results in increasing their motivation to work on their substance abuse.

Conversational and Friendship Skills

Substance use often occurs in social situations. Simply refusing offers to use substances in these situations is a difficult task, especially since such refusals may meet with disapproval or downright rejection. For many clients, success in cutting down on substance use or achieving abstinence requires developing alternative social outlets with people who do not use substances. Conversational and friendship skills are needed to help these clients develop new and meaningful relationships in their lives.

Developing new relationships requires basic skills in conversation, such as beginning and ending conversations, identifying high-interest topics, and monitoring the level of self-disclosure (e.g., not disclosing too much personal information to a new or casual acquaintance). Friendship skills involve learning how to spend enjoyable times with another person, sharing positive feelings, and (for intimate relationships) expressing affection. Examples of conversational and friendship skills that can be targeted for clients with dual disorders are provided in Table 11.3. The specific steps of these skills, as well as suggestions for establishing the rationale for each skill, examples of role-play situations, and hints to

leaders in teaching each skill, are provided in Bellack and colleagues (1997).

Assertiveness and Conflict Management Skills

Clients with dual disorders often experience problems in asserting themselves and handling conflicts with others. *Assertiveness* generally refers to the ability to "stick up for oneself," including making requests of others and responding to requests from others in a manner that is consistent with one's own preferences and respectful of the other person. *Conflict management* skills are aimed at facilitating a mutual exchange of views with another person without allowing negative feelings to escalate, and, when appropriate, striving to reach a compromise that is satisfactory to both parties. Problems with assertiveness and conflict management may contribute to substance abuse, as described in the two clinical vignettes below.

CASE EXAMPLE

Charlotte had decided that she wanted to stop drinking, but she had difficulty turning down offers to go to parties with her friends. Her friends were sympathetic to her goal of not drinking, but saw no problem with her coming to parties and "just saying no." However, when Charlotte came to a party, she often changed her mind and started drinking. Social skills training focusing on assertiveness enabled Charlotte to resist her friends' invitations to go to parties, and thereby to avoid difficult drinking situations.

CASE EXAMPLE

Julio had disagreements with his wife, which would often lead to shouting matches and even occasional pushing and shoving. Julio would often end the conflict by walking out. He would then engage in a retaliatory bout of smoking crack or snorting speed. Improving Julio's skills at managing conflicts with his wife helped him decrease his binges of drug use.

TABLE 11.3. Conversational and Friendship Skills

Conversational skills	Friendship skills
Listening to others	Expressing positive feelings
Starting conversations	Giving compliments
Maintaining conversations by asking questions	Accepting compliments
Maintaining conversations by giving information	Finding common interests
Maintaining conversations by expressing feelings	Asking someone for a date
Ending conversations	Expressing affection

Assertiveness and conflict management skills are summarized in Table 11.4. Further details about these skills can be found in Bellack and colleagues (1997).

Problem-Solving Skills

Good social skills increase the chances of being successful in social encounters, but even the most skillful person may be confronted with situations in which good skills appear not to work. In addition, people, including clients with dual disorders, often experience problems in which an important part of their task is to decide *what* to do before determining *how* to do it. Teaching problem-solving skills provides clients with a standard, structured format for handling any of the wide variety of problems they may face. Clients can use problem solving on their own to deal with problems in the social skills group, with their clinicians, or with significant others (such as family members).

The sequence of problem-solving skills is outlined in Table 11.5, and a problem-solving form is provided in Appendix C (see Form C.20). When problem-solving skills are taught to a group, the rationale for these skills is established in the same manner as with other social skills. However, instead of conducting role plays, the leader introduces the group to the sequence of skills, leading the group members through solving a problem shared by some of the group members. Homework assignments can involve having clients identify suitable problems and work on them independently. Although some clients are successful in this, others benefit more from working on problems in the group, where they can receive feedback and suggestions from others.

There is an extensive clinical literature on training problem-solving skills. More information about problem-solving training (in a the family format) is contained in Chapter 14 of this book. Other useful references about problem-solving training include D'Zurilla and Nezu (1999), Mueser (1998), Nezu and Nezu (1989), and Nezu, Nezu, and Perry (1989).

TABLE 11.4. Assertiveness and Conflict Management Skills

Assertiveness skills	Conflict resolution skills
Making requests	Expressing negative feelings
Refusing requests	Compromise and negotiation
Making complaints	Disagreeing without arguing
Responding to complaints	
Asking for information	
Making apologies	

TABLE 11.5. Sequence of Problem-Solving Skills

1. Defining the problem
2. Brainstorming possible solutions
3. Evaluating each solution
4. Selecting the best solution (or combination of solutions)
5. Planning how to implement the solution, and implementing it
6. Following up the success of the solution, and conducting additional problem solving if necessary

SOCIAL SKILLS TRAINING PROCEDURES

Social skills training groups usually follow a standard set of procedures. Several group sessions are usually devoted to teaching each particular skill. The first session in which a skill is introduced begins with a discussion of the importance of learning that skill, followed by a review of the specific behavioral components of that skill. Then the leaders model the skill in a role play. After the skill has been demonstrated, each participant practices it in several role plays. Each role play is followed by positive feedback from the group and constructive suggestions for improvement. After each client has practiced the skill, the clients are assigned homework to practice the skill on their own.

The next group session begins with a review of homework. Each participant is asked to identify situations in which he or she tried to use a skill, or could have used a skill but forgot. These situations are then enacted in role plays, in which clients practice the skills and receive feedback after each role play as before. Between one and three follow-up social skills training sessions are typically spent helping clients master a specific skill.

The Steps of Social Skills Training: Introducing a New Skill

The specific steps of introducing a new skill in a social skills training session are summarized in Table 11.6 and are described below.

Establishing a Rationale for the Skill

In order to motivate clients to learn a particular skill, a rationale for that skill must first be established. Because members often share a great deal of collective wisdom, the rationale can be elicited by stimulating a discussion with open-ended questions, such as "Why do you think it might be important to be able to make requests of another person?" or "What typically happens when you make a demand of someone, or when someone else de-

TABLE 11.6. Steps for Introducing a New Social Skill

1. Establishing a rationale for the skill
   - Elicit reasons for learning the skill from group participants.
   - Acknowledge all contributions.
   - Provide additional reasons not mentioned by group members.

2. Discussing the steps of the skill
   - Break down the skill into three or four steps.
   - Write the steps on a board or poster.
   - Discuss the reason for each step.
   - Check for understanding of each step.

3. Modeling the skill in a role play
   - Plan the role play in advance.
   - Explain that you will demonstrate the skill in a role play.
   - Use two leaders to model the skill (when possible).
   - Keep the role play simple.

4. Reviewing the role play with the members.
   - Discuss whether each step of the skill was used in the role play.
   - Ask group members to evaluate the effectiveness of the role model.
   - Keep the review brief and to the point.

5. Engaging a client in a role play
   - Start with a client who is more skilled than others or is likely to be compliant.
   - Request the client to try the skill in a role play of the same (or a similar) situation with one of the leaders.
   - Ask the client questions to make sure he or she understands the goal.
   - Instruct group members to observe the client.

6. Providing positive feedback
   - Elicit positive feedback from group members about the client's performance.
   - Encourage specific feedback.
   - Postpone corrective feedback, and cut off any negative feedback.
   - Praise effort and provide hints to group members about good performance.

7. Providing corrective feedback
   - Elicit suggestions for how the client could do the skill better next time.
   - Limit the feedback to one or two suggestions.
   - Strive to communicate the suggestions in a positive, upbeat manner.

8. Engaging the client in another role play of the same situation
   - Request that the client change one behavior in the role play.
   - Ask the client questions to check on his or her understanding of the suggestion.
   - Work on behaviors that are most salient and changeable.

9. Providing additional feedback
   - Be generous but specific when providing positive feedback.
   - Focus first on the behavior that the client was requested to change.
   - Engage client in two to four role plays, with feedback after each one.
   - Use other behavior-shaping strategies to improve skills, such as coaching, prompting, and supplemental modeling.

(Steps 5–9 are repeated for each client.)

10. Assigning homework
   - Give an assignment to practice the skill.
   - Tailor the assignment to each individual client.
   - Ask group members to identify situations in which they could use the skill.

mands something from you?" Leaders can offer any reasons for learning the skill that clients do not volunteer.

Social skills training groups for clients with dual disorders may include members at different stages of treatment with different levels of motivation to work on their substance abuse. Therefore, when the rationale for learning an interpersonal skill is being established, it is useful to prompt group members to consider the relevance of that skill to improving their social relationships (for clients at all stages of treatment), as well as to reducing substance use or maintaining abstinence (for clients in the active treatment or relapse prevention stages). We provide a brief example below of establishing the rationale for the skill of starting a conversation.

LEADER: Why do you think it might be helpful to be able to start a conversation with someone you don't know?

DUANE: It's a way of getting to know people.

LEADER: Right! What's so good about getting to know other people?

JULIE: Making friends. Everyone needs friends.

LEADER: That's a good point, Julie. Being able to start conversations is the first step toward making friends, and everyone needs friends.

SHARON: I feel lonely because I don't hang out with my friends much these days. I found it just too hard since I stopped using—we always used to drink and get high together.

LEADER: I see. How do you think starting conversations might help you with your goal of remaining abstinent?

SHARON: Maybe I could make some new friends.

Discussing the Steps of the Skill

After the rationale for the skill has been developed, the leaders break it down into component steps and discuss each step. These steps are displayed on a poster, blackboard, or flipchart. For example, the skill of starting a conversation can be broken down into the following four steps: (1) choosing the right time and place; (2) introducing yourself or greeting the person you want to talk with; (3) making small talk (e.g., about the weather, sports); and (4) deciding whether the other person is listening or wants to talk.

The leaders can elicit from group members the importance of each step of the skill by asking questions, similar to the manner in which the rationale for the skill is developed. This process involves the members in considering the basic elements of the skill, while breaking it down into manageable steps. We continue with

our example of the group learning the skill of starting conversations.

LEADER: I have found that it can be helpful to break a difficult skill down into smaller steps. The steps of starting a conversation can be broken down into four steps. The first step is choosing the right time and place (*pointing to the flipchart*). Why is do you think this step is so important?

SHARON: So you don't blow it.

LEADER: Yes, trying to start a conversation at the wrong time or place can be unsuccessful because it's not convenient for the other person. Does anyone want to add to what Sharon said?

EDDIE: I find it hard to start conversations, because I'm never sure what's a good time, and I never know what to say.

JULIE: Me too.

LEADER: I understand. That's a pretty common problem that we can work on here. Let's spend a little time talking about good times and places where you can start conversations with people. I'll make a list of the different ideas on the flipchart. . . . (*After the leader identifies good times and places to start conversations, he reviews the other steps of the skill, generating high-interest topics for conversation starters.*)

Modeling the Skill in a Role Play

Demonstrating the skill in a role play brings life to the individual steps of the skill. In modeling the skill, it is important for the leaders to make it clear that a role-play demonstration will be conducted, as well as to indicate when the role play begins and when it ends. These things can be accomplished with explicit statements; in addition, it is helpful if the leaders get out of their seats and go to a place in the room designated for role playing (e.g., in the center of the circle of chairs). Then, when the role play is completed, the leaders can return to their chairs to discuss the demonstration with the group members. Before the role play commences, members are instructed to observe the leaders to see the different steps of the skill.

In selecting role-play situations, the leaders should take care to choose plausible, everyday situations that group members are likely to encounter. The leaders should be prepared to demonstrate a preplanned situation, although this can be changed, depending on the group discussion preceding the role play. Most role plays should be short, lasting 1 or 2 minutes, although longer role plays are warranted as members' skills develop and more complex skills and difficult situations are addressed (e.g., conflict management skills, dealing with pressure to use drugs, problem solving).

We continue with our group as the leaders model the skill of starting a conversation.

LEADER A: We are now going to demonstrate the steps of starting a conversation in a role play. Let's pretend that I am a member of the local drop-in center, and I've noticed that a new person has begun to attend the center. I am interested in starting a conversation with her. Yvonne [Leader B] will be the other person in this role play. Let's say that Yvonne is in the dayroom, she came in a few minutes ago, and she's reading a magazine. Do you think that would be a good situation for me to try and start a conversation?

DUANE: Sure, she's not too busy.

LEADER A: Okay. We're going to move into the middle of the circle to do the role play. I'd like everyone in the group to watch me and see which of the steps of "starting a conversation" you see me doing.

JULIE: All right.

LEADER A: Good. Let's start the role play now. (*The leaders move into the center of the room and begin the role play.*)

LEADER A: (*Walks up to Leader B.*) Hi, my name's Jim. I come here sometimes, but I haven't met you before.

LEADER B: Hello, I'm Selma. I just moved here, and someone mentioned that this would be a good place to visit.

LEADER A: I think there are some nice things about this center. Sometimes I come here just to hang out, but there's other things to do here as well.

LEADER B: Like what?

LEADER A: Like taking trips. And the food's pretty good, too! It's fun to help out cooking the meal sometimes.

LEADER B: Sounds good. Thanks for filling me in.

LEADER A: Sure. Okay, let's stop the role play here. (*The leaders resume their seats.*)

Reviewing the Role Play with the Members

After the role play is completed, each step is reviewed (one leader points to it on the flipchart), and the overall effectiveness of the leader modeling the skill is evaluated. The review of the role play can be quite succinct, lasting just a few minutes. Group members are encouraged to be as specific as possible when giving feedback

to the leaders. Leaders can prompt particular members by asking them specific questions about steps of the skill, to ensure their attention to the demonstration.

LEADER A: What did you like about how I did that role play? Which of the steps of starting a conversation did you see me doing?

EDDIE: You said who you were.

LEADER A: Yes, I introduced myself with something like, "Hi, my name's Jim." What else? Did I make small talk?

SHARON: Yes, you did.

LEADER A: Right. What was the topic that I actually talked about? (*Leader A then reviews the rest of the steps of the role play, and asks the group members to rate his overall effectiveness in starting the conversation.*)

Engaging a Client in a Role Play

Immediately after the leaders model the skill in a role play and everyone reviews the performance, a leader engages a client in a similar role play. It is best to use the same situation for this role play as the one just modeled by the leaders, or a very similar situation. The advantage of using the same situation rather than a different one is that it places the least load on clients' cognitive capacity to learn the skill. As clients gain familiarity with the skill, role-play situations can be selected from their own experiences.

A leader tells clients that he or she would like to give them a chance to practice the skill, and then selects a client (or asks for volunteers). The client is instructed to try to use the skill in the role play, just as the leader demonstrated it in the preceding role play. Minor adjustments can be made to the situation for each client to make it more realistic, based on input from the client.

LEADER A: I'd like you to have a chance to practice this same skill in a role play. Sharon, how about if we start with you?

SHARON: Okay.

LEADER A: Good. Let's use the same situation. For this role play we will pretend that you sometimes attend the local drop-in center, and that you have recently noticed a new person at the center, Yvonne [Leader B]. Does this seem like a realistic situation to you?

SHARON: I guess so. I've gone to the drop-in center a few times.

LEADER A: That's fine. Let's stick with that situation. In this role play, your task is to start up a conversation with Yvonne, following the steps you just saw me demonstrate. Yvonne will pretend to be reading a magazine a few minutes after coming into the center. Any questions?

SHARON: Nope.

LEADER A: Okay, let's get you and Yvonne into position for the role play. (*Sharon and Leader B move into position.*) Let's start the role play now.

SHARON: (*Approaches Leader B.*) Hello, how are you? (*Avoids eye contact.*)

LEADER B: Okay. How about you?

SHARON: I'm okay, I guess. Are you new around here?

LEADER B: Yes. I moved here a few months ago, and my case manager suggested I check this place out.

SHARON: It's a decent place. What do you think about the weather?

LEADER B: I'm glad that spring has finally arrived.

SHARON: Yes, the winter seems to last forever around here . . . (*Sharon and Leader B talk a little more about the weather, and the role play ends.*)

Providing Positive Feedback

Role plays are always followed by providing positive feedback to the client about which aspects of his or her performance were done well. Giving positive feedback immediately after the role play reinforces the client for his or her effort in trying the skill. Providing specific feedback lets the person know exactly which component behaviors were performed best.

Positive feedback can be elicited from group members by asking questions and reminding them of the steps of the skill. Corrective feedback is postponed until the positive feedback has been given. After the first few sessions of social skills training, clients usually learn that positive feedback always precedes corrective feedback, and little prompting is required to maintain this norm. (*Purely negative feedback, of course, should be avoided altogether.*)

LEADER A: (*Addressing the group*) What did you like about the way Sharon started a conversation in her role play with Yvonne?

DUANE: She just went right in and said "Hi."

LEADER A: I agree, Duane. Sharon, you did a nice job of greeting Yvonne just then. What else did you like about Sharon's performance? Julie, what did you think?

JULIE: (*Talking to Sharon*) I thought you talked about a good topic. The weather. There's always something to say.

LEADER A: Yes, that got the conversation going . . . (*The leader elicits more praise from other group members about the steps of the skill that Sharon performed well.*)

Providing Corrective Feedback

After positive feedback has been provided, the leader elicits (or directly provides) constructive suggestions to the client about how to improve his or her skill performance. (Again, outright criticism is avoided.) These suggestions may refer to specific steps of the skill, or to paralinguistic features or nonverbal behavior that would contribute to the overall effectiveness of the person in the social encounter. Suggestions for improvement need not be exhaustive, and should be limited to a few key points. Sometimes group members may disagree about a particular suggestion, which can prompt a brief discussion, with group consensus determining the importance of the point.

LEADER A: Does anyone have any suggestions for how Sharon could improve her performance of the skill "starting conversations"?

EDDIE: She looked kind of shy.

LEADER A: That's a good point, Eddie. Could you be a little more specific for Sharon? What did Sharon do in that role play that made her look shy?

EDDIE: (*Speaking to Sharon*) You didn't look at Yvonne very much.

SHARON: I know. I always feel awkward when meeting people.

LEADER A: Yes, avoiding eye contact is a common difficulty people have when they're meeting someone. Any other suggestions? Julie, did Sharon introduce herself?

JULIE: I don't think so.

LEADER A: I don't think so, either. Sharon, in this role-play situation, you had never met Yvonne, so introducing yourself is another suggestion for how you could do this skill even better.

SHARON: Yes, I forgot to do that.

Engaging the Client in Another Role Play of the Same Situation

The primary objective of providing corrective feedback is to give the client an opportunity to improve his or her skill in a subsequent role play. After obtaining suggestions from other group members for improvements, the leader asks the client to try the role play again, and this time to make one or two changes based on the corrective feedback. The request is made by the leader in an upbeat, encouraging manner.

The decision as to which behavior(s) to focus on changing is based on how salient the behavior (or its absence) is, and how changeable the behavior appears to be. The *salience* of a behavior refers to how critical the behavior is to the overall performance of the skill. For example, if the client speaks so quietly that he or she can barely be heard by the other person, focusing on improving the loudness of his or her voice tone is a crucial next step. However, some behaviors are less changeable than others. For example, blunted affect (diminished facial expressiveness and lack of tonal variation in the voice) is a common symptom of schizophrenia that is difficult to improve through social skills training (Matousek et al., 1992).

LEADER A: Sharon, you got some good feedback from the other members. I'd like you to try this same role play with Yvonne again, and this time to work on your eye contact.

SHARON: Okay, but I feel uncomfortable looking at someone's eyes, and I get flustered and don't know what to say.

LEADER A: I see. One helpful hint is that you don't have to look right into the other person's eyes when you're talking, but just in the general direction. For example, looking at the person's forehead or nose is close enough.

SHARON: I'll try. (*Sharon and Leader B get up and conduct another role play of the same situation.*)

Providing Additional Feedback

Like the first role play, the second role play (and any others that ensue) are followed by providing additional positive and corrective feedback. In eliciting positive feedback, special attention is given to feedback about component skills that the leader requested the client to modify, if some improvements were evident. Positive feedback is also given about other components of the skill that were performed well.

Clients sometimes have difficulty improving their social skill performance on the basis of verbal feedback alone. In such cases, the leader has several options to help the client learn the targeted skills. First, the leader can use additional *modeling* to demonstrate the skill for the client, this time instructing the client to pay special attention to a particular behavior. This is followed by the client's trying the skill again in a role play. Second, the leader can use *coaching* (i.e., whispering verbal prompts to the client during the role play) to help the client use the skill, and then fade the coaching in subsequent role plays.

Third, the leader can arrange with the client to provide *nonverbal prompts* during the role play, in order to remind him or her to focus on a particular component skill (e.g., motioning his or her thumb up to instruct the client to speak more loudly). Fourth, the leader can illustrate the importance of a particular component skill by *discrimination modeling*, in which two role plays are performed by the leader in quick succession—the first highlighting a poor performance of the skill, and the second highlighting a good performance. Following a brief discussion of the difference between the role plays, the client is encouraged to try the role play again, paying special attention to improving that component skill. Further information on techniques for improving social skills can be found in Bellack and colleagues (1997).

Between two and four role plays are usually done with each client. The most important considerations are that each client demonstrate at least some improvement in skill from the first to the last role play, and that all clients' experience of role playing is a positive one. Thus clients feel good as their skills improve over successive role plays.

LEADER A: You did a great job in that role play, Sharon. I especially liked your good eye contact with Yvonne.

SHARON: Thanks,

LEADER A: (*Addressing other group members*) What else did you like about Sharon's performance just then?

DUANE: She seemed a little more comfortable this time. And she talked about a good topic, the weather. (*Other group members give Sharon feedback, and both leaders thank her for her participation in the role plays.*)

When one client has completed some role plays, a leader engages another client in a similar role play (step 5). Just as with the first client, a series of role plays is conducted, with each role play followed by positive and corrective feedback and, if necessary, the use of additional behavior-shaping strategies (e.g., coaching, additional modeling) (steps 6–9). This process is conducted until all clients have participated in at least two role plays.

Assigning Homework

At the end of the session, the leaders give the members an assignment to practice the skill in situations which they encounter in their own lives. Homework assignments are most likely to be followed through when the leaders (1) ask clients to anticipate possible situations in which they could use the skill, and (2) individualize the assignment for each client. For example, at the end of the first session on "starting conversations," the leaders could ask each group member to identify one or two situations in which he or she could practice this skill, and make note of each situation in order to follow up the assignment in the next session.

Consolidating Social Skills in Follow-up Sessions

After a skill has been introduced, follow-up sessions on the same skill begin with a review of the homework assignment. Clients are asked to describe situations they encountered in which they had an opportunity to try to use the skill. Clients who did not remember to use the skill in an appropriate situation are encouraged to identify and describe situations in which they could have used the skill.

When a situation has been identified and briefly described by a client, the leader asks him or her to help set up a role play to show the group what actually happened. In setting up this role play, the client is given freedom and help to recreate the situation. This may include choosing someone else to participate in the role play who reminds the client of the other person, rearranging furniture, or the like. The client should also give enough information to the other person in the role play so he or she knows how to play the part correctly. When the situation has been recreated, the client is asked to show what happened in the role play. A client who forgot to use the skill can be instructed to demonstrate in the role play how he or she could have used the skill.

The role play is completed; then, just as in the session in which a new skill is introduced, specific positive feedback is provided, followed by corrective feedback. Usually the client participates in one or two more role plays, each followed by feedback (and, if necessary, other teaching strategies). A discussion is also held with the client about the success of his or her attempt to use the skill (i.e., whether it achieved the desired consequence). When the client describes and shows appropriate use of the skill, but reports not being successful in achieving his or her goal, group members are involved in a problem-solving discussion to explore possible reasons for the lack of success, and to determine whether other options exist. Clients are informed that although better social skills improve one's chances for success, they do not guarantee success. Often this discussion leads to alternative solutions to the situation that end up being successful.

Some clients have great difficulty identifying personal situations in which they can practice a skill. For such a client, a leader (in conjunction with the client) can either use a situation described by another client, or use a situation that the client anticipates might happen in the future. The important goal of follow-up sessions is to give each client ample opportunity to practice the social skill in a variety of role plays, based on situations that have high personal relevance. As some clients become very adept at using skills, the leaders can make the situations even more challenging to help them hone the skills further. For example, a client who has learned skills for refusing offers to use alcohol can be engaged in a role play in which he or she is repeatedly badgered to drink by a "friend" who just won't take "no" for an answer.

The decision to move on to another skill is based on two main considerations. First, have most of the group members demonstrated significant progress toward acquiring the skill? And second, are group members becoming restless, suggesting that it is time to move on? Regardless of the exact number of training sessions spent on a skill, it is helpful to review skills previously taught, and to prompt clients to use those skills in later sessions when they describe appropriate situations.

STRATEGIES FOR ENHANCING GENERALIZATION

In addition to prompting and encouraging clients to follow through on their homework assignments, several strategies can be used to enhance generalization of skills from the training session to clients' real lives. First, community trips can be organized to give clients opportunities to practice their skills in natural settings, but with support and feedback from other group members. Second, other clinicians (e.g., case managers), residential workers, or significant others (e.g., relatives) can be informed about the nature and purpose of the skills training group and the specific skills being taught, so that they can prompt clients to use the skills in appropriate situations. In order for these individuals to prompt skills in appropriate situations, they need to be familiar with the skills that are taught in the group. This can be accomplished by conducting regular meetings in which the skills are reviewed, and appropriate situations for using the skills are discussed. Research shows that involving significant others in helping clients practice skills outside training sessions improves skills generalization and overall social functioning (Tauber, Wallace, & Lecomte, 2000).

Community trips, staff members, and significant others are useful for facilitating the generalization of basic conversation skills and sometimes conflict management skills. However, these strategies are less useful with substance abuse situations, which tend to occur privately, in the absence of others involved in a client's treatment. Extensive practice of skills for dealing with substance use, combined with exploring ways of avoiding such situations, is the best way of helping clients manage these situations.

CASE EXAMPLE

We provide a case example of a client whose participation in a social skills training group played a critical role in her recovery from substance abuse.

Claudia was a 42-year-old woman with a psychiatric diagnosis of major depression with psychotic features, as well as an extensive history of cocaine and alcohol abuse. During her depressive episodes (which were frequent and severe), she often experienced auditory hallucinations of a voice telling her to join her deceased mother, which led to several suicide attempts. Claudia used cocaine daily, often with a circle of friends who also used cocaine; she tended to use alcohol on her own. Her substance abuse precipitated her depressive symptoms, resulting in hospitalizations, and contributed to high levels of conflict with her relatives, especially when she was living with them. Claudia sometimes lived with her sister, sometimes with her brother, and at other times with friends.

Following a suicide attempt and hospitalization, Claudia was referred to a specialty dual-diagnosis service at her mental health center. During the first 2 months, assertive outreach was used to engage her in treatment and to help her develop a working relationship with her treatment team. Then, in the third month after her referral, Claudia began participating in a persuasion group (Chapter 9). A month later, she also began participating in a social skills training group for clients with dual disorders.

Within a month of joining the social skills group, Claudia had become an active participant. She often volunteered for role plays, and expressed a strong interest in improving her skills for handling a range of social situations. Claudia worked in the skills group on two situations related to substance abuse: dealing with pressure to buy or use cocaine from former dealers, and responding to pressure to "join in" when she was around her old friends with whom she had used cocaine or alcohol. Claudia also worked on improving her skills in several situations not directly related to substance abuse, including handling difficulties with family members (e.g., compromise and negotiation, problem solving) and expressing her feelings more openly, including both positive and negative feelings. In addition to participat-

ing in many role plays to improve her own skills, Claudia encouraged other members to practice their skills, made suggestions for how to handle difficult situations, and offered to play the other person in role plays. Her active participation added much to the group as a whole, and inspired other clients to learn new skills for dealing with the social challenges they faced related to substance abuse.

Claudia began to decrease her cocaine and alcohol use within 2 months of joining the social skills group, and over the next 6 months she achieved abstinence from cocaine. She continued to use alcohol occasionally, but experienced no problems related to it. A year and a half after Claudia joined the skills group, her cocaine and alcohol use disorders continued to be in remission; her insight and judgment were improved; and she was motivated to maintain her abstinence from cocaine. Claudia's recovery from addiction also helped her psychiatric illness; she did not have a relapse of her depression or a hospitalization for more than a year after going into recovery.

SUMMARY

Social skills are the perceptual, cognitive, and behavioral skills necessary to be effective in social situations. Clients with dual disorders can benefit from improved social skills for several reasons. They may use substances in social situations because they have difficulty resisting offers to use substances, because they lack the skills needed to establish relationships with people who do not use, or because they have few other outlets for recreation and leisure. Skills training is used to help clients improve their skills in all of these areas. Clients who are in the persuasion, active treatment, or relapse prevention stage can benefit from social skills training groups. Clients in skills training groups can also participate in other dual-diagnosis groups, such as stage-wise groups (persuasion or active treatment groups) or self-help groups.

Social skills training groups are highly structured, usually meet more than once a week, are organized around preplanned curricula, and focus on teaching skills based on the principles of leaning. Skills training sessions use extensive modeling by the leaders, role playing by members, and positive and corrective feedback to members to help them improve their skills. Homework assignments are given for clients to practice the skills on their own. Generalization is facilitated by community trips to practice skills *in vivo*, and by involving significant others and treatment staff members so that they can prompt clients to use the skills in appropriate situations.

12

Self-Help Groups

Self-help groups, such as Alcoholics Anonymous (AA), have a long tradition of helping people recover from substance use disorders. Furthermore, many treatment programs for substance abuse have the goal of linking clients to self-help organizations available in their communities. Although self-help approaches are widely accepted as useful for people with addictive disorders, attempts to involve clients with dual disorders in these groups pose a variety of problems. For example, early in treatment many clients do not endorse abstinence as a personal goal, in conflict with the membership expectations of most self-help organizations. In addition, clients with dual disorders often feel uncomfortable at self-help meetings, and they may have difficulty relating to other group members. Despite these and other problems, many clients can benefit from participating in self-help groups, provided that appropriate steps are taken to link them to such groups.

This chapter begins with a discussion of the role of self-help groups in recovery from dual disorders. We then describe the history and nature of AA (and similar *Twelve-Step approaches*), since AA is the best-known and most widely available self-help group in the world, and the one to which clients with a dual disorder have the greatest access. Then we discuss common difficulties clients with dual disorders experience in AA and similar Twelve-Step self-help groups; this is followed by a description of self-help groups that are alternatives to the traditional Twelve-Step approach. We conclude with practical guidelines for involving clients in self-help groups, and with a case description of a woman whose recovery was assisted by such a group.

THE ROLE OF SELF-HELP GROUPS IN DUAL-DISORDER TREATMENT

Self-help groups play a unique role in the recovery of many clients from dual disorders. Much as stage-wise treatment groups (Chapters 9 and 10) and social skills training groups (Chapter 11) do, self-help groups capitalize on the social nature of substance abuse by creating a social milieu that is conducive to understanding the destructive effects of substances on people's lives, and to developing skills and supports for establishing a sober lifestyle. In contrast to other group interventions, self-help groups by their very nature are not professionally run, and often they are operated independently of mental health or substance abuse agencies. Therefore, the primary function of self-help groups is to provide a vehicle for social support to clients who are already committed to eliminating substance abuse from their lives.

Participation in self-help groups requires that clients be motivated not to use substances, because most such groups are abstinence-oriented. Therefore, attempts to involve clients in self-help groups should usually not begin before the active treatment stage, when they have demonstrated their motivation by cutting down or stopping substance use. These groups are also clearly appropriate for clients in the relapse prevention stage of treatment. During the engagement stage, a clinician lacks a strong therapeutic relationship with a client and there is no evidence that the client wants to stop using substances, so referral to self-help groups is clearly inappropriate. During the persuasion stage, a therapeutic relationship has been established between the client and clinician, but the client's motivation to address substance abuse is either nonexistent or tenuous at best. Clients who are in the persuasion stage may be appropriate for self-help groups if they have made significant progress in cutting down on substance use or developing abstinence as a goal, and if they are willing to explore or have an interest in exploring such groups. This may be a particularly useful strategy for clients with strong social skills who shun association with mental health treatment or peers with mental illness.

Involvement in self-help groups must be voluntary, with a clinician's role limited to helping a client consider the possible benefits of participation in a self-help group, helping him or her identify and try available self-help groups, and processing the experience with the client. Many clients with dual disorders have little or no experience with these groups, and there are few guidelines as to who benefits the most from them. Therefore, clinicians should explore participation in self-help groups with all clients in the active treatment or relapse prevention stage, and may selectively explore such groups with clients in the persuasion stage. However, clinicians should be aware that a significant number of clients do not like self-help groups, and they should respect the choices their clients make about attending these groups. In our experience, clients with major mood disorders are more likely to benefit from participation in self-help groups than clients with schizophrenia-spectrum disorders (Noordsy et al., 1996); nevertheless, participation in self-help should be explored with all appropriate clients.

Participation in self-help groups is usually reinforcing, because clients receive positive feedback about their decision to become abstinent from others with similar experiences. Clinicians can also reinforce participation in self-help groups, as well as the principles of self-help, by incorporating self-help concepts into their psychotherapeutic work with clients—especially in the context of case management (Chapter 6) or during cognitive-behavioral substance abuse counseling (Chapter 8), active treatment groups (Chapter 10), or family interventions (Chapters 13–15). Self-help groups are an important adjunctive treatment for dual disorders that can be incorporated with other components of integrated treatment, and that may help clients sustain abstinence as their involvement in professional services declines.

Among self-help groups, AA is the most well-known and most widely available/accessible group, as noted at the beginning of this chapter. In the next section, we describe the rise of the self-help movement, the history and philosophy of AA, and the nature of AA and similar Twelve-Step groups.

AA AND THE SELF-HELP MOVEMENT

Since the 1960s and 1970s there has been an explosive growth in the number and variety of self-help groups for individuals with different life challenges, ranging from fear of public speaking to addictive disorders to coping with mental illness (or coping with a relative who has a mental illness). For people with addictive disorders, self-help organizations have been especially important, and numerous individuals credit these groups with helping them stop their substance abuse and regaining control over their lives. Among self-help groups for addictive disorders, the largest and oldest such organization is AA—whose basic philosophy and structure have been emulated by numerous other self-help groups, such as Narcotics Anonymous (NA).

As the term *self-help* implies, these groups are not professionally run. Rather, they are a group of people who come together with a common problem, and who help one another with that problem by sharing their experiences and offering support. The core philosophy of AA and similar groups is embodied in the *Twelve-Steps*, which are the principles that members follow to guide them into recovery.

The History of AA

The birth of AA dates back to 1935, when Bill Wilson, a salesman from New York, and Bob Smith, a surgeon from Akron, Ohio, first met to discuss their problems with alcohol (AA, 1990). Bill had suffered for many years with a severe drinking problem. He had been through many "drying-out" processes, but it was during a detoxification program in 1934 that he began his permanent sobriety. It was here that Bill had what is referred to in AA as a "spiritual awakening." In a desperate moment, Bill prayed for help; he related that the room filled with light, and he knew he had been saved. When Bill left the hospital, he set out on a mission to save other alcoholics. (Note that although we have avoided using the term *alcoholics* in this book in general, it is the term commonly used in AA.) In his efforts to help alcoholics, he would bring them to his home, nurse them back to health, and try to convince them to stop drinking. However, despite his good intentions, Bill did not have much success with this approach.

In 1935, Bill was on a sales trip in Akron, Ohio. Still sober, but away from home and lonely, he began to crave a drink. Bill made several desperate phone calls and finally linked up with a local surgeon, Bob Smith, who was a notorious drinker. Bill and Bob stayed up all night long talking about themselves, the role that alcohol use had played in their lives, the terrible consequences they and others had suffered, and their commitment to end the power of alcohol over their lives. After that encounter, both Bill and Bob stayed sober for the remainder of their lives.

Bill and Bob started visiting other alcoholics in hospitals and explaining to them the importance of getting together to talk and explore the effects of alcohol, in order to maintain their own sobriety and get back their lives. Gradually, they began to convince a few men to join them, and to meet regularly to talk about staying sober. As more people joined the meetings, word spread, new meeting groups were established, and the organization of AA was eventually founded. Although official records of membership in AA are not maintained (because of its emphasis on anonymity), it has been estimated that about 3.5 million people attend AA or similar Twelve-Step group meetings each year (Room, 1993).

THE PRINCIPLES AND GUIDELINES OF AA

As noted earlier, the foundation of the AA philosophy for gaining control over one's drinking and maintaining abstinence is a set of core steps called the Twelve Steps; these were first published in the book *Alcoholics Anonymous* in 1939 (AA, 1953). These steps emphasize that one must accept the essential nature of one's alcoholism (i.e., admit that one is powerless over one's drinking); humble oneself and embrace the spiritual centrality of God (or at least a "higher power") to one's life; take and maintain an honest inventory of oneself; and make amends to others for the wrongs one has done. The Twelve Steps are provided in Table 12.1.

The Twelve Steps of AA are principles designed to be followed by alcoholics as they work to maintain sobriety. Following the identification of these principles,

the *Twelve Traditions* of AA were developed and first published in 1946 (AA, 1953). These traditions are guidelines for groups and individuals as they deal with maintaining the AA organization and relating to others outside the group. The Twelve Traditions are provided in Table 12.2. Because of Bill Wilson's "spiritual awakening," the principles and guidelines of AA have a spiritual foundation. Reliance on a "higher power," which many people in the meetings do call "God," is seen as fundamental to recovery; however, no specific theology is endorsed by AA, and members are free to construe the meaning of a "higher power" in their own terms.

AA Meeting Types and Formats

The typical AA meeting runs 60–90 minutes in length. There are several different types of meetings, and the specific type determines the format. There are so-called "step meetings," where one of the Twelve Steps is read and discussed. There are "Big Book meetings," where a chapter from the book *Alcoholics Anonymous* is read and discussed. There are also "speaker–discussion meetings," where one member tells his or her story of drinking and recovery, and the meeting is then opened up for general discussion among the members. Most meetings are opened by the chairperson's reading a brief AA reading or a prayer, and closed by members' joining together in the Lord's Prayer. Meetings may be *open* (anyone interested may attend) or *closed* (only for people with a desire to stay sober).

Benefits of AA and Similar Twelve-Step Groups

The basic structure and principles of AA have been adapted for individuals who abuse other substances (e.g., narcotics, cocaine, marijuana). The AA approach

---

TABLE 12.1. The Twelve Steps of AA

1. We admitted we were powerless over alcohol—that our lives had become unmanageable.
2. Came to believe that a Power greater than ourselves could restore us to sanity.
3. Made a decision to turn our will and our lives over to the care of God *as we understood Him.*
4. Made a searching and fearless moral inventory of ourselves.
5. Admitted to God, to ourselves and to another human being the exact nature of our wrongs.
6. Were entirely ready to have God remove all these defects of character.
7. Humbly asked Him to remove our shortcomings.
8. Made a list of all persons we had harmed, and became willing to make amends to them all.
9. Made direct amends to such people wherever possible, except when to do so would injure them or others.
10. Continued to take personal inventory and when we were wrong promptly admitted it.
11. Sought through prayer and meditation to improve our conscious contact with God *as we understood Him,* praying only for knowledge of His will for us and the power to carry that out.
12. Having had a spiritual awakening as the result of these steps, we tried to carry this message to alcoholics, and to practice these principles in all our affairs.

Note. From Alcoholics Anonymous (1953).

TABLE 12.2. The Twelve Traditions of AA

1. Our common welfare should come first; personal recovery depends upon AA unity.
2. For our group purpose there is but one ultimate authority—a loving God as He may express Himself in our group conscience. Our leaders are but trusted servants; they do not govern.
3. The only requirement for AA membership is a desire to stop drinking.
4. Each group should be autonomous except in matters affecting other groups or AA as a whole.
5. Each group has but one primary purpose—to carry its message to the alcoholic who still suffers.
6. An AA group ought never endorse, finance or lend the AA name to any related facility or outside enterprise, lest problems of money, property and prestige divert us from our primary purpose.
7. Every AA group ought to be fully self-supporting, declining outside contributions.
8. Alcoholics Anonymous should remain forever nonprofessional, but our service centers may employ special workers.
9. AA, as such, ought never be organized; but we may create service boards or committees directly responsible to those they serve.
10. Alcoholics Anonymous has no opinion on outside issues; hence the AA name ought never be drawn into public controversy.
11. Our public relations policy is based on attraction rather than promotion; we need always maintain personal anonymity at the level of press, radio and films.
12. Anonymity is the spiritual foundation of all our traditions, ever reminding us to place principles before personalities.

Note. From Alcoholics Anonymous (1953).

has also been used to help family members cope with a relative who has a substance use problem (e.g., Al-Anon, Alateen, Children of Alcoholics). The AA model has even been adapted to help people manage and overcome other problem behaviors, such as compulsive eating, shopping, and sexual activity.

Research on AA and similar Twelve-Step groups has been limited by the anonymous nature of participation in such groups. However, a growing body of evidence provides modest support for their beneficial effects (e.g., Emrick, Tonigan, Montgomery, & Little, 1993; Morgenstern, Labouvie, McCrady, Kahler, & Frey, 1997; Thurstin, Alfano, & Nerviano, 1987). Several key elements of AA and similar groups appear to have made them useful to so many people.

First, there is the element of identification. When members attend a group meeting, they identify themselves as having a problem, and meeting with others who have similar problems helps them realize that they are not alone. This normalizes the experience of substance abuse, resulting in social validation. Second, many people seem to benefit from *sponsorship*. A new person in a group chooses a mentor with some experience, from whom he or she can learn and receive individual support. Such mentors are called *sponsors*, and they can help new members both inside and outside the group meetings.

A third key to the popularity and success of AA in particular is the widespread availability of its meetings. A member of AA may attend any meeting that is available, anywhere. Because alcoholism is so common, AA meetings can be found in numerous locations throughout the United States and the world, every day, and often at multiple times throughout the day and night. Local AA meetings can be identified by either looking up AA in the telephone book, consulting a local newspaper, or checking the Internet. Thus active AA members

never have to go far or wait long to attend a meeting, even when they are away from home.

Fourth, AA and similar Twelve-Step groups promote reaching out to and maintaining contact between members. Groups frequently offer phone lists so that members can stay in touch with one another. The availability of social support can help people resist urges to use substances, and can lead to developing a social network of abstinence supporters.

Fifth, the anonymous nature of AA and other traditional Twelve-Step approaches has broad appeal. People attending meetings of such groups do not feel stigmatized by their addiction, nor does such attendance amount to a public disclosure of their problems. In fact, because many successful people have had problems with addiction and have sought help in AA and similar organizations, participation has the benefit of normalizing addiction, while providing members with access to positive role models who have regained control over their lives by accepting their addiction and making a personal resolve to end their use of alcohol or drugs.

Sixth and last, for people who are receiving professional care for their addiction problems, self-help groups can be a useful adjunct to their treatment. Clinicians who treat persons with addictions can incorporate the Twelve-Step principles in their work with clients. This can reinforce clients' decision to remain abstinent, their ability to use the Twelve Steps in their own lives, and their continued involvement in AA or similar groups.

The advantages of AA and other traditional Twelve-Step groups for people with substance use disorders are summarized in Table 12.3. Despite these advantages, clients with dual disorders encounter several common problems with these groups. These problems are described in the next section.

TABLE 12.3. Advantages of AA and Similar Twelve-Step Groups

- No cost—attendance at Twelve-Step groups is free.
- Diverse membership—people from all walks of life attend these groups, so that a person can usually find someone with whom to identify.
- Accessibility, particularly of AA groups—wherever a person goes, he or she can find an AA meeting.
- Acceptance—everyone is welcome to attend these groups.
- Value system—these groups offer a way for people to think about and structure their lives.
- Consistency—groups are basically the same wherever a person goes.
- Support—phone lists and sponsors provide support outside groups.

PROBLEMS WITH TRADITIONAL TWELVE-STEP GROUPS FOR CLIENTS WITH DUAL DISORDERS

AA and similar Twelve-Step groups have a broad appeal for people with substance use problems (Westermeyer, Myott, Aarts, & Thuras, 2001), but they also involve some disadvantages for clients with dual disorders (Noordsy et al., 1996). By being aware of these potential problems, clinicians can increase the chances that their clients with dual diagnoses will benefit from this valuable treatment option. In addition, clinicians will appreciate that not all such clients benefit from participation in traditional Twelve-Step groups.

AA and similar Twelve-Step groups are strongly abstinence-oriented, and any argument by a member that he or she can continue to use substances in a "controlled" fashion is met with strong opposition from other group members. Some clients with a dual disorder may find this degree of rigidity difficult to accept, especially those who have begun to decrease their use of substances but have not yet endorsed abstinence as a personal goal, and for whom additional motivational work is in order (see Chapter 7). In a similar vein, it is difficult for many clients with dual disorders to accept the fundamental tenet of AA and similar Twelve-Step groups that people with substance use problems must admit that they are "powerless" over their substance use; however, such an admission is a prerequisite for participation in these groups. Referral to AA-like groups is not likely to persuade clients with dual disorders that they cannot control their substance use. Such clients often come to believe that they are indeed powerless over their addictions through extensive trial and experience, rather than through interpersonal confrontation.

Another problem that clients may have with AA and similar groups is their large size. Groups with more than 10 or 15 people may contribute to social anxiety, feelings of paranoia, or delusions of reference (e.g., the belief or conviction that others are talking about a client when they are not). Clients may also have various difficulties with the strong spiritual orientation of traditional Twelve-Step groups, including the importance of God or a "higher power." Some clients who do not have strong spiritual convictions may object to the religious flavor of these groups. Other clients with religious delusions may feel uncomfortable with the frequent references to God, which may become entwined with their delusional convictions. However, it is also important not to ignore the fact that many clients with dual disorders emphasize the importance of spirituality to their recovery (McDowell et al., 1996).

Clients with dual disorders may have difficulty relating to the types of losses that other members in traditional Twelve-Step groups typically describe. For example, members may describe such experiences as the loss of a good job, the dissolution of a marriage or family, or the forfeiting of possessions such as cars and houses due to their substance abuse. Many clients with dual diagnoses have never had a good job, have never married, and lack the resources to own a car or a house. These clients may thus feel different and alienated from other members of the Twelve-Step group, by virtue of their different personal experiences.

Yet another problem with AA and similar Twelve-Step groups is that some clients with dual disorders may act and look differently from other members of the group because of their mental illness. Individuals with schizophrenia often have poor social skills, including diminished expressiveness, slower processing of social information, trouble identifying appropriate and interesting conversational topics, and difficulty being responsive to other people (Mueser & Bellack, 1998); these impairments can interfere with fitting into a group meeting. Although social skills training may rectify some of these problems (see Chapter 11), clients may be aware of their social difficulties and feel uncomfortable because of them, making them reluctant to participate in these groups.

A further problem can arise for clients with a dual diagnosis who are taking psychiatric medications. Although the principles of traditional Twelve-Step groups do not address the use of medications (such as antipsychotics, mood stabilizers, antidepressants), some members believe that medications are unnecessary, compromise sobriety, or even serve as a "crutch." This can lead them to pressure clients with a dual disorder to stop using such medications. Most of these clients need pharmacological treatment for their mental illness, however, and stopping their medication can lead to symptom relapses and re-hospitalizations. Although some group members hold negative attitudes about clients who take psychiatric medications, a recent survey of AA contact persons indicated that the vast majority did not disapprove such medications for people with addictive disorders (Meissen, Powell, Wituk, Girrens, & Arteaga, 1999).

Table 12.4 contains a summary of the common problems associated with participating in traditional self-help groups for clients with dual disorders. These problems underscore the importance of exploring, preparing, and supporting these clients' participation in self-help groups.

SELF-HELP APPROACHES OTHER THAN TRADITIONAL TWELVE-STEP GROUPS

Some of the problems with traditional Twelve-Step groups described in the preceding section are unique to persons with dual disorders (e.g., some members' disapproval of persons who take psychiatric medication), while others are not (e.g., dislike of the emphasis on a "higher power"). Several alternative self-help group approaches have been developed, some specifically for persons with dual disorders and others for anyone with an addiction. We discuss these programs below.

Of the alternatives to traditional Twelve-Step approaches developed specifically for people with dual disorders, the two best-known groups are *Dual Recovery Anonymous* (Hamilton & Sample, 1994) and *Double Trouble in Recovery* (Vogel, Knight, Laudet, & Magura, 1998). These groups are based on the Twelve Steps of AA, but incorporate advice and hope for coping with and managing one's psychiatric illness within the Twelve-Step framework. Both of these organizations appear to be valuable sources of social support for clients with dual disorders.

As is the case for AA, little research has been conducted on the clinical effects of participation in Double

Trouble in Recovery or Dual Recovery Anonymous. However, one study, using a cross-sectional design, found that participation in Dual Recovery Anonymous groups was correlated with lower mental health and substance abuse symptoms, as well as higher levels of personal well-being; by contrast, participation in traditional Twelve-Step groups was not associated with better functioning in these areas (Laudet, Magura, Vogel, & Knight, 2000). Thus connecting clients with Dual Recovery Anonymous or Double Trouble in Recovery appears to be a viable alternative to traditional Twelve-Step groups when these groups are available. Local groups can be identified through newspapers, the phone book, or the Internet.

Aside from special groups for dual disorders based on the Twelve Steps of AA, alternative self-help groups have been developed that deemphasize the importance of spirituality, while maintaining a focus on mutual support for the goal of maintaining sobriety. The best-known such group is Rational Recovery (Trimpey, 1992, 1996), which is based on the principles of rational–emotive therapy (Ellis & Harper, 1975). Rational Recovery takes the focus off spirituality and places it on encouraging members to assume responsibility for their own behavior, to challenge self-defeating and irrational beliefs they have about themselves, and to provide social support to other members accomplishing these tasks. In contrast to Twelve-Step groups, Rational Recovery does not require an abstinence goal. In addition, rather than encouraging members to follow the AA adage of taking "one day at a time," members in Rational Recovery are encouraged to think farther into the future and to articulate personal goals to keep them motivated and aware of how alcohol and drugs can interfere with achieving those goals. Rational Recovery programs may be a viable alternative to traditional Twelve-Step programs, but, like Dual Recovery Anonymous and Double Trouble in Recovery groups, they are less widely available than AA.

GUIDELINES FOR INVOLVING CLIENTS IN SELF-HELP

Here, we provide clinical guidelines for helping clients choose whether self-help groups should be a part of their recovery from dual disorders.

Introducing Clients to Self-Help Groups as a Possible Treatment Option

All clients who reach the active treatment stage, and some who remain in the persuasion stage, should be engaged in a discussion of the potential benefits of attending self-

---

TABLE 12.4. Disadvantages of Traditional Twelve-Step Groups for Clients with Dual Disorders

- These groups focus on abstinence from the start.
- The groups have a strong spiritual orientation.
- Clients may have difficulty relating to the losses experienced by other group members.
- Some members of self-help groups are hostile to psychiatric medications.
- Clients may experience anxiety in large groups.
- Clients may have difficulty assimilating with other group members, due to social skill deficits.

help groups for their disorders. Clinicians cannot predict which clients will or will not benefit from self-help. Therefore, rather than making the choice for clients, clinicians should give them the option of choosing for themselves whether to participate in a self-help group.

When clients are being introduced to the idea of self-help groups, they need to have an understanding of both what the groups' purposes are and what to expect at a typical meeting. Clinicians can help by explaining the routine of a meeting and attending several meetings with clients. Clinicians can also help clients overcome social barriers to group participation by assisting them in introducing themselves to people at the meeting, and helping them build a new social network. Developing such a network is critical; research has found that among clients with dual disorders, frequency of contacts with members of AA/NA is predictive of better substance abuse outcomes (Trumbetta et al., 1999). When more than one group is available, clients have the opportunity to decide which group feels the most comfortable to them, and clinicians are able to review with the clients the experience of participating in the group. By processing meetings together, clinicians and clients can make an informed decision about which group is best and where problems might arise.

Another way of introducing clients to self-help groups is to use role plays to enact part of a typical group. This can be accomplished most readily in an active treatment group (Chapter 10)—in which some clients may already have familiarity with self-help groups and may even be attending local groups—or a social skills training group (Chapter 11). The general structure of self-help groups can be reviewed and role-played, with a focus on the beginning (first 15–20 minutes) of a typical group meeting.

We provide an example of introducing a client (John) to self-help groups in the persuasion stage of treatment, followed by reintroducing him to self-help at a later time, during the active treatment stage.

CLINICIAN: John, we've been talking about how your drinking seems to be causing some problems for you. You have been having trouble getting to work on time, and you have been missing your doctor's appointments. You have a hard time getting out of bed in the morning when you've been drinking the night before.

JOHN: Yes. A few friends have been dropping by my apartment a couple of nights a week, and we have a few beers. Then I don't want to get out of bed the next morning. But I'm not sure that's the beer. I think it might be my medication.

CLINICIAN: I see. How about if I take you to a support group where the people who attend have problems with drinking? We'll go to a few groups and see what you think.

(John agrees, and the clinician explains in detail what an AA meeting is like and what John can expect. They attend several meetings, but then John loses interest and stops attending. The clinician tries to engage John again at a later time, when he has entered the active treatment stage.)

CLINICIAN: John, do you remember several months ago when we attended a few AA meetings?

JOHN: Yes, but I didn't like them very much. Everybody was talking about all these problems they were having with drinking, and I didn't feel like my drinking was a problem.

CLINICIAN: What do you think about that now?

JOHN: Things have changed. I think some of the trouble I was having was because I was drinking beer and smoking some pot.

CLINICIAN: Now that you're thinking about your substance use a bit differently, it might be helpful for us to try a few more AA meetings. You might find them helpful as you work on your recovery.

JOHN: All right, I'll try it again. Maybe I'll find someone I can talk to there about my problems.

Treating Psychiatric Symptoms and Social Skill Deficits That May Interfere with Participation in Self-Help Groups

Persistent psychiatric symptoms need to be stabilized—both to motivate clients to participate in self-help groups, and to avoid problems in the groups themselves. Clients with fixed delusional beliefs despite optimal psychopharmacology may benefit from cognitive-behavioral therapy aimed at reducing these symptoms or their impact on clients' behavior (Garety, Fowler, & Kuipers, 2000; Gould, Mueser, Bolton, Mays, & Goff, 2001). Clients with social skill deficits may need adjunctive skills training (Chapter 11; Bellack et al., 1997) in order to help them communicate more effectively with other self-help group members and feel at ease in the group. It is important to help clients feel as comfortable as possible in self-help groups, because comfort level is related to the frequency of attendance at these groups for clients with a dual disorder (Kurtz et al., 1995). In short, treatment of psychiatric symptoms and skills deficits will enable such clients to function more successfully and more independently in self-help groups.

Supporting Clients' Involvement in Self-Help Groups

Once a client has become engaged in a self-help group, the clinician can support his or her involvement in several ways. One strategy is to refer to self-help concepts when doing other work with the client—for instance, during case management (Chapter 6), cognitive-behavioral counseling (Chapter 8), active treatment groups (Chapter 10), or family therapy (Chapter 14). Such references can serve to reinforce clients' participation in self-help by helping them generalize the Twelve Steps or other self-help principles to their own personal lives. Clinicians can also process meetings with clients and help them interpret experiences that were confusing or difficult to understand.

Backing Off if a Client Does Not Want to Participate in Self-Help

Clients need to be aware that self-help groups are an option, but the decision to participate in them should remain their own. If clinicians push clients too hard to get involved in self-help, the clients may reject both the self-help groups and the clinicians themselves. Furthermore, the strategy of pressuring clients to participate in self-help groups may backfire by inducing *psychological reactance*—a motivational state that can develop when a person perceives a threat to his or her personal freedom, and reacts by opposing that perceived threat (Brehm, 1966). Above all, clinicians need to preserve their therapeutic alliance with their clients; if clients reject self-help, the clinicians should accept this, and look for opportunities at a later time to gently raise the topic again. If a client is not choosing to participate, it is not *self*-help.

The guidelines for involving clients in self-help groups are summarized in Table 12.5.

TABLE 12.5. Guidelines for Involving Clients in Self-Help Groups

1. Introduce clients to self-help groups as a possible treatment option.
2. Offer to accompany a client to a self-help group meeting (or meetings).
3. Treat psychiatric symptoms and social skill deficits that may interfere with participation in self-help groups.
4. If a client does not want to participate in self-help, back off.

CASE EXAMPLE

We provide a case example of a woman whose participation in a self-help group played an important role in her recovery.

Lisa was a 26-year-old woman with a diagnosis of schizophrenia, paranoid type. She was first hospitalized at the age of 20, because she reported hearing the voices of Satan and his followers ordering her to kill herself. She became paranoid about these voices, and was hospitalized because she posed a threat to herself. In the hospital, Lisa received the diagnosis of schizophrenia and was given antipsychotic medication. For the next 6 years she was a client of the local mental health center, where she received case management services. Lisa did well on her medication, and did not hear voices or have delusions except when she drank alcohol.

Lisa tended to binge on alcohol, consuming 10 to 15 drinks over a period of several hours, several times a week. When she would have these binges, she would also stop taking her medication, and her hallucinations and delusions would return. Because of Lisa's problematic drinking, she was assigned to a special case management team for clients with dual disorders.

When Lisa's case manager had developed a therapeutic alliance, she began to talk with Lisa about her use of alcohol, including some of the problems (e.g., symptom relapses, rehospitalizations, fights with family members). Lisa acknowledged some of the problems related to her substance abuse, but was ambivalent about stopping. Her case manager then talked to Lisa about AA meetings, and suggested that they try attending a meeting to see what it was like; Lisa agreed, and they went to some meetings. Because Lisa was still drinking and hearing voices, however, she believed that people at the AA meetings were part of a Satanic cult, and that their talk of God and a "higher power" were just ways of fooling her. Because of the voices she heard and her beliefs about the group members, Lisa refused to go back to AA.

Several months later, Lisa began to cut down her use of alcohol, and then decided to try a period of abstinence. After a month of not using alcohol, Lisa's mental illness had become stable, and her case manager suggested giving AA another try. Lisa agreed and began attending meetings. She went to the first two meetings with her case manager, and said that she felt "okay" going to more alone. Her case manager suggested to Lisa that any time she felt uncomfortable she could leave the meeting, and they could talk about it the next time they met. At the first several AA meetings Lisa attended alone, she needed to leave early; however, each meeting she was able to stay longer than the previous one, and she was eventually able to sit through an entire meeting. She also met some other women in the meetings who talked to her, took her out for coffee, and encouraged her to stay sober. Lisa continued attending two AA meetings per week, and was able to maintain her sobriety for over 2½ years.

SUMMARY

Self-help groups modeled after the Twelve-Step approach, such as AA, are commonly used for helping people in the general population cope with their alcohol and drug problems. The widespread availability of these groups makes them an important potential resource for clients with dual disorders as well. However, there are some common problems with traditional Twelve-Step groups for such clients, such as the groups' emphasis on abstinence and spirituality, clients' difficulty relating to the losses of other self-help group members, and clients' social awkwardness related to psychiatric illness. By being aware of these potential problems, clinicians can successfully link many of their clients with self-help groups.

Self-help groups are most helpful for clients in the active treatment or relapse prevention stage of treatment, because of the focus of these groups on abstinence. Clinicians can facilitate clients' involvement in self-help groups by raising it as a possibility, while avoiding pressuring reluctant clients to participate. Other strategies clinicians can use to assist clients in joining self-help groups include attending some self-help meetings together, addressing problematic symptoms or social skill deficits that can interfere with participation in self-help groups, and using and explaining self-help concepts in their work with clients. Not all clients with a dual diagnosis are interested in or able to participate in self-help groups. However, with the support and encouragement of clinicians, many clients are able to find a self-help group that they feel comfortable attending, and are able to reap the benefits of the social support and shared philosophy that such a group can provide.

V

Working with Families

13

Family Collaboration

Families play an important role in the lives of all people with severe mental illness, but especially in the lives of those with dual disorders. Families can buffer the effects of stress on these clients, whereas the loss of family support can have devastating effects on their lives and the course of their disorders. However, families can also unintentionally contribute to or maintain clients' ongoing substance abuse. Working with families of clients with a dual diagnosis is crucial to their involvement and support, and ultimately to the outcome of the dual disorders.

This chapter provides general guidelines to clinicians about forming collaborative relationships and working with families of clients with dual disorders. In Chapter 14, we describe a specific model for working with single families—*behavioral family therapy (BFT)*, which is based on structured psychoeducation and problem-solving training. In the last chapter of this section (Chapter 15), we describe how to conduct multiple-family groups aimed at providing psychoeducation and social support to families of clients with a dual disorder. Throughout all three chapters of this section, we recommend including a client along with his or her relatives in family work whenever possible.

We begin this chapter with a discussion of the role of family collaboration in the integrated treatment of dual disorders. This is followed by discussions of who the family members of clients are, and the importance of working with families. We then describe the general goals of family intervention, as well as the principles of engaging and working with families. Next, we address the importance of helping families find solutions to common substance-abuse-enabling situations. We then discuss how the stages of treatment can be used to guide clinicians in involving families in the integrated treat-

ment of dual disorders. We conclude by considering other sources of social support for families.

THE ROLE OF FAMILY COLLABORATION IN DUAL-DISORDER TREATMENT

Family interventions constitute one of the three major groups of psychotherapeutic treatment strategies described in this book for dual disorders, in addition to individual and group interventions. All clients who are in regular contact with family members, as ascertained during the functional assessment (Chapter 4), can benefit from some form of family intervention at any or all of the different stages of treatment. Family collaboration is aimed at developing a strong working relationship between the client's family and the treatment team; it is the most basic type of family intervention. Such collaboration is achieved by reaching out to families, establishing a mutually trusting relationship, providing them with necessary information about dual disorders, and involving them in treatment planning. In contrast to this relatively unstructured approach, BFT (Chapter 14) is a structured family intervention program aimed at teaching family members information and skills that are critical to the treatment of dual disorders. Informal family collaboration may be sufficient for clients who have irregular contact with their family members, or who are making substantial progress in their recovery through participation in individual or group treatment modalities and whose families are supportive of these gains. BFT may be appropriate when a client lives with family members; when the client's dual disorders have a substantial negative impact on the family; when there are high levels of tension in the family; when family members face multiple challenges other than coping with the dual disorders (e.g., poverty, other members with mental illness or substance abuse problems); and/or when the client has not made substantial progress through participation in other modalities.

Family collaboration may be provided to clients as the primary psychotherapeutic treatment modality, or as an adjunctive intervention in combination with individual or group treatments. In most cases, family collaboration is provided at a minimum in combination with case management (Chapter 6), although many of the functions of case management may be provided in the context of family work, with relatively few individual contacts for case management purposes. Family collaboration can be combined with motivational interviewing (Chapter 7) and cognitive-behavioral counseling (Chapter 8); in these cases, family meetings are used to reinforce gains made in the individual work. Family collaboration can similarly be combined with group work, including persuasion groups (Chapter 9), active treatment groups (Chapter 10), social skills training groups (Chapter 11), and self-help groups (Chapter 12). When this is the case, family meetings are oriented to informing relatives about a client's progress in whichever of these treatment modalities are being employed, and supporting the gains made.

WHO ARE THE FAMILY MEMBERS OF CLIENTS WITH DUAL DISORDERS?

The families of clients with dual disorders include relatives who are already involved with the clients or those who could be involved through professional outreach but are not. Involved relatives include those with whom a client lives or has regular contact (e.g., weekly or monthly contact). Relatives sometimes deliberately decrease their contact with a family member who has a dual disorder because of the effects of the substance abuse, but are willing to become more involved if help is provided. Family members are those persons who can provide care and support to the client, who can help manage the mental illness, and who can collaborate with the treatment team to help the client work on his or her substance abuse problem.

Broadly speaking, *family members* can include any persons a client defines as such. Often family members include parents, although mothers are typically more involved than fathers. Siblings are often involved, especially as clients grow older and parents are less able to provide caregiving and support. A client's spouse (or boyfriend/girlfriend, partner, significant other, companion, etc.) is a very important family member to involve in treatment. Without this person's active engagement, the treatment of the dual disorders is often undermined

(e.g., when a couple abuses alcohol or drugs together) and the relationship is prone to conflict and dissolution, with the concomitant loss of social support to the client. Finally, a client's children may be an important source of social support, and the involvement of adolescent or adult children in treatment can be crucial to recovery from dual disorders.

THE IMPORTANCE OF FAMILY INTERVENTIONS FOR DUAL DISORDERS

There are several reasons for attending to and strengthening the bonds between clients with dual disorders and their relatives, whether through informal family collaboration, BFT, multiple-family groups, or a combination of these strategies. First, between 25% and 50% of clients with a dual disorder live with family members, and even more see their families on a regular basis (Clark, 1996; Mueser et al., 2000). These families help clients meet a wide range of needs, including basic care and nutrition, response to crises, and involvement with the service system. The high level of family contact and involvement in the lives of clients with dual disorders indicates that family-based interventions have considerable potential for influencing the disorders' course.

Second, family stress, reflected in such problems as a tense family atmosphere, frequent conflict among family members, and poor communication, has a significant negative effect on the course of both psychiatric and substance use disorders. Numerous prospective studies have found that clients with severe mental illness who are exposed to high levels of family stress are much more likely to have relapses or hospitalizations than are similar clients with less stressful family relationships (Butzlaff & Hooley, 1998). Similarly, familial stress can contribute to a poorer course of substance abuse (Fichter, Glynn, Weyer, Liberman, & Frick, 1997).

Among the important sources of stress in families are the challenges of caregiving for a relative with a psychiatric illness (Lefley, 1996). These difficulties include both financial burden and emotional distress, both of which are partly determined by the severity of the client's illness. The added strain of substance abuse can contribute further to family conflict and burden (Dixon et al., 1995; Salyers & Mueser, 2001). If these issues are not addressed, the end result is an increase in family stress, which in turn can worsen the dual disorders.

Third, families of clients with a dual diagnosis express a strong interest in learning more about psychiatric illness, factors which influence it, and the principles of its management (Bernheim & Lehman, 1985; Mueser, Bellack, Wade, Sayers, & Rosenthal, 1992). Table 13.1 summarizes what families want from professionals. Considering the high level of contact between relatives and clients, improved knowledge about the symptoms of mental illness and substance abuse can help families understand the impact of substance abuse on the psychiatric illness (and vice versa), improve their ability to monitor the course of dual disorders, and take corrective action to address problems soon after they develop. The educational handouts provided in Appendix B can address many of families' needs for information about dual disorders. The importance of family collaboration with the treatment team is illustrated by the success of numerous family intervention programs for clients with severe mental illness (Dixon, Adams, & Lucksted, 2000) and substance use disorders (Stanton & Shadish, 1997).

Fourth, dual diagnosis increases the risk of problems for clients and their families beyond the risk posed by severe mental illness alone. Dual disorders result in more relapses and rehospitalizations, poorer medication compliance, increased violence (especially toward family members; Steadman et al., 1998), and more time in jail (see Chapter 1). Clients with dual disorders sometimes exploit family members to obtain money for substances. These consequences can strain family relationships to the point where the family members' ability to cope is often overwhelmed; the loss of family support, and ultimately the loss of housing, may follow (Caton et al., 1994, 1995). If unaided, therefore, families of clients with a dual diagnosis are often unable to provide the necessary buffers between stress and the clients, and the clients' disorders may worsen as a result (Clark, 1996).

In a family where one spouse or partner has a dual disorder, the failure to intervene and work with the couple can result in the eventual dissolution of the marriage and the family, and the loss of valued parenting responsibilities for the ill member (Fox, 1999). Such losses can be upsetting and demoralizing to all involved. Furthermore, clients with a dual disorder are often highly motivated to preserve their families and their roles as parents, which can facilitate their involvement in treat-

TABLE 13.1. What Families Want from Dual-Disorder Clinicians

- Help in working with the mental health or substance abuse system in getting their needs met
- Information about symptoms of mental illness
- Information about medications and other treatments for mental illness
- An understanding of the interactions between mental illness and substance abuse
- Knowledge about the nature of addiction
- Specific strategies for coping with common symptoms and problem behaviors
- Ways of promoting the client's independence
- Decreased stress and caregiving strains on themselves

ment. Intervention aimed at educating both members of such a couple about the disorders, reducing stress, and collaborating with the treatment team can have a profound effect on both the mental illness and the family as a whole.

In a family where both spouses or partners have dual disorders, one client's substance use and/or mental illness management may have a profound effect on the stability of the other person. Living in an apartment full of alcohol, drugs, and substance-abusing individuals can make it extremely difficult for a client who has reached active treatment or relapse prevention to stay sober. Clients are also vulnerable to being taken advantage of for their money, sex, or medications. In these situations, careful consideration of care for both partners is essential; such care should perhaps even be delivered by the same clinician. Frequent joint meetings between both clients and their clinician(s) are usually necessary as well.

The short-term benefits of family interventions for clients with dual disorders thus include decreased family stress and improved monitoring of the disorders, resulting in fewer relapses, fewer rehospitalizations, and less housing instability. The long-term benefits of working with these families are even more profound. As family members develop their resources and skills for maintaining their relationships with an ill relative and fostering his or her recovery, the family bonds are strengthened, as is their contribution as members of the treatment team.

THE GOALS OF WORKING WITH FAMILIES

Family interventions for dual disorders are aimed at achieving several goals. These goals can be accomplished through work with single families, through multiple-family groups, or a combination of the two. The primary goals of family work include improving family members' understanding of dual disorders, decreasing family stress, improving clients' adherence to treatment recommendations, improving communication between the family and the treatment team, coordinating efforts of the family and treatment team, and reducing substance abuse and its effects on family members.

Fostering Understanding of Dual Disorders

Family members often know little about mental illness, less about substance abuse, and close to nothing about the interactions between the two types of disorders. Educating family members (including the client) about the nature of dual disorders and the principles of their treatment decreases the sense of isolation many families feel when attempting to cope with their predicament (again, the educational handouts in Appendix B can be used to help inform families about dual disorders). When clinicians work with family members and teach them how to recognize the signs and symptoms of both types of disorders, the relatives become able to monitor the disorders' course more effectively, and can immediately alert the treatment team when potentially significant changes have been observed. Furthermore, educating family members about the effects of substance abuse on the psychiatric illness can motivate them to work on the problem of substance abuse.

Lowering Family Stress

As noted earlier, the stress that is so common in these families can worsen the course of dual disorders, weaken family bonds, and threaten clients with the loss of important social support. Therefore, an important goal of family work is to decrease stress in the entire family, including stress impinging on the client from relatives, as well as the impact of the client on his or her relatives. In addition to improving the course of the dual disorders, lowering stress enhances the well-being of all family members, enhancing their capacity to function effectively.

Improving Adherence to Treatment Recommendations

Treatment nonadherence is common in clients with severe mental illness, and even more common in those with dual disorders. This problem is of particular concern regarding compliance with medications, which clients often discontinue when they abuse alcohol or drugs. Furthermore, the combination of substance abuse and medication noncompliance can contribute to interpersonal violence (Swartz et al., 1998b). Collaborating with family members, and educating them about the principles of treating dual disorders, can increase their understanding and willingness to endorse these principles. When relatives are given the opportunity to learn about the components of treatment, to ask questions and raise concerns, and to understand the underlying rationale for treatment recommendations, they can be active in encouraging and supporting a client in adhering to his or her treatment plan.

Improving Communication between the Family and the Treatment Team

Treatment providers often dismiss family members' efforts to contact and have input into the treatment team, and many families have little or no contact with treatment providers. There are several problems associated with the lack of such contact. First, family members tend to have more contact with a client than treatment providers do, and they may be able to detect subtle changes in the client's condition and adherence to treatment long before team members are aware. Family members have often experienced the longitudinal pattern of the client's disorders and may have an acute awareness of early warning signs of relapse. Poor communication between the family and treatment team makes it difficult for the team to respond to such changes in the client in a timely fashion; this delay in response may result in unnecessary relapses and other negative consequences.

Second, inadequate communication between the family and treatment team can result in family members' not supporting, or actually undermining, the treatment goals. Third, lack of contact can impede the treatment team's ability to identify and address family factors that may influence the course of the dual disorders, such as family stress or substance abuse in other members. Therefore, improved communication between the family and treatment providers, to the point where the family members become active members of the treatment team, is an important goal of family collaboration.

Coordinating Efforts of the Family and Treatment Team

Family members sometimes appear to be working at cross-purposes with the treatment team. For example, they may support a client's decision to stop medication, offer the client alcohol to manage agitation, or give the client money when his or her payee limits access to Social Security funds (to prevent them from being used to purchase substances). Treatment providers may become frustrated with the family or encourage separation. Family members typically have the same ultimate goals as the treatment team (to help the client get better), but may lack knowledge of current treatment approaches. Educating the family about the rationale behind recommended treatments can help members align their efforts to help the client with those of the treatment team.

Decreasing Substance Abuse and its Effects on Family Members

A major goal of family work is to reduce substance abuse in a client with dual disorders. However, an equally important goal is to reduce the impact of the client's substance abuse on family members. Before there is a reduction in the use of substances, it can take a heavy toll on the family. Common effects on the family members include the stress of responding to crisis situations resulting from substance-induced relapses; threatened or actual physical violence; increased expenditures due to legal expenses, theft, or coercive tactics on the part of the client; high levels of interpersonal conflict; and upsetting interactions with law enforcement and the legal system related to the client's substance use and its consequences. If not attended to, these consequences can overwhelm the coping resources of family members, eventually resulting in the withdrawal of support and its associated benefits to the client. Thus both working to reduce substance abuse and minimizing its effects on the family are important goals of family interventions.

We provide below a brief clinical example of an intervention aimed at reducing the immediate effects of substance abuse on a family member.

CASE EXAMPLE

Early in the course of family treatment, the long-standing girlfriend of Tony, a man with bipolar disorder and polysubstance abuse, expressed her distress when he would get drunk and call her to yell and complain about his other family members. The girlfriend, Josie, who herself was recovering from alcoholism, felt that Tony was leaning on her for social support when he drank, and that he was placing her between himself and his family. Josie found these calls very upsetting and didn't want to take them, although in the past she had passively accepted them. The clinician talked over the situation with the couple and encouraged Josie to express her feelings to Tony. With the support of the clinician, Josie explained that she felt uncomfortable talking with Tony on the phone after he had drunk or used drugs. She asked him not to call after using, and said that she would hang up if he did. The plan worked, and after several attempted calls while intoxicated, Tony stopped trying to call her after using substances. The solution reduced the immediate impact of Tony's substance abuse on Josie, and over the next several months significant improvements were made both in his substance use problems and in their relationship.

PRINCIPLES OF FAMILY COLLABORATION

Collaboration with family members is guided by several general principles. These principles apply to the engagement and ongoing work with all families, including both short-term and long-term interventions, and both single-family work (including BFT) and multiple-family groups. Following these general principles will improve clinicians' ability to reach out and establish good working relationships with the families of clients with dual disorders.

Engaging Family Members on Their Own Terms

In order to develop a collaborative relationship with family members, clinicians need to engage them on their own terms. This often requires outreach, in which a clinician meets with family members in their own home or another location that is convenient to them. Although the setting of family sessions for some families may eventually shift to the clinic, meeting relatives in their home is easy; it provides the clinician with useful information about the environment in which the client lives; and it conveys to family members that the clinician cares about them and values their involvement.

In addition to outreach, successful engagement requires that clinicians be sensitive to the needs of family members, and offer help aimed at addressing their most immediate (and most clearly perceived) needs. Common concerns among family members of clients with dual disorders include reducing relapses and rehospitalizations, improving client independence, and reducing caregiving responsibilities and family stress. In the process of engagement, it is important to demonstrate to family members an understanding of their concerns, and to explain how family collaboration will help address these issues.

Some family members recognize the problem of a client's substance abuse, while others do not. If relatives do not express concern about the client's substance abuse, it is often best to wait until they are engaged in a working relationship with the treatment team before beginning to educate them about substance abuse. Attempting to persuade relatives of the importance of substance abuse before they are engaged in treatment runs the risks of alienating them by not validating their concerns, and of placing the clinician's agenda before that of the relatives.

Providing Ongoing and Interactive Psychoeducation

An important goal of family treatment is to educate clients and relatives about the nature of mental illness, the principles of treatment, the effects of drugs and alcohol, and strategies for decreasing substance use in persons with severe mental illness. Once again, various educational handouts covering the information families need is included in Appendix B. Although educational material can be covered in specific family sessions devoted to psychoeducation, family members often require long periods of time to absorb and integrate the pertinent information. Therefore, a clinician must be aware of this and must always be alert for opportunities to help family members understand important information. For example, some education may take place during the process of engaging family members (e.g., during an initial contact when a parent asks, "What caused my son's mental illness?").

In addition to the fact that psychoeducation needs to be ongoing, it also should be interactive, in order for family members to process information actively and understand how it relates to their own circumstances. To facilitate this, the clinician needs to ask frequent questions to assess members' understanding, and to identify specific examples, rather than only presenting information in a didactic manner. It is through interactive discussions about mental illness and substance use problems that the clinician is able to help family members understand and assimilate the educational material. More information about psychoeducational teaching strategies is provided in Chapter 14.

Minimizing Tension and Conflict in Family Meetings

In order for family members to learn basic information and address family issues, a safe and supportive working environment must be established in the family meetings. It is imperative that the clinician create a comfortable working environment with the family in which criticism, stress, and arguments are minimized. Family members must feel free to express their opinions to each other without fear of censure or reprisal. In all family work, the clinician strives to develop an atmosphere in which different opinions can be aired, while maintaining respect for others and avoiding emotionally charged interactions.

In order to establish and maintain a supportive working environment, the clinician must be alert to criticisms, blaming of family members, raised voices, or pejorative "put-downs," and take steps to stop these behaviors as soon as they occur. In most cases, intervening and requesting family members to express opinions more constructively, to speak in a quieter tone of voice, or to return to the focus of the meeting are sufficient to contain strong conflict in the family. If necessary, the clinician can take a break to allow family members to compose themselves again. However, the clinician should not cancel a family meeting because of strong conflict among members, because this conveys the message that the clinician cannot help the family in dealing with its most pressing problems.

Keeping Family Work Collaborative

Effective family work involves genuine collaboration between family members and the clinician. Although the clinician has special expertise to offer (e.g., knowledge about dual disorders and their treatment), family members (including the client) also have unique expertise, based on their knowledge, contact, and concern for each other. The clinician works on developing a relationship with the family that is based on the mutual sharing of information, and genuinely values the input and experiences of family members. The more family members feel they are important members of the treatment team, the more likely they will be to support the goals of intervention, and to be open to discussing any disagreements with or concerns about these goals with the clinician. Likewise, the more the treatment plan is informed by family input, the more likely it will be to be relevant and on target.

Keeping Family Work Oriented toward the Future

The focus of working with families is on improving the future, not on looking into the past or assigning blame. Many families of clients with dual disorders tend naturally to slip into arguing about the past, creating hard feelings and preventing the resolution of problems. When a clinician is educating family members about a client's psychiatric and substance use disorders, it can be helpful to encourage the members to identify examples of symptoms and problem behaviors, in order to illustrate specific points and to clarify the pattern of the client's illness over time. However, relatively little time is spent focusing on or attempting to understand the past.

People often interpret the purpose of psychotherapy as gaining insight, rather than as working to improve the future. Family members may need to be refocused onto the future and dissuaded from dwelling extensively on the past. On the other hand, many family members appreciate this constructive approach to family sessions, and are relieved not to talk about the past.

Addressing the Needs of the Whole Family, Not Just the Client

Working with families of clients with dual disorders is aimed at improving both the disorders' course and the families' overall functioning. Since decreasing the overall stress level in a family is an important goal of treatment, family work is aimed at helping *everyone* in the family, not just the client. In addition to improving stress in the whole family, focusing on all family members has the advantage of removing the exclusive focus of family work on the client, and thus reducing uncomfortable pressure on that individual.

Sometimes family members can be quite articulate about expressing their needs and goals. At other times the clinician may need to be on the lookout for changes in the family that will either decrease burden or otherwise improve the quality of life for relatives. Throughout family collaboration, the clinician should look for opportunities to help all members improve their personal lives. The better the overall functioning of the family, the more effective it will be at buffering stress on the client, and the more able members will be to reinforce improvements in the client's functioning (including decreases in substance abuse and increases in capacity for independent living).

Avoiding Blame of the Family

Relatives often feel guilty or concerned that they may have contributed to a client's psychiatric illness and substance abuse problems. Conversely, some family members are guarded in their interactions with mental health and substance abuse professionals, for fear that they will be blamed for their relative's problems. Such concerns are not completely unrealistic, considering that in recent history families have been blamed by professionals for causing even severe psychiatric disorders, such as schizophrenia (Terkelsen, 1983). The "nature versus nurture" debate continues today, and some clinicians still blame families for clients' problems.

It is best to avoid casting blame or judgment on family members for a client's disorders, and to look instead for ways of alleviating feelings of blame or guilt in the family. Blaming the family members interferes with the clinician's ability to develop a trusting and collaborative relationship with them, since it implies that the relatives either lack concern for the client's welfare or have malevolent intentions toward him or her. The clinician should use basic psychoeducation to help family members understand that they are not to blame for their relative's problems, and that improved understanding of the disorders and close work with the treatment team can help them play an important role in helping the client recover. Even when relatives appear to have a negative or destructive effect on the client, it is more helpful to construe their behavior as "doing the best they can," and to focus on helping them learn better ways of showing their concern and dealing with their frustrations.

ADDRESSING FAMILY MEMBERS' ENABLING BEHAVIORS

Psychoeducation and Problem Solving

Although clinicians must be careful to avoid blaming the family for the client's difficulties, they should also be mindful of enabling behaviors that can contribute to the client's substance abuse. Some family members inadvertently enable a relative's substance abuse because they are unaware of its effects on the client's mental illness; if so, psychoeducation combined with problem solving can often correct the situation. We provide a case example below.

CASE EXAMPLE

David, a 35-year-old man with schizophrenia and chronic alcohol abuse, lived at home with his parents. David had persistent hallucinations, was very socially withdrawn, and had few hobbies or activities other than drinking. The functional assessment of his drinking habits and his parents' attitudes indicated that he drank alone almost daily, and that his father supplied him with his favorite beverage, beer. His parents did not believe that David's drinking was a problem, although they were concerned that he occasionally became belligerent after drinking too much. His father felt strong empathy for his son's illness, especially his auditory hallucinations, which were a source of much distress. The father explained that he viewed David's drinking as one of the few pleasures in his life, and that the least he could do for him was to buy him his beer.

After engaging with the family and understanding the parents' perceptions concerning David's drinking, the clinician provided them with basic psychoeducation about schizophrenia and its interactions with alcohol, using educational handouts similar to those in Appendix B. This helped the parents to understand that David's alcohol use probably worsened the symptoms of his schizophrenia, including his hallucinations. Problem-solving discussions followed; these focused on developing new recreational activities for David, while beginning a gradual program of cutting down on alcohol use. Various new activities were identified and followed through on (e.g., the father and son's going fishing together), and over a period of several months David became abstinent from alcohol.

Solutions to Common Enabling Situations

Family members sometimes enable substance use behaviors because they are unable to identify suitable alternatives, they fear the consequences of not enabling, or they are responding to direct coercion by the client. Addressing situations that result in the family's enabling the client's substance abuse, and helping members identify alternative solutions to those situations, is a core element of family collaboration. We provide several examples of resolving common enabling situations in families.

Problem 1: The Client at Risk during a Family Holiday

The wife of a client with alcohol abuse says, "On holidays our family celebrates at my sister's house. Everyone is drinking, so how can I help my husband avoid joining in with everyone else? His doctor has told him he shouldn't drink with his medications."

Common enabling solutions include the following:

- Join in as usual, knowing it's only this one special day.
- Tell him he should skip a day of medication.

Here are some alternative solutions the clinician can suggest:

- Ask other members not to drink.
- Hold the celebration at your house to limit drinking.
- Hold a separate family celebration without drinking.

Problem 2: The Client's Smoking Marijuana before a Date with a Family Member

The brother of a client who abuses marijuana says, "When I go to my sister's apartment to pick her up for grocery shopping, she frequently has been smoking marijuana and seems 'out of it.' We usually get into an argument."

Common enabling solutions include these:

- Argue about it, and then go shopping as usual.
- Offer to do the grocery shopping for her.

The clinician can suggest these alternative solutions:

- Arrive early in the morning.
- Make an arrangement—and stick to it—that you'll leave any time you arrive and find she's been smoking.
- Bring a friend along to support you in doing the most appropriate thing.

Problem 3: The Client's Spending All His or Her Money on Alcohol and Drugs

The mother of a client with polysubstance abuse says, "My son spends all of his money on alcohol and drugs, so we end up paying for his groceries."

Common enabling solutions include the following:

- Continue to buy his groceries while he spends his money on substances.
- Give him more money, so he can "meet his own needs."

The clinician can propose these alternative solutions:

- Refuse to buy his groceries.
- Shop with him when he gets his checks.
- Arrange for him to have a representative payee or some other "guardian" over his money management.

Directly addressing family enabling behaviors in ways such as these, and helping the family develop constructive alternative solutions, can bring the actions of the family and of the treatment team into alignment. The results will be consistent behavioral responses and reinforcement, greater effectiveness, and a collaborative, unified support system.

STAGE-WISE FAMILY TREATMENT

Just as the stages of treatment provide the clinician with a framework for formulating treatment goals and identifying appropriate interventions for individual clients, they also provide useful guidelines for family collaboration (Mueser & Fox, 2002). We briefly review the stages of family treatment below, and include a discussion of goals and interventions at each stage.

Engagement

At the initial stage of family collaboration, a clinician needs to reach out and establish a good working relationship with the family, as described earlier. Outreach may include helping the family resolve a pressing problem or crisis, providing short-term psychoeducation, or listening empathically in order to understand and validate relatives' concerns. Sometimes the treatment team makes its first contact with family members, who facilitate engagement with the client. The client's substance abuse is not emphasized as an important focus of treatment in the engagement stage, unless family members express concern about it. A summary of the engagement stage of family treatment is provided in the first section of Table 13.2.

Persuasion

Once the family has been engaged, the focus shifts in the persuasion stage to helping family members appreciate the importance of the client's dual disorders, in order to motivate them to address the substance use problem. Interventions at this stage include psychoeducation about the interactions between psychiatric illness and substance abuse, solving family problems not directly related to substance abuse, and exploring with family members how substance abuse may have interfered with achieving other valued goals. A summary of the persuasion stage of family treatment is provided in the second section of Table 13.2.

Active Treatment

During active treatment, the emphasis of family work is on helping the client further reduce his or her substance use, or maintain a recently achieved abstinence. At this stage, family collaboration focuses on practical ways to help the client either avoid substance abuse situations or manage those situations more effectively; for example, family meetings can focus on helping the client improve his or her skills for refusing offers to use substances, or on developing problem-solving strategies for dealing with cravings. In addition, family work at this stage can focus on teaching the family how to set limits. A summary of the active treatment stage is provided in the third section of Table 13.2.

TABLE 13.2. The Four Stages of Recovery for Families of Clients with Dual Disorders

Stage	Description	Goal	Examples of clinical strategies
Engagement	The family members are in contact with a case manager or counselor; they are beginning to develop a working alliance.	To establish regular contacts with the family and develop a therapeutic relationship.	• Meet family members on their own turf (e.g., at home). • Provide empathic listening and support. • Convince the family that the clinician has something to offer, and instill hope that change is possible. • Educate family members about psychiatric illness and its management. • Help resolve the most pressing problems.
Persuasion	The family members are engaged in a relationship with a case manager or counselor, are discussing the client's substance use, and may be participating in monitoring and helping the client to begin to reduce use.	To persuade family members that clients' substance abuse is a problem and needs to be addressed.	• Educate families about effects of substance abuse on mental illness. • Encourage family members to develop external social supports. • Begin problem solving on family issues that may or may not be related to substance abuse. • Explore how substance abuse may interfere with achieving other family goals.

Active treatment	The family members are engaged in treatment, are discussing the client's substance use, and are helping the client work toward abstinence (or controlled use without associated problems). The family members may be helping the client avoid high-risk situations and reduce stressors.	To help family members develop strategies for reducing substance abuse in the dually diagnosed client.	• Modify stressful communication styles that may contribute to substance abuse.
			• Teach problem-solving skills so that family members can help the client do the following:
			  • Refuse offers to use substances.
			  • Avoid high-risk situations.
			  • Develop alternative leisure activities.
			  • Cope with persistent symptoms.
			  • Structure daily time (e.g., find part-time work).
			• Teach family how to set limits.

Relapse prevention	The family members are engaged in treatment, and have acknowledged that the client's substance use is a problem. The client has achieved abstinence (or controlled use without associated problems) for at least 6 months, and the family members continue to offer support and practical assistance.	To help family members maintain an awareness of the client's vulnerability to relapses, and to build on the client's successes by facilitating improvements in other areas as well.	• Periodically review progress made by the family, and risk factors associated with relapse of substance abuse.
			• Help families enhance other areas of client functioning:
			  • Relationship skills.
			  • Work or education.
			  • Self-care and independent living skills.
			  • Enjoyment of leisure activities.

Relapse Prevention

At the relapse prevention stage, the client has succeeded in becoming free of substance use (or has experienced no problems) for a sustained period of time; the focus of family work thus shifts to providing support for the gains made in treatment and addressing other areas of functioning. Problem solving may be used to help the client make progress toward other desired goals, such as improved relationships, work, education, or more independent living. A summary of the relapse prevention stage is provided in the final section of Table 13.2.

RESOURCES FOR FAMILIES

Because family collaboration is critical to improving the course of dual disorders, family members need to have contact with and become members of the treatment team, to ensure that a client's illnesses are effectively monitored and that all stakeholders are involved in consensus building and treatment planning. In addition to this collaboration, many families benefit from receiving social support from other families with similar experiences. There are several possible resources available to these families.

First, as described in more detail in Chapter 15, families of clients with a dual disorder can support each other through participation in multiple-family groups. Although this is an ideal service for these families, such groups need to be organized and conducted as part of a comprehensive mental health and substance abuse treatment service.

A second alternative is that relatives may receive support from other families with a member who is mentally ill through self-help organizations of such families. The best-known of these organizations in the United States is the *National Alliance for the Mentally Ill* (NAMI), which has numerous state and local affiliates. Local NAMI chapters typically meet on a monthly basis and involve a combination of shared support and guest speakers. Although NAMI is principally aimed at relatives of persons with mental illness, clients themselves are also invited to participate in meetings. Local chapters of NAMI can be identified through consulting a local phone book or searching on the Internet.

Third, families may benefit from participating in support groups for relatives of persons with substance use disorders, such as Al-Anon. Al-Anon is similar to NAMI in its emphasis on providing opportunities for relatives to share their coping experiences. It differs from NAMI with respect to its stand on advocacy and lobbying work. Al-Anon—like its counterpart for persons with alcohol use disorders, Alcoholics Anonymous—is apolitical and is not involved in advocacy work. In contrast, NAMI (and its local affiliates) is actively involved in advocacy work and lobbying of national and local politicians concerning legislation with implications for the treatment of psychiatric disorders. Clinicians should be familiar with local chapters of NAMI, Al-Anon, and other self-help organizations for relatives.

SUMMARY

Family members—including parents, siblings, children, spouses/partners, and other relatives—play an important role in the lives of clients with dual disorders. These persons are often vital sources of economic and social support to clients, but their own lives can be dramatically affected by the dual disorders. Without collaboration with professionals, the strain of coping with a dually disordered relative can take a huge toll—often overwhelming family coping, and leading to the breakup of families, the loss of support, and housing instability for many clients. The goals of family collaboration include fostering an understanding of dual disorders, lowering family stress, improving the client's adherence to treatment recommendations, improving communication between the family and treatment team, coordinating efforts of the family and treatment team, and decreasing substance abuse and its effects on family members.

In this chapter, we have also reviewed the general principles of family collaboration for clients with a dual disorder: engaging families on their own terms, providing ongoing and interactive psychoeducation, minimizing tension in family meetings, addressing substance abuse when a family is ready, keeping family work collaborative and future-oriented, improving the lives of everyone in the family, and not blaming the family. In working with families, clinicians need to help families find solutions to common situations that enable clients' substance abuse. We have then described how the stages of treatment are applied to family work, and we have concluded by considering additional sources of social support for families.

14

Behavioral Family Therapy

In Chapter 13, we have emphasized the importance of collaborating with families of persons with a dual disorder, and have reviewed the goals and general principles of family work. This chapter describes a specific model of working with single families—*behavioral family therapy* (BFT). BFT is aimed at systematically teaching family members information about dual disorders and their treatment, and helping them develop more effective communication and problem-solving skills. These skills can be used by families to address substance abuse, to work on other problems, and to make progress toward individual and shared goals.

We begin the chapter by describing the role of BFT in the treatment of dual disorders. Next, we provide an introduction to the BFT model, including its goals and treatment components. We then discuss logistics, such as the setting, timing, and duration of sessions, and who should be involved in BFT. Following this, we address the importance of a family meeting held between BFT sessions, in which family members can review information learned in sessions and practice skills. Next, we consider how crises should be handled in family sessions. We then describe the specific phases of BFT for dual disorders: *connecting* with the family, *assessment*, *psychoeducation*, *communication skills training*, *problem-solving training*, and *termination*. We conclude by providing a fairly detailed case example of a client treated with the BFT model, and a postscript on addressing substance use and abuse in the relatives of clients.

The BFT model has been widely applied to both psychiatric and substance use disorders, and there is extensive research supporting its effectiveness (Falloon et al., 1985; Fals-Stewart, Birchler, & O'Farrell, 1996; Miklowitz et al., 2000; O'Farrell, Cutter, Chouquette,

Floyd, & Bayog, 1992; O'Farrell, Cutter, & Floyd, 1985; Randolph et al., 1995; Xiong et al., 1994). Further information about BFT—including assessment instruments, numerous clinical vignettes, and a comprehensive review of the BFT research literature—can be found in Mueser and Glynn (1999).

THE ROLE OF BFT IN DUAL-DISORDER TREATMENT

BFT is a standardized approach to working with couples and families that helps all members to participate actively in the treatment of psychiatric and substance use disorders, to communicate more effectively with one another, and to resolve problems and achieve goals through cooperative work. As described in Chapter 13, family intervention is a critical psychotherapeutic treatment strategy for clients with dual disorders. All clients who have regular contact with family members (e.g., every other week) should receive at least some form of family collaboration with the treatment team. It is possible for clinicians to collaborate actively with families without providing formal BFT by following the guidelines in Chapter 13; such collaboration can be quite beneficial in the treatment of the dual disorders. The primary advantage of BFT over informal family collaboration is that the BFT model provides a theoretical framework for understanding the influence of family members on dual disorders, which leads to a systematic and structured approach to single-family intervention. This framework is useful in work with all families, but it is crucial in work with families that pose special challenges—such as high levels of tension and criticism between members; family members' intentional or unwitting reinforcement of a client's substance abuse; chaotic family life; or multiple family hardships in addition to the client's dual disorders, such as mental illnesses or substance abuse problems in other members, health problems, poverty, or ongoing exposure to violence. In addition, BFT can be useful when other approaches to treating dual disorders have met with minimal success, and the clinician elects to harness family resources in the treatment of the disorders. Information about all these family factors is obtained during the functional assessment and functional analysis of the client's substance use problems (Chapters 4 and 5), and is incorporated into treatment planning and updated regularly (Chapter 5).

Like informal family collaboration, BFT may be provided to clients as the primary psychotherapeutic treatment modality, or as an adjunctive intervention in combination with individual or group treatments. When BFT is provided, the amount of individual case management (Chapter 6) is usually decreased, with case management tasks being addressed in the context of family sessions. BFT can be combined with motivational interviewing (Chapter 7) and cognitive-behavioral counseling (Chapter 8); in these instances, family sessions are used to reinforce gains made in the individual work. However, because the first several months of BFT are relatively intense, with weekly family sessions, it is often preferable not to initiate individual motivational interviewing or cognitive-behavioral counseling during this early phase. Instead, the clinician or team should wait until the frequency of BFT sessions has decreased to biweekly or monthly before evaluating the need for these individual approaches. BFT can also be combined with group work, including persuasion groups (Chapter 9), active treatment groups (Chapter 10), social skills training groups (Chapter 11), and self-help groups (Chapter 12). In such cases, family sessions occasionally touch on issues raised or gains made during participation in these group activities.

OVERVIEW OF THE BFT MODEL

BFT is designed to equip family members with the information and skills they need to collaborate with the treatment team and effectively manage the dual disorders. According to the BFT model, all family members (including the client) need specific information about psychiatric illness, substance abuse, their interactions, and their treatment; they need to be able to communicate effectively and with a minimum of stress; and they need to be able to work together to solve problems and achieve goals. Therefore, the focus of BFT is on teaching information and skills to the family, with

the specific teaching tailored to the unique problems and goals of each family, and treatment often delivered on a time-limited basis (e.g., 1–2 years). The total number of sessions may very from 15 to over 30, with their frequency declining as the family learns the requisite skills. From the beginning of BFT, the clinician prompts the family members to have weekly meetings on their own, and to focus these meetings on reviewing material covered in sessions or conducting family problem solving. BFT can be divided into six phases: connecting with the family, assessment, psychoeducation, communication skills training, problem-solving training, and termination.

The six phases of BFT should be distinguished from the four stages of dual-diagnosis treatment. The stages of treatment, as described in Chapter 2, are based on a client's motivation to work on substance use problems. Knowing the client's stage of treatment throughout the intervention is critical for the clinician to determine how material should be presented in BFT, which problems to work on, and whether or not to target substance abuse directly as a goal of treatment. The phases of BFT, on the other hand, are the order in which the family work unfolds. The phases describe the nature of the clinical activities performed, which are tailored to the client's stage of treatment. The connecting phase of BFT often overlaps with the engagement stage of treatment, when dual-disorder treatment is initiated with both the client and relatives. After the connecting phase of BFT, the clinician works through the remaining phases of family treatment, tailoring the family work to the client's stage of treatment.

In the *connecting* phase (1–3 sessions), the clinician reaches out to the family and lays the groundwork for developing a collaborative relationship with all members, including the client. The primary goal of this phase is to develop a willingness among family members to work together with the clinician. The idea of family work is first presented to the client, and the client's approval is solicited. Then family members are contacted, and a brief orientation meeting is arranged.

In the *assessment* phase (2–5 sessions), the clinician forges relationships with each family member through individual interviews to evaluate each member's understanding of the psychiatric and substance use disorders, and to explore personal goals that may be the focus of family work. The assessment phase is thus a continuation of the connecting phase; it also yields crucial information concerning the family's motivation to work on issues related to substance use, as well as other issues. The family assessment information is used to formulate a functional analysis of the client's substance abuse problems (or to modify a functional analysis, if one has already been completed based on individual work; see Chapter 5). This analysis is then refined during the next phase.

In the *psychoeducation* phase (6–7 sessions), family members learn basic information about psychiatric illness, medications, substance use and abuse, and the treatment of dual disorders, as well as ways to improve their communication. This information is particularly critical to helping family members understand the role of substance use in worsening the course of psychiatric illness, and the importance of medication for the management of the psychiatric disorder. For many families, simply learning about the interactions between psychiatric illness and substance use is enough to convince them that substance abuse is an important problem to address. The functional analysis formulated earlier is re-evaluated at the end of psychoeducation, and a treatment plan is developed that guides the remainder of BFT.

Communication skills training (4–8 sessions, if included in BFT) is provided to families whose members interact in a stressful manner marked by frequent criticisms, lack of acknowledgment for what others have said, frequent interruptions, speaking for others and invalidating their feelings, or angry outbursts (including shouting or storming out of the room). Without the ability to communicate clearly, directly, specifically, and with a minimum of tension, families will be unable to engage in the communication necessary to solve problems cooperatively. Families that do not have these communication problems can skip this phase of BFT and progress directly to problem-solving training. Families that receive communication skills training are taught a core set of skills for communicating effectively, including active listening, expressing positive feelings, making positive requests, and expressing negative feelings; the principles of social skills training are employed.

Problem-solving training (5–15 sessions) involves teaching a sequence of skills designed to help families identify effective solutions to problems or goals while minimizing stress and tension. Family problem solving is used to address a wide range of different problems, including both those related to substance abuse and other family problems or goals. As families become more adept at solving problems on their own, the need for the clinician to lead the family problem solving decreases, as does the members' reliance on the clinician. In the *termination* phase, the clinician reviews with the family members their accomplishments in working together; potential problems are discussed; and plans are reviewed for responding to relapses in psychiatric symptoms or substance abuse. The phases of BFT, the corresponding stages of client substance abuse treatment, and the approximate number of sessions for each phase are summarized in Table 14.1.

LOGISTICAL CONSIDERATIONS

In this section, we discuss the logistics of providing BFT to clients with a dual diagnosis and their families, including the location, frequency, and length of sessions, as well as who should participate.

Location of Sessions

BFT sessions can be provided at the family home, at the clinic, or in another mutually agreed-upon location. Although the effectiveness of this family intervention does not depend on where it is provided, it is easier to engage some families (and more family members) by offering sessions at home. Clinicians may find it useful to provide the first several treatment sessions at the home, and then to shift the locus of treatment to the clinic.

Frequency of Sessions

BFT sessions are usually provided on a declining-contact basis over 8–12 months, and longer if necessary. After the connecting and assessment phases have been completed, sessions are held on a weekly basis for about the first 12 weeks, followed by biweekly sessions for

TABLE 14.1. Phases of BFT, Corresponding Client Stages of Substance Abuse Treatment, and Approximate Number of Sessions for Each Phase

Phase of BFT	Client stage of treatment	Number of sessions
1. Connecting	Engagement	1–3
2. Assessment	Engagement or persuasion	2–5
3. Psychoeducation	Persuasion or active treatment	6–8
4. Communication skills training (if necessary)	Persuasion, active treatment, or relapse prevention	4–8
5. Problem solving training	Persuasion, active treatment, or relapse prevention	5–15
6. Termination	Active treatment or relapse prevention	1

about 6 months, followed by monthly sessions for 3 or more months. The specific frequency of sessions can be tailored to meet the family's particular needs. Weekly sessions should be conducted at least until all of the core BFT material has been covered (psychoeducation, communication skills if necessary, and problem solving), and weekly sessions may be extended if the family faces multiple stressors that interfere with the learning of the information and skills. On the other hand, families that find meeting on a weekly basis to be too difficult (e.g., due to scheduling conflicts or travel time) may benefit from a BFT program delivered mainly on a biweekly basis.

Many families benefit from time-limited treatment, and are able to maintain their collaborative relationship with the treatment team after formal BFT sessions have ended. However, some families require sessions on an ongoing, time-unlimited basis. Such continued family sessions (e.g., once every 2–4 weeks) may be particularly helpful for families that are prone to frequent crises, that live in impoverished or otherwise very stressful conditions, or that include a client whose substance abuse or mental illness is severe and chronic.

Length of Sessions

Family sessions are usually 1 hour long, but this can be modified depending on members' attention span, interest level, and involvement in the issues. Some clients have significant attention problems, requiring breaks during sessions or briefer sessions. Some families have no difficulty participating in longer sessions, and 75- to 90-minute sessions may be optimal for them.

Participants in Sessions

The participants in BFT include the client and any key relatives with whom he or she has regular contact. A general rule is that at least one participating relative should have weekly contact with the client (or be willing to have weekly contact). Although BFT can help when there is less contact, diminished benefits are to be expected.

The question of which family members should be included in family sessions depends on the role they play in the client's life. Some relatives play a major role, whereas others are more peripheral. It may be helpful to engage the more peripheral family members in some, but not all, of the family sessions. For example, if a client lives at home with his or her parents, and has occasional contact with brothers and sisters who live elsewhere, the parents and client could participate in all of the family sessions, while the siblings participate in just

the psychoeducational sessions and a few problem-solving sessions.

The decision about whether (and, if so, how much) to involve relatives who have less contact with the client is also based on their interest and motivation to participate in the family sessions. Sometimes concerned relatives decrease their involvement because they do not know how to help, yet they are motivated to work actively with the client when aided by the clinician. A successful outcome of family intervention with such relatives may include increased contact between the client and relatives, and greater progress toward shared goals.

Participants in BFT need not be limited to blood relatives or members of the same household; they can include other persons who are concerned about the client. For example, a legal guardian, a member of the clergy, a close friend, or a non-live-in boyfriend or girlfriend can be involved in family sessions if they express a commitment to working with the client and family.

It is best to engage in treatment as many family members who have regular contact with the client as possible. Some relatives are difficult to engage initially, and the clinician may need to proceed without a key family member. In these situations, the clinician should make direct contact with the reluctant relative, and to establish an open-door policy regarding his or her participation in sessions. The clinician can then be on the lookout for an opportunity to engage this member in family sessions at a later point in treatment.

BETWEEN-SESSION FAMILY MEETINGS

Because BFT is a learning-oriented intervention, families need to review the requisite information and practice the targeted skills on their own, in order to become familiar and proficient with them. To accomplish this, from the beginning of regular BFT sessions, the clinician sets the expectation that the family will conduct a weekly family meeting to review information or practice skills taught in sessions. This is accomplished by reviewing the rationale for such meetings with the family, and then helping them to set a regular weekly time to meet.

At the beginning of BFT, family meetings can be quite brief (e.g., 15 minutes) and should be highly structured, with clear instructions to family members about what they should do in each meeting. During the psychoeducation phase of BFT, family members can be instructed to review the most recently covered educational handout together (e.g., by taking turns reading sections of it to each other, and noting any questions that arise). For families that receive communication skills training, family meetings can involve practicing the targeted communication skills. During problem-solving training, members use family meetings to practice the problem-solving skills on their own—gradually taking on more and more of these skills, and tacking increasingly difficult problems.

In order to get the family into the habit of conducting regular family meetings, the clinician must follow up in each session by asking whether the family met as planned, and, if so, by providing ample positive feedback. If the family meeting did not take place, the clinician should explore with the family members the obstacles they encountered, and work with them to develop a plan for overcoming them. Common obstacles to having family meetings include forgetting the meeting time, not fully understanding the purpose of the meetings, scheduling conflicts, and not assigning anyone the responsibility to call the meeting. At times, having the family conduct a brief family meeting at the beginning of the BFT session, in which the clinician sits back and does not contribute anything, can stress to family members the importance of these meetings; it can also provide the clinician with useful information about what happens when a family meeting occurs. If the clinician sticks to the goal of getting the family members to meet on their own between BFT sessions, in most cases he or she will be successful, despite problems with follow-through early in the course of BFT.

RESPONDING TO CRISES AND STRESSORS IN FAMILY SESSIONS

Family members often look to the clinician to help them deal with stressors or crises in family sessions. When a family presents with a "crisis" early in the course of BFT, the clinician must determine the urgency of the problem and ascertain whether the failure to address it will significantly hamper the family's ability to learn the information and skills taught in BFT. Problem situations can be divided into two types; different strategies are used to respond to each kind.

Long-Standing, Noncrisis Problems

Some problems are chronic and are unlikely to be solved in a single meeting, especially early in treatment. For these problems, it is best to acknowledge the family's concern; to explain that because the problem has been present for a long time, it will take a concerted effort to resolve it; and to state that the clinician will return to it later in the family sessions, after members have learned problem-solving skills. Examples of these

types of problems include conflict over the client's spending money on substances or not working, or major disagreements over household responsibilities.

Crises That Need to be Addressed in the Session

Acute problems require immediate attention to avoid negative consequences and maintain relatives' involvement in treatment (e.g., an impending relapse, potential loss of housing, health problem). When such a problem is identified at the beginning of the session, the clinician evaluates whether it needs to be addressed at the beginning of the session or whether it can wait to the end. If the problem is so great that family members will not be able to focus on learning the information or skills covered in the session before a tentative resolution has been reached, the clinician sets aside 10–20 minutes to work on the problem at the beginning of the session, and then returns to the planned agenda after completing work on the problem. If the problem can wait until the end of the session, time is set aside to address it after the planned agenda is covered.

The clinician can use problem solving to help families deal with problems early in the course of family treatment. In this situation, the clinician assumes the role of the chairperson and leads the family through the sequence of problem-solving skills, recording progress on the Problem-Solving or Goal-Setting Sheet (see Appendix C, Form C.20). The clinician tries to reach a resolution to the problem as quickly as possible, so that the family can to get back to work on learning the relevant material. A focused discussion of a problem, led by the clinician using the problem-solving skills, can usually be accomplished in 10 or 15 minutes.

THE SIX PHASES OF BFT

In this section, we describe in detail the six phases of BFT for dual disorders: *connecting* with the family, *assessment*, *psychoeducation*, *communication skills training*, *problem-solving training*, and *termination*.

Connecting (1–3 Sessions)

The connecting phase is crucial, since no family work can take place without successful engagement. In this first phase, the clinician reaches out to the family—first to the client to explain the importance of working with his or her family, and second to the relatives to stimulate their interest and enlist their involvement. A brief orientation meeting is then arranged and carried out. Most of the obstacles to engaging family members can be overcome if the clinician is attentive to addressing their concerns, enthusiastic about the benefits of the family program, and flexible in accommodating family needs.

Presenting Family Work to the Client

In order to initiate BFT, the client must first be motivated to participate in family sessions and give the clinician permission to contact his or her relatives. The most critical ingredient to convincing the client that family work is in his or her own best interest is the *clinician's own belief* in the importance of such work. Clinicians who understand that working with families is helpful, even when families appear to have a negative effect on clients' adjustment, will be successful in engaging most clients and their relatives in family treatment. Clinicians who fear that family work will unnecessarily burden relatives, will worsen stress on clients, or will interfere with other types of psychotherapeutic work may unintentionally convey their doubts to the clients, preventing them from connecting with relatives.

When one is presenting BFT to a client, it is helpful to describe it as a program to help family members work together and achieve personal and shared goals. Common goals of family work that a client usually values include providing information about psychiatric illness and medications, helping relatives understand the nature of the client's difficulties, reducing stress and tension, reducing hospitalizations, and helping everyone (including the client) become members of the treatment team. Clients who are in the active treatment or relapse prevention stage of dual-disorder treatment can also be motivated to participate in BFT in order to address their substance abuse problems. Clients should understand that the goals of the family program are to work on improving the future, not to dredge up the past. If a client agrees, key relatives are identified who can be contacted about participation. In addition, the clinician can solicit suggestions about who should be contacted first.

Clients often readily give permission to contact and work with their relatives. However, some clients have misgivings about family work. In order to deal with these concerns, the clinician must understand the basis for the client's reluctance. Two concerns are most common: worry about the stress of family sessions, and concern about burdening relatives.

Concern about Stress in Family Sessions. A client may be worried that family sessions may increase stress, including exposure to criticism from relatives. The clinician can respond to this concern by explaining that BFT is intended to educate and support the entire family, and to lower stress on everyone. The positive, future-oriented nature of family work should be emphasized, to assure the client that sessions will be learning experiences for everyone involved. For clients who have had negative experiences with other approaches to family therapy, the clinician should highlight the differences between these other approaches and BFT, including BFT's focus on education and reducing family conflict.

Concern about Burdening Relatives. Some clients are painfully aware that their illness has been a source of strain to their relatives, and they prefer not to involve them in treatment to avoid burdening them further. These concerns can be assuaged by letting clients know that the goals of BFT are to reduce stress on *all* family members, including relatives. Clients also benefit from hearing that relatives appreciate the opportunity to learn more about psychiatric illness and ways to work more closely with the treatment team, which will actually alleviate their burden.

Connecting with Relatives

The clinician initiates contact with the relatives after the client has given permission. The goal of the first contact is to describe the purposes of the family program and, if the contact is made over the phone, to arrange for an in-person meeting with family members to discuss the program in more detail. During the first contact with each relative, the clinician explains that the overall goal of the BFT program is to help relatives become members of the client's treatment team, and to work closely with the team to manage the psychiatric illness. More specific goals include decreasing relapses and rehospitalizations, and increasing the client's capacity for independent living. The clinician should not assume that relatives will view the client's substance abuse as a problem (Mueser, Bellack, et al., 1992). However, the clinician should be prepared to discuss this as a focus of the program if relatives express concern or if it is known that the relatives view substance abuse as a problem.

After briefly describing the goals of BFT, the clinician describes the format of family sessions, emphasizing that the main ingredients of sessions are education about the client's psychiatric disorder, substance abuse, their interactions, and other topics; helping families communicate effectively; and teaching family members problem-solving skills for dealing with common situations. Brief psychoeducation about the nature of the psychiatric illness or substance use disorder and their treatment may be helpful with some families in the connecting phase. Sometimes several meetings are needed to motivate families to participate; these meetings may include various members of the family, and provide members with opportunities to ask further questions about the program.

Relatives may be reluctant to participate in family sessions for two common reasons: burnout, and fear of stress and conflict. Strategies for responding to these concerns are described below.

Burnout. Some relatives have a long history of trying to cope with an ill member and doubt that family work will help. The primary obstacle for these relatives is mustering the energy to participate in the family sessions. There are two general strategies for motivating such relatives: instilling hope, and encouraging relatives to give the program a try.

In order to instill hope, the clinician must first validate relatives' experiences by empathizing with the challenges they have faced. Relatives are often surprised and relieved to learn that other families have had similar experiences. Relatives are also encouraged to hear that other families who have experienced years of frustration have been able to benefit from BFT, and that it is never too late to work on improving for the future.

Relatives may not want to make a long-term commitment to participating in the BFT program. The clinician can encourage these relatives to try participating in family sessions, and stop if they do not find them helpful. With such relatives, it may also be helpful to convey the idea that they risk little by trying the program, and stand to gain much.

Fear of Stress and Conflict. Like some clients, some relatives are afraid of stress and conflict in family sessions. These concerns can be addressed using the same strategies for responding to clients' concerns, such as emphasizing BFT's orientation toward the future, and distinguishing it from other approaches to family therapy.

Family Orientation Meeting

After all the family members have agreed to participate in the program, an orientation meeting is scheduled to solidify their decision to work together and to set positive expectations for participation. This meeting is arranged as soon as possible after the last family member has agreed to participate. The orientation takes place in a single meeting, usually lasting 15–20 minutes, and involves all relevant family members (including the client). At the beginning of the meeting the clinician hands out to each family member an Orientation to Behavioral Family Therapy sheet (see Appendix C, Form C.15), which is used to guide the family through the discussion of BFT. Each component of this sheet is briefly reviewed by the clinician, who answers questions as they arise.

At the end of the orientation, the clinician arranges individual meetings with each person, and establishes a time to convene the family for the first session. The individual assessments are completed as soon as possible to minimize delay before beginning family sessions.

Assessment (2–5 Sessions)

Individual interviews form the basis for the clinician's initial assessment of the family. The Family Member Interview and the Functional Assessment Interview (with the client) guide the clinician through the information-gathering process (see Appendix C, Forms C.16 and C.4, respectively). It is important to make each person feel as comfortable as possible; to establish good rapport; not to rush the person; and to allow him or her to deviate from the major focus of the questions, but eventually to guide the person back to the topic. This assessment is then treated as a hypothesis through the next phase (psychoeducation) as additional information is gathered.

The initial meetings with each family member serve three general purposes. First, they are used to gather information about each member's understanding of the client's mental illness and substance use problems, their perceptions of factors that may maintain the substance abuse, and obstacles to change. Second, the individual meetings help to develop a personal relationship between each family member and the clinician. All members should feel free to contact the clinician outside the session, and should perceive the clinician as not taking sides with specific members, but instead as being interested in the welfare of the whole family. Third, the individual meetings can be important in identifying information that might not otherwise be revealed during family sessions. For example, members may be reluctant to acknowledge physical or sexual abuse, or their own substance abuse problems, during family sessions. Knowing such information may be important in planning family sessions.

Hints on Conducting Individual Interviews

When discussing the client's use of substances, the clinician should avoid trying to persuade family members that it is a problem. The most important goal is to get an unbiased understanding of each family member's perception of the client's substance use and its associated problems. The opportunity to convince family members that the client's substance use has negative effects will come later, mainly during psychoeducation and problem-solving training.

During the inquiry about social and leisure activities, the clinician should explain that the purpose of these questions is to help the clinician know about positive experiences in family members' lives, as well as areas in which change is desired. The clinician seeks to understand the "whole person"—including strengths and interests, and not just the challenges the individual faces.

In the section of the interview about goals, the clinician should explain that the focus of the program is on improving the lives of *all* family members, not just the client. Because some relatives have difficulty identifying goals in the individual interview, the clinician can briefly explain the purpose of establishing goals, and ask each member to think of some goals over the next several weeks. The clinician can then check with members during the psychoeducational sessions to make sure that each one identifies at least one personal goal on which to work.

When exploring each family member's goals, the clinician should bear in mind that goals need to be for that individual, rather than another member. When one member expresses concern about another's behavior, the clinician can explore how that behavior affects the first person. For example, a client who abuses alcohol, stays up late, and misses appointments may inconvenience a relative by contributing to a disruptive home environment and requiring more of the relative's time (so that missed appointments can be rescheduled and the client can be transported to them). It is best if goals are behaviorally specific.

Functional Analysis

When the individual interviews with family members have been completed, a functional analysis of the client's substance use behavior is conducted—or, if one has been performed already as part of individual work with the client, it may be modified. (See the Payoff Matrix [Form C.6 in Appendix C] and Chapter 5 for more details.) As with individual treatment, the functional

analysis serves as an initial hypothesis about the most important factors that need to be modified over the course of BFT in order to address the client's substance abuse. For example, a client's substance use may be motivated by social factors and a need for something to do. For this client, family sessions may partly focus on developing other social outlets and structuring the person's time in order to help him or her cut down or eliminate substance use. Figure 14.1 shows an example of a Payoff Matrix completed following a family assessment. The information is based on family interviews with a client (Bob Smith), his mother, and his stepfather, who have been engaged in BFT.

Summary of Family Assessment

The Summary of Family Assessment (see Appendix C, Form C.17) succinctly describes the most relevant information to guide the clinician in conducting the initial family sessions. This information includes a brief description of the family; the client's psychiatric disorder and substance use problems; the impact of the substance abuse on the client and relatives; critical factors hypothesized in the functional analysis to be maintaining the client's substance abuse (or to pose a risk for relapse); the observed degree of supportiveness or tension among family members; the client and relatives' motivation to improve management of the psychiatric disorder and to address the substance abuse; and the client's stage of treatment. This summary is used to formulate treatment goals (see below). Figure 14.2 shows a Summary of Family Assessment completed for the case of Bob Smith and his family.

Family Treatment Plan

Drawing from the individual family member interviews and the Summary of Family Assessment, the Family Treatment Plan (see Appendix C, Form C.18)

	Using Substances	Not Using Substances
Advantages	• Hangs out with friends when smoking marijuana • Enjoyable "buzz" from drinking • Looks forward to drinking as something to do at end of day	• Better relationship with mother and stepfather • Less severe psychotic symptoms • Might be able to return to school and complete college degree
Disadvantages	• Conflict with mother and stepfather; sometimes belligerent after drinking • Worsens symptoms and self-care skills, leading to relapses and rehospitalizations • Concentration problems interfere with work or going to school	• Nothing fun to do or to look forward to • Turning down offers to use marijuana with friends

FIGURE 14.1. Payoff Matrix for Bob Smith, completed during BFT assessment.

Instructions: Summarize and integrate the pertinent information from the functional assessment interview (with the client) and individual family member interviews on this form.

Description of family (e.g., living arrangement and family contacts):

Bob has a large family with several siblings and stepsiblings who live in another state. Bob presents for treatment with his mother and stepfather. Bob lives with his parents, with whom he has daily contact. He sees his siblings and stepsiblings several times per year, often at family gatherings.

Client's psychiatric disorder and substance abuse problems:

Bob has schizophrenia, which was diagnosed during his second year of college. Bob began using substances in high school—mainly drinking and smoking marijuana with friends. When he entered family treatment, he was drinking daily (usually alone) and smoking marijuana weekly (most often with friends).

Impact of substance abuse on client and relatives:

Bob's substance use often worsens his symptoms and leads to rehospitalizations. When Bob is using substances, it also interferes with his personal hygiene and self-care skills, and he sometimes becomes angry and belligerent with his parents. These problems cause a great deal of tension in the family.

Critical factors identified on functional analysis:

Bob often uses marijuana with friends, and sometimes drinks with them as well. In order to give up using substances, Bob will need to develop new social outlets for spending time with other people who do not abuse substances. Bob also likes to drink when he's alone sometimes, because he enjoys the "buzz" he gets from alcohol. In order for Bob to give up alcohol, he will need to develop other recreational activities. In addition, helping Bob pursue his educational goals (completing college) and obtain work might structure his time and give him something other than alcohol and marijuana to focus his energy on.

Degree of supportiveness or tension among family members:

Bob's mother and stepfather are very supportive of him, and he is currently living with them. There is some tension between Bob and his stepfather, who doesn't understand very much about schizophrenia, and sometimes thinks that Bob is just lazy. However, Bob's stepfather has expressed an interest in learning more about schizophrenia and participating in family sessions.

Client and relatives' motivation to improve management of psychiatric disorder:

Both Bob and his parents would like to see him get better control of his symptoms and stay out of the hospital. The parents would also like Bob to learn more about how to manage his illness, so that he can live independently and they are not required to monitor his symptoms and medication adherence.

Description of family's strengths (as gathered from individual interviews and observations of the family):

Bob and his family have several strengths. They are a close family, committed to helping each other and maintaining each other's support. Family members have good communication skills; they listen to each other, rarely raise their voices, and attempt to express their feelings directly. Bob's mother has been actively involved in helping Bob get the treatment he needs and monitoring his illness, and she has attended to her own needs by joining a local affiliate of the National Alliance for the Mentally Ill. Bob's stepfather is extremely supportive of his wife, and wants to learn more about Bob's mental illness so that he can be more supportive of Bob and communicate more effectively with him. Bob has a very close and loving relationship with his mother, and tries hard to get along with his stepfather. Thus family members show significant respect and concern for each other.

Client's stage of treatment (from the substance abuse treatment scale—Revised):

___ Preengagement	___ Early Active Treatment
___ Engagement	___ Late Active Treatment
_X_ Early Persuasion	___ Relapse Prevention
___ Late Persuasion	___ Recovery

Overall family stage of treatment (taking into consideration all family members):

___ Preengagement	___ Early Active Treatment
_X_ Engagement	___ Late Active Treatment
___ Early Persuasion	___ Relapse Prevention
___ Late Persuasion	___ Recovery

FIGURE 14.2. Summary of Family Assessment, completed for Bob Smith and his family.

identifies the specific goals of family intervention that guide the clinician in the BFT work. Included in the Family Treatment Plan are individual goals set by each family member; shared family goals; goals based on the functional analysis of the client's substance use behavior; and goals based on the client's stage of treatment. When BFT is the primary psychotherapeutic intervention provided to the client, the Family Treatment Plan replaces the Individual Dual-Disorder Treatment Plan (Appendix C, Form C.9; see Chapter 5). When BFT is not the only intervention provided to the client, both the Individual Dual-Disorder and Family Treatment Plans should be completed. An example of a Family Treatment Plan completed for the case of Bob Smith and his family is provided in Figure 14.3.

Reassessment of the Family

Reassessments of individual and family-based goals should be conducted every 3–6 months. These assessments evaluate progress toward goals, modify old goals, and establish new goals. Reassessment can be conducted either in a meeting involving all family members or in brief meetings with each family member, followed by a family discussion concerning shared goals. Reevaluation of the functional analysis should also be conducted every 3–6 months, depending on progress (or

---

Family Treatment Plan (Bob Smith)

I. Client's Individual Goals

  1. Complete college
  2. Find part-time work
  3.

II. Family Member 1's Individual Goals (Mom)

  1. Join an aerobics class
  2. Attend monthly meetings of National Alliance for the Mentally Ill
  3.

III. Family Member 2's Individual Goals (Stepfather)

  1. More vacation time with wife
  2. Attend Rotary Club breakfast meetings regularly
  3.

IV. Family Member 3's Individual Goals

  1.
  2.
  3.

V. Shared Family Goals

  1. Spend time together every weekend, having dinner and watching videos
  2. Independent living for Bob
  3.

VI. Factors Identified by Functional Analysis

  1. Help Bob get involved in new social and recreational activities
  2. Help Bob get part-time work
  3. Enroll Bob in college class

VII. Stage-Wise Treatment Goals

  1. Regular family meetings
  2. Education about interactions between mental illness and substance abuse

FIGURE 14.3. Family Treatment Plan, completed for Bob Smith and his family.

the lack of progress) in addressing substance abuse and other goals.

Psychoeducation (6–8 Sessions)

The psychoeducation phase of BFT has two main purposes. The first is to provide family members with basic information about mental illness, substance abuse, their interactions, and their treatment. The second is to provide the family members with information they need to work together, as well as with strategies for improved communication. At the same time, these sessions allow the clinician to gather more information about specific factors that maintain the substance abuse and interfere with achieving a healthier lifestyle.

Content of Psychoeducational Sessions

The 16 educational handouts included in Appendix B can be used in the psychoeducational sessions. Most families receive psychoeducation on at least eight different topics (the Appendix B handouts used for these topics are indicated in parentheses):

1. Psychiatric Diagnosis (Handout B.1, B.2, B.3, B.4, B.5, or B.6, depending on a client's diagnosis)
2. Medication (Handout B.7, B.8, or B.9, depending on the type of medication a client is taking)
3. The Stress–Vulnerability Model of Psychiatric Disorders (Handout B.10)
4. Role of the Family (Handout B.11)
5. Basic Facts about Alcohol and Drugs (Handout B.12)
6. Alcohol and Drugs: Motives and Consequences (Handout B.13)
7. Treatment of Dual Disorders (Handout B.14; Handout B.16, on Infectious Diseases, may also be covered with some families)
8. Communication Skills (Handout B.15)

Each of the educational topics can be reviewed in one family session, with the exception of The Stress–Vulnerability Mode of Psychiatric Disorders and Role of the Family, which may be combined in a single session. More than one session may be spent on some topics if warranted. The educational topics are usually presented in the order listed above. The usual way of moving through these topics is first to establish the validity and nature of the client's mental illness, followed by the principles of its treatment and the role of the family (educational topics 1–4). Discussion of the stress–vulnerability model of psychiatric disorders introduces families to the fact that alcohol and drug use can interact with mental illness. This discussion paves the road for providing more in-depth information about substance abuse and dual disorders, concluding with a discussion of treatment options (educational topics 5–7). When family members have been educated about dual disorders, the last topic addresses communication skills (educational topic 8), in order to prepare the family for training in cooperative problem solving. Families that need formal communication skills training can skip this last topic.

Psychoeducational Strategies

Five basic strategies, described below, are used in conducting psychoeducational sessions.

Two Ways of Using Educational Handouts. Handouts can be used in two ways. A handout can be given to family members at the beginning of the session and reviewed over the course of the session, or the clinician can summarize the main points of the handout, and then give it to members to review as a homework assignment at the end of the session. If the handout is not used during the session, it is helpful to use a flipchart, poster, or blackboard to summarize the main points.

Interactive Psychoeducation. To ensure that family members understand the relevance of educational material, the clinician asks frequent questions and engages the members in understanding how information is related to their own experiences. Truly effective psychoeducation is interactive, rather than purely didactic. Another reason for using an interactive teaching style is that the clinician can assess family members' understanding of the material by asking open-ended questions. After an educational topic has been covered in a family session, the clinician can ask family members questions to evaluate their comprehension of the material and provide corrective information before moving on to the next topic. Examples of review questions for each of the educational topics are provided in Table 14.2. Although seven sessions are usually sufficient to cover the educational material, more time can be allotted if necessary. If the review questions about a topic reveal that some family members have not grasped the information, repeating that topic may be important before moving on.

Treating the Client as the "Expert." During the psychoeducational sessions, the clinician can refer to the client's experience with mental illness as making him or her the "expert" on the topic (Falloon, Boyd, & McGill, 1984). Acknowledging the client as the expert gives him or her a positive role to play during the educational sessions, and recognizes that the client is able

TABLE 14.2. Review Questions for Educational Topics

Psychiatric Diagnosis
- What is the client's diagnosis?
- What are some examples of symptoms of this diagnosis?
- How common is this disorder?

Medication
- What type of medication is the client receiving?
- What are the effects of this medication?
- What medication side effects have been noticed by the client?
- If side effects have been noted, what strategies have been used to try to deal with them?

The Stress–Vulnerability Model of Psychiatric Disorders
- What causes mental illness?
- What are some of the factors that can improve mental illness?
- What are some of the factors that can make the mental illness worse?

Role of the Family
- How do families respond when a member develops a psychiatric illness?
- What are the early warning signs of relapse of the client's psychiatric illness?
- What are the steps of the relapse prevention plan family members need to take if early warning signs of a relapse are detected?

Basic Facts about Alcohol and Drugs
- What are the different substances that people sometimes use?
- What are the effects of alcohol? Marijuana? Stimulants, such as cocaine? Sedatives?
- How do these substances affect a person with a mental illness?

Alcohol and Drugs: Motives and Consequences
- What are some of the reasons the client uses alcohol or drugs?
- What are some of the negative consequences associated with drug or alcohol use?
- What is substance abuse?
- What is substance dependence?
- Why are clients with psychiatric illnesses more likely to have problems with alcohol and drug use than people in the general population?

Treatment of Dual Disorders
- What are the different stages of treatment?
- What are some examples of ways of treating persons with a dual disorder?
- How can family members help a person with a dual disorder?

Infectious Diseases (if necessary)
- How are HIV, hepatitis B, and hepatitis C spread from one person to another?
- What organ of the body is hurt by hepatitis B and hepatitis C?
- How does HIV lead to AIDS?
- What treatments are available for HIV, hepatitis B, and hepatitis C?
- How can you take care of yourself if you have one of these infectious diseases?

Communication Skills
- Why is good communication important in families?
- What are some strategies for communicating effectively with family members?

to speak with authority about the experience of mental illness. Relatives also have expertise in mental illness by virtue of their familiarity with the client, and this fact is also acknowledged during the educational sessions. Communicating these roles to family members helps them to see that everyone in the family has had valuable experiences, and that these can contribute to better understanding and care of the client's mental illness and substance abuse.

Respecting Differences in Opinion. The clinician strives to create an atmosphere in the sessions in which family members are free to disagree with one another, and with the educational material presented, without fear of criticism. Despite any disagreements, the clinician still reviews the material, while acknowledging the different points of view. For example, when the client Bob Smith and his family are discussing the client's psychiatric illness, Bob may state that he does not believe that he has schizophrenia, while his mother and stepfather attempt to persuade him that he does. Rather than provoking a debate on this topic, the clinician can acknowledge that the family members differ in their opinions, and point out that what is most important is that they are willing to work together as a family to achieve goals.

Structure of Psychoeducational Sessions

Psychoeducational sessions follow a simple three-part structure. They begin with a brief check on the family meeting and a review of questions on the last session's topic. The bulk of the session is spent presenting and discussing a new topic. The session concludes with an assignment of homework: to review that week's handout at the family meeting. Psychoeducational sessions are conducted by the clinician, who weaves back and forth between presenting information and eliciting family members' perceptions and experiences about the material. The general structure for each session is summarized in Table 14.3. When this structure is maintained and the discussion is kept focused on the educational material, members learn that they can talk about mental illness and substance abuse without major conflict.

A Brief Summary of Psychoeducational Sessions

We provide a brief description of seven psychoeducational sessions below. Note that these sessions are numbered beginning with the first psychoeducational session, and do not include sessions devoted to the connecting and assessment phases of BFT (see Table 14.1). See Mueser and Glynn (1999) for more information about leading psychoeducational sessions, as well as clinical vignettes.

Psychoeducational Session 1: Psychiatric Diagnosis. In the first session, the clinician informs the family about the client's psychiatric diagnosis—how the diag-

nosis is established, what the characteristic symptoms are, and what its longitudinal course is likely to be. Each family member's understanding of the illness is elicited; misunderstandings are clarified; and the client's role as the "expert" in the illness is introduced. Disagreements among members, such as on the issue of the psychiatric diagnosis or the client's symptoms, are acknowledged without attempting to resolve them. This first psychoeducational session often serves as a "rallying point" in motivating a family to work together to improve the client's and each member's lives.

Psychoeducational Session 2: Medication. The second session summarizes the main medication(s) used by the client. It includes information on the effects of medications on the symptoms and course of psychiatric illness; the common side effects of medications and strategies for dealing with them; and misconceptions about many medications, such as the belief that they are addictive. The session is intended to improve adherence to medication due to such problems as the failure to understand the purposes of medication, side effects, and misunderstandings about the interactions between medication and substances. It is important to check with the client's psychiatrist about any possible interactions between currently abused substances and prescribed medication (see Chapter 19), in order to inform family members about adherence to medication when substance abuse is still active.

Psychoeducational Session 3: Stress–Vulnerability Model of Psychiatric Disorders, and Role of the Family. The two educational handouts reviewed in the third session (Handouts B.10 and B.11 in Appendix B) cover two topic areas: a major theoretical model of psychiatric disorders, and common reactions in families to mental illness in one member. Discussion of the stress–vulnerability model helps family members understand that the psychiatric illness is biological in nature, but that its severity and course can be affected by environmental factors (such as stress and coping), as well as by biological factors (such as medication and substance abuse).

The handout on the role of the family explains how family members can help the client manage his or her disorder, based on the stress–vulnerability model. In addition, many of the reactions family members have in response to a relative's illness, such as anxiety or overprotection, are discussed as common and normal reactions. At the end of the session, the clinician helps the family develop a relapse prevention plan (see Appendix C, Form C.11) for responding to the early warning signs of a relapse of the psychiatric illness. This plan can be posted somewhere prominent in the family's home (e.g., on the refrigerator). If the client and rela-

TABLE 14.3. Structure of Psychoeducational Sessions

Time period	Clinical activity
First 5–10 minutes	Check on family meeting and ask review questions about preceding session's topic. Evaluate understanding; answer questions; troubleshoot if no family meeting occurred.
Next 40–50 minutes	Present and discuss new educational topic.
Last 5 minutes	Assign homework to read handout together during family meeting and note any questions that arise.

tives live separately, the plan can be posted in more than one location.

Psychoeducational Session 4: Basic Facts about Alcohol and Drugs. The fourth session is aimed at facilitating a frank discussion of alcohol and drug use by the client and other family members. The goal is not to persuade members that the client's use of substances is a problem, but rather to encourage an open discussion that is free of stress and tension. This is accomplished by first normalizing substance use as a common human behavior, and then discussing different types of commonly used substances and their effects (both positive and negative). In this session, it is often easier to talk with families about alcohol and drug use without using such terms as *addiction, substance abuse,* or *substance dependence.* During this educational topic and the next one, the clinician is alert to any member's willingness to discuss his or her own use of substances, including relatives of the client. The clinician does not push family members to talk about their substance use, even if such use is obvious, but strives to create an atmosphere in the family sessions in which members feel safe talking openly with one another.

Psychoeducational Session 5: Alcohol and Drugs: Motives and Consequences. The fifth session focuses on the different reasons people use alcohol and drugs, and the major consequences of use. The clinician facilitates a balanced discussion of substance use, including some of the reasons the client uses substances, as well as some of the disadvantages of using. By recognizing that people use substances for specific reasons, the clinician validates some of the client's experiences while also opening the door to consideration of the disadvantages of substance use.

Psychoeducational Session 6: Treatment of Dual Disorders (and Infectious Diseases, if Necessary). The sixth session introduces family members to the stages-of-treatment concept, and encourages them to evaluate their own motivation to work together on the client's substance use problems. Different strategies for treating clients with dual disorders are discussed, with an emphasis on the role of family problem solving. For family members who view the client's substance use as a problem, this session serves to identify the most promising strategies. For other members who are not yet convinced that the client's use of substances is a problem, or for whom there is conflict, this session can help them discuss options and exchange viewpoints without a commitment to action.

An additional educational handout (Handout B.16

in Appendix B) provides information about infectious diseases in persons with dual disorders. Depending on the extent of the client's high-risk behaviors for such diseases (e.g., unprotected sex, intravenous or intranasal drug use) and the relationship of a relative to a client (e.g., spouse or girlfriend/boyfriend vs. other family member), the clinician may choose to cover this handout with the entire family or privately with the client. The decision about whether the family should participate in the educational session on infectious diseases needs to weigh privacy concerns for the client against the need for family members (e.g., spouses) to know, and the potential role the family members can play in helping clients reduce high-risk behaviors or obtain treatment for the disease. If a client is assessed to be at low risk for infectious diseases, this handout can be omitted altogether.

Psychoeducational Session 7: Communication Skills. Good communication is an important prerequisite for training families in problem solving. Without adequate communication skills, problem solving can easily become mired in arguments, criticism, and blaming; frustration and family disengagement may be the results. The educational handout on communication skills (Handout B.15 in Appendix B) covers some of the basics of good communication, and is intended for families whose members have adequate or good communication skills and do not require formal training in communication (see below). When the basics of good communication have been reviewed with all family members, the clinician can prompt them to adhere to the rules in later sessions when problems occur.

Communication Skills Training (4–8 Sessions, if Necessary)

In some families, communication between members is a significant problem that psychoeducation alone cannot correct. Such families may benefit from specific training in communication skills before proceeding to problem-solving training. Indications that family communication is stressful, and that training in communication skills is in order, include frequent criticisms or pejorative putdowns (e.g., "You're lazy!"); failure to listen to what others say; frequent interruptions; speaking for another person and assuming that one knows "what's best" for that person; invalidating others' feelings; or angry outbursts.

When communication skills training is undertaken, four to eight sessions are spent teaching the five specific skills outlined in the Communication Skills handout: expressing positive feelings, making a positive request, expressing negative feelings, compromise and negotiation, and requesting a time out. The principles of social skills training (see Chapter 11) are adapted for this work, with one to two sessions spent per communication skill. After each skills training session, family members are instructed to practice the skills on their own, in their day-to-day interactions with each other, and to note their efforts to use the skill on homework sheets. These homework sheets can be reviewed at family meetings, and are followed up at BFT sessions. The steps of communication skills training with families are summarized in Table 14.4. More information about communication skills training is provided in Mueser and Glynn (1999).

Problem-Solving Training (5–15+ Sessions)

Training in problem solving involves teaching a standard sequence of six skills to family members; these skills are designed to minimize conflict and to maximize the identification of successful solutions. Individuals and families can use the skills to address a wide range of both problems and goals, including those related to substance use. It is through the teaching of problem-solving skills that family members become empowered to solve their own problems rather than always relying on the clinician to solve their problems for them.

TABLE 14.4. Steps of Communication Skills Training with Families

1. Establishing a rationale for learning the skill
   - Elicit comments from each family member about why the skill is important.
   - Provide additional reasons as necessary.

2. Presenting the component steps of the skill
   - Review each step of the skill, using posters or handouts.
   - Briefly discuss why each step is important.

3. Modeling (demonstrating) the skill for the family
   - Explain that you will give an example of how to use the skill.
   - Choose an everyday situation to demonstrate.
   - When the skill has been modeled, ask family members which steps of the skill they have observed you do.

4. Engaging a family member in a role play to practice the skill
   - Choose a situation that recently happened.
   - Simulate the physical conditions of the original situation (e.g., have family members stand or sit facing each other), rearranging furniture if necessary.
   - Instruct the family member to try the skill in a role play.
   - Request other family members to monitor performance.

5. Providing positive feedback about the role play
   - Elicit positive feedback from family members about specific behaviors in the role play.
   - Provide additional positive feedback as necessary.
   - Cut off any criticism from family members, and postpone corrective feedback until positive feedback has been given.

6. Providing corrective feedback
   - Point out one specific behavior in which the family member could improve.
   - Explain what the person could do differently to be more effective in using the skill.

7. Engaging the family member in another role play of the same situation
   - Request the person to do the role play again, this time making one change in behavior based on the corrective feedback.
   - Use additional modeling, coaching, and/or prompting to help the person further improve his or her ability to do the skill.

8. Providing additional positive and corrective feedback about the role play
   - Always provide (and elicit from family members) positive feedback first, then give corrective feedback.
   - If improvements can still be made and the person is willing, do one or two more role plays of the same situation.

9. Engaging another family member in a different role play, followed by feedback and more practice (steps 4–8)
   - Have every person practice the skill in at least two role plays of a specific incident, eliciting feedback from family members.
   - Provide ample encouragement and reinforcement for effort and improvement.

10. Assigning homework to practice the skill
   - Explain the rationale for homework, give out homework sheets, and review how they should be completed.
   - Elicit and answer questions about the assignment.
   - Ask family members when they can complete their assignment each day and how they will remember to do it.

Sequence of Problem-Solving Skills

The specific sequence of problem-solving skills is briefly described below.

1. *Defining the problem.* To solve a problem or achieve a goal, family members must first agree on what the problem is. To accomplish this, all members should express their opinions about the problem, arrive at a definition acceptable to everyone, and record the definition on the Problem-Solving or Goal-Setting Sheet (Appendix C, Form C.20). It is important that all family members agree on the definition of the problem. When disagreement exists, the clinician can help the family members creatively define the problem so that all members agree. For example, if Bob Smith's mother is upset that her son spends all his money on alcohol, and he resents the fact that his mother berates him for drinking, the problem could be defined as "Mother gets upset with Bob's frequent drinking of alcohol."

2. *Brainstorming possible solutions.* Family members generate as many possible solutions to the problem as possible, without evaluating their advantages and disadvantages. Each possible solution is written down, and every family member is encouraged to contribute at least one solution.

3. *Evaluating all solutions.* After at least five solutions have been generated, each solution is evaluated. The evaluation of solutions need not be exhaustive, but should be sufficient to identify which solutions offer the most promise for resolving the problem. The advantages and disadvantages of different solutions are recorded; family members may find it helpful to put stars or asterisks next to those solutions judged to be most promising.

4. *Determining the best solution(s).* After all the solutions have been evaluated, family members select which solution or combination of solutions is most likely to solve the problem. Often the best solution is obvious after all of the solutions have been evaluated. Sometimes more than one solution appears viable, or family members disagree as to the best solution. In such cases, more than one solution may be selected, different solutions may be combined into a composite solution, or competing solutions may be tried sequentially.

5. *Planning on how to implement the solution(s), and doing so.* When a solution has been selected, a plan is needed for implementing it. This plan should include information about roles ("Who is going to do what?"), the time frame ("When are the different parts of the solution going to be implemented?"), and resources ("What information, money, or skills are needed to implement the plan?"). Because some plans involve several people, it may be helpful if family members elect a coordinator who follows up on whether each person has fulfilled his or her role.

6. *Scheduling a time to follow up, doing so, and conducting additional problem solving if necessary.* Problem solving is sometimes successful after the first attempt. However, many problems require multiple attempts before progress is made. Setting up a time to follow up on problem solving ensures that unsolved problems will continue to be addressed by the family. The follow-up meeting should be scheduled as soon as possible after family members have had a chance to implement the plan, preferably within a week.

At the follow-up meeting, the chairperson determines whether the problem has been solved. There are many reasons why a problem may not be solved after the first attempt. If the solution has been successfully implemented and the problem is improved but not resolved, additional problem solving may be conducted on the problem, or the family may decide to move on to another problem. If the problem has not improved, it must be determined whether the plan was implemented correctly. If the plan was not implemented, a new plan needs to be made. If the plan was implemented, but the solution did not improve the problem significantly, family members need to reconsider whether another solution might be more effective for dealing with the problem, and then to develop a new plan for implementing that solution.

If repeated problem-solving efforts have been unsuccessful or minimally successful, it is useful for families to attempt to define the problem differently to make it easier to solve. With such problems, it may be helpful to break the problem down into smaller steps that may be tackled one at a time, or to attempt to minimize the negative consequences associated with the problem (e.g., if the client is prone to driving while intoxicated and efforts to address the drinking have so far been unsuccessful, problem solving about not driving after drinking or not driving at all may be productive).

Selection of Problems for Problem Solving

The selection of which problems to address in problem-solving training is determined by a combination of factors, including the specific goals identified in the family assessment (both individual and family goals), the client's stage of treatment, and the functional analysis of the client's substance use behavior. At least some of the problem-solving sessions should address the client's substance use behavior, while others should address different family goals.

Family problem solving can be used in different ways to address the client's substance abuse, depending on the client's stage of treatment. We discuss later how problem solving can be used with clients who are in the persuasion stage of treatment, as well as those in the active treatment and relapse prevention stages.

Format

Problem-solving skills are first demonstrated by working on a relatively easy problem or goal. The clinician walks the family through the sequence of skills, working together on a problem so that family members are able to participate and see how the process works. After the clinician leads them through the sequence, they gradually assume the primary responsibility for leading the problem solving, with the assistance and intervention of the clinician as necessary. Assignments are given to family members to practice the problem-solving skills during their own weekly meetings held outside of the sessions. Gradually, they become more adept at solving problems. Although the ultimate goal is for family members to solve problems on their own, the clinician remains involved in helping families solve problems as long as necessary.

The problem-solving efforts are coordinated by a chairperson (chosen by consensus), who assumes the responsibility of keeping family members on task and following the sequence of problem-solving skills. For many families, it is convenient if the chairperson keeps track of the different skills on the Problem-Solving or Goal-Setting Sheet (Appendix C, Form C.20). Some families like to have one person chair the problem-solving discussion and another person be the secretary who records the family's efforts.

During the initial teaching of problem solving, the use of each skill in the sequence is recorded on the Problem-Solving or Goal-Setting Sheet. Keeping a written record has the advantage of slowing down the problem-solving process, which can be useful when people have strong feelings about the problem. In addition, recording the problem solving ensures that a more thorough job of addressing the problem is done. Family members are given homework assignments to practice the problem-solving skills on their own. Although families are often quite capable of doing this, most gravitate away from keeping written records. Therefore, as the family members become more competent at problem solving, the clinician can wean them from keeping written records, while still adhering to the basic structure.

A Brief Description of Problem-Solving Sessions

We describe the first several sessions of problem-solving training below. (Note that, similar to the pscyhoeducational sessions described earlier, these sessions are numbered beginning with the first problem-solving session.)

Problem-Solving Session 1: Introduction. In the first session, the clinician explains the rationale for problem solving, reviews with the family the sequence of problem-solving skills, and illustrates the skills by working on a problem with the family. At the end of the session, the family is given an assignment to follow up on the agreed-upon solution.

The clinician can introduce the family members to problem solving as follows:

"All families experience a variety of problems that they want to solve and goals that they want to achieve. Some of these problems or goals are shared by everyone in the family, and others may be more individually based. In our individual and family meetings, we have already talked about some of the changes you would like to make. As a clinician, I can help you work on some of these problems and goals. However, I will not always be around to help you find the best solutions. For that reason, we are going to work together for the next several weeks to improve your ability to solve problems as a family."

After the rationale for problem solving has been explained, the clinician hands out copies of the Problem-Solving or Goal-Setting Sheet. The clinician explains that the problem-solving process is led by a chairperson and progress is recorded. The clinician then provides a brief review of the sequence of problem-solving skills. Establishing the rationale for problem solving and reviewing the six skills requires 10–15 minutes. See Mueser and Glynn (1999) for examples of introducing and teaching the problem-solving method.

After the problem-solving skills have been reviewed, the clinician illustrates the process by working through a problem or goal with the family. During the demonstration, the clinician takes the roles of both chairperson and secretary, explaining what he or she is doing at each point along the way. The problem that is worked on is selected jointly by the clinician and family members. The primary goal of this demonstration is to familiarize family members with the problem-solving method. This is best accomplished by working on a relatively simple problem or goal, and avoiding long-standing or emotionally charged problems until the family members have improved their skills.

If the family does not identify a suitable problem or goal, the clinician suggests one. One good family goal that can be addressed in a first problem-solving session is spending leisure time together. For example, the clinician can suggest:

"When I met with each of you individually, you indicated you did not do very many things together in your spare time. How about if we take a problem-solving approach to the goal of identifying an activity you can do together as a family?"

If the family members agree to this, the clinician leads them through the problem-solving sequence. At the end of the session, the clinician gives the family the completed Problem-Solving or Goal-Setting Sheet, and an assignment to meet together during the week to review the plan for implementing the agreed-upon solution. The clinician prompts the family members during the session to select their meeting time for the forthcoming week, and to determine who will convene the meeting.

Problem-Solving Session 2: Continued Work. At the beginning of the second session, the clinician follows up with the family to determine whether they met during the week to review their problem-solving plan and, if so, how the plan went. The clinician then prompts the family to produce the Problem-Solving or Goal-Setting Sheet. If a family meeting was not held but the plan was successfully implemented, the clinician briefly explains that follow-up meetings are important to ensure that unsolved problems are not forgotten, and then proceeds to work on a new problem. If a family meeting was not held and the problem was not resolved, the family is prompted to hold a meeting then, at the beginning of the session. The clinician allows the family 5–10 minutes to discuss the problem-solving plan. Then the clinician joins in the discussion and helps the family members modify their plan accordingly.

When the previous Problem-Solving or Goal-Setting Sheet has been reviewed, work begins on a new problem, with family members taking the roles of chairperson and secretary. As this problem is the first in which family members lead themselves through the problem-solving sequence, it is best if a manageable problem is chosen (e.g., a very narrowly defined problem or one that is unlikely to evoke significant conflict). The family then goes through the sequence of skills, with the clinician assisting to help members engage in the different skills and to clarify questions about the process. As in the first session, the family members are prompted to review the problem-solving plan on their own before the next session.

In principle, it is preferable for the clinician to limit his or her feedback to the family during the problem-solving sessions to issues of process rather than content, since the goal of problem-solving training is to teach family members the process required for effectively solving problems (i.e., the sequence of skills). Furthermore, if the clinician becomes too actively involved in determining which solutions are best, the family members will become dependent on the clinician.

On the other hand, not all families learn all the problem-solving skills, and the resolution of problems may be critical to improving the dual disorders. Therefore, the clinician strikes a balance between teaching the family members how to solve problems and working with them to solve their problems.

Problem-Solving Sessions 3+. The same format for conducting the second session is followed for the third and subsequent problem-solving sessions. The clinician begins with a review of the family's progress on the previous problem or goal, including the family meeting held between the sessions. The rest of the session is spent either continuing work on a problem or goal that has not yet been completed, or working on new ones. To the extent possible, the clinician focuses on helping the family members improve their problem-solving skills, while becoming sufficiently involved in solving specific problems to ensure progress toward their resolution. With many families, it is important for all members to have experience chairing family problem-solving meetings. In some families, however, there is a member who naturally falls into this leadership role, and the clinician can increase the chances that problem solving will be incorporated into such a family by accepting this person's role and focusing on helping him or her learn how to chair problem-solving meetings.

Problem Solving in the Persuasion Stage

There are two general strategies for using family problem solving to address substance abuse in clients at the persuasion stage of treatment: the functional-analytic approach and the motivational interviewing approach. Although each approach is different, they are compatible with each other, and either or both can be used.

The functional-analytic approach involves applying problem solving to the factors that maintain substance abuse, such as the socialization, coping, or recreational needs that clients are currently meeting by using substances (see Chapter 5 for an in-depth discussion of the functional analysis). As clients learn alternative ways of getting their needs met, their desire to continue using substances weakens; the disadvantages of substance abuse become more apparent; and they become more motivated to stop using substances. For example, if the primary functions of alcohol use are to help a client cope with persistent hallucinations and to facilitate socializing with peers, problem solving can be used to help the client develop different strategies for managing hallucinations and other outlets for social interaction, and thereby reducing his or her need for alcohol to achieve these aims.

The motivational interviewing approach is based on the principles outlined in Chapter 7, except that these are applied in family sessions rather than individual ones. The essence of motivational interviewing is that people are only motivated to change behaviors they see as problems. Rather than trying to convince clients that their substance abuse is a problem, motivational interviewing emphasizes identifying and working on goals that a client (or family) chooses, while exploring the degree to which substance abuse interferes with achieving these goals. When clients begin to perceive substance use as interfering with personally valued goals, then they become motivated to change their substance use.

CASE EXAMPLE

Isabelle and her family were motivated to work on helping her obtain a job, and this became a focus of problem solving. In the course of working on this, it became apparent that Isabelle's use of alcohol interfered with her ability to get up in the morning and follow up potential job leads. In a problem-solving session, the family identified cutting down on drinking and scheduling drinking for designated times of the week as possible solutions (among others) to the goal of obtaining employment. Isabelle first chose the solution of scheduling her drinking for a certain time of the week (weekends). This solution helped in getting a job, but she still found that her drinking over the weekend was a problem for her job performance early the next week. In further problem solving, she chose to cut down on her weekend drinking by setting a goal of not having more than one drink on any day over the weekend. This solution proved effective, and her job performance improved markedly.

Problem Solving in the Active Treatment and Relapse Prevention Stages

Once the family endorses reduction of substance abuse as a primary treatment goal, problem solving can be used to help the client make progress toward further reducing substance use, and ultimately toward abstinence. As in the persuasion stage, the functional analysis of substance abuse behavior can be used to identify reinforcers of substance use (or factors that pose a risk for relapse). For example, if a client in the active treatment stage has succeeded in reducing his or her use of marijuana, but still occasionally uses it during periods of boredom, problem solving can be used to identify alternative activities for the client to engage in during such periods.

Aside from addressing reinforcers of substance use, problem solving can be used to work on other goals related to the reduction of substance use or maintenance of abstinence. For example, problem solving can be used to develop a plan to familiarize the client with dual-disorder treatment groups (Chapters 9–11) or local self-help groups (Chapter 12); to help him or her cope with cravings or withdrawal symptoms; to bolster social networks of abstinent peers; or to identify meaningful ways of structuring free time.

Termination (1 Session)

The exact timing and duration of family treatment are negotiated with all participants, and so families are prepared for the termination in advance. Although some families require ongoing sessions in order to avert crises and maintain gains, most families can benefit from a time-limited course of treatment. The termination session is focused on reviewing past accomplishments and planning for the future.

The session begins with a discussion of past accomplishments. The clinician prompts each member to describe the improvements he or she has observed since the initiation of family work. If family members are unsure of what to discuss, the clinician can make suggestions. Examples of areas in which BFT may have helped include improved understanding of dual disorders and their treatment; communication between family members; the family's ability to solve problems together; decreased substance abuse; better social relationships (either within or outside the family); work; self-care skills; and new social and leisure activities. All family members are encouraged to share their perspectives about how they or the family as a whole has benefited from participation in BFT.

After each person has contributed a comment, the clinician provides his or her observations. These comments should focus on positive changes and be as specific as possible. The overall message is one of validating the family members' efforts to work together, while maintaining an awareness of the challenges that lie ahead.

When the family has reviewed its past accomplishments, attention turns to planning for the future. If the family attends a multiple-family support group—either a group conducted by professionals (see Chapter 15) or a local chapter of the National Alliance for the Mentally Ill—this should be noted as a valuable way of obtaining support from other families and strategies for coping. If the family does not attend such a group, the clinician can discuss the purposes of both types of groups (education and support) and explore whether family members are interested in trying such groups now that BFT has ended.

Planning for the future also involves determining

how to respond to an impending relapse into acute psychiatric symptoms, or into substance abuse for clients whose substance abuse is in remission. Family members are informed of the significant risk of such relapses, and are reminded that rapid response to an impending relapse can prevent a full-scale one from occurring. Developing a relapse plan for substance abuse follows the same basic methods as the relapse plan for psychiatric illness (described at the end of psychoeducational session 3; see also Chapter 8), but employs a different relapse prevention form (Appendix C, Form C.12). After introducing the goal of developing a relapse plan, the clinician leads the family in a discussion of the client's most recent relapse. This discussion is then followed by identifying key signs of an impending relapse (including resumption of substance use in a formerly abstinent client), and determining the steps that the family should follow in responding to these signs. These steps are recorded on the relapse prevention sheet. The specifics of the plan will vary from family to family, but should include most of the following elements:

- Talking about the concern with the client and relatives
- Evaluating any immediate dangers to the client or others (e.g., suicidal thinking or behaviors)
- Calling the client's case manager (or other team member) to discuss signs of the relapse
- Arranging for an evaluation with the appropriate team member (e.g., case manager, doctor, nurse)

When the plans for responding to relapses have been completed, the clinician asks family members to anticipate any possible stresses they may face in the forthcoming months, and to consider how they might manage those challenges. It is preferable if the clinician is able to be available to family members if they have concerns, if either psychiatric symptoms or substance use problems reemerge, or if a crisis occurs. With some families, the clinician may opt to offer the family members regular meetings after the end of BFT to check up on their progress, identify and work on problems, and provide support. In such cases, family sessions may be conducted on a monthly or bimonthly basis, and follow a loose "check-in" and problem-solving structure. Alternatively, the clinician may work out an agreement with family members to stay in telephone contact after BFT sessions have ended, and to arrange special family sessions as needed. Regardless of the specific arrangement, family members should feel comfortable and confident with the prospect of ending BFT sessions, and should be aware of the resources at their disposal for responding to an impending relapse or handling other stresses they may experience.

CASE EXAMPLE

Iris was a 38-year-old woman with schizoaffective disorder who shared a mobile home with her mother, who ran a cleaning business. Iris's substance abuse was severe; it included daily drinking (resulting in alcohol dependence), as well as weekly marijuana and cocaine abuse. Iris was very socially withdrawn, spending much of the day sleeping, and staying up most of the night. She had not worked in a long time and depended heavily on her mother, which her mother complained about.

Iris and her mother were engaged in BFT, with sessions conducted at their home. The assessment of the family revealed that Iris often allowed her mother to speak for her, was passive, and frequently retreated from her mother to her room during arguments, where she would drink or sometimes use drugs. Iris expressed some awareness that her drinking and use of marijuana and cocaine made her symptoms worse. However, she said that these substances provided some of the few pleasures in her life, and she was accordingly ambivalent about working on her substance use problems. Iris did express an interest in getting along better with her mother and finding something interesting to do with her time. Iris's mother understood little about either her psychiatric illness or the effects of Iris's substance use on her symptoms and relapses. The mother's major goal for the family sessions was to get more help around the house from Iris.

Over the course of the psychoeducational sessions, both Iris and her mother became actively involved in learning about schizoaffective disorder and its interactions with substance use. These sessions helped them talk directly for the first time about the psychiatric illness and its effects on them. In addition, Iris became interested in cutting down on her substance use, for which she received encouragement from her mother. The clinician observed that Iris and her mother communicated relatively well, and elected to review the Communication Skills handout rather than to conduct formal communication skills training.

As problem solving became the focus of the family sessions, Iris began to express herself more openly, to voice her opinions, and not to allow her mother to out-talk her. Problem solving provided a structured format for the mother and daughter to resolve many conflicts, including disputes about money, time the mother devoted to helping her daughter, and the daughter's contribution to the running of the household. Problem solving was also used to help Iris begin cutting down on her substance use; these efforts were initially focused on alcohol, but then later shifted to marijuana and cocaine. As progress was made in the relationship between the mother and daughter, Iris began spending less time alone, and her sleep–wake cycle normalized. Her substance abuse decreased, and the focus of problem solving shifted to Iris's goal of going back to work. Iris obtained work for the first time in many years, and her substance use disorders went into remission.

Iris and her mother participated in BFT for 8 months. Halfway through the BFT, they also began attending a monthly multiple-family group held at the mental health center, in which they continued to participate after BFT had ended. One and a half years after Iris and her mother began BFT, Iris's substance abuse continued to be in remission; she was still working; and she reported a good relationship with her mother. Iris's mother concurred that Iris had begun to help around the house more and was more independent, and added that she now enjoyed their relationship.

POSTSCRIPT: ADDRESSING SUBSTANCE USE AND ABUSE IN RELATIVES

Substance use disorders are more common in the relatives of clients with a dual disorder than in those of clients with only severe mental illness (Noordsy et al., 1994; Tsuang et al., 1982). Thus clinicians may expect to encounter other family members with substance use problems when doing family work in the dual-disorder population. Even when relatives do not have substance use problems, their substance use may become an issue if it contributes to a client's substance abuse. Clinicians need to look for opportunities to address substance abuse in other family members, while not alienating relatives who do not wish to become the focus of attention. The BFT format is flexible and can be tailored to address substance abuse in multiple family members.

Substance use problems in other family members often become evident early in BFT work, during the assessment and psychoeducation phases. Nevertheless, the clinician must be cautious about trying to address substance abuse in relatives too early, before a strong relationship has been developed. The clinician can invite family members to share their experiences, without specifically prompting them to do so. Directly focusing on another family member's substance use during the psychoeducational sessions without his or her permission can drive the person away from treatment. On the other hand, if a member talks freely about substance abuse during the psychoeducational sessions, this can set the stage for working on these problems later.

During problem solving, there are several ways in which another family member's substance use may be addressed in family work. We briefly describe four strategies below.

Addressing Substance Use as a Shared Activity

Problem solving can be used to address substance use in a relative when it is an activity shared by the client and the relative, as illustrated below.

CASE EXAMPLE

Jared was a 28-year-old man with major depression and alcoholism. He lived in his own apartment, but often spent weekends with his father, who lived on a farm outside of town. When Jared visited his father, he would spend much of the day helping him with farm work. In the evenings, the two of them would relax by drinking together. This drinking often destabilized Jared's major depression, contributing to relapses. After reviewing the interactions between alcohol and major depression in the psychoeducational sessions, Jared and his father were willing to work on their drinking together in family problem solving. They succeeded in identifying some alternative activities for spending time together, including playing cards, watching TV, and going to local square dances.

Taking a Motivational Interviewing Approach

In line with motivational interviewing, substance abuse in a relative may become a topic of family problem solving when that person begins to perceive it as interfering with a personally valued goal, as illustrated below.

CASE EXAMPLE

Joel and Jim were twins who lived together with their mother. Joel had severe major depression and polysubstance abuse (mainly marijuana and cocaine abuse). Jim also used marijuana heavily, and occasionally smoked crack as well. During the psychoeducational sessions, Joel talked openly about his substance use, but Jim was more guarded. Over the course of problem solving, attention turned to one of Jim's personal goals—working on his general equivalency diploma (GED) so that he could enroll in a school for chefs. As family sessions began to address this goal, Jim enrolled in a GED course. He had particular difficulty with the math, and found studying difficult in general. The clinician encouraged him to monitor his substance use to explore whether it interfered with his ability to study. When Jim followed through on this, he saw that his regular marijuana use (often with Joel) interfered with his ability to study. Jim stopped smoking marijuana on weekdays, and his concentration improved. The progress Jim made was encouraging to Joel, who also began cutting back on his crack and marijuana use.

Sharing Concern with a Relative Who Uses Substances

When the clinician has developed a good rapport with a relative who has a substance use disorder (usually well into problem-solving training), the clinician can approach the person directly and share his or her concerns. This is often most tactfully accomplished by approaching the relative privately and exploring his or her willingness to address the problem. The case example below illustrates this.

CASE EXAMPLE

Samantha had schizophrenia, and her sister, Ella, had schizoaffective disorder. Both of them had cocaine and alcohol dependence. BFT was initiated to address the dual disorders in both sisters, with their mother (Barbara) and brother (Dallas) also involved in the family sessions. During the psychoeducational sessions, it became apparent that Barbara often had difficulty attending to the information and appeared sedated. During these sessions, Barbara indicated that she took medications for her "nerves," including both benzodiazepines and hypnotics. However, she was not aware of any negative consequences of taking these medications. During problem solving, it became increasingly clear to the clinician that Barbara was addicted to tranquilizers, and that her own addiction made it difficult for her to participate actively in the management of her daughters' dual disorders or in family problem solving. The clinician followed up with Barbara privately and expressed her concern about Barbara's heavy use of tranquilizing medications. Barbara listened, and agreed to talk with the clinician more about it the next week. In the next meeting Barbara expressed her willingness to work on this problem, and to allow it to be raised during the next problem-solving meeting.

Addressing Substance Abuse That Disrupts Family Sessions

When active substance abuse in a family member is disruptive to conducting BFT sessions (e.g., the member is coming to sessions intoxicated), the clinician can lead a problem-solving discussion with the family. In this situation, the problem can be defined as the clinician's problem, because he or she cannot teach the family the skills they need in order to manage the dual disorders. The clinician can then lead a problem-solving discussion aimed at minimizing the chances of family members' coming to sessions after using substances.

SUMMARY

In this chapter, we have described the BFT model for working with an individual family that includes a member with a dual disorder. The BFT model is a time-limited intervention that focuses on teaching families information about dual disorders and their management, and problem-solving skills for dealing with common problems and achieving shared or personal goals. The model can be divided into six phases: connecting, assessment, psychoeducation, communication skills training, problem-solving training, and termination. Although the provision of BFT unfolds in the order of the phases, family treatment itself is tailored to the client's stage of substance abuse treatment. Educational handouts covering the material taught in the psychoeducation phase are provided in Appendix B, and forms for use with families are provided in Appendix C.

15

Multiple-Family Groups

Behavioral family therapy (BFT), described in Chapter 14, is an approach to working with single families to help them overcome the problem of dual disorders. *Multiple-family groups* are interventions provided by professionals in which several families (including the clients) meet together to learn and share about the management of dual disorders and to provide social support to each other. This chapter presents a specific model for conducting such groups, which was originally developed for the Treatment Strategies for Schizophrenia study (Mueser, Sengupta, et al., 2001; Schooler et al., 1997), and has since been adapted for clients with dual disorders and their families (Mueser & Fox, 2002).

We begin with a discussion of the role of multiple-family groups in the treatment of dual disorders. Next, we describe the logistics of organizing and conducting these groups, and the structure of group meetings. Then we consider therapeutic strategies employed in conducting multiple-family groups, as well as educational and discussion topics for the groups. We conclude by providing a case example of a family's participation in a multiple-family group.

THE ROLE OF MULTIPLE-FAMILY GROUPS IN DUAL-DISORDER TREATMENT

Because of the importance of working with families of clients with dual disorders (Clark, 1996), it is useful to have more than one model of family intervention available within a service delivery system. Multiple-family groups can be provided either as an alternative to BFT or in addition to it. Both approaches have advantages and disadvantages. The unique advantages of multiple-family groups include the greater availability of social support to clients and relatives from other families; less potential disruption due to staff turnover; increased opportunities for input from other families; and the more economical nature of the group format. The unique advantages of BFT include the greater ease of engaging family members in the single-family format; the ability to devote more time to solving individual family problems; and the ability to provide outreach to family members in their natural living environments, in order to keep them involved in treatment.

Multiple-family groups alone may be sufficient for clients who have irregular contact with their family members, or for clients who are making substantial progress in their recovery through participation in individual or group treatment modalities and whose families are supportive of these gains. As previously discussed, BFT may be appropriate when a client's dual disorders have a substantial negative impact on the family, when there are high levels of tension in the family, when family members face challenges other than coping with the dual disorders, or when the client has not made substantial progress through participation in other modalities. BFT is usually provided on a time-limited basis, whereas multiple-family groups are not; for this reason, it is often useful to involve family members in BFT first, and then to introduce them to a multiple-family group (Mueser & Fox, 2002). When this sequence is followed, the multiple-family group can help maintain the continuity of family collaboration with the treatment team over the long term, while requiring a much lower level of service intensity.

Clients in any stage of treatment, and their relatives, can benefit from participating in multiple-family groups. However, actual attendance at groups is most likely to occur in the persuasion, active treatment, and relapse prevention stages. If a client is in the engagement stage, and there is no regular contact between the client and the clinician, outreach and other engagement strategies can be employed to engage both the client and relatives. The strategies for engaging family members in multiple-family groups are the same as those outlined for the connecting phase of BFT in Chapter 14.

Families of clients at different stages of treatment benefit in different ways from participating in multiple-family groups. Families of persuasion-stage clients can receive support for exploring the effects of substance abuse on their lives. They can also learn from the experiences of other families where clients have progressed to later stages of treatment. Persuasion-stage clients and their relatives also have the opportunity to learn about how other families have handled common problems related to dual disorders—such as interpersonal conflict, money problems, and a tense, unstable home environment—without being pressured to acknowledge the substance abuse problem.

When clients are in the active treatment and relapse prevention stages, families share the goal of helping all the clients in the group further reduce their use of substances or achieve and maintain abstinence. Family members sometimes find it easier to mentor clients unrelated to them, with whom they do not have complicated family ties. Discussing coping skills for dealing with high-risk substance abuse situations and the elements of relapse prevention plans in the group enables families to benefit from each other's ideas, to enjoy the success of others, to be complimented on their own successes, and to receive social support during setbacks. For clients in the relapse prevention stage, family participation in the group results in relatives' being continually reminded of the possibility of a relapse, while also acting as positive role models to other families with clients at earlier stages of treatment. The awareness of vulnerability to relapse, and the positive regard and respect from other group members, help to buffer clients and their relatives against relapses into substance abuse.

LOGISTICAL CONSIDERATIONS

In this section, we discuss the timing, composition, and leadership of multiple-family groups. We also review other details for conducting successful groups, such as the use of reminder letters, refreshments, and educational handouts.

Timing and Location

Multiple-family groups can be conducted either monthly or biweekly (every 2 weeks). Because one of the primary goals of these groups is to provide family members with social support, they can be expected to benefit from this support as long as they continue to play a caregiving role to a client, or simply maintain a relationship with him or her. Thus these groups should be provided on a time-unlimited basis. The duration of multiple-family group meetings is usually 60–90 minutes.

Groups should be conducted in a physical space large enough to accommodate from 10 to 25 people. The space should be well-lit, publicly accessible, and reasonably quiet. The space should also permit chairs to be arranged in a circle or semicircle (not around a table), to facilitate direct interaction among the participants. It is also convenient if the space has facilities that permit the use of overhead projectors, blackboards, or posterboards, which can be used by leaders/presenters when talking about educational topics.

Conducting multiple-family groups at the local community mental health center or substance abuse treatment setting has several advantages over using other settings in the community. First, as the leaders are themselves professionals, conducting groups at the local clinic is convenient for them. Second, bringing families into the clinic reinforces to them that these groups are a clinic activity and are an integral part of the client's overall treatment program. Third, the mental health or substance abuse treatment center will be at least somewhat familiar to most clients and their relatives; this may be advantageous for families whose members are reluctant to travel to other places in the community. This familiarity can be especially useful for clients who are prone to agitation during group discussions, and may choose to leave the meeting for a few minutes and return at a later time.

Group Composition

Both relatives and clients are invited to participate in the groups. If either relatives or clients decline to join, the other family members are nevertheless free to participate. Family members may participate regardless of whether they are also participating in BFT. In some instances, it may be especially useful for family members who are peripherally involved with a client to attend a multiple-family group (while *not* participating in the more intensive BFT), in order to learn more about the client's dual disorders and the ways other families manage similar problems.

It is preferable if at least three to five families can

participate in a group from the outset. The recommended minimum initial size is 6–8 individual participants. The maximum number of participants in a group should generally not exceed 25–30. When a group reaches this size, it is best to begin a new group as more families become eligible, rather than to split the existing group into two smaller groups, in order to preserve cohesion.

There are no special rules for the inclusion of symptomatic clients. Clients who are hospitalized at the time of a group meeting can participate if they are interested and their clinical condition permits. The most critical factors determining participation are a client's interest, motivation to attend, and ability to follow group norms.

Group Leaders

The optimal leaders for the group are two professionals—one with a background in mental health, and the other with a background in substance abuse treatment. The leaders should either be personally involved in working with some of the participants or maintain direct and regular contact with clients' treatment teams, in order to stay informed about clients' progress. Leaders should also alert treatment teams about impending relapses, medication side effects or nonadherence, or other clinically relevant information that emerges in group meetings. The following qualities are important for group leaders:

- Empathy, interest, responsiveness, and caring
- Ability to structure group interactions so as to facilitate supportive discussion and sharing among families
- Knowledge about dual disorders and family experiences in coping with mental illness
- Ability to communicate effectively with other mental health professionals

Other Details

The group meetings should be held at a standard time and location (e.g., the second Tuesday of each month, if a group meets monthly). Evening meeting times are usually most convenient for family members who work during the daytime. Groups should not be canceled if a leader is on vacation. If the usual group date falls on a major holiday, the group should be rescheduled for an alternative week of that same month.

Each month (again, if a group meets monthly) reminder letters should be sent out to all group participants about 2 weeks before the next meeting. These letters should specify the date, time, and location of the next group, as well as the topic that will be the focus of the meeting. Leaders should follow up with family members who unexpectedly miss group meetings, in order to express their concern, to evaluate whether any current problems need attention, and to troubleshoot obstacles that may interfere with future participation.

Refreshments should be served at all multiple-family group meetings. Juices, coffee, cookies, and fruit are all favorite refreshments. Refreshments should be available to participants from the beginning of the group. When group members are familiar with one another, holding a holiday potluck (e.g., around Christmas and Chanukah time) in which each family brings a dish can be a nice variation to the usual refreshments, and provides a novel way for each family to contribute to the overall group.

Educational handouts summarizing the main points covered in the brief educational topic at the beginning of each group are often appreciated by families. These handouts can be as short as one or two pages (or larger if desired), should be written in plain language, and should be given to families at the beginning of the group. The leaders may either prepare the handouts themselves, use the handouts in Appendix B of this book, or use other materials (books chapters, articles, etc.).

STRUCTURE OF GROUP MEETINGS

Each multiple-family group meeting follows the same basic structure, which is summarized in Table 15.1. It consists of a 5- to 10-minute greeting period, followed by presentation of an educational topic, a group discussion, and a session wrap-up. Educational topics may overlap with those in the psychoeducation phase of BFT (Chapter 14), but may also encompass a broader range of issues. The discussion group portion of the session can be loose in structure, but if appropriate can include problem solving and practice.

TABLE 15.1. Structure of Multiple-Family Group Sessions

Time	Activity
First 5–10 minutes	Greetings, introductions, and sharing
Next 20–35 minutes	Presentation of the educational topic
Next 20–35 minutes	Group discussion
Final 5–10 minutes	Wrap-up and discussion of future topics for groups

Greetings, Introductions, and Sharing

After the initial greetings at the beginning of the session, the leaders introduce any new family members who have just joined the group. Previous members of the group can introduce themselves at this time as well. Following greetings and introductions, the leaders can facilitate brief informal discussion among families about how things have been going for them since the last group meeting. The purpose of this conversation is to warm up the group members, to identify any critical issues that the leaders may need to address later in the group meeting or after the meeting, and to set the stage for ongoing interaction among family members for the remainder of the group. The total length of the introductory period should not exceed 10 minutes.

Presentation of the Educational Topic

When the introductions have been completed, the leaders shift the focus to the presentation of the educational topic selected for that meeting. This presentation can provide useful information to families about the nature of mental illness, substance abuse, and ways of dealing with common problems. In addition, it can stimulate a group discussion that serves both to encourage the sharing of different coping strategies among families, and to validate the experiences of members struggling to meet the challenges of dual disorders.

For the first several multiple-family group sessions, one of the leaders should give the presentation on the educational topic. Presentations by the leaders in the formative stages of the group help to build the cohesion necessary for an effective multiple-family group. After several group meetings have been conducted, the leaders can invite outside speakers to come and present educational topics, interspersing these presentations with others done by the leaders. When invited speakers present topics, the leaders act as group facilitators to stimulate discussion and sharing among family members.

The presentation of an educational topic should be prepared in advance and supplemented during the session with visual aids, such as posters, overhead transparencies, flipcharts, or blackboards. It is most helpful if the visual aids contain brief summaries of major points, key words, and concepts to which the speakers refer. These aids are useful in addition to handouts.

The educational material is presented in a semididactic fashion, with the presenter frequently pausing to solicit questions from group members. Like psychoeducation in BFT (again, see Chapter 14), psychoeducation in multiple-family groups is most effective when the participants are actively involved in talking about the material and understanding its relevance for their own experiences. To accomplish this, presenters may ask open-ended questions designed to engage family members in talking about a particular topic, and to stimulate focused discussion on that topic. For example, when beginning a presentation about coping with depression, the presenter might ask group members to name as many different symptoms or signs of depression that they can think of, while the presenter records the different answers on a blackboard.

Group Discussion

The presentation of educational material generally lasts between 25 and 45 minutes, depending on the amount of material presented and the extent of discussion throughout. The transition from the didactic presentation into the group discussion is gradual, often without a formal demarcation. This group discussion can be facilitated by both the presenter (if the presenter is an outside speaker) and the group leaders.

The main goal of the group discussion is to encourage family members to share their thoughts, feelings, experiences, doubts, successes, and coping strategies regarding the educational topic. As long as an active discussion among the different families is underway, the facilitator's job is easy; it is primarily limited to acknowledging, validating, and reinforcing contributions among the participants. Even if the discussion veers off the topic, the leader need not bring the group immediately back to the topic if group members are engaged and the discussion appears productive.

In order to stimulate discussion, it may be useful to ask probe questions about what experiences family members have had with a particular problem, how they have coped with the problem, and so on. One way of acknowledging the contributions of participants and facilitating further discussion is to write down lists of ideas, coping strategies, symptoms, or other relevant points suggested by family members on a blackboard. Reviewing the list, adding more items, and inviting family members to contribute additional suggestions can further aid discussion.

Sometimes during the discussion, conflict among the members of a family becomes evident—for instance, a disagreement between a client and his or her relatives about the causes or consequences of the client's substance abuse. A leader can explore with other families their experiences with similar situations, and elicit suggestions or examples of how they have dealt with those problems. When facilitating a discussion of a specific problem or conflict, a leader strives to maintain a mutually respectful, solution-focused atmosphere in the group, while acknowledging the frustrations of the members who are involved. Ultimately, the leader should both validate the negative feelings experienced by the family members and get input from other group members on their own experiences and how they have handled those situations in the past.

The leaders may opt to use group-based problem solving to address some common problems or goals shared by many families, or a problem raised by a single family. To facilitate such problem solving, the leader should lead the group through the sequence of problem-solving skills outlined in Chapter 14, taking the role of the chairperson. As when working with single families, the leader (chairperson) keeps track of the problem-solving efforts by recording the pertinent information at each point in the sequence, using overhead transparencies, a blackboard, or flipchart.

Problem solving in a group can be useful for identifying a variety of different solutions to a problem or goal, while allowing each family to make its own choices as to which specific solutions appear most promising. In order to accomplish this, the leader (chairperson) can identify several solutions that group members perceive as most promising, without singling out a single "best" solution. If a copy machine is available, the leader can make copies of the completed Problem-Solving or Goal-Setting Sheet (or summary of solutions) and distribute it to the group members. Alternatively, the leader may make blank copies of the Problem-Solving or Goal-Setting Sheets (or pads of paper) and pens available, so that participants can keep their own notes. When group-based problem solving is used, the leader should follow up with the group at a subsequent meeting and, if necessary, conduct additional problem solving to address continuing problems. Further information about problem solving in multiple-family groups is available in McFarlane (1990, 2002).

Wrap-Up

The last several minutes of each group session are devoted to a wrap-up of the meeting and planning later meetings. At the beginning of the wrap-up, it is helpful if the leader briefly summarizes some points about the topic and group discussion. The leader may also elicit the comments of a few members about the meeting. Then a brief discussion can be held to discuss possible topics for future meetings. The leader should have several topics to suggest to members, and should encourage members to suggest other possible topics.

During the first several group meetings, members may have few suggestions, so it is important that the leader not rely on input until the members have become more accustomed to the group format. When considering possible topics, the leader should acknowledge all suggestions, seek clarification when necessary, and ask questions of other members to determine whether a topic is of general interest. A suitable topic need not be endorsed by all group members, but its popularity provides an indication to the leader about the participants' level of interest in the topic.

After talking about possible topics and invited speakers, the leader informs the group that he or she will explore those topics for the next session, including the possibility of arranging for a special speaker to present a topic to the group. Group members will be informed about the chosen topic for the next group in the reminder letter they receive before each group session. At the end of the wrap-up, the leader also reminds members about the date and time of the next meeting.

THERAPEUTIC STRATEGIES WITH MULTIPLE-FAMILY GROUPS

The facilitation of multiple-family groups is based on some core principles drawn from psychoeducational work, traditional group psychotherapy, and support groups. Leaders strive to make multiple-family groups educational, emotionally supportive, rewarding, and practically useful. More information about conducting multiple-family groups for persons with severe mental illness can be found in Atkinson and Coia (1995), Kuipers, Leff, and Lam (1992), Mueser, Sengupta, and colleagues (2001), and McFarlane (2002). The strategies described below are common in different types of multiple-family groups.

Psychoeducation

Some families may have been exposed to information about mental illness, substance abuse, and their treatment in single-family intervention (e.g., BFT) or elsewhere, while others may have not. Regardless of family members' knowledge of dual disorders, multiple-family groups provide valuable opportunities for learning more about these and other topics, as well as for sharing personal experiences. Family education is an ongoing process that is not limited to a time period or set number of sessions, and multiple-family groups provide a format for continued education.

Like psychoeducation conducted in BFT, psychoeducation in multiple-family groups is most effective when it is interactive, when it helps family members to understand the information by identifying examples from their own experiences, and when opportunities are provided for previously covered material to be reviewed. In the multiple-family context, psychoeducation takes place both during the part of a session when an educational topic is presented, and later in the session during the more general discussion. During the discussion, leaders may help family members process previously covered educational material by asking pertinent questions and pointing out relevant material when the opportunity arises. In addition to the leaders' or presenters' providing information to family members, group members may educate each other over the course of the general discussion. Thus the leaders are always on the lookout for new opportunities to help family members understand the nature of dual disorders and their treatment.

Here is an example of a client involved in a discussion of recovery:

CLINICIAN: Tonight we're going to talk about recovery and the things that we can do to help us move into recovery.

CLIENT: It was really hard when I got sick. I had to give up everything, like going to school. Now I'm working, and that really is important to me.

CLINICIAN: Work is a good example of something that can aid people in the recovery process. Does anyone else have things that have moved them into recovery?

Sharing Coping Strategies

An important feature of multiple-family groups is the sharing of different coping strategies. There is tremendous variation in the extent to which families try different strategies for coping with common problems, as well as in the effectiveness of those strategies. One goal of multiple-family groups is to encourage family members to share coping strategies and their perceived efficacy with each other, as in this example:

FAMILY MEMBER 1: I know when John got sick, I used to spend every day worrying about him, and I felt so helpless.

FAMILY MEMBER 2 (NOT RELATED): Yes, I remember feeling that way too, but after a while I realized I had to get on with my life, so I went back to school.

The leaders can facilitate discussion of coping by periodically asking group members what strategies they have used to manage a particular problem and what the results of their efforts were. In general, coping strategies may have one of two different aims (although some strategies may have both aims). First, they may focus on altering the nature of the problem itself, such as trying to reduce the frequency and/or intensity of a disruptive behavior (e.g., working toward reducing a client's use of alcohol, which leads to family conflicts about money). Second, coping strategies may be aimed at reducing the negative effects of the problem on one or more family members, without directly changing the problem behavior itself (e.g., developing strategies to prevent a client from stealing money from relatives to support his or her drug addiction). When repeated attempts to change a problem behavior are unsuccessful, alternative efforts at minimizing the negative effects of those problem behaviors are a more productive focus of coping efforts.

Validation

A crucial therapeutic benefit family members derive from participation in multiple-family groups is validation and understanding of their experiences and feelings from others with similar difficulties. This validation is important for both clients and relatives. Leaders can inquire about which group members have had certain experiences, to facilitate discussion among families. Family members benefit simply from understanding that they are not alone, and that their reactions and hardships are shared by others in similar situations.

Communication between Families

Sometimes in a multiple-family group one member of a family is able to communicate more effectively with a member of a different family than with his or her own relatives. Facilitating communication between members of different families, especially *intergenerational communication* (e.g., between the mother of one family and the son of another family), can be a powerful way of helping members understand their own families. For example, it is common for the offspring of one family to be able to say something to the parents of another family, and for those parents to listen more attentively than when their own children speak. The leaders take advantage of the therapeutic benefits of communication between families by encouraging and highlighting such communication.

CLIENT: It's really hard to have a mental illness. Everyone looks at you differently, and I feel like people at work look down on me.

FAMILY MEMBER (NOT RELATED): I think it is so great that you have a job and are sticking with it. I know it is hard, but you just have to hang in there.

CLIENT: Thank you. That makes me feel proud that I am working.

Problem Solving

Problem solving (see Chapter 14 for a detailed description) can be used to address a common problem or goal shared across several families. As noted earlier in this chapter, the leader plays the role of the chairperson when group-based problem solving is conducted to keep families focused on the core steps of the method. Problem solving may be especially helpful for dealing either with unanticipated problems or with problems that have previously been the focus of group discussions of common coping strategies. If group-based problem solving is conducted, it is helpful to follow up the success of the solutions in a subsequent meeting, which may serve to reinforce the efforts of the group work.

CLINICIAN: Everyone seems to have identified feeling uncomfortable in social situations as a problem. Let's work on that. Who can come up with an idea that might help with this problem?

CLIENT 1: Well, you might go with a friend.

CLINICIAN: That's a great idea! Let's write that down on this flipchart. (*Writes solution down.*) What else?

CLIENT 2: You might go somewhere where there are only a few people.

CLINICIAN: That's a good one too. (*Records solution.*) What other ideas can you think of for how to deal with feeling uncomfortable in social situations? We can make a list of solutions and then talk about the advantages and disadvantages of each one. . . .

TOPICS FOR MULTIPLE-FAMILY GROUPS

As described earlier, each multiple-family group meeting includes education and general discussion among members on a topic of relevance to coping with a dual diagnosis, reducing the consequences of substance abuse, or maintaining sobriety. Topics are selected in advance and prepared by a presenter (either a group leader or an outside speaker). The educational presentation need not be lengthy, but should both provide some basic information which serves to stimulate discussion among group members. Examples of topics for multiple-family groups are provided in Table 15.2.

Many different sources of information can be tapped to help leaders develop the curriculum for educating family members about a particular topic. These include books for families about coping with mental illness or substance use disorders, self-help books, books and periodicals for professionals, and educational videos. A list of references containing information that can be adapted for topics is provided in Table 15.3.

CASE EXAMPLE

James was a 24-year-old man diagnosed with schizophrenia, paranoid type. In addition to his schizophrenia, James had problems with alcohol and marijuana abuse. He struggled with negative symptoms, such as social isolation and difficulty following through on plans, which got worse when he drank. He also smoked marijuana, which tended to increase his paranoia. James lived on his own in an apartment near the mental health center, but he maintained regular contact with his mother, who lived about 10 miles away. They had phone contact at least once a week, and tried to get together over the weekends and on holidays.

Despite James's participation in motivational interviewing sessions with his clinician (Chapter 7) and sporadic attendance at persuasion groups (Chapter 9), his substance abuse continued unabated. James's clinician had occasional contact with his mother, who voiced her concerns about his situation and his substance abuse. The clinician met with James and his mother twice to explain the nature and purposes of a multiple-family group, which they agreed to attend.

The multiple-family group was conducted monthly at the local mental health center where James received his other treatment. After inconsistent attendance for

TABLE 15.2. Examples of Topics for Multiple-Family Groups

Dealing with cravings	Resolving conflicts
The biology of addiction	Recreational and leisure activities
Improving communication	Substance use: Positive and negative effects
Managing stress	Work: Finding and keeping jobs
Coping with holiday stress	Household rules
Dealing with high-risk situations	Reducing family burden
Coping with depression	Planning for the future
Self-help groups (e.g., Alcoholics Anonymous)	New advances in medication treatment
Dealing with anxiety	Money management
Finding and improving relationships	Coping with negative symptoms
Recovery	Coping with positive symptoms

TABLE 15.3. Resources for Educational Topics of Multiple-Family Groups

Atkinson, J. M., & Coia, D. A. (1995). *Families Coping with Schizophrenia: A Practitioner's Guide to Family Groups*. Chichester, UK: Wiley.

Berger, D., & Berger, L. (1991). *We Heard the Angels of Madness: A Family Guide to Coping with Manic Depression*. New York: Morrow.

Bockian, N. R. (2002). *New Hope for People with Borderline Personality Disorder*. New York: Prima.

Burns, D. D. (1999). *Feeling Good: The New Mood Therapy* (rev. ed.). New York: Avon.

Catalano, E. (1990). *Getting to Sleep*. Oakland, CA: New Harbinger.

Charlesworth, E. A., & Nathan, R. G. (1984). *Stress Management: A Comprehensive Guide to Wellness*. New York: Ballantine Books.

Copeland, M. E. (1994). *Living without Depression and Manic Depression: A Workbook for Maintaining Mood Stability*. Oakland, CA: New Harbinger.

Davis, M., Eshelman, E. R., & McKay, M. (1988). *The Relaxation and Stress Reduction Workbook*. Oakland, CA: New Harbinger.

Fanning, P., & O'Neill, J. (1996). *The Addiction Workbook: A Step-by-Step Guide to Quitting Alcohol and Drugs*. Oakland, CA: New Harbinger.

Fletcher, A. M. (2001). *Sober for Good*. Boston: Houghton Mifflin.

Foa, E. B., & Wilson, R. (2001). *Stop Obsessing! How to Overcome Your Obsessions and Compulsions* (rev. ed.). New York: Bantam.

Glasser, W. (1976). *Positive Addiction*. New York: Perennial Library.

Gorski, T. T. (1989). *Understanding the Twelve Steps: An Interpretive Guide for Recovering People*. New York: Simon & Schuster.

Gorski, T. T. (1992). *The Staying Sober Workbook: A Serious Solution for the Problem of Relapse*. Independence, MO: Herald House/Independence Press.

Gorski, T. T., & Miller, M. (1986). *Staying Sober: A Guide for Relapse Prevention*. Independence, MO: Herald House/Independence Press.

Greenberger, D., & Padesky, C. A. (1996). *Mind over Mood: Change How You Feel by Changing How You Think*. New York: Guilford Press.

Herbert, C., & Wetmore, A. (1999). *Overcoming Traumatic Stress: A Self-Help Guide Using Cognitive-Behavioral Techniques*. New York: New York University Press.

Jamison, K. R. (1995). *An Unquiet Mind: A Memoir of Moods and Madness*. New York: Vantage Books.

Jeffers, S. (1992). *Feel the Fear and Do It Anyway*. New York: Fawcett Books.

Jeffers, S. (1998). *Feel the Fear and Beyond: Mastering the Techniques for Doing It Anyway!* New York: Fawcett Columbine.

Lewinsohn, P. M., Muñoz, R. F., Youngren, M. A., & Zeiss, A. M. (1978). *Control Your Depression: Reducing Depression through Learning Self-Control Techniques, Relaxation Training, Pleasant Activities, Social Skills, Constructive Thinking, Planning Ahead, and More*. Englewood Cliffs, NJ: Prentice-Hall.

Marsh, D. T., & Dickens, R. (1997). *How to Cope with Mental Illness in Your Family: A Self-Care Guide for Siblings, Offspring, and Parents*. New York: Tarcher/Putnam.

McKay, M., Davis, M., & Fanning, P. (1983). *Messages: The Communication Skills Book*. Oakland, CA: New Harbinger.

Miklowitz, D. (2002). *The Bipolar Disorder Survival Guide: What You and Your Family Need to Know*. New York: Guilford Press.

Mondimore, F. M. (1999). *Bipolar Disorder: A Guide for Patients and Families*. Baltimore: Johns Hopkins University Press.

Mueser, K. T., & Gingerich, S. L. (in press). *Coping with Schizophrenia: A Guide for Families* (2nd ed.). New York: Guilford Press.

Neugeboren, J. (1999). *Transforming Madness: New Lives for People Living with Mental Illness*. New York: Morrow.

O'Keefe, R. (1980). *Sober Living Workbook*. Center City, MN: Hazelden.

O'Neill, J., & O'Neill, P. (1992). *Concerned Intervention: When Your Loved One Won't Quit Alcohol or Drugs*. Oakland, CA: New Harbinger.

Papolos, D., & Papolos, J. (1999). *Overcoming Depression* (3rd ed.). New York: Harper/Perennial.

Prochaska, J. O., Norcross, J. C., & Diclemente, C. C. (1994). *Changing for Good: A Revolutionary Six-Stage Program for Overcoming Bad Habits and Moving Your Life Positively Forward*. New York: Avon.

Rosen, L. E., & Amador, X. F. (1996). *When Someone You Love Is Depressed: How to Help Your Loved One without Losing Yourself*. New York: Fireside.

Secunda, V. (1997). *When Madness Comes Home: Help and Hope for the Children, Siblings, and Partners of the Mentally Ill*. New York: Hyperion.

Sheffield, A. (1998). *How You Can Survive When They're Depressed: Living and Coping with Depression Fallout*. New York: Three Rivers Press.

Weiden, P. J., Scheifler, P. L., Diamond, R. J., & Ross, R. (1999). *Breakthroughs in Antipsychotic Medications: A Guide for Consumers, Families, and Clinicians*. New York: Norton.

Whybrow, P. C. (1997). *A Mood Apart: Depression, Mania, and Other Afflictions of the Self*. New York: Basic Books.

Woolis, R. (1992). *When Someone You Love Has a Mental Illness: A Handbook for Family, Friends, and Caregivers*. New York: Tarcher/Perigee.

Yapko, M. D. (1997). *Breaking the Patterns of Depression*. New York: Doubleday.

several months, and encouragement from James's clinician and the group leaders, James and his mother began to participate regularly in the group.

Over 2½ years of participation in the group, both James and his mother experienced significant benefits. James's mother appreciated the support and validation she received from other families struggling with the same issues. For example, she learned from educational presentations that James's difficulty on following through on plans was a common symptom of his schizophrenia, which was exacerbated by his substance abuse. She also learned from other group members strategies for helping her son pursue personal goals (e.g., meeting weekly to plan and review progress toward goals; writing down with James specific steps to be taken and posting them in his apartment) and preventing his substance abuse from interfering with their relationship (e.g., informing James that she would not meet with him when he was high or inebriated).

James also benefited from exposure to other clients who had struggled with and made progress on their substance use problems. At first, James spoke little, and on several occasions he left group meetings early. However, he gradually warmed up over time and eventually began sharing with other group members his ambivalence about using substances. Several people were able to point out to James that his substance use tended to worsen his symptoms and contributed to his overall state of loneliness. James listened to these comments and decided to give up marijuana. To fill up his time, James decided to get a part-time job. With the help of an employment specialist from a supported employment program (Chapter 18), James obtained a job in a florist's shop. As James worked, he found that he enjoyed the social aspects of the job, and that he did not miss marijuana as much as he thought he would. However, his drinking remained problematic and led to several unexplained absences. When James's employer put him on probation for his job, he decided to stop drinking altogether. With advice from other group members and support from his mother, he became abstinent from alcohol. Two years after joining the group, James had achieved sobriety for 8 months; he was continuing to work; and he and his mother reported an improvement in the quality of their relationship.

SUMMARY

Multiple-family groups conducted by professionals are efficient and effective for providing social support, continued education, and hope to families of dual-disorder clients. Families can be engaged in multiple-family groups, BFT (Chapter 14), or both; each approach has its own unique advantages. We have reviewed the logistics of conducting multiple-family groups, including the setting, duration, and frequency of sessions, as well as group composition and leadership. Groups are structured to combine didactic presentations on educational topics selected by group members with discussion and problem solving by families. We have also discussed different topics for group presentations. The chapter has concluded with a case example of one family's participation in a multiple-family group.

VI

Other Treatment Approaches

16

Residential Programs and Other Housing Options

Safe and protective living environments are important features of effective integrated dual-diagnosis treatment programs. Clients who live in environments where substance abuse is common, and whose primary social contacts include others who habitually use and abuse substances, experience great difficulty in decreasing their substance use and developing a healthier, substance-free lifestyle. Although family interventions (or other social-network-based treatments) may be effective in reducing the impact of such environments on clients with dual disorders, many clients do not have relatives or friends who can be engaged in treatment. In addition, some clients' substance use problems are so severe that even family or social-network-based interventions are insufficient to bring their substance use under control. Therefore, there is an important role for residential programs and various other housing options in the treatment of clients with a dual disorder.

We begin this chapter with a discussion of this role, and then consider the causes of housing instability and homelessness in clients with a dual diagnosis. Next, we discuss possible housing options, with emphasis on an optimal continuum of housing alternatives based on clients' stages of treatment. We then review clinical issues pertinent to developing residential programs for clients with severe dual disorders; this is followed by description of a specific residential program for such clients, the Gemini House program. Finally, we discuss strategies for assisting clients with severe dual disorders and housing problems when residential treatment is not available.

THE ROLE OF RESIDENTIAL PROGRAMS IN DUAL-DISORDER TREATMENT

Loss of housing is a major problem in clients with dual disorders. It can interfere with the ability not only to engage them in treatment, but to protect them from the ravages of life on the street. As described in the discussion of treatment planning (Chapter 5), attaining stable housing must often take priority over other treatment goals. Accordingly, guidelines are needed for clinicians working with clients who are currently beset by these problems.

In this book, we have previously described three general approaches to improving housing instability in clients with dual disorders. First, as part of the advocacy function of stage-wise case management (Chapter 6), clinicians can assess clients' housing problems, identify needs, coordinate access to appropriate housing options, and provide necessary supports to help maintain desired housing. Second, because the loss of family support is a critical determinant of housing instability, family collaboration (Chapter 13) and behavioral family therapy (BFT; Chapter 14) are strategies for either addressing potential housing crises before they occur or dealing with crises that occur when family members are still involved with clients. Third, motivational interviewing (Chapter 7) may focus on achieving stable housing if it is a significant client goal, and a client can develop motivation for reduction in substance abuse to support this goal.

However, despite clinicians' best efforts, community-based treatment of dual disorders—including assertive outreach, intensive case management, supported housing, and family services—is sometimes unsuccessful in preventing the cycle of housing instability and homelessness that pervades the lives of some clients. For these clients, specialized residential programs may represent a crucial service that enables them to make initial progress on their dual disorders and to return eventually to the community. Thus, throughout the assessment process (Chapters 4 and 5), residential programs should be considered for clients who have been persistently unable to maintain stable housing in the community, provided that they have had sufficient prior access to stage-wise case management and family services.

One major goal of residential programs is to stabilize clients' housing in order to gain ready access to them and to engage them in treatment. According to the stages-of-treatment concept, engagement is a critical prerequisite to helping clients develop the motivation, skills, and follow-through necessary to address substance abuse and establish a sober lifestyle. Therefore, individual work, including motivational interviewing (Chapter 7) and cognitive-behavioral counseling (Chapter 8); group work (Chapters 9–12); and family interventions (Chapters 13–15) can all be effectively combined with residential programming for dual disorders. The incorporation of psychotherapeutic dual-disorder work into residential programs is particularly critical for developing the necessary motivational and skills base that clients will need to survive in the community after the most intensive residential supports are removed.

HOUSING INSTABILITY IN PERSONS WITH DUAL DISORDERS

Numerous studies have shown that among the most common consequences of substance abuse in persons with severe mental illness are housing instability and homelessness (Caton et al., 1994; Drake, Wallach, & Hoffman, 1989; Olfson, Mechanic, Hansell, Boyer, & Walkup, 1999). An understanding of how substance abuse leads to housing instability can inform the development of housing options and residential programs for clients with dual disorders. Osher and Dixon (1996) have identified three types of factors that may account for the link between substance abuse and housing problems: *system issues*, *legal issues*, and *clinical factors*. We describe each set of factors below.

System Issues

Supported housing and other residential services are especially scarce for clients with dual disorders because of restrictive eligibility criteria. Osher and Dixon (1996) point out that, traditionally, neither the mental health system nor the substance abuse system has taken responsibility for the housing of clients with a dual diagnosis. As a result, many substance abuse residential programs exclude clients with severe mental illness, and many housing programs for people with severe mental illness exclude clients who also have substance use disorders. This lack of viable housing options naturally contributes to the common problem of homelessness in these clients.

Legal Issues

Osher and Dixon (1996) point out several legal issues that may further contribute to housing instability in clients with dual disorders. First, clients with substance use disorders are not eligible for public housing unless they can document that they are currently receiving treatment for these disorders. Without enrollment in a substance abuse or dual-diagnosis treatment program, these clients have no access to the most affordable housing suitable to their incomes. Second, disability payments to persons with primary substance use disorders were severely limited by the U.S. Congress in laws enacted in 1994. It is unclear what impact these laws have had on clients with dual disorders, but they have undoubtedly limited the ability of at least some such clients to afford housing. Third, many clients with dual disorders have experienced legal problems—some related to their substance abuse, and others stemming from their psychiatric illness. Regardless of the cause of these problems, many landlords are reluctant to rent to people with criminal records.

Clinical Issues

Behavioral problems—whether related to clients' psychiatric symptoms, to their substance abuse, or to the interaction of the dual disorders—can act as a barrier to securing and maintaining stable housing. Clients may appear socially awkward; they may act on psychotic symptoms (e.g., talking back to voices); and they may have poor hygiene, making them less desirable as tenants. In addition, many clients with psychiatric disorders sleep much of the day and are awake much of the night, disregard common social conventions or rules (e.g., they smoke in nondesignated areas or leave the door to a locked apartment complex open), and are socially avoidant. These qualities may be further impediments to maintaining stable housing. Finally, violence in people with severe mental illness is strongly related to substance abuse (Swartz et al., 1998b), and such violence is often directed at people in clients' most immediate living environments, especially family members (Steadman et al., 1998). Thus a history of aggressive behavior may also lead to housing problems.

HOUSING OPTIONS

For the reasons described above, many individuals with a dual diagnosis experience persistent problems with their housing. Without appropriate residential supports, these problems are barriers to their recovery. Such clients need access to a continuum of housing options that are sensitive to their individual stages of treatment. Osher and Dixon (1996) recommend that housing options vary in terms of their so-called "wetness"—that is, with respect to their tolerance for substance use.

"Wet" housing is most appropriate for clients in the engagement and early persuasion stages, where the primary purpose of housing is to provide shelter and safety without the requirement that clients reduce substance use. "Damp" housing is most appropriate for the persuasion and early active treatment stages, where some expectations can be placed on clients' substance use behavior, without the assumption that they have fully accepted abstinence as a goal. In damp housing, the expectation can be established that substance use will not occur at the site of the housing itself, but may occur off the premises. "Dry" housing assumes that clients endorse abstinence from substance use as a goal, and is most appropriate for clients in the later active treatment and relapse prevention stages. Dry housing stipulates that clients will not use substances, either on the premises or off.

In the early stages of treatment, the simple provision of shelter and basic protection may be critical to engaging clients in treatment. In the intermediate stages of treatment, housing options provide the same protection, but also begin to focus on addressing issues related to substance abuse. In addition to establishing basic rules for when substance use will not be tolerated (in the residence), damp housing provides an ideal opportunity for doing persuasion work. Residential programs for clients at the intermediate stages of recovery can offer persuasion groups, social skills training groups, family work, and motivational interviewing as strategies for helping clients understand the effects of substance use on their lives, and encouraging them to begin to view substance abuse as a problem.

In the later stages of treatment, clients benefit from housing options that are clearly supportive of their own personal goals of remaining substance-free. The treatment offerings mentioned above for damp housing options should also be provided in dry housing; in addition, dry residences should include programming oriented toward relapse prevention. Table 16.1 summarizes the different characteristics of wet, damp, and dry housing for persons with a dual disorder.

When a treatment team is considering a client's housing needs, it is important to have residential options that do not impose arbitrary time limits on the duration of stay at the residence (Kline, Harris, Bebout, & Drake, 1991). Such time constraints are unrealistic for many clients, and fail to appreciate the individual differences either among clients as individuals or in their progression through the stages of treatment. In addition to the need for a continuum of housing options that is oriented toward clients' stage of treatment, residential treatment must take into consideration the severity of clients' dual disorders. Some severely impaired clients may require special residential programs in order to avoid repeated or long-term institutionalization. Although these programs must also work with individuals at their different stages of treatment, expectations and

TABLE 16.1. Continuum of Housing Needs for Clients with Dual Disorders

Type of housing	Tolerance of substance use	Stage of treatment	Primary functions of housing
Wet housing	Relatively tolerant	Engagement–persuasion	• Shelter and safety • Stable housing (i.e., minimization of homelessness) • Tolerance of substance use to facilitate engagement of the client
Damp housing	Somewhat tolerant	Persuasion–active treatment	• Stable housing that imposes some limits on substance use • Support for clients in exploring effects of substance use on their lives • Limits on substance use to facilitate early efforts toward reduction and abstinence
Dry housing	Relatively intolerant	Active treatment–relapse prevention	• Stable housing that helps clients sustain an abstinent lifestyle • Freedom from substance-abusing peer group • Availability of social support from others who choose to be substance-free • Facilitation of work on other areas of living, such as employment and social relationships

tolerance concerning substance abuse can be tailored to individual clients within such a program, rather than requiring the clients to move through different residential programs with different degrees of wetness.

CLINICAL ISSUES IN RESIDENTIAL PROGRAMMING

When teams are determining the residential programming needs of clients, a number of factors require consideration.

Clients' Stages of Treatment

As described earlier in this chapter, residential programming decisions need to be based on clients' stages of treatment. Clients who are motivated not to use substances, and who have made progress toward reducing their substance use or achieving abstinence, benefit from residences that include clients at similar stages of treatment (i.e., active treatment or relapse prevention). Exposure to ongoing substance abuse for clients in these stages of treatment may increase their risk of relapse, and the presence of other clients who are not yet motivated to address their substance use problems may frustrate them.

On the other hand, clients in the engagement and persuasion stages of treatment need safe and protective housing that acknowledges their premotivational state, and that does not place unrealistic expectations on their behavior (which are likely to result in their expulsion from the residence). Although individual expectations of clients may vary within a given residential program, different housing options may be necessary to meet the needs of clients at different stages of treatment. Naturally, the quality and attractiveness of residences may vary with respect to the stage of treatment for which they are designed. Although all housing must assure that clients are safe (and thus must offer some protection from infiltration by drug dealers and substance-abusing individuals with no mental illness), the quality of housing, the amenities available, and the opportunities for greater self-sufficiency may increase in residences for clients in later stages of treatment.

Clients' Levels of Functioning

Clients with severe dual disorders are often impaired in their psychosocial functioning, especially their independent living skills. Residential programs for dual disorders thus need to evaluate clients' psychosocial functioning, and to provide rehabilitation in areas where deficits are present. Areas in which clients need sys-

tematic training may include self-care skills, cooking, cleaning, apartment maintenance, and establishing and improving social relationships. Improvements in these areas of functioning will decrease the risk of housing instability and substance abuse relapse when clients make the transition to more independent living.

Access to Self-Help Groups

Self-help groups are widely available in most communities. Although not all clients benefit from self-help approaches, residential programs provide unique opportunities for exposing and engaging clients in such groups. Involvement in self-help groups in residential programs should be encouraged and facilitated—but not required, because coercion to participate in self-help is contrary to the very principles by which self-help operates (see Chapter 12).

Residential programs may help clients gain access to self-help programs available in their immediate communities, and may facilitate their participation in various ways (providing transportation, accompanying clients to groups, etc.). In addition, residential programs may develop self-help groups specifically focused on the needs of clients with dual disorders (e.g., Dual Recovery Anonymous) and provide these groups as part of their program. Such groups may be offered both to clients who are residing within the program and to other clients, such as former residents or other clients from the local mental health or substance abuse treatment center who are not residents.

Family Involvement

Clients with a dual diagnosis often continue to see family members regularly and to be involved in their lives after moving into a residential program (see Chapter 13). Family relationships are important to clients, but they may be rife with conflict, misunderstandings, stress, and tension. Relatives of clients with dual disorders often have many concerns. They may want to help but may not know how, and their involvement may be perceived as problematic by staff members. Residential facilities need to recognize the importance of families in the lives of their clients, and develop ways of including rather than excluding them from being involved in the clients' treatment.

Relatives of clients participating in residential treatment benefit from contact with treatment providers who respect their concerns for the clients. In addition to the importance of validating their feelings and acknowledging the difficulties they have experienced, families also benefit from basic education about dual disorders and social support from others who have had similar experiences. Time-limited psychoeducation and family consultation (Chapter 13), behavioral family therapy (Chapter 14), and ongoing multiple-family support groups (Chapter 15) are all strategies for positively involving families in the treatment of relatives in a residential program.

GEMINI HOUSE

Gemini House is a residential and rehabilitation program for clients with a dual disorder who have histories of either long-term or repeated institutionalization in hospitals or jails. The program is available to clients for whom efforts to provide community-based treatment have been unsuccessful or minimally successful in reducing institutionalization. The program is operated as a part of the Greater Manchester Mental Health Center in Manchester, New Hampshire, and was initially partially funded through the U.S. Department of Housing and Urban Development. In this section of this chapter, we provide an in-depth description of Gemini House, which illustrates how the principles of integrated dual-diagnosis treatment can be incorporated into a residential program.

Structure and Staffing

The Gemini House program includes both a residential program (with capacity for 15 clients) and a day program (which serves both clients in the residential program as well as other clients, including some who are making the transition in or out of Gemini House, and graduates who are living in the community). In addition to clients who are residents at Gemini House, 5–10 more clients participate in the day program.

Twenty-four-hour staffing is provided at the residence, with 11 staff members covering the residence, day program, and community outreach. The staffing pattern includes a director of the program, two nurses, three master's-level clinicians, a rehabilitation counselor, four bachelor's-level clinicians, and a quarter-time psychiatrist. Most of the clients participating in the program are from the Manchester area, and an important goal of the program is to reintegrate them into their community living environments. When clients participate in the program, they maintain ongoing contact with their dual-disorder treatment case managers, while the preponderance of their care is provided by the Gemini House program.

Philosophy

Gemini House is an action-oriented program suited for clients who are motivated to work on their substance use problems. It is thus most appropriate for clients in

the persuasion or active treatment stages, and successful completion of the residential part of the program occurs some time after clients have reached the relapse prevention stage. Because the program is aimed at clients who view substance abuse as a problem, but who have had difficulty reducing their substance use in the community, it serves a group of clients interested in joining with others to make a change in lifestyle. Orienting the program toward individuals motivated to address their substance abuse also limits the natural tension that develops in a residential program when some clients view substance abuse as a problem but others do not.

In Gemini House, clients develop the rules of the program (within reasonable limits), based on regular meetings with all the residents at the house and the staff members. Involvement in setting the rules that govern the conditions upon living at the residence ensures that clients are active members of the Gemini House community. It also promotes self-efficacy by showing clients that they are able to influence and shape their own living environment.

Gemini House is located in a community, and residents continue to be involved in the community through such activities as going to work and attending school. A natural consequence of the location of Gemini House is that clients can gain access to alcohol and drugs while in the program, and some slips and relapses do occur. There is a moderate tolerance for substance abuse slips and relapses at Gemini House. On the one hand, slips and relapses are viewed as natural parts of the recovery process from dual disorders, and therefore as events to be expected. On the other hand, clients are also expected to demonstrate some commitment to working on their substance abuse problems as a condition for living at the residence. Clients who show a pattern of repeated and frequent slips or relapses, or who continue to use substances and lie to staff members about their use, are not sufficiently motivated to benefit from participation at Gemini House. They are thus usually asked to leave the program, with an invitation to return when they are more motivated to work on their substance abuse.

There are some similarities and some dissimilarities between the Gemini House program and therapeutic communities developed for primary substance use disorders. Like therapeutic communities, Gemini House has frequent meetings among the staff members and residents, and it places significant emphasis on the relationships among individuals. Unlike therapeutic communities, Gemini House does not emphasize direct confrontation, because affectively charged challenges can lead to disorganization or social withdrawal in many clients with dual disorders. Even though confrontation is avoided, however, high expectations are placed on clients, and extensive facilitation is provided to ensure that clients are successful in meeting these expectations.

Programming

Active programming is a central feature of Gemini House. Two basic conditions for living at the residence are that clients cannot spend time during the day in their rooms and that they are expected to work or attend school. No matter how severe clients' depression, negative symptoms, or positive psychotic symptoms may be, they are not permitted to spend time during the day in their rooms. In addition, all clients are assumed to be capable of working or continuing their education at some level, and involvement in such constructive and normalizing activity is viewed as an important therapeutic part of the treatment of their dual disorders. The specific programming provided at Gemini House is designed to help clients meet these expectations, and to make progress in other areas of functioning as well.

Programming at Gemini House is provided in five main areas: psychiatric stabilization, training in drug and alcohol abstinence, independent living skills, community reintegration, and vocational rehabilitation.

Psychiatric Stabilization

Many clients come to Gemini House following long histories of severe mental illness and substance abuse. For clients who are living in the community before referral into the program, their substance abuse often continues up to the point of admission to Gemini House. As a result, many clients' psychiatric symptoms are exacerbated when they first come to Gemini House, and it is often difficult to discern which symptoms are due to their psychiatric disorders and which are related to their substance use disorders. Therefore, psychiatric stabilization is an important treatment priority during the first several months following admission into the program.

Because the acute effects of alcohol and drugs can either mimic or exacerbate psychiatric symptoms, and because withdrawal from substances can lead to depression or anxiety, as few changes as possible are made in clients' pharmacological treatment during the first several weeks of the program. Clients who are physically addicted to substances when they come to the program are detoxified at the community mental health center's crisis stabilization unit prior to admission to the residence. After the clients have been substance-free in the program for more than a month, a careful evaluation of their persisting psychiatric symptoms can be conducted, and modifications in their treatment regimens can be undertaken.

Training in Drug and Alcohol Abstinence

The Gemini House program espouses a philosophy of abstinence from alcohol and drug use, and clients who participate in the program are expected to endorse this principle of treatment. Specific programming is provided at Gemini House both to reinforce clients' belief in the importance of an abstinent lifestyle, and to help them develop skills for maintaining their sobriety when they move from the program back into independent living in the community. Awareness of the importance of abstinence is fostered through persuasion groups that combine psychoeducation about the interactions between psychiatric disorders and substance abuse with exploration of the effects of substance abuse on clients' lives (see Chapter 9).

Clients are helped to develop skills for maintaining an abstinent lifestyle through evaluations of their individual high-risk situations for relapses into substance abuse. On the basis of these evaluations, clients may be helped to develop better social skills for establishing relationships with non-substance-abusing peers (see Chapter 11), to learn strategies for dealing with persistent symptoms, and to identify and practice alternative leisure and recreational pursuits. In addition, clients are helped to develop their own personal relapse prevention plans; these include their personal triggers for relapse, contingency plans for responding to those triggers, and strategies for preventing a slip into substance use from leading to a full-blown relapse (see Chapter 8). Finally, clients are encouraged to participate in self-help groups offered both at Gemini House and in the community (see "Self-Help," below).

Independent Living Skills

Problems in self-care and independent living skills are common in clients with severe psychiatric disorders, and these difficulties are often worsened by years of substance abuse interspersed with periods of institutional care. The ultimate goal for clients in the Gemini House program is independent, substance-free living in the community. In order to accomplish this, clients must acquire the requisite community living skills.

An important focus of the day treatment program at Gemini House is building clients' independent living skills. Attention is given to the broad range of client needs in this area, including hygiene and grooming, laundry, shopping, food preparation, cleaning, use of public transportation, personal health care (e.g., management of the psychiatric disorder [including medications and plans for preventing or responding to psychiatric relapse], safe sex, etc.), self-management of finances, and using resources in the community. Independent living skills are taught through a combination of skills training, *in vivo* practice, and community trips. As clients make the transition to more independent living in the community, careful assessments of their needs are conducted so that additional skills can be taught.

Community Reintegration

Although limited research has examined the effectiveness of residential programs for clients with dual disorders, the evidence suggests that programs segregated from the community result in rapid relapse rates when clients are discharged and suddenly reintroduced into the community (e.g., Bartels & Drake, 1996). It appears that the effects of the environment on vulnerability to relapse are not significantly altered by long periods of time spent in separate, controlled living environments, whether these are residential programs, hospitals, or jails/prisons. Thus residential programs are most likely to be successful when they are located within clients' natural communities, and when they provide opportunities for community reintegration.

Programmed community reintegration is an important goal for all clients at Gemini House. The integration of clients with their larger community outside the program starts at the beginning of their participation at Gemini House. From the time of their admission, clients participate in some activities in the community, such as work or continuing their education. As clients work on developing their independent living skills, excursions into the community are regularly planned, as are trips to participate in leisure and recreational activities. As clients make progress in developing their sobriety skills, they can participate in self-help groups conducted in the community, and begin spending more of their time in the community than in the program. In order to facilitate successful transitions into the community, the process of moving out of Gemini House is quite gradual, taking place over many months. Even after clients have moved out of Gemini House and into apartments in the community, they may continue to be involved in the outpatient program, and may even spend some nights back in Gemini House in order to ensure the ultimate success of the transition. Clients continue to have contact with and receive support from the program staff as they resume living in the community. Thus the goal of reintegrating clients into their local community is accomplished by never completely severing their connection to the community.

Vocational Rehabilitation

An important prerequisite for participating in the Gemini House program is the willingness to be involved in either work or education outside the program. The expectation that clients are involved in some constructive activity outside Gemini House connotes to clients that no matter how challenged they are by their psychiatric and substance use problems, they are capable of pursuing life goals and contributing to society. Work and education have normalizing effects on individuals with dual disorders, since they can participate in these activities side by side with nondisabled persons. Furthermore, the focus of school or work is not on psychiatric or substance abuse issues, but on either continuing education or producing something that has financial and practical value. Reestablishing life roles and responsibilities is the essence of the recovery process (Noordsy et al., 2000).

Vocational rehabilitation of clients at Gemini House is accomplished by using the individual placement and support (IPS) model of supported employment (see Chapter 18). The IPS model emphasizes rapid search for competitive jobs based on clients' preferences, and deemphasizes extensive prevocational assessment or training. Once clients secure jobs, they are provided with assistance in keeping those jobs. This may include any of a variety of supports, such as on-the-job coaching, supportive counseling, negotiating reasonable accommodations with employers, or social skills training for interacting with coworkers. When job transitions occur, past experiences are viewed as "learning experiences" rather than "failures," with an eye toward applying what has been learned to obtaining a better or more satisfying job.

Some clients are less interested in working than in continuing their education, such as pursuing the goal of getting a general equivalency diploma (GED) or an advanced degree. Other clients, after working on one or several jobs for a few months, become discouraged by the lack of future prospects in that area of work, and choose to return to school in order to improve their position in the labor market. Still other clients prefer working to attending school, because a job gives them something meaningful to do; it provides them with additional money; and it is respected by peers, professionals, and family members.

Self-Help

Participation in self-help groups (see Chapter 12) is accomplished in several ways in the Gemini House program. First, in order to introduce clients to self-help concepts and to familiarize them with the typical structure and nature of these groups, pre-self-help groups are provided. These groups provide clients with an opportunity to learn about the self-help approach, without the obligations of endorsing fundamental self-help principles or conforming to the rules of self-help group participation.

Second, self-help groups are provided at Gemini House. Clients who have attended pre-self-help group meetings, and who are interested in participating in self-help, are encouraged to participate in these self-help group meetings. The meetings follow the same basic principles and format of self-help groups in the community, with the main difference being that all the participants in the groups have a dual diagnosis. Other clients with dual disorders who are not current residents at Gemini House may also attend.

Third, to help integrate clients into the local community, they are encouraged to participate in self-help groups available there. Gemini House staff members provide transportation to local meetings on a regular basis. Helping clients explore different available self-help groups in the community can provide the support necessary for them to identify a group they feel comfortable with and that will be convenient for them when they have moved out of the program. Although participation in self-help groups is strongly encouraged, it is not a strict requirement of the program. Nevertheless, most clients participate in at least some self-help-oriented activities.

Case Example

Leo was a 33-year-old man with chronic paranoid schizophrenia and a long history of alcohol dependence, plus occasional bouts of drug abuse. He had dropped out of high school in the 11th grade and had never married. Leo's primary psychiatric symptoms included severe hallucinations and delusions, accompanied by social withdrawal. He had poor skills for interacting with others, few friends, and minimal contact with a sister who lived in the area. Leo's drinking often led to his becoming disruptive and violent.

Leo received community-based, integrated dual-diagnosis treatment. Through assertive outreach, his treatment team was able to keep Leo engaged in treatment, to oversee his adherence to antipsychotic medications, and to protect him from the legal consequences of his violent outbursts. However, outreach, individual counseling, and persuasion groups had minimal impact on Leo's alcoholism over a 4-year period. As a result of his drinking and severe symptoms, Leo lost his housing on multiple occasions, spent numerous days in respite care, and was frequently hospitalized.

Leo was referred to Gemini House following a 2-month stay at the state hospital. With extensive prompting, Leo participated in the various aspects of psychosocial programming provided at Gemini House. Soon after coming to the program, he was engaged in a social skills training group aimed at improving his interpersonal skills, and an educational/persuasion group that focused on helping him to explore the impact of his drinking on his life. With regular prompting and support, Leo became a regular participant in these groups. In addition, he was closely monitored to minimize his access to alcohol in the community. After several months in the program, Leo began to verbalize some understanding of the effects of alcohol on his ability to live in the community. He began to attend self-help groups provided at Gemini House, and showed some improvement in his ability to initiate and follow through on conversations with others. Leo also started working at a local coffee shop, where he swept and cleaned up after closing for 1 hour each night.

After about 15 months at Gemini House, Leo had made sufficient progress to begin making plans for his transition back into the community. Over the next 3 months, Leo spent gradually more time outside the program and in the community, increasing his hours of working at the coffee shop to 15 per week. In preparation for moving out of Gemini House, the program staff helped him explore possible housing options. Eighteen months after coming to the program, Leo moved out of Gemini House and into a supported housing program; he also continued working at the coffee shop, expanding his hours to 22 per week. Leo maintained contact and received support from the program staff following his move into supported housing, and he continued to participate in the Gemini House outpatient dual-diagnosis program.

A 6-month follow-up after discharge from the Gemini House residential program indicated that Leo had had two bouts of alcohol abuse, but that a major relapse into alcohol dependence had not occurred. In each case, Leo's alcohol abuse had been interrupted by his treatment team; he was refocused on the importance of not drinking to maintain his stable housing; and major negative consequences were averted. With the encouragement of his outpatient treatment team, Leo continued to participate in self-help groups at Gemini House, and was helped to view his "slips" as a normal part of the recovery progress. A 5-year follow-up after discharge from the program indicated that Leo had achieved abstinence from alcohol and drugs for 2 years. He had continued to maintain his stable housing, uninterrupted by any psychiatric hospitalizations, during the entire follow-up period. Leo had moved on to another job, working 25 hours per week as a janitor at a local restaurant. Although still experiencing psychotic symptoms, Leo had made gains in his social functioning by establishing some friendships with other clients in his outpatient program. Leo talked openly about his own accomplishments in gaining control over his alcoholism, and continued to be an occasional participant in self-help groups for persons with dual disorders.

STRATEGIES FOR ASSISTING CLIENTS WHEN RESIDENTIAL TREATMENT IS NOT AVAILABLE

The availability of residential treatment programs for clients with a dual disorder is limited in many settings. In such cases, clinicians must take other steps to create living environments that are less conducive to continued substance abuse, and that are as generally safe and protective as possible. There are several options for developing such environments.

Finding an Alternative Living Situation

First, an alternative living situation can be sought that removes a client from the immediate temptations of substance use with peers. For example, an apartment in another part of town can be secured, with assistance provided to help the client adjust to the new neighborhood, develop new social relationships, and so forth. The primary advantage of this approach is that it offers clients a "fresh start" on their lives, and gives them an opportunity to break undesirable habits, including alcohol and drug use. Leaving the environment in which much substance abuse occurred reduces exposure to environmental cues that trigger craving and substance use. This strategy is most effective with highly motivated clients whose substance use is closely intertwined with their social relationships, and who are willing to take on the challenges of moving to a new location and beginning new relationships. One problem with changing living arrangements is that it may be difficult to identify affordable alternatives in which there is less access to drugs and alcohol. In addition, many clients are reluctant to leave their familiar surroundings, or may be dependent upon others for meeting their basic needs (which will preclude more independent living).

Providing Structured Activities in Another Setting

Second, the impact of a client's environment can be decreased by arranging for the client to spend less time there, while maintaining his or her residence. Unstructured time increases the opportunities for substance use and abuse. Identifying structured, meaningful activities in which to engage can decrease free time and hence substance use, especially if those activities take place in a setting in which substance use is outside the norm. For example, continuing one's education, pursuing work, joining a club, participating in a consumer drop-in center, volunteering, or developing a hobby or sport can temporarily remove people from their immediate living environments; it can also give them something else to look forward to and from which to derive pleasure. This strategy is usually helpful in the development of a new social network as well.

Forming Allegiances with Social Network Members

A third strategy for lessening the negative impact of the environment on substance abuse, or for improving the management of severe dual disorders, is to reach out and form allegiances with individuals who are in contact with a client or with whom the client lives. Many of the same strategies involved in family collaboration can be used to work with others in clients' social networks (including friends, non-live-in girlfriends/boyfriends, etc.). In addition to friends, landlords may be in a unique position to help clients with a dual diagnosis (Kloos, Zimmerman, Scrimenti, & Crusto, 2002). Landlords are naturally invested in having good tenants who pay their bills and are not nuisances. At the same time, landlords are often concerned about the welfare of their tenants with disabilities, and may be useful allies in their treatment. We provide a case example below of how a treatment team working with a severely impaired client with a dual diagnosis developed a close working relationship with the client's landlord, thereby stabilizing his housing and making the first inroads into the treatment of his disorders.

Case Example

Jerome was a 38-year-old man with schizoaffective disorder, cocaine dependence, and marijuana abuse. At the time of Jerome's referral to a dual-disorder program, he had been recently discharged from a psychiatric hospital for treatment of a relapse of psychiatric symptoms. Over the prior year, he had experienced multiple psychiatric hospitalizations. Jerome was often guarded and socially isolated when his symptoms were stable; he had minimal contact with a sister who lived in the area, and he reported often feeling depressed and hopeless. Jerome tended to stop taking medication when he was using drugs. He described the effects of crack cocaine and marijuana as providing a temporary escape from his feelings. However, this substance use, combined with not taking his medication, often resulted in symptom relapses in which he would become paranoid, hostile, belligerent, and sometimes disorganized. On one occasion he was arrested for stealing ornaments off the lawns of homes (for which he had no use). On another occasion he was hospitalized after crawling on the street and howling like a dog. Jerome's substance abuse, together with his social withdrawal or bizarre behavior, often led to problems in maintaining housing (and thus to intermittent homelessness).

When Jerome began receiving dual-diagnosis services, he had been living in an apartment for several months. Two recent hospitalizations, during which his behavior had been disruptive, were threatening the stability of this living arrangement. The treatment team reached out to Jerome by conducting numerous home visits. When he would permit it, team members would take him shopping, help him pay bills, informally chat, and attempt to reestablish contact between him and his sister. However, Jerome's psychiatric symptoms were only tenuously stabilized, and his cocaine dependence and marijuana abuse continued unabated. In order to facilitate Jerome's adjustment in his apartment, and to avoid possible eviction due to his unpredictable behavior, the treatment team obtained Jerome's permission to make direct contact with his landlord. The landlord expressed concern over Jerome, including both his problematic behavior and his need for treatment, and appreciated the involvement of clinicians from his treatment team.

Over the next several months, a good working relationship developed between the landlord and the treatment team. The landlord enjoyed a closer relationship with Jerome than did the clinicians on his team, and Jerome trusted him more fully as well. The clinicians recognized that the landlord cared about Jerome; they provided him with basic information about his mental illness, as well as the effects of drug use on that illness. This enabled the landlord to help in monitoring the dual disorders when team members could not. On several occasions, the landlord was able to provide information to the team about Jerome's functioning when he refused to be seen by the team. The landlord also used his relationship with Jerome to ease his anxiety and suspiciousness about the treatment team, and sometimes invited team members to join him and Jerome to have something to eat and to talk. Jerome gradually became more comfortable with the clinicians, and he started taking his medication again. During the next several months, Jerome had only one psychiatric hospitalization; while he was in the hospital, his landlord visited him and brought him his mail.

Although Jerome's drug abuse continued, over the next 6 months he began to see team members regularly, and to look to them (in addition to his landlord) for support and assistance. Of equal importance, his housing remained stable, despite occasional problems due to continuing substance abuse and bizarre behavior. As Jerome became engaged in treatment, his clinicians began persuasion work. He was invited to participate in weekly persuasion groups, which he attended irregularly. After several months, while he was still in the persuasion stage of treatment, team members involved Jerome in a social skills training group aimed at improving his ability to socialize with others. Jerome liked the skills training group and began attending it on a consistent basis. He continued to have a close relationship with his landlord, who encouraged his involvement in the dual-diagnosis groups at the mental health center.

Approximately 8 months after beginning to participate in the persuasion and social skills training groups, Jerome began to talk openly with his landlord and clinicians about wanting to work on his drug abuse. Four months later, after several unsuccessful attempts, Jerome succeeded in cutting down on both his cocaine and marijuana use. Thus, 18 months after referral to the dual-diagnosis team, Jerome entered the active stage of treatment. Through establishing a close, collaborative relationship with Jerome's landlord, the treatment team was successful in stabilizing his housing, improving medication adherence, and averting hospitalizations. These gains provided a foundation for work on substance abuse, enabling Jerome to make progress toward his recovery.

SUMMARY

Clients with a dual diagnosis need safe and protective living environments. In this chapter, we have reviewed the reasons why substance abuse in persons with severe mental illness leads to housing instability, and have stressed the importance of safe housing for the long-term treatment of dual disorders. The need for housing options that vary on the continuum of "wetness" (i.e., permissibility of substance abuse) and are tailored to meet the needs of clients at different stages of treatment has been addressed. We have next addressed clinical issues that require consideration in determining the residential needs of clients with dual disorders. We have then described Gemini House, a long-term residential program designed for clients with severe dual disorders who have not benefited from other community-based interventions. We have concluded with a discussion of strategies for addressing severe dual disorders and housing problems when residential programs are not available.

17

Involuntary and Coerced Interventions

In this chapter, we discuss the use of involuntary and coerced interventions in the treatment of clients with dual disorders. *Involuntary interventions* can be defined as strategies that involve the physical or legal restriction of clients, their property, or their authority to make decisions. Civil commitment to a psychiatric hospital, payeeship, and guardianship are all commonly used involuntary interventions. *Coerced interventions* are strategies used to engage people in mental health or substance abuse treatment by threatening the loss of personal choice and freedom if individuals do not comply with treatment recommendations. For example, an individual with dual disorders who is convicted of a crime may be mandated by the criminal justice system to receive treatment for his or her disorders, or someone with multiple psychiatric hospitalizations and admissions to inpatient detoxification units may be civilly committed to outpatient treatment. In either case, the failure to receive the appropriate outpatient treatment can result in imprisonment or involuntary hospitalization.

Many techniques are available for assisting clients to engage and comply voluntarily in dual-disorder treatment. However, like other clients with severe mental illnesses, clients with dual disorders may sometimes require involuntary or coerced interventions because they appear likely to harm themselves or others, or because their substance abuse has resulted in legal transgressions. Involuntary interventions by definition restrict personal choice and freedom, and coerced interventions threaten the loss of freedom. Involuntary interventions take away clients' self-control, and both involuntary and coerced interventions can undermine clients' motivation. Since motivation and self-control are strengths that dual-disorder treatment aims to cultivate, the use of involuntary and coerced interventions requires particular care.

We begin this chapter by discussing the role of involuntary and coerced interventions in dual-disorder treatment. We then provide a background description of such interventions for persons with psychiatric or substance use disorders, followed by a discussion of attitudes toward these interventions. We next briefly review the research on such interventions in the mental health system, and then consider the important role of close monitoring in dual-diagnosis treatment. Specific guidelines are suggested for determining the need for involuntary and coerced interventions for clients in community-based settings. We then describe how to provide integrated treatment to clients in institutional settings. Special issues regarding the treatment of people involved in the criminal justice system are considered, including jail and prison diversion programs, outpatient work with clients on parole or probation, and work with inmates with dual disorders. We conclude the chapter with recommendations for a synthesis: achieving a balance between necessary structure and constraints on the one hand, and client self-determination and liberty on the other. The ideal results of such a balance are shared responsibility and enhanced client motivation to address the problem of substance abuse.

THE ROLE OF INVOLUNTARY AND COERCED INTERVENTIONS IN DUAL-DISORDER TREATMENT

Psychiatric disorders often impair individuals' reasoning and judgment, contributing to potential danger to themselves and others; these impairments are often worsened by substance abuse. Involuntary hospitalization is a legal mechanism for safeguarding clients during these times of crisis, and for providing treatment that might otherwise not be given. Substance abuse, on the other hand, frequently involves or leads to illegal behaviors (e.g., the possession of illicit substances, disorderly or aggressive behavior, or driving under the influence of alcohol). These illegal behaviors often result in contact with the criminal justice system and various sanctions, such as incarceration, probation, or parole. Because the rates of both hospitalization and incarceration for clients with dual disorders are high (Mueser, Essock, et al., 2001; Swofford et al., 1996), providing either involuntary or coerced interventions under these and similar circumstances is a crucial aspect of integrated dual-disorder treatment.

Clients with dual disorders who are prone to relapses and rehospitalizations, or who become involved in the criminal justice system, are frequently in and out of treatment—and are often not well engaged even when they are in treatment. Hospitalization or incarceration represents a valuable opportunity to engage clients in treatment who might otherwise be inaccessible to clinicians; either intervention may permit the development of a working alliance and progression along the stages of treatment. Other coerced or involuntary interventions, such as court-mandated outpatient treatment or financial payeeships (Rosen et al., 2002), may afford similar engagement opportunities. Therefore, a critical function of involuntary and coerced interventions with clients with a dual disorder is to accomplish the first stage of treatment—engagement, defined as establishing regular contacts between a client and a clinician (or treatment team).

In addition to the opportunity to engage clients in treatment, important psychotherapeutic work can be achieved under such conditions, depending on the duration of the coerced or involuntary interventions. On an individual basis, motivational work can be conducted to establish personal life goals (including termination of the involuntary conditions), and to explore the interference of substance abuse with achieving these goals (Chapter 7). For clients who already view their substance abuse as problematic and are motivated to stop it, individual cognitive-behavioral substance abuse counseling (Chapter 8) is useful for identifying high-risk situations, for preparing alternative behaviors or skills to use in such situations, and for formulating and rehearsing relapse prevention plans. Because of the ready access to multiple clients, different types of group work can also be facilitated in coerced or involuntary intervention settings—including persuasion (Chapter 9), active treatment (Chapter 10), social skills training (Chapter 11), and self-help (Chapter 12) groups. Family interventions can often be initiated in coerced or involuntary

settings, in part because of the safety inherent in those settings (Chapters 13–15). Finally, involuntary or coerced interventions may provide other opportunities for treating dual disorders more effectively, such as optimizing psychopharmacological treatment (Chapter 19) or providing vocational rehabilitation (Chapter 18).

Although involuntary and coerced interventions thus represent valuable opportunities to engage and work with clients, clinicians must bear in mind the importance of treatment continuity that extends beyond the duration of those interventions. As described in Chapter 2, shared decision making is a crucial value of integrated dual-disorder treatment, and involuntary or coerced interventions by their very nature lack such a collaborative process. In order to empower clients with the decision-making authority they will eventually have in the community when they are free of constraints, clinicians need to join with clients in working to develop the skills they will need to move beyond involuntary or coerced interventions to voluntary treatment, and assuming ownership and responsibility for making their own treatment decisions.

BACKGROUND DESCRIPTION

Involuntary and coerced interventions raise a number of legal, political, ethical, moral, and clinical questions that are important to both administrators and clinicians of dual-disorder programs. The legal mandate for such interventions is essentially a *paternalistic* action taken by society. A paternalistic approach is justified if certain moral rules are fulfilled (Culver & Gert, 1982):

1. The harm to the person that would be prevented by the action is so significant that the person could not rationally prefer the alternative.
2. The person does not have an adequate reason for suffering the harm that the paternalistic act is designed to prevent.
3. The harm is likely to occur if the paternalistic act is not done, and the act will significantly diminish the probability of such harm.

Justification therefore hinges on (1) the seriousness of harm to be avoided, (2) the extent of the person's rational responsibility, (3) the likelihood of harm, and (4) the likelihood that the involuntary intervention will diminish the chances of harm.

In mental health care, involuntary and coerced interventions are legally mandated mechanisms for limiting a person's choices. The mechanisms fall into three categories: *protections for person and property, man-*

dates for treatment, and *orders associated with illegal behaviors* (e.g., court orders, conditions of probation, parole, pretrial release). Protections for person and property take the form of payeeships for Supplemental Security Income, Social Security Disability Insurance, and other funds, as well as guardianships or conservatorships over the person, the person's medical care, or the person's property. Mandates for treatment include orders for emergency inpatient or outpatient treatment, involuntary hospitalization, conditional discharge from a hospital, and inpatient or outpatient commitments. Orders associated with illegal behaviors, which can be tailored to address dual-disorder treatment goals, encompass restraining orders, conditions for avoiding prosecution, detention, conditions of sentencing, and stipulations or conditions associated with probation or parole.

Outside the mental health system, involuntary or coerced interventions are frequently used in substance abuse treatment when a person's addiction has placed that person or others in jeopardy. Indeed, many substance abuse treatments are coercive in the sense that family members, employers, courts, police, or others push clients into treatment. For example, an individual arrested for a nonviolent offense may be court-ordered to receive outpatient or residential substance abuse treatment. In the mental health system, involuntary and coerced interventions are widely sanctioned by laws, but are quite negatively regarded by clients and client advocates. Many clinicians and administrators are reluctant to use involuntary interventions, and to a lesser extent coerced interventions, except when necessary to prevent serious harm.

The laws of every state sanction the coercion or involuntary admission of people with mental illnesses into treatment, usually with the requirement that a person is likely to harm self or others if treatment is not mandated. The actual use of involuntary hospitalization varies from place to place. Although 27% of psychiatric hospital admissions are involuntary across all states, the rate is as high as 75% in some states (Monahan et al., 1995). Procedures and criteria vary from state to state as well, with some states having separate procedures for brief emergency commitment, for longer observational commitment, and for longer-term extended commitment. Similarly, states vary widely in the availability of, and laws governing, civil outpatient commitment to psychiatric treatment (Torrey & Kaplan, 1995).

Some states have civil statutes permitting the coercion of people with substance use disorders into treatment, and others do not. When substance abuse leads to legal transgressions, however, coerced or involuntary treatment for the substance use disorder may be legally mandated in all states. For example, individuals who are arrested for driving while intoxicated may be required to participate in substance abuse treatment in order to get their licenses back (coercion); if they are arrested a second time for drunken driving, they may be involuntarily committed to an inpatient treatment program for alcoholism.

ATTITUDES TOWARD INVOLUNTARY AND COERCED INTERVENTIONS

Few issues in the care of persons with severe mental illness have generated as much active debate as the role of involuntary and coerced treatments. Prior to the reform of U.S. laws in the 1970s regarding involuntary mental health interventions, the rights of clients with psychiatric disorders were practically nonexistent; all decisions regarding their care, including long-term confinement, were left to the control of physicians (Hiday, 1996). Civil rights reforms formally recognized the rights of mental health clients to refuse treatment, limiting coerced or involuntary treatment to situations in which a client presents a clear danger to self or others (Winick, 1997). Despite these changes in legal policies, the use of involuntary and coercive interventions continues to be a controversial topic. Mental health consumers have been eloquent in describing the negative, often traumatic effects of such interventions on their lives (Beale & Lambric, 1995; Deegan, 1990; Millett, 1991). Family members, on the other hand, who often bear the brunt of managing relatives' psychiatric relapses and are most likely to be the victims of any violence that ensues (Steadman et al., 1998), have been vocal in their frustrations about trying to get treatment for resistant relatives (Torrey & Kaplan, 1995).

Although from a legal perspective involuntary and coercive interventions refer to compelled or forced treatments, coercion may also be involved in obtaining so-called "voluntary" treatment for a client. At the same time, some clients who are legally involuntarily hospitalized actually express a preference for hospitalization. In a summary of research on client perceptions of treatment involuntariness or coercion, Hiday, Swartz, Swanson, and Wagner (1997) reported that about half of voluntarily hospitalized clients described their treatment as actually involuntary or described coercion as playing a significant role, whereas between one-fifth and one-third of involuntarily hospitalized clients stated that they really wanted to be hospitalized. Thus legal status and perceptions are not necessarily the same.

From the standpoint of the therapeutic relationship, the client's perception of coercion or involuntariness may be more critical than the extent to which legal pressure is actually employed (Monahan et al., 1995).

Clients often attach more importance to the admitting staff's attitudes and interactions than to the legal status of an involuntary hospital admission (Lidz, Mulvey, Arnold, Bennett, & Kirsch, 1993). Clients are more likely to perceive coercion or involuntariness when they believe that they are not mentally ill; when they think that others are not acting in good faith, or are being deceptive, unfair, or disrespectful; or when they feel forced, criminalized, or otherwise poorly treated in the process (Bennett et al., 1993; Monahan et al., 1995).

Hiday and colleagues (1997) have discussed two distinct concepts that contribute to clients' perceptions of involuntariness or coercion: *negative pressures* and *fair process*. Negative pressures are threats of force that would result in undesired consequences if the person does not comply with the treatment. Negative pressures are more than persuasion; they involve the potential loss of something of value, such as personal freedom or some material goods. Fair process refers to the extent to which an individual has a voice in actions concerning him or her, and perceives others as acting in good faith and with impartiality. Hiday and colleagues point out that a fair process does not necessarily mean that a client is successful in influencing the outcome of a potentially involuntary or coercive treatment process. However, if clients perceive the process as fair, and view others as believing they are acting in the clients' best interests, they are less likely to view themselves as having been pressured (Monahan et al., 1995).

Stone (1975) has suggested that many psychiatric clients, whose mental illness clouds their judgment at the time of a symptom exacerbation, are eventually thankful to clinicians who compel them to receive treatment. Research supports Stone's theory by indicating that the majority of clients who resisted psychiatric hospitalization and were involuntarily hospitalized held positive views of their treatment at discharge (Hiday, 1996; Lucksted & Coursey, 1995). Similarly, clients with dual disorders often express their appreciation for what they have gained from such external controls as involuntary payeeships or supervised living arrangements that they entered involuntarily.

An involuntary or coerced intervention sometimes "breaks the ice" of treatment refusal and resistance, and engages clients with their treatment teams. In addition, the experience of such an intervention can awaken a client to the physical peril caused by years of substance abuse. Some clients looking back on these circumstances report that experiencing this type of intervention gave them a powerful message of caring that enhanced their engagement, insight, and personal control, and that also engendered their trust in the treatment team.

RESEARCH ON INVOLUNTARY AND COERCED INTERVENTIONS

Few studies have evaluated the effects of involuntary or coerced interventions on clients with a dual disorder, and the research questions continue to be framed (Monahan et al., 1996; Munetz, 1997). An uncontrolled study in Manchester, New Hampshire, showed clinical improvements for 26 clients with severe mental illness, many with substance use disorders, who received mandated community treatment under conditional discharge from the hospital (O'Keefe et al., 1997). After 1 year, clients had improved their adherence to medication, housing stability, and vocational activity, and they had reduced their substance abuse, violent behaviors, and days in the hospital. At 2 years, positive effects remained for medication compliance, substance abuse, and violent behavior, but not for housing stability, vocational activity, and days in the hospital.

Several other uncontrolled studies also suggest positive outcomes associated with outpatient mental health commitment. Compared either with other clients who were not committed or with themselves prior to commitment, clients who were legally mandated to receive outpatient mental health services attended more outpatient appointments, were more adherent to medication (Greenman & McClellan, 1985; Hiday & Scheid-Cook, 1987, 1990), and were hospitalized less and for a shorter duration of time (Fernandez & Nygard, 1990). In addition, even after the time limits of outpatient commitment had expired, clients who had been court-committed to treatment tended to have better attendance at their outpatient treatment (Hiday & Scheid-Cook, 1987, 1989). A limitation of these studies is that none were controlled or focused exclusively on clients with a dual disorder.

One controlled study used a randomized design to evaluate the effect of involuntary outpatient commitment on treatment outcomes for 142 clients with severe mental illness discharged from Bellevue Hospital in New York City (Policy Research Associates, 1998). All clients received intensive community treatment, as well as enhanced assessment and discharge planning. The experimental group received supervision under a court order, while the controls received the same supervision without a court order. Results showed that all clients improved on symptoms, quality of life, treatment continuation, arrests, days in the hospital, and violent behavior, but that the court order itself had no differential effect on outcomes. Unfortunately, the number of clients with substance abuse problems was too small to test the effects of the court order on substance abuse.

A second controlled study compared the outcomes

of 264 clients who were involuntarily admitted for inpatient psychiatric treatment. Upon discharge, they were randomly assigned to either outpatient mental health commitment for 30–60 days or no outpatient commitment, and were then followed for 1 year (Swartz et al., 1999). Clients assigned to outpatient commitment could have their commitment extended if clinicians petitioned the court. Hospitalization outcomes did not differ between the two groups. However, clients who received more than 180 days of commitment were less likely to be hospitalized and spent less time in the hospital than clients who received fewer days of outpatient commitment or were not committed at all. This effect was only present in clients with psychotic disorders who received higher levels of outpatient psychiatric service. This study provides support for the effects of outpatient mental health commitment, but suggests that extended periods (at least 6 months) of commitment may be necessary in order for benefits to accrue. In the broader sample of clients, extended commitment was also related to higher levels of medication adherence (Swartz et al., 2001), and lower levels of violence (Swanson et al., 2000) and victimization (Hiday et al., 2002). These benefits were achieved partly through reduction of substance abuse.

Although more research is needed, evidence across studies indicates that clients with severe mental illness often experience improvements in outcomes following involuntary or coerced interventions (Hiday, 1992). In the related field of substance abuse treatment, it has been shown that involuntariness or coercion is unrelated to substance abuse treatment outcomes across an array of programs (McLellan et al., 1994). Thus those who do not enter treatment of their own free wills seem to do as well as those who enter voluntarily.

THE ROLE OF CLOSE MONITORING IN DUAL-DISORDER TREATMENT

In dual-disorder services, coercive or involuntary interventions fit into a broader array of strategies for close monitoring. *Close monitoring* refers to intensive supervision in the community, which at times is provided with a client's consent and at other times is provided involuntarily. Close monitoring and involuntary/coerced interventions are more likely to be necessary early in the course of dual-disorder treatment, before clients are motivated to work on their substance abuse and when the likelihood of harm is greatest. As clients become more involved in treatment, and their self-control and adherence to treatment grow, the intensity of close monitoring can be gradually decreased.

The stages-of-treatment model provides a useful framework for understanding the role of close monitoring in the course of recovery from dual disorders (see Chapter 2). During the engagement stage, when a client's symptoms are often poorly regulated and he or she does not yet have a working alliance with a clinician, coerced or involuntary interventions are more often justified than during other stages of treatment. Monitoring compliance with prescribed medications is a common form of close monitoring at this stage, since substance abuse is not yet a focus of treatment. During the persuasion stage, when the clinician has a working alliance with the client but substance abuse continues to be problematic, urine drug screens (or other substance-testing methods, such as Breathalyzer tests or hair analysis) are a helpful form of close monitoring. Clients usually consent to these tests and can collaborate with their clinicians in using their findings. Clinicians may also closely monitor attendance at persuasion groups (Chapter 9), psychiatric visits, and other rehabilitation or therapy appointments.

In the active treatment stage, when the client has made progress in reducing substance abuse, the likelihood of harm diminishes; close monitoring therefore focuses on supporting the client in achieving his or her action goal. Examples of close monitoring during this stage include living in supervised "dry" housing, screens for substance use, frequent individual sessions and/or home visits, and monitored disulfiram treatment (see Chapter 19). During the relapse prevention stage, when the client's substance abuse is in sustained remission, the intensity of close monitoring decreases as treatment focuses on supporting the client's development of additional skills and strengths for preventing relapses and coping with setbacks. Close monitoring at this stage may involve a regular check-in with a group or an individual clinician, and/or use of a self-help group sponsor, as in Alcoholics Anonymous (AA).

Most strategies for close monitoring of clients with dual disorders who are receiving treatment from community mental health centers are voluntary and relatively nonrestrictive. In many cases, the careful use of voluntary close monitoring strategies can prevent the need for coerced or involuntary interventions. Clinically, close monitoring provides structure in a person's social environment and supervision over patterns of daily living. Urine and other substance use screens are forms of close monitoring that give a clinician and client feedback on actual substance use and form a basis for work at the persuasion stage, during which the client begins to appreciate the connections between use and consequences. For many individuals with dual disorders, close monitoring enables community-based treatment to progress while motivation is still developing. Ideally, a client and a treatment team work together to negotiate structures and limits, and to monitor their effects.

Community supervision of clients in the criminal justice system by probation and parole officers involves a variety of close monitoring strategies, both involuntary/coerced and voluntary. These strategies can include mandated random urine screens or other tests for substance use; monitoring of adherence to prescribed medications; required participation by clients in substance abuse and mental health treatment groups; and participation by officers in case reviews and treatment team meetings. Regular, ongoing collaboration with the treatment team is crucial to ensure that criminal justice concerns and the management of the dual disorders are attended to simultaneously and in a coordinated fashion. Probation and parole officers benefit from special training designed to enable them to become active members of clients' treatment teams, and to maximize their involvement in helping clients with a dual diagnosis remain successfully in the community.

As we describe below, involuntary or coerced mental health interventions are morally and clinically justified in situations where grave danger of harm is present. But otherwise, such interventions are considered only after all voluntary options for close monitoring and engagement in treatment have been exhausted, and/or when a client has actually participated in the choice of the intervention. We find, for example, that a payeeship can often be pursued with the client's active involvement.

Voluntary Options

A client's voluntary or coerced participation in a carefully designed close monitoring program can in many cases prevent the need for coercive or involuntary interventions. Many voluntary options are available for engaging clients in treatment and for supporting treatment adherence. These include frequent visits, outreach, counseling, treatment plan contracts, informal agreements, behavioral contracts, and consent to restrictions. Table 17.1 summarizes the voluntary mechanisms that can be used in close monitoring.

Clients can also consent to have legal or programmatic restrictions for a time. Clients can participate in many different ways to show their adherence to such plans. They can keep regular appointments, check in, participate in a drug-screening program, enter a supervised living arrangement, and hold to agreements with family members and significant others. Other clinicians and providers, family members, and friends can play important roles as collaborators and supporters for a client's success in a plan.

TABLE 17.1. Voluntary Mechanisms for Close Monitoring

What types of voluntary arrangements are made:
- Person-to-person agreement
- Treatment plan
- Behavioral contract
- Rewards for short-term successes (e.g., praise, going out for a treat)
- Bonus rewards for longer-term successes (e.g., special time with caregivers or family, shopping trips for new clothes associated with recovery-oriented activities, extra spending money from family, special meal with family)
- Power of attorney
- Consent for legal protections of property or person
- Consent for more personal supervision (e.g., housing program)

What is monitored:
- Drug and alcohol use
- Severity of psychotic symptoms
- Compliance with taking psychotropic medications
- Psychotropic medication levels
- Attendance at treatment meetings (group and individual)
- Attendance at structured activities (e.g., program, school, or competitive employment)
- Level of participation in structured activities
- Avoidance of risky situations
- Thoughts/impulses to harm self or others

How client participates in monitoring:
- Logging or charting behaviors on a calendar (e.g., medication doses, symptoms, grooming tasks)
- Meeting in town with provider as scheduled
- Being home to meet with provider as scheduled
- Making scheduled visits to office for appointments
- Participating in laboratory testing for substances or medication levels
- Checking in by phone or in person when having a problem
- Checking in on a schedule, by phone or in person
- Cooperating in a supervised program (e.g., housing or home-based outreach services)

Who collaborates with client in monitoring:
- Client's case manager
- Client's individual counselor (if different from case manager)
- Treatment team
- Individual team members
- Family members
- Significant others or friends
- Other providers (e.g., housing outreach team, vocational specialists, community integration specialist)

Rules of Thumb

Since many close monitoring mechanisms and coercive strategies—and all involuntary interventions—take some responsibility away from clients and give it to others, consideration of such interventions places a special burden on counseling to identify and maximize clients' awareness of their ultimate responsibility for themselves. Table 17.2 provides rules of thumb that guide clinicians in closely monitoring their clients with a dual disorder. For most such clients, much time will pass before they develop dependable motivation and reliable self-control.

Paying close attention to a client's preferences helps with motivation and self-control, and encourages a sense of ownership over the treatment. If the client suggests an alternative that the counselor believes to be less promising than his or her own suggestion, the two can agree to try the client's alternative first, using the model of an empirical trial. Expectations must be made clear, measurable, and time-limited. Any restrictive measure—voluntary, coerced, or involuntary—can and should be time-limited.

Restrictions should be shaped for gradual reductions, beginning as soon as a period of sustained stability has been achieved, so that the client gradually assumes increased responsibility (e.g., time out of hospital, management of money). Small increments can ensure success and thereby sustain motivation for recovery and self-control. Even when the odds of success for voluntary engagement are low, it is important to try voluntary means. Sometimes clinicians find that it is necessary to allow clients to experience failures of their own chosen plans before they are willing to agree to a close monitoring strategy (e.g., a payeeship).

EVALUATING THE NEED FOR A COERCED OR INVOLUNTARY INTERVENTION

The principal treatment goals in dual-disorder programs include control of symptoms; clients' acquisition of skills; preservation of clients' safety and that of others; and cultivation of clients' motivation and determination to develop self-control for recovery. A proposed coerced or involuntary intervention may help to achieve a treatment effect such as the control of symptoms or reduction of harmful behavior. The intervention may also have an effect, either positive or negative, on the client's growing motivation and self-control. The decision to employ a coerced or involuntary intervention can be based on the consideration of three questions. Together, the questions illuminate the clinical indications and contraindications for coerced and involuntary interventions with a given client and situation.

1. Is a coerced or involuntary intervention necessary and likely to prevent harm?
2. How will the coerced or involuntary intervention affect the client's motivation and determination for recovery?
3. How will the coerced or involuntary intervention affect the client's self-control?

Each question highlights the impact of coerced or involuntary interventions on different goals of dual-disorder treatment. The first question expresses a traditional societal goal: *to assure safety.* The second question expresses goals that are typical in mental health and substance abuse treatment services: *to cultivate motivation and determination for recovery.* The third question expresses a goal that is particularly important in recov-

---

TABLE 17.2. Rules of Thumb in Close Monitoring

- Do everything possible to preserve trust in the therapeutic relationship.
- Maintain unconditional acceptance and positive regard for the client; if blame is necessary, blame the disorder.
- Confine the use of involuntary or coerced interventions to dangerous situations.
- Work with the client to try all voluntary options before considering involuntary or coerced restrictions.
- Consider both the risks and benefits of restrictions, focusing on the consequences for motivation and self-control.
- Always involve the client in evaluating and choosing the options.
- Never surprise the client (e.g., having the police appear at the client's door to take him or her to the hospital).
- Be clear about expectations and consequences.
- Write a contract.
- Limit restrictions as much as possible.
- Provide choices within the restrictive arrangements, so that the client has some ownership and self-control.
- Plan to reduce the restrictions as soon as possible (i.e., after a reasonable period of sustained stability suggests improved likelihood of success in self-management).
- Impose behaviorally linked time limits on the restrictions.
- Build in steps to freedom, loosening restrictions in stages, so that the client can demonstrate capabilities (e.g., after 1 month of full medication compliance, reduce medication monitoring to every other day).
- Become convinced with the client that the plan is the best option under the circumstances and that the restrictions are required.
- Always identify successful illness self-management as the ultimate goal.

ery-oriented dual-disorder treatment: *to help clients develop self-control.*

Is the Intervention Necessary and Likely to Prevent Harm?

Much of the thinking about coerced or involuntary interventions in mental health care (e.g., involuntary psychiatric hospitalization) follows a conceptual framework in which the goal of assuring safety justifies such interventions (Group for the Advancement of Psychiatry, 1994). This is consistent with ethical guidance in medical care (Culver & Gert, 1982). Again, the consideration of a coerced or involuntary intervention related to harm and safety follows the logic of the moral rules: (1) seriousness of the harm to be avoided; (2) extent of the person's rational responsibility; (3) likelihood of harm; and (4) likelihood that the coerced or involuntary intervention will significantly diminish the chances of harm.

The clinician and treatment team, with the client whenever possible, should evaluate any imminent risks of harm to the client and others. In exploring voluntary alternatives to the intervention, the team may decide that the costs of restricting the client's liberties are less than the costs of the present danger of harm, and that the benefits of a coerced or involuntary intervention outweigh the costs. When the client cannot actively participate in examining the options, the clinician may have to decide with the family (and/or other members of the client's support network) and with the treatment team whether or not to pursue such an intervention. With either choice, the stakes are high. Personal safety and legal liabilities are at stake.

Even those clinicians who most honor individual rights and self-determination are concerned for safety, and they are duty-bound under the legal principles of the Tarasoff decision (i.e., *Tarasoff v. Regents of the University of California*, 1976; for discussions of this decision, see Stone, 1984, and Applebaum, 1994) to warn people who are potentially endangered by a client's behavior. Clinicians also have a duty to protect their clients' well-being. Having seen the painful results of untreated dual disorders (e.g., destroyed relationships, lost identities, incarcerations, increased incidence of HIV and other infectious diseases, physical degeneration, deaths), many clinicians see restrictive measures as morally imperative. In addition, restrictions of one kind may prevent the necessity of employing even more restrictive measures. Conservatorship, for example, may forestall recourse to involuntary hospitalization. For clients with very severe dual disorders, whose lives are in shambles, conservatorship can improve the quality of life by assuring safety, attending to basic needs, and reducing chaos (Lamb & Weinberger, 1993).

Clinicians must not confuse coerced or involuntary interventions with treatment. We encourage clinicians to view a coerced or involuntary intervention as a structure that assists in assuring safety and access to a client during the delivery of treatment for dual disorders. The clinician who must consider a paternalistic act is in the middle ground between society and the client. He or she must stand on this middle ground and examine how the moral rules apply to the adoption of a paternalistic stance. The coerced or involuntary intervention should be kept distinct from treatment and the therapeutic relationship. Clients are much more likely to perceive the coerced or involuntary intervention as motivating if they view their treatment team as working collaboratively with them to help overcome the need for it. The intervention is best placed in the context of the need for people to obey the mandates of the state and the requirements of society. Treatment, on the other hand, is for the client—something that he or she needs in order to gain or regain self-control. The clinician's message to the client is this: "We are fighting with you against the need for coerced or involuntary intervention, and trying to help you overcome it."

How Will the Intervention Affect the Client's Motivation and Determination for Recovery?

The lack of motivation for treatment occupies a central place in the target problems of clients with dual disorders. The client's motivational state must change for substance abuse treatment goals to be achieved. Individual counseling in dual-disorder services therefore focuses on evoking, cultivating, and supporting motivation (see Chapter 7). The counseling process and motivational development depend on a relationship of trust and empathy between the client and his or her counselor. In this context, any coerced or involuntary intervention would seem to undermine the therapeutic endeavor except in situations of grave danger. Table 17.3 summarizes the potential impact of coerced or involuntary interventions on motivational development in clients with a dual disorder.

Early in dual-disorder treatment, most clients lack hope—the wellspring of motivation. Clients frequently inhabit a culture of demoralization where social norms sustain disorder and abuse, and where the very idea of hope is foreign. With such a client, external motivators may be necessary to kindle hope and motivation. Medication to control psychiatric symptoms, for example, or a comfortable and well-structured living situation with supports, may provide the spark. A coerced or involuntary intervention can also give the client the opportunity to experience temporary abstinence—an experience that he or she can contrast with otherwise

TABLE 17.3. Motivational Development versus Involuntary or Coerced Interventions

Motivational development requires . . .	Involuntary or coerced intervention may provoke . . .	
	Negative response	Positive response
Trust in the counselor and in the relationship	Feeling of violation and betrayal; anger at not being trusted	Feeling that the counselor cares enough to do something effective
Unconditional acceptance by the counselor	Anger over being infantilized and judged when counselor resorts to an authority outside the relationship	Continued nonjudgmental acceptance through the involuntary or coerced process, with encouragement to grow beyond it
Belief in the possibility of change	Sense of failure over efforts already made; loss of self-confidence for making changes; loss of optimism and of the desire for change	Experience of positive change
Willingness to try change	Defensiveness and resistance to change	Greater sense that success is possible
Self-efficacy	Perception that others have taken away responsibility; feeling of dependency on others	A sense of control and participation through the involuntary or coerced process

unabated substance use. Nevertheless, such interventions can damage trust and impair the therapeutic process.

For this reason, *how* a coerced or involuntary intervention is approached is just as critical as *whether* such an intervention is used. The fullest possible participation of the client is recommended. When a coerced or involuntary intervention is implemented in which the client has absolutely no role and exerts no control, the intervention may well exacerbate the client's sense of hopelessness and despair, thereby damaging the working alliance. Conversely, when the intervention is approached with respect and a collaborative stance, the therapeutic alliance is often strengthened, and the client's motivation is sustained or improved.

Clinicians can often discuss openly with clients the benefits and risks of using coerced or involuntary interventions. Many clients see some benefit in such interventions (e.g., staying alive, being cared about and cared for, being safe without substances), and most will see the risks (e.g., having responsibility taken away, feeling paranoid about the loss of control, losing trust in their clinicians, wanting to rebel). The probability of clients' perceiving these interventions as fair and caring is increased by involving them in the process as early as possible.

The working alliance and a client's sense of self-determination can be maximized by placing a coerced or involuntary intervention not within a clinician's control as a therapeutic tool or punishment, but rather within the legal system as a parameter defined by society that applies to everyone. When situations occur where society requires this limit to be set, clinicians

should clearly communicate their willingness to use the therapeutic alliance to help clients overcome the need for the coerced or involuntary restriction.

We recommend a stepwise approach to implementing a coerced or involuntary intervention, starting as soon as the possibility of harm appears:

1. If possible, give the client an opportunity to avoid the coerced or involuntary intervention by trying to control the dangerous behavior on his or her own.
2. When planning a coerced or involuntary intervention, always communicate clearly and specifically with the client about why the intervention is being used and exactly what will happen.
3. After clearly identifying the possible harm and the problems leading to the intervention, talk with the client about the parameters both for initiating it and for discontinuing it.
4. Maintain an open dialogue with the client; use such strategies as making contingency contracts, talking about responsibilities, and planning from the start how to build the client's responsibility, skills, and self-control.
5. Provide intensive training in the skills needed to discontinue the intervention or to minimize the need to use it again in the future (e.g., budgeting skills for a payeeship).

These steps can place coerced and involuntary interventions clearly within context of building client motivation and determination for recovery.

How Will the Intervention Affect the Client's Self-Control?

Learning to be in control of oneself, including one's treatment and use of substances, is a primary objective for clients in the active treatment and relapse prevention stages. Clinicians are frequently challenged to balance the value of self-directed controls with the value to the clients of learning to experience and practice control. Either a major mental disorder or a substance use disorder can cause impaired judgment, disordered behavior, and the loss of self-control. Like motivation, reliable self-control may be foreign to a person with dual disorders. Not knowing self-control, clients may benefit from a temporary experience of external controls, whether they receive these controls voluntarily, under coerced conditions, or involuntarily.

On the other hand, when clients only experience abstinence as a result of to external controls, they may not develop a sense of self-control. They may resent the external controls and rebel against them just to be defiant or to express their free will. The freedom from external controls itself may become a trigger for relapsing into substance use. Typically, external controls are only temporarily successful in enforcing abstinence, as clients who have not developed motivation to abstain from substances are resourceful enough to elude coercive or involuntary controls at some point. This often leads to a pattern of escalating use over time, as clients become more proficient at working around the attempts to control their behavior externally.

In summary, when the question arises as to whether external controls should be initiated, the clinician must consider three issues: how the external control might assure safety and prevent harm; how it might impair or enhance motivational development and the working alliance; and how it might improve or detract from the client's learning of self-control.

Case Example

Jon was a 39-year-old divorced male. He had a 20-year history of schizophrenia marked by hallucinations, ideas of reference, and delusions of persecution. He had also abused alcohol, marijuana, and cocaine heavily in his life, resulting in multiple adverse consequences. One spring Jon became threatening toward family members and ultimately assaulted one of them; this led to a 2-month involuntary hospitalization and a long-term (5-year) outpatient commitment to dual-disorder treatment. Jon's community treatment team initiated the hospitalization and negotiated the criteria for the outpatient commitment. During the hospital stay, a guardian was appointed for Jon. His guardian approved involuntary treatment with antipsychotic medication (eventually including clozapine), and a partial hospital program at the community mental health center following his discharge from the hospital. These programs gradually resulted in a 2-year period of sustained abstinence from substances, freedom from threatening or hostile behavior despite continued delusions, and sustained employment in a supported environment. Close monitoring through medication monitoring, urine drug screens, and frequent visits with the clinical team were gradually tapered as Jon demonstrated increasing capacity for self-control and an ability to be responsible for abstinence, medication adherence, and keeping appointments.

As the 5-year term of the outpatient commitment drew to a close, the treatment team met with Jon, his guardian, and his family. A mutual decision was reached not to apply to the court for an extension of Jon's commitment, but to allow it to expire. Jon's payeeship had been terminated earlier by agreement, as he had shown he could independently manage his money for his daily living needs.

Over the course of the next 6 months, Jon gradually began to drop some of the structures that had supported his stability. He quit his job, became isolated at home, missed occasional doses of medication, and had a few slips into substance use (which were detected on urine screens). The team pointed out this pattern to Jon and worked with him to prevent a full-blown relapse, to boost his motivation, and to maintain his determination for recovery. However, he became increasingly paranoid toward the treatment team, blamed team members for his difficulties, and once again made threats toward family members and other acquaintances.

At this point, the team psychiatrist and case manager met with Jon and advised him that his clinical condition was meeting criteria for an involuntary hospitalization or a renewal of his outpatient commitment to treatment. He was advised that the treatment team did not favor such an action and preferred to develop a voluntary treatment plan that would help him to regain control. Jon agreed to reenter the community mental health center partial hospitalization program temporarily; to resume home-based medication monitoring and urine drug screens; and to begin working with a vocational specialist to identify an appropriate vocational activity that would provide daily structure. By the following morning, when he was to start the partial hospital program, Jon began to waver in the decision he had reached with his treatment team. Jon's case manager supported him in following through with the agreement by accompanying him to the program and by visiting with him again at lunch hour, to give him further support and to remind him of his goal of regaining stability.

Jon quickly became acclimated to the program. He resumed taking his antipsychotic medications, which stabilized his psychiatric symptoms, and he stopped all threatening behaviors. He also stopped using substances, as verified by clean urine screens. Jon began to interview for jobs, and resumed initiating appropriate contacts with family members and others.

TREATMENT IN INSTITUTIONAL SETTINGS

Some clients with a dual disorder spend significant periods of time in psychiatric hospitals, jails, or prisons—as a consequence of the dual disorders, of criminal thinking tendencies that predispose some individuals to criminal behavior, or of both. *Criminal thinking* refers to a pattern of beliefs that may predispose individuals to engage in illegal or sociopathic behaviors. Examples of criminal thinking tendencies include habitually viewing oneself as a victim and blaming others (e.g., childhood, family, social conditions); thinking of oneself as better than others; emphasizing one's own positive attributes, while being unwilling to acknowledge one's own destructive behavior; and being unable or unwilling to learn from the past and make plans for the future. The time that a client spends in an institution can provide an important opportunity to initiate and make progress toward treatment goals, as the client is literally a captive audience and may clearly experience the consequences for behaviors that have led to relapse. However, the involuntary nature of the treatment setting, and the difficulties inherent in establishing an open dialogue with clients about any covert substance use that may be occurring in this setting, requires consideration of the design of integrated dual-diagnosis treatment in an institution.

From the stages-of-treatment perspective, working with individuals who are either hospitalized or incarcerated assures easy access to clients. Although engagement is defined as regular contact between a dual-diagnosis clinician and a client (Chapter 2), careful attention must be given in institutional settings to forming a working alliance based on honesty and trust. Techniques for developing a working alliance with clients in these settings may differ from those used with outpatients, such as respecting clients' need to control the frequency and timing of interactions with clinicians.

In work with outpatients, the progression from the persuasion stage to the active treatment and relapse prevention stages is based on clients' success in reducing substance abuse and achieving a remission of their substance abuse. When clinicians are assessing progress in outpatient treatment, they assume that clients have continued access to substances *and* that the clinicians have accurate information about clients' ongoing use of substances. In such circumstances, and in the absence of powerful coercive or involuntary interventions, decreased substance use is a critical behavioral indicator of the clients' motivation to work on their substance use problems.

However, there are several obstacles to accurately determining a client's motivation to work on substance use problems in an institutional setting. First, clients in a psychiatric hospital usually have restricted access to alcohol and drugs. When access to substances is limited by the environment, reduction in substance use is a poor indicator of motivation to work on substance abuse. Second, although many clients in prisons and jails continue to have access to substances (albeit at higher prices), the prohibited nature of such covert substance use makes it difficult or impossible for clients to be honest with their clinicians about their current use of substances. Treatment providers working in institutions are viewed by clients as allies of the forces that resulted in their incarceration or hospitalization, whether or not the clinicians actually choose to be such allies. This difficulty in fostering an open dialogue with clients about their ongoing use of substances interferes with determining their motivation to change. Third, by their very nature, institutional settings differ from the communities in which clients reside outside of the hospital, jail, or prison. Motivation to work on substance use problems in the institution does not necessarily translate into motivation to avoid substance use once the clients have been released into their communities. Thus "true" motivation may be situation-specific.

The difficulty distinguishing among the persuasion, active treatment, and relapse prevention stages of clients in institutional settings has a number of clinical implications for dual-disorder treatment. We discuss four of these implications below: the importance of engagement- and persuasion-stage work; the role of psychosocial rehabilitation; the use of incentives for participation in dual-disorder treatment; and the need for treatment follow-up in the community.

The Importance of Engagement- and Persuasion-Stage Work

Engagement strategies are important for people in institutional settings, who may only superficially comply with court-ordered treatment. Engagement may be especially difficult in prison programs unless inmates can identify potent consequences for not participating in treatment. Many prison systems are now turning to mandated treatment—placing inmates in treatment as the equivalent of work assignments, and penalizing nonparticipants through methods such as not providing "gain time" or sentence reduction.

As described above, once clients are engaged in treatment in an institutional setting, it is difficult to determine their true motivation to work on their substance abuse. Consequently, meaningful distinctions among the persuasion, active treatment, and relapse prevention stages cannot be made with confidence. The inability to distinguish among these stages means that an important focus of institution-based treatment is on the persuasion stage, since it is not assumed in persuasion that clients view their substance abuse as problematic.

A variety of persuasion-stage interventions can be conducted in institutions. Like many outpatients, clients in institutional settings frequently know little about their psychiatric illness, the principles of its treatment, and its interactions with stress or with alcohol and drugs. Psychoeducation—conducted either individually, in groups, or with family members—provides a vehicle for helping clients understand how substance use contributes to psychiatric disorders (and vice versa), as well as the steps needed to better manage their psychiatric illness and take control of their substance use problems (see Appendix B for educational handouts). Psychoeducation can also help clients learn more about substance use disorders by systematically reviewing the symptoms used to diagnose substance abuse and dependence.

Persuasion groups can be conducted in institutional settings, following many of the same procedures as with outpatients (see Chapter 9). These groups can informally integrate educational material, while serving the primary goal of encouraging participants to examine the effects of substance use on their lives. With institutionalized clients, such effects often include exacerbations of their psychiatric illness; disinhibition and impulsiveness, resulting in violent or other antisocial behaviors; unsafe drug use or sexual practices; and criminal behavior in order to support a habit. These behaviors have often led to their current hospital admission or imprisonment. Discussion of the negative effects of substance use can be balanced by an understanding of the individual motivating factors that have contributed to clients' use of substances. Helping clients explore the meaning of substance use and the roles it has played can enable them to consider how they can develop a new sense of purpose in their lives, and to identify alternative strategies for getting their needs met.

The Role of Psychosocial Rehabilitation

Psychoeducation and persuasion groups approach the problem of substance abuse directly, by providing pertinent information about dual disorders and encouraging clients to explore the effects of substance use on their lives. Psychosocial rehabilitation, on the other hand, addresses substance abuse indirectly, by building compensatory skills and activities that undercut clients' need and desire to use substances (see the "Functional Analysis" section of Chapter 5 for more discussion of these two approaches to reducing substance use). By focusing some efforts on the psychosocial rehabilitation of clients in institutional settings, clinicians may be able to increase clients' motivation to work on their substance use problems in a controlled setting with limited access to substances. Furthermore, rehabilitation-based strategies support the goals of institutional management and safety, which are very important to facility administrators.

Broadly speaking, psychosocial rehabilitation can address client needs in the areas of social functioning, coping with psychiatric symptoms, education, and work. Social skills training can be used to help clients improve various aspects of their social functioning, such as initiating and maintaining conversations, expressing affection, making friends, asserting themselves, and managing conflicts (Bellack et al., 1997; Liberman et al., 1989; see Chapter 11). Clients can also be taught coping strategies for a wide variety of problematic symptoms. Possible methods include cognitive restructuring or cognitive therapy for depression (Beck, Rush, Shaw, & Emery, 1979), anxiety (Beck & Emery with Greenberg, 1985; Foa & Rothbaum, 1998), substance abuse (Beck et al., 1993), or psychosis (Fowler, Garety, & Kuipers, 1995; Sensky et al., 2000; Tarrier et al., 1999); relaxation and exposure for anxiety disorders (Barlow, 2002; Foa & Rothbaum, 1998); problem solving as a general tactic (D'Zurilla & Nezu, 1999); dialectical behavior therapy for self-destructive and parasuicidal behavior (Linehan, 1993); sleep hygiene skills for sleep problems (Catalano, 1990); self-management of mood swings (Copeland, 1994); and training in recognition and response to early warning signs of relapse into any disorder (Herz et al., 2000; Perry, Tarrier, Morriss, McCarthy, & Limb, 1999). Engaging clients in a discussion of strategies for managing problematic psychiatric symptoms may also encourage them to consider that they may have used substances to cope with symptoms, and to acknowledge the problems that have resulted from such coping efforts.

Longer-term confinement, such as incarceration, can provide opportunities for clients to pursue educational objectives or to learn new vocational skills. Improved educational level or job skills may increase clients' interest in and desire for work, and thus decrease vulnerability to substance abuse. Longer-term confinement may also help some clients with very severe psychiatric disorders to develop more effective social and self-regulatory skills.

In addition to addressing the common needs of persons with dual disorders, rehabilitation in jail and prison settings should teach skills designed to counter criminal thinking tendencies (Andrews & Bonta, 1994; Gendreau, 1996; Lösel, 1995). This approach uses cognitive restructuring or cognitive therapy to assist offenders in identifying and challenging the maladaptive thinking patterns that support criminal and antisocial behaviors. Correcting these patterns may also create opportunities to address the interactions between substance abuse and criminal behavior.

The focus of rehabilitation efforts is on the use of cognitive-behavioral approaches for teaching new skills and more adaptive behaviors, and supported education and employment methods for furthering schooling and developing work experience. This emphasis is consistent with the use of social learning approaches to teaching social and independent living skills to long-term psychiatric inpatients (Paul & Lentz, 1977). Similarly, meta-analyses of the research literature on rehabilitation methods for incarcerated persons has supported the effectiveness of cognitive-behavioral approaches for reducing criminal recidivism (Andrews et al., 1990; Lipsey, 1995).

Incentives for Participation in Dual-Disorder Treatment

Incentives (e.g., snacks) are often used to encourage attendance at persuasion and education groups in outpatient settings, since clients in the early stages of treatment are not motivated to attend these activities by a desire to address their substance abuse problems. In an institutional setting, similar incentives can be used, as well as the expectation that participation in such groups is a part of the clients' treatment plan while they are in the institution. Furthermore, small incentives can be provided to encourage clients to move voluntarily from persuasion work into active treatment and relapse prevention work. For example, providing incentives to prison inmates who progress in their dual-disorder treatment—such as transitional housing, employment, status recognition, or small privileges—can reinforce their involvement in treatment in an environment otherwise not conducive to self-improvement.

It should be noted, however, that the most important role for external incentives is in engaging clients and beginning the persuasion process. As clients progress toward the active treatment and relapse prevention stages, it becomes critical for their internal motivation to become a driving force in their participation, and for the role of external incentives to fade. It is important, therefore, for an institution to have at least some active treatment and relapse prevention activities (e.g., partici-

pation in self-help groups) that are purely voluntary and are not associated with powerful incentives. These activities provide clients with opportunities to act on their internal motivation to work on their substance abuse. This also means that it is important for programs in institutions to be flexible in moving clients from interventions suitable for the earlier stages of treatment to ones suitable for the later stages, rather than to rigidly standardize the progression of treatment from one stage to the next, regardless of clients' apparent motivation (or lack thereof) to work actively on their substance abuse.

How can clinicians determine when clients are ready to move on to active treatment and relapse prevention work? The most useful insights into clients' motivational states are based on their spontaneous behavior, including verbalizations to both clinicians and others involved in their treatment or incarceration. Examples of behavioral indicators that a client is ready to begin active treatment work are provided in Table 17.4.

Follow-up Treatment in the Community

The primary advantages of institution-based treatment are the easy access to clients, the time available for treatment, and the ability to work with clients who are not under the influence of alcohol or drugs (primarily in psychiatric hospitals). The main disadvantage is that an institution is a controlled setting that is very different from the community. In addition, competing activities in prison (e.g., work assignments, ongoing security "counts" that can interfere with ongoing treatment activities, and lack of incentives for treatment participation) can be obstacles to treatment. However, once integrated treatment is provided in an institution, continued

---

TABLE 17.4. Behavioral Indicators of Potential Readiness for Active Treatment and Relapse Prevention in Institutionalized Clients

- Consistent participation in persuasion groups or individual motivational interviewing sessions
- Expressed desire to learn more about coping with high-risk situations and relapse prevention
- Interest in participating in voluntary self-help groups, such as Alcoholics Anonymous
- Spontaneous sharing of personal experiences in self-help groups
- Repeated spontaneous discussion and elaboration of negative consequences of substance use
- Identification of personal goals incompatible with substance abuse, and plans to pursue those goals
- Talking to others not directly involved in dual-diagnosis treatment about desire to work on substance abuse
- Unprompted expression of desire to make amends for consequences of substance abuse
- Verbalized acceptance of responsibility for substance use

and coordinated treatment in the community is necessary if even state-of-the-art intervention and improved client motivation are to have effects on longer-term substance abuse following discharge or release.

Hospitalization or incarceration provides an important opportunity to identify community treatment resources that can be harnessed in order to continue treatment initiated in the institution. Treatment providers and other stakeholders (e.g., family members, probation officers) can be identified prior to clients' discharge or release from the institution, and plans to continue dual-diagnosis treatment in the community can be formulated. Clinicians in the institution need to reach out to individuals who will be involved in clients' treatment in the community by inviting them to participate in treatment team meetings in the institution, meeting with them in the community, and valuing their input and insights into treatment. Outreach activities into the community prior to clients' release or discharge may be critical in regard to such issues as housing, medical needs, medication, financial needs, and employment or education.

Although clients may have made significant progress while in the institution—including motivation to work on substance abuse, new skills for dealing with or avoiding high-risk situations for substance use, and a relapse prevention plan—the community presents novel challenges to them. Even the most motivated and prepared clients are confronted with previously established environmental cues, urges, and social situations in the community that pose a serious risk for resuming their prior substance use habits. In order to minimize the chances of a relapse into substance abuse, it is helpful to conceptualize clients who have recently been discharged from an institution as temporarily returning to the persuasion stage of treatment. Thus treatment following discharge should involve at least some persuasion work.

Unique stressors are associated with community reentry for clients with dual disorders, such as moving from a structured to a less structured or an unstructured daily schedule, requirements or expectations to gain and hold employment, and reunion with family members. Because of these stressors, as well as the temptations to which clients will be exposed following a hospitalization or incarceration, close monitoring of substance use in the community is important. Close monitoring can be facilitated if a client has been conditionally discharged from a hospital, is committed to outpatient treatment, or is on parole or probation. However, close monitoring should be attempted even in the absence of such conditions. Several options for enhanced community supervision exist for offenders with dual disorders, such as house arrest, electronic monitoring, specialized caseloads for parole or probation officers trained in mental illness/substance abuse, and reduced caseloads.

Persuasion work following discharge should also involve reviewing and exploring with the client how substance use has affected his or her life, and reestablishing motivation for working toward personal goals. Clients who have progressed to active treatment and relapse prevention work in the institution should have their strategies for dealing with high-risk situations and relapse prevention plans reviewed periodically after discharge or release into the community. Clients who have begun to participate in self-help groups (e.g., AA, Dual Recovery Anonymous) in the institution should be connected with similar groups in the community, and, if possible, should attend some community meetings before they leave the institution.

CLIENTS WITH DUAL DISORDERS IN THE CRIMINAL JUSTICE SYSTEM

Special attention is needed to the growing problems of clients with a dual disorder in the criminal justice system. There are several reasons for developing specific services that target these clients' needs, and for reducing their significant levels of recidivism. First, rates of incarceration for people with mental illness are high, and the percentages of severely mentally ill persons in jails or prisons are increasing as beds and lengths of stay in psychiatric hospitals have decreased (Teplin, 1983, 1985). Second, substance abuse in persons with severe mental illness is an important factor contributing to incarceration (Mueser et al., 2000), and large numbers of prison inmates have dual disorders (Peters, Greenbaum, Edens, Carter, & Ortiz, 1998). For example, in a survey of 391 clients receiving dual-disorder services in New Hampshire or Connecticut, 70% had been charged with a crime, 53% had been convicted, and 47% had been incarcerated at some time in their lives (Mueser, Essock, et al., 2001).

Third, inmates with dual disorders tend to be more impaired than inmates with only substance abuse (Peters, Kearns, Murrin, & Dolente, 1992) and to benefit less from traditional substance abuse treatment in prison settings (Peters & Bartoi, 1997). Fourth, involvement in the criminal justice system for a client with dual disorders can present another obstacle to effective community integration. Having a mental illness is stigmatizing, as is substance abuse. The additional stigma associated with criminality and its consequences can impede the ability of such clients to find adequate housing or employment, and to repair or renew relationships with family and friends.

In recent years, new programs and treatment strategies have been developed to address the needs of persons with dual disorders who are involved in the criminal justice system. We discuss these strategies below, including jail diversion programs and drug or mental health courts, community treatment of offenders with dual disorders, and treatment in prisons.

Jail Diversion Programs and Drug or Mental Health Courts

Jail diversion programs are specifically designed to help persons with severe mental illness (and often co-occurring substance abuse) whose behavior has resulted in legal transgressions and contact with law enforcement to avoid or minimize involvement in the criminal justice system (Steadman et al., 2001). These programs are based on findings that persons with severe mental illness who receive minimal psychiatric care often come into contact with law enforcement for relatively minor legal incursions (e.g., inappropriate and threatening behavior, destruction of property, and petty theft). The likelihood of these behaviors increases when such a person also has a substance use disorder, and there is the added potential for legal problems due to intoxication, possession of drugs, and selling drugs. A major goal of jail diversion programs is to ensure that vulnerable clients receive the mental health and substance abuse services they need to stem inappropriate and illegal behaviors that can result in arrest and incarceration.

Jail diversion programs vary in the location, staffing, and specific services they provide. Typically, such programs include formal or informal partnerships between the mental health and criminal justice systems, with some programs also involving the substance abuse system. For example, Project Link in Rochester, New York, includes a core of case advocates who minimize the chances of jail recidivism and connect clients with necessary medical, psychiatric, and housing services (Project Link, 1999). The Project Link team includes the advocates, a nurse, a coordinator, and a forensic psychiatrist who work in close collaboration to provide 24-hour coverage (and mobile treatment when necessary). Referrals to the team come from a variety of sources, including correctional facilities, police departments, public defenders, psychiatric hospitals, and emergency rooms. A major role of the program is to educate the general public, the police, and those in the criminal justice system (including judges, prosecutors, public defenders, and probation and parole officers) about mental illness and substance abuse. Team members meet with clients and criminal justice personnel in courts and jails, and explore options for avoiding incarceration by referral to the treatment team or releasing clients from jail to

the team. An evaluation of Project Link indicated that participation in the program was associated with a significant reduction in days in jail as well as in the hospital.

An overlapping approach to avoiding incarceration due to substance abuse and increasing involvement in treatment has been the emergence of *drug courts* in the U.S. judiciary system (Cooper & Trotter, 1994; Deschenes & Greenwood, 1995). In contrast to most jail diversion programs, which are organized by mental health systems, drug courts are organized by the judiciary. The primary goal of drug courts is to involve clients in community-based treatment and court supervision for their substance abuse, and to retain them in treatment by enabling them to avoid time in prison (Inciardi, McBride, & Rivers, 1996).

Drug courts, as well as more recently evolved *mental health courts* (Watson, Hanrahan, Luchins, & Lurigio, 2001), provide an opportunity for coerced supervision and control over clients' mental health and substance abuse treatment needs. In recent years, some drug courts have added mental health or dual-disorder tracks to meet the special needs of this population. Other specialty mental health courts have been established to divert nonviolent offenders with psychiatric disorders from jail into appropriate community treatment. These drug courts and mental health courts also offer ongoing supervision through regularly scheduled status hearings in front of a judge or magistrate to review a client's progress, in contrast to the episodic nature of review hearings provided by most forensic review boards.

A growing body of research suggests that drug courts are successful in retaining many clients in substance abuse treatment, and in reducing criminal recidivism (Belenko, 1998). Interestingly, in one study of two treatment-based drug courts, Peters and Murrin (2000) found that they were most effective when clients remained involved in the courts for at least 1 year. This finding is consistent with Swartz and colleagues (1999), who found that outpatient mental health commitment was effective only when provided over longer periods of time (over 180 days). Although the effects of drug courts for clients with dual disorders are unclear, legally mandated treatment is an important strategy for avoiding incarceration of these persons.

Treatment of Offenders in the Community

The provision of treatment to offenders with a dual disorder living in the community is complicated by several factors, including the difficulty of accessing services and the potential for conflicts among the different professionals and agencies.

Offenders with dual disorders often have difficulty accessing the services they need in the community. Many of the obstacles faced by offenders are similar to those experienced by others with dual disorders, but may be worse because of the unique stigma associated with involvement in the criminal justice system. Peters and Hills (1999) have noted that some of the most common barriers to community-based treatment for offenders include discontinuity of services between the institution and the community; long waiting lists for counseling or residential services; exclusionary criteria; limited availability of specialized dual-disorder services; limited awareness of dual-disorder treatment programs; and confidentiality issues that limit the sharing of information between different treatment providers. Individuals and agencies responsible for overseeing and coordinating community-based treatment for offenders need to be aware of these barriers, and to develop strategies that ensure offenders timely access to substance abuse and mental health treatments. Successful engagement and continuation of dual-disorder treatment in the community may require the active involvement of different service providers, including officials in the criminal justice system, in order to minimize the chances of dropouts or recidivism.

The involvement of different individuals from different agencies in working with these offenders has significant potential for creating conflicts. Such conflicts can arise quite naturally between individuals from the criminal justice system (whose primary responsibilities are enforcing the law and protecting society) and mental health and substance abuse professionals (whose primary responsibility is to their clients). For example, conflict may arise between a dual-disorder clinician and a parole officer concerning how a minor violation of parole involving substance use should be responded to (e.g., a stern warning plus increased community monitoring, or reincarceration). In order to minimize conflict, multidisciplinary treatment teams need to include individuals from all the different agencies involved with an offender, and should meet regularly in order to plan treatment, monitor progress, and respond to problem behaviors—whether these are relapses of psychiatric or substance use disorders, criminal recidivism, or both (Peters & Hills, 1999).

Dual-Disorder Programs in Prisons

Special programs in prisons that focus on offenders with a dual disorder are a recent innovation. In a survey of seven dual-disorder programs for offenders, Edens, Peters, and Hills (1997) noted a number of common modifications to substance abuse programs. These modifications are summarized in Table 17.5.

TABLE 17.5. Common Features of Dual-Disorder Programs in Prisons

- High level of program structure
- Endorsement of psychoeducational, self-help, cognitive-behavioral, and relapse prevention strategies
- Phased treatment: (1) assessment and orientation, (2) intensive treatment, and (3) relapse prevention and transition
- Reduced caseloads compared to primary substance abuse treatment
- Briefer, simpler meetings to accommodate psychotic symptoms and cognitive impairment
- Addressing "criminal thinking" and values (e.g., using cognitive-behavioral strategies to identify and challenge "thinking errors" that lead to substance abuse and crime)
- Education about medication, and distinguishing between it and commonly abused substances
- Minimizing confrontation
- Specialized training of correctional staff about dual disorders
- Planned transition and linkage to aftercare services

Note. From Edens, Peters, and Hills (1997).

In addition to the strategies discussed earlier in this chapter for providing integrated dual-disorder treatment in an institutional setting, several other issues unique to the prison setting merit consideration. These include comprehensive mental health screening of inmates with identified substance use disorders; addressing issues of trust and safety; and preparing offenders for mandated participation in self-help substance abuse treatment when they leave prison.

Comprehensive Mental Health Screening

In inpatient and outpatient treatment of dual disorders, severe mental illness is often identified first, followed by substance abuse. When psychiatric symptoms are acute, they may also be detected first in prison and jail settings. However, in these settings substance abuse is often identified first, especially if the mental health problems are not flagrant (e.g., symptoms of major depression). An important implication of this is that mental illness needs to be routinely screened for in all inmates with identified substance use disorders. Self-report screening instruments (Zimmerman & Mattia, 2001) or structured clinical interviews are useful for identifying psychiatric disorders in offenders (e.g., Peters et al., 1998).

Addressing Issues of Trust and Safety

Offenders with dual disorders often face survival in a hostile environment. Aside from following stringent rules imposed by the prison system, offenders must live in a harsh social environment in which they are on constant guard against exploitation and abuse at the hands of other offenders. In such settings, there is little incentive for inmates to expose their personal weaknesses to others, including difficulties with substance abuse or mental health. Indeed, offenders who openly seek substance abuse treatment may be ridiculed by other inmates for "not being able to handle their drugs." In order to facilitate the engagement in treatment of offenders with dual disorders, and to protect them from the general prison population, it can be helpful to isolate those inmates into specialized treatment units.

Even in special programs, inmates may have difficulty establishing trust with one another and talking openly about their disorders in group settings. This may be especially problematic in process-oriented groups such as persuasion groups (Chapter 9), where the primary goal is to foster honest and open communication among the participants about the impact of dual disorders on their lives. Two strategies may be helpful in addressing trust. First, persuasion groups with closed membership from the beginning may be effective in developing group cohesion and promoting trust among offenders over long periods of time, as group members learn more about each other and become more willing to share their experiences. On the other hand, open-ended groups have the advantage of using senior group members as role models, who can confront members who do not yet recognize the impact of substance abuse. These senior group members are often a clinician's best ally in eliciting motivation for change and treatment adherence from offenders in the engagement and persuasion stages.

Second, the problem of establishing trust can be addressed by lessening the importance of group process and increasing the focus on learning in the group. In contrast to mainly process-oriented groups such as persuasion groups (Chapter 9), learning-based groups such as active treatment groups (Chapter 10) or social skills training groups (Chapter 11) are less dependent upon establishing high levels of trust within the group; however, they provide opportunities for participants to share with one another in a limited, structured fashion. Offenders may benefit from more structured persuasion groups that provide psychoeducation and/or skills training, while also giving participants opportunities to explore the effects of substance abuse and poor management of their psychiatric illness on their lives (see Table 9.5).

Preparing Offenders for Self-Help Groups in the Community

Based on the stages of treatment approach, we recommend self-help groups such as AA for clients in the active treatment or relapse prevention stages of treatment (see Chapter 12). Furthermore, we have emphasized that participation in self-help should be voluntary, not involuntary or coerced, in order to support clients' internal motivation to change their substance abuse behavior. However, it is common practice in the criminal justice system to mandate attendance at self-help groups for offenders released from prison into the community, regardless of their motivation to participate. Therefore, some work needs to be done in the prison to prepare offenders with dual disorders for participation in community self-help groups.

While all such offenders may benefit from preparation for self-help groups in the community, it can be useful to offer self-help groups in the prison on a voluntary basis. One solution is to provide two different levels of these groups in the prison: a traditional AA or Dual Recovery Anonymous group that is offered on a purely voluntary basis, and an "AA-Lite" or "Dual Recovery-Lite" group that is required for all offenders who do not participate in the traditional self-help groups. The goal of AA-Lite or Dual Recovery-Lite groups is to orient offenders to the Twelve Steps, to familiarize them with the structure and nature of group meetings, and to provide them with an opportunity to ask questions and prepare themselves for participation in community self-help groups.

An alternative solution is to offer self-help groups on a voluntary basis, but to mandate attendance at a limited number of meetings during the several months prior to release from the prison. This approach does not require two levels of self-help groups. However, it involves combining offenders who are motivated to use self-help and offenders who are not so motivated into a single group.

A SYNTHESIS

Clients with dual disorders frequently require involuntary or coerced interventions. These interventions provide a structure that assists in assuring safety during the delivery of dual-disorder treatment. Coerced or involuntary interventions are strategies for close monitoring that can be necessary and justified in situations where grave danger of harm is present or a person presents a threat to self or others. Empathy, unconditional positive regard, and nurturance are critical for developing motivation, and at the same time disciplines and structures are necessary for developing self-control. In order to address the goals of developing self-motivation and self-control, it is best to offer liberty and structure together. With a thoughtful balancing of interventions and shared responsibility, clinicians can assist clients to internalize liberties and nurture on one side, and discipline and constraints on the other. As indicated in Table 17.6, the dialogue be-

TABLE 17.6. Reframing Strategies for Developing Clients' Motivation and Self-Control

Black or white (either . . . or)	Shades of grey (both . . . and)
Directive or facilitative	Suggesting directions and listening for reflective self-instructions
Coercive or evocative	Providing a structure and asking for further ideas
Judgmental or accepting	Giving opinions and yielding to decisions
Critical or empathetic	Sharing accurate feedback and listening fully
Punitive or permissive	Following through with expected consequences and providing freedom
Withholding or nurturing	Helping to keep valued assets safe and giving freely to help concretely
Out of control or in control	Losing control completely in some areas and keeping reliable control in others
Consensual or involuntary	Providing many options to choose from and insisting on a few behaviors

tween clients and clinicians leads to a synthesis in which the apparent conflicts between liberty and constraint are reframed and resolved over time.

SUMMARY

Coerced and involuntary interventions should be considered only after other options for close monitoring and engagement in treatment have been exhausted. Various coerced or involuntary interventions are available, ranging from representative payeeships and outpatient commitment to involuntary hospitalization or incarceration. Evaluation of a proposed coerced or involuntary intervention for a client with dual disorders requires addressing several treatment goals simultaneously: the assurance of safety, the encouragement of the client's motivation, and the development of the client's self-control. Close monitoring of clients' substance use can avoid the need for coerced or involuntary interventions, or prevent the need for greater restrictions on their personal freedoms.

Dual-disorder treatment in institutional settings requires special considerations. Because of the restricted access to substances in institutions, as well as the lack of accurate information concerning substance abuse, much dual-disorder work in institutions focuses on persuasion-stage interventions. For clients in institutions who do show motivation to work on their substance use, interventions for active treatment and relapse prevention can be provided. Careful follow-up treatment in the community after discharge or release from an institution

is essential, and regardless of progress made in the institution, some persuasion work should be provided after discharge and release.

Special consideration is also needed regarding the treatment of dual disorders in persons involved in the criminal justice system. Programs designed to divert clients with dual disorders away from jails and prisons have been developed, including programs run by community mental health centers, as well as drug courts and mental health courts run by the judiciary. Adaptations are needed in these programs for the engagement and persuasion stages of treatment for persons with dual disorders, and specialized dual-disorder tracks or services are emerging. Within prisons, where substance abuse is often identified first, comprehensive screening of mental disorders is needed to identify offenders with dual disorders. Treatment groups in prisons need to attend to fostering trust among offenders, and some work is needed to prepare offenders for participation in self-help groups in the community (which they may be required to participate in as a condition of their parole or probation). Accessing community-based treatment often requires additional effort in order to overcome barriers against offenders receiving services, and to coordinate the efforts of criminal justice system personnel and dual-disorder treatment providers.

When clinicians balance a sensitivity to clients' desire for personal liberty with a need for constraints to protect them and others, involuntary and coerced interventions can lead to shared responsibility for the treatment of dual disorders, and can cultivate client motivation to address problems related to substance abuse.

18

Vocational Rehabilitation

This chapter focuses on *vocational rehabilitation* and its role in the process of recovery for clients with dual disorders. A central principle of such rehabilitation is that it is often more helpful to build up the positive aspects of clients' lives than to attempt to reduce their negative behaviors. As people develop and experience more worthwhile and more positive ways of spending their time, their negative behaviors tend to decrease, including their abuse of substances.

Previous chapters have described how clients progress from abusing substances to cutting down use and often achieving abstinence as they develop an awareness of the impact of substances on their lives and the advantages of avoiding them. Learning to lead a lifestyle that is not dependent upon substances is the crux of recovery for clients with a dual disorder. For many clients, these changes in lifestyle precede significant progress in reducing substance abuse and achieving abstinence. Vocational rehabilitation is an important approach to helping clients pursue personal goals and develop motivation to address their substance use problems.

We begin this chapter with a discussion of the role of vocational rehabilitation in integrated dual-disorder treatment. This is followed by a review of the merits of supported employment for persons with severe mental illness, and then consideration of issues regarding provision of supported employment to clients with dual disorders. We next describe a specific approach to supported employment, the *individual placement and support (IPS)* model, and conclude with a detailed case example of a client whose participation in IPS played a key role in his reducing substance abuse and working toward abstinence.

THE ROLE OF VOCATIONAL REHABILITATION IN DUAL-DISORDER TREATMENT

At the beginning of dual-disorder treatment, as the client weighs the pros and cons of substance use versus sobriety, the balance is often tipped toward continued substance use. At this point, the typical client's view is something like this: "My life is a wreck. It is painful. I don't have anything constructive to do. I don't have any talents. I don't have good friends, and using substances is the only thing that gives me some pleasure in life, some friends, and something I look forward to doing every day." In short, the costs of giving up substances for an uncertain life of sobriety often appear too great, and such clients naturally seek the solace and familiarity of continued substance use, despite its devastating consequences. When the functional assessment (Chapter 4) and functional analysis (Chapter 5) reveal that a client has few positive and meaningful activities in his or her life, vocational rehabilitation should be considered as a treatment strategy.

In the long-term process of rehabilitation and recovery, clinicians help clients explore and develop additional reasons for reducing their use of substances, such as through motivational interviewing (Chapter 7). Recovery involves a huge change for people: envisioning a better, more satisfying life without drugs; having the faith and courage to pursue such a life; and building the skills and supports needed to sustain a new life. It involves the transformation of clients' identity, habits, and daily activities, as well as the ways they deal with anxiety, depression, frustration, and the other challenges life offers. People who struggle to gain control over their substance abuse often say, "When I don't drink [or use drugs], my life is lonely and boring, and I feel anxious and depressed. There is not much there for me." These sentiments make it clear that recovery from substance abuse involves helping clients find more satisfying and meaningful things to do with their time than being chronic mental patients or continuing the endless pursuit of getting high or obliterating their feelings.

In most societies, work is what the great majority of people do for much of the day; it is how they support themselves, how they organize their days, how they meet people, and part of how they define themselves. In short, it is one of the main bases of their self-esteem. Persons with psychiatric disabilities attach the same importance to work. The majority of clients with severe mental illness report that work is an important personal goal (Mueser, Salyers, & Mueser, 2001; Rogers, Walsh, Masotta, & Danley, 1991). Many others are young people who want to return to school, older people who consider themselves retired but would like to volunteer or work part time, or people who want to resume child care responsibilities or some other important role. Ethnographic studies have found that people with mental illness feel stigmatized by their disorders and do not want to think of themselves as "mental patients"; they want to see themselves as normal people who have an illness that they need to manage (Alverson, Becker, & Drake, 1995; Estroff, 1981). Work is a normalizing activity for most people, including those with mental illness.

Work is equally important for clients with dual disorders. Contrary to common assumptions, long-term remission of substance abuse is not a prerequisite for such clients to participate in and benefit from vocational rehabilitation. Provided that the clients are interested in work, they can be referred to vocational rehabilitation soon after they have developed a working alliance with their clinicians, during the persuasion stage of treatment. Available research suggests that clients with dual disorders do as well as those with only severe mental illness in vocational programs (Bell, Greig, Gill, Whelahan, & Bryson, 2002; Lehman et al., 2002; Sengupta et al., 1998).

In addition, work can help clients reduce their use of substances and achieve abstinence. For example, clients often make comments such as this: "I cut down on my alcohol [or drug] use because I like going to work, and I can't work very well if I'm stoned during the day. So now I drink [or smoke dope] only at night, because I stay sober during the day while I'm at work." Cutting down alcohol and drug use in order to work more effectively and pursue goals is a natural step in the recovery process. As clients develop motivation and enter the active stage of treatment, the treatment goal becomes helping them develop strategies to further reduce their

substance use or stop altogether. Thus vocational rehabilitation is a major strategy for helping clients get on the road to recovery from their dual disorders, and abstinence is not a prerequisite for participation in a vocational rehabilitation program.

SUPPORTED EMPLOYMENT

The most effective approach to helping people with disabilities get to work is *supported employment* (Bond, Becker, et al., 2001). Vocational rehabilitation approaches that preceded supported employment were fundamentally different because they were based on the train–place model. In this model, clients were viewed as needing some type of testing, training, or experience before being placed in a work setting. The training could be for work skills, work habits, or personal hygiene and appearance; it could be teaching them interviewing skills; it could be experience in sheltered workshops to accustom them to regular work, but at a slower pace; and so on.

In the 1970s and 1980s, people in the developmental disabilities field concluded that the train–place model was not effective because people became stalled in a variety of preemployment experiences. For example, clients placed in sheltered employment jobs continued working at those workshops and rarely progressed on to real jobs paying competitive wages in regular community settings. The place–train model was developed as an alternative; in this second model, a person with a disability is placed directly in a competitive job paying regular wages in a community setting, and is then provided with the services needed to learn to do the job and retain the job (Wehman, 1981, 1986). Thus the supported employment approach is based on this change to a place–train sequence.

According to the federal definition (*Federal Register*, 1987), *supported employment* refers to a program in which a person with severe mental illness is provided with assistance that enables him or her to rapidly acquire a job paying competitive wages in community-based work settings. This means that clients work in jobs located in the community with people who do not have disabilities. In addition, clients receive ongoing support, either on or off the job, to help them succeed at the workplace.

In the 1980s, supported employment programs began to be developed and implemented in the mental health field (Bond et al., 1997). The *individual placement and support (IPS)* model was one of the first types of programs to tailor the supported employment approach specifically for people with severe mental illness, and it is the most standardized and well-studied.

The IPS model was developed to be implemented in community support programs for clients with severe mental illness at community mental health centers. Within the community support program, IPS functions by integrating vocational services with clinical services in the day-to-day work of the treatment team. Vocational services in IPS are provided by employment specialists, with each specialist assigned to a multidisciplinary treatment team. The employment specialist attends all team meetings, and provides the full array of vocational services to the clients on his or her caseload (e.g., job search, negotiating reasonable accommodations, job support). A supervisor of the IPS program oversees the employment specialists and conducts regular meetings with the employment specialists to share job leads, arrange cross-coverage, and problem-solve challenging situations. The IPS model is described in a manual that clinicians and vocational specialists can easily follow (Becker & Drake, 1993). Furthermore, the effectiveness of IPS for improving employment outcomes has been demonstrated in several controlled research studies (Drake, Becker, Clark, & Mueser, 1999).

In addition to the IPS model, other types of programs have been developed that incorporate the principles of supported employment. For example, practitioners of the assertive community treatment (ACT) model have incorporated the principles of supported employment into their service model (Becker, Meisler, Stormer, & Brondino, 1999; Meisler & Williams, 1998). Researchers in Madison, Wisconsin, have developed and redefined supported employment within the ACT approach; they found that by including the vocational service within their multidisciplinary team model, they dramatically improved vocational outcomes, even compared to their outcomes in the first 10 years of the ACT program (Test, Allness, & Knoedler, 1995).

DUAL DISORDERS AND SUPPORTED EMPLOYMENT

We have emphasized that rehabilitation and recovery are often based on employment, and have described the IPS approach to supported employment. How is supported employment modified for people with dual disorders? The simple answer is that there is very little change in the basic approach. Work is a natural part of the recovery trajectory for people with severe mental illness, including clients with comorbid substance abuse.

The more subtle answer to how the IPS model is modified for clients with dual disorders is that changes related to substance abuse are built into the individualized approach of the model. As employment specialists help individuals find the right jobs, they consider their clients' dual disorders, just as they consider other personal strengths and weaknesses. We consider below some of the typical modifications or pertinent issues related to providing supported employment to clients with dual disorders. With these issues in mind, we review the key characteristics of the IPS model.

Job Match and Vulnerability to Substance Abuse

Finding the right job for a client with a dual disorder must take into account the person's vulnerability to substance abuse. Employment specialists need to know about potential employers and job settings, and avoid placing individuals in jobs with high exposure to alcohol (e.g., many restaurants jobs) or to drugs (e.g., some construction work). Other cues for substance use are more individual and must be avoided until a client has achieved sufficient sobriety to ignore them.

CASE EXAMPLE

Steve had obsessive–compulsive disorder and a recent history of alcohol and cocaine abuse. He had worked successfully as a waiter in the past, and enjoyed working with other people. However, on several occasions Steve's tenuous sobriety had been interrupted by alcohol and cocaine binges brought on by his work. Steve reported that he found it difficult to serve alcohol to customers when he was trying to remain abstinent. Steve and his employment specialist explored other job options, and he was able to get a job working as a salesperson at a local department store. This job was also consistent with Steve's preferences, but did not involve exposure to alcohol. Steve was successful at the new job, and he was able to stick to his goal of being abstinent from alcohol and cocaine.

Disclosure of Information about a Client's Dual Disorders

The decision as to whether to disclose information about a client's psychiatric and substance use disorders is based on the client's preference. When the client permits disclosure of his or her mental illness to prospective employers, the employment specialist can play a more active role in securing a job and providing follow-along supports in close coordination with the employer. However, the question remains about the desirability of disclosing information concerning the client's substance use disorder.

There are no clear "rights" and "wrongs" as to whether employers should be informed about a client's substance use problems, and the decision must be made jointly by the client and employment specialist. However, in general, most employment specialists in IPS programs do *not* find it helpful to disclose to prospective employers information regarding problems clients are currently having with substance abuse. Whereas disclosure to employers of clients' psychiatric disabilities often evokes feelings of sympathy and a desire to help out, clients (and people in general) tend to be held more responsible for their substance abuse problems, especially when these latter problems are ongoing. Thus disclosing to prospective employers information about a client's current or recent substance abuse can make it more difficult to obtain a desired job. However, there may be situations in which the client and employment specialist decide that disclosure about substance use problems may be in the client's best interest: It may prevent potential surprises for the employer, and the employer may even consent to help monitor signs of substance abuse.

For some clients who have achieved sobriety, there may be advantages to disclosing past problems with substance use. For example, the employer may be able to monitor the client for signs of a possible relapse into substance abuse, such as unexplained absences or falling asleep on the job. Occasionally, employers may be in recovery from alcohol or drug abuse themselves, and may be able to serve as mentors or sponsors. However, in making the decision about whether or not to disclose past substance abuse, the client and counselor need to weigh the potential advantages of improved monitoring with the possible disadvantages of stigmatizing the client and raising fears that a relapse is likely to compromise the client's ability to perform the job. Regardless of whether or not the client's substance use disorder is disclosed to an employer, the client should be treated like other employees in terms of rules and regulations (including drug and alcohol screens, warnings, probation, suspension, and dismissal).

Money

Money is an important issue, both for clients contemplating work and for those returning to work. Many clients with dual disorders have their money managed by another person, such as a representative payee or a family member. In order to limit their ability to buy alcohol or drugs, clients may receive a daily or weekly allowance that is just sufficient to meet their living needs.

When clients control their own money, a very common problem is how to handle their paychecks. Money is often a cue for using substances, and many clients with dual disorders recognize their need for help in dealing with this situation. For a client in active treatment or relapse prevention, the support plan developed by the employment specialist, the case manager, and the client needs to address how payday will be handled in order to avoid a relapse into substance abuse. Plans may include such strategies as having pay directly deposited into the client's account, arranging for the clinician to accompany the client on the way home after receiving a paycheck, helping the client plan a special activity for payday that does not involve using substances, or role-playing situations in which the client is confronted with coworkers or friends who suggest using drugs or alcohol.

Even most clients with a representative payee have full access to their paychecks, as the payee has authority over benefit checks only. Therefore, returning to work can represent a substantial increase in available cash, which may trigger increased substance use. A clinician or payee can plan with a client how to handle this situation to reduce potential harm. The payee may eliminate the allowance, so that the client can use his or her own earnings for spending money. The client may take over responsibility for paying certain bills (e.g., phone bill, cable TV) from his or her paycheck, or begin saving for a larger goal (i.e., putting down a security deposit on an apartment, buying a used car, paying off a debt).

CASE EXAMPLE

Yvonne was a 41-year-old woman with schizoaffective disorder and a history of cocaine dependence and marijuana abuse. Over the past 3 years, she had no time in which she had not used drugs for more than a few days. She had also experienced various forms of victimization (including sexual and physical assault), due to prostitution and spending time with other drug-using individuals. Yvonne had recently been arrested for theft, and she was placed by the court in a halfway house for rehabilitation of her substance abuse. An expectation of staying at the halfway house was that Yvonne not use drugs. Despite her long history of drug abuse, Yvonne expressed a desire to become abstinent— partly in order to become a better mother for her two children, who were being raised by her mother. With the help of her employment specialist, Yvonne got a job working at a local fitness center. Yvonne wanted to increase her spending money, but she and her employment specialist also knew that this money would make it easier for her to relapse back into drug use. They worked out an agreement in which Yvonne would start out with $10 of extra spending money per month from her job, and that for each month she was clean, her spending money would be increased by $10. If she relapsed at any time, she would return to the original amount of $10. She was supported in using the extra money to buy things for her children. The agreement eventually worked. Although Yvonne had several relapses over the first year, she succeeded in gradually increasing her sober time, and enjoyed the benefits of working by earning more spending money.

Role of the Employment Specialist in the Substance Abuse Treatment Plan

As clients become involved with work, it is important that their substance use disorders continue to receive the attention they need. The employment specialist monitors the warning signs of substance abuse, and supports treatment and recovery. For a client in the persuasion stage of treatment, when substance abuse continues to be problematic and motivation to work on it is lacking, the employment specialist is always on the lookout for opportunities to process and explore with the client the interactions among substance use, job performance, and the pursuit of vocational goals. The employment specialist helps the client process and understand problems in vocational functioning caused by substance abuse, such as getting to work late, coming to work intoxicated, frequent absences, poor quality of work, attention problems, poor hygiene and grooming, and fatigue; the principles of motivational interviewing (Chapter 7) are employed. The vigilance and support of the employment specialist, combined with the client's commitment to achieving specific goals, are often sufficient to motivate the client to work on reducing substance use or achieving abstinence without losing the job.

Job Loss Due to Substance Abuse

Despite the best efforts of clients and employment specialists, job losses due to substance abuse do occur, and these experiences must be processed in order to learn and profit from them. Usually, it is best for an employment specialist to avoid directly blaming a client's loss of a job on substance abuse. Rather, it is more effective to use the Socratic method (Chapter 7)—that is, asking the client questions and evaluating the possible factors that led up to the job loss, including substance abuse. When the specialist asks questions rather than giving answers, the client is more likely to "own" the conclusions that are reached, and not to view the specialist as an adversary or someone on a mission to curtail his or her substance abuse.

The awareness of how substance abuse affects job performance and retention may develop slowly in some clients, over the course of obtaining and losing several jobs. Each vocational experience provides a valuable learning opportunity about the type of job the client most wants, and the changes he or she needs to undertake in order to succeed at the workplace—including changes in substance use habits. By remaining upbeat, optimistic, and problem-solving-oriented, the employment specialist keeps the hope that work is possible alive, while providing new opportunities for understanding the interactions between work and substance abuse. At the same time, if substance abuse repeatedly contributes to job losses, the employment specialist can discuss this openly with the client, and at some point inform the client that he or she will not continue to recommend new jobs unless the client takes some steps to address the substance abuse problem.

With these issues in mind, we next review the IPS model in more detail, illustrating its application to clients with dual disorders.

THE IPS MODEL

The Practical Approach of IPS

IPS is a model of vocational rehabilitation aimed at finding or creating natural opportunities for persons with severe mental illness, including those with dual disorders, to work at real jobs in community settings. Several practical issues arise when a treatment team is developing and implementing an IPS program, including eligibility, benefits, and assessment/job development.

Eligibility

Anybody with a major mental illness is eligible to work with an employment specialist in the IPS model, regardless of whether a client also has an active substance use disorder. The only criterion for participating in an IPS program is that the client wants to work. A client may have never worked a competitive job, and may be homeless, addicted to crack cocaine, and psychotic. Nevertheless, that client is eligible for supported employment as long as he or she expresses a desire to work. Because of these minimal requirements for participation in an IPS program, most clients with dual disorders are eligible for vocational rehabilitation, as illustrated in the case example below.

CASE EXAMPLE

Jim was a 31-year-old man with schizophrenia marked by persistent hallucinations. He would often drink large quantities of alcohol with friends or alone, often to the point of passing out. He said that alcohol provided him with a temporary respite from his hallucinations. Even though Jim acknowledged that in the long run his alcohol abuse was probably worsening his symptoms, he said that it was helpful in the short term, and he didn't have anything else to do with his time.

Through close collaboration with Jim, his treatment

team found that he was interested in working. However, Jim was not sure he would be able to work competitively, since he had not worked since developing schizophrenia 10 years before; he preferred a low-stress job that would provide him with contact with others. Jim was helped to land a job as a dishwasher working 2 hours per night, 5 days per week. Jim found that he enjoyed his work, that he liked working around other people, and reported that his hallucinations were less troublesome when he was working. He gradually increased his time on the job to 18 hours per week. As Jim spent more time working, he felt good about himself and his accomplishments, and his alcohol use decreased substantially. Jim's success on the job encouraged him to begin pursuing other goals, so he began taking classes to complete his high school education, while continuing to work.

Benefits

The rules for such benefits as Supplemental Security Income (SSI), Social Security Disability Insurance (SSDI), welfare, Medicaid, and others are complex. Most clients are afraid that if they go to work, they will lose their benefits. This is the greatest disincentive to working. Despite these concerns, clients can actually work quite a bit without losing Medicaid, which is the key benefit for most people with severe mental illness.

Many mental health centers use computer programs to calculate benefits, so that a client can determine how much to work and what the effects on his or her benefits will be. Depending on how much they work, clients may lose some of their SSI or SSDI benefits. However, clients usually become willing to lose some disability income because they want to work, and most clients who work experience an increase in their total income.

Assessment and Job Development

The assessment process is individualized. Clients are asked what they have done in the past and what they would like to do. Employment specialists also try to find out what activities, mental tasks, and supports help a person to function optimally. The whole team is involved, because the clinicians often know what clients' strengths are, what is stressful for clients, and what they do to manage their symptoms. An outline of the vocational assessment conducted in the IPS model is provided in Table 18.1.

Job development is driven by a client's needs, preferences, interests, skills, and talents. There are many different approaches. Some clients want to find and interview for jobs themselves. By and large, however, the traditional approaches of sending out resumés, looking at newspaper ads, and calling about jobs do not work very well. Effective employment specialists get to know their clients, the kinds of jobs they want, and their needs, and then the specialists themselves go looking for those jobs. Often an employment specialist finds an employer with the desired type of job and talks him or her into hiring a client. Many employers are interested in hiring people with disabilities, and they are willing to

---

TABLE 18.1. Outline of Vocational Assessment in the Individual Placement and Support (IPS) Program

Sources of information
- The client, the treatment team, and clinical records
- Family members and previous employers (with client's permission)

Work goal
- Client's long-term work goal or life dream for work
- Client's short-term work goal

Work background
- Education and work history
- Most recent job: Reason for leaving job, positive experiences, problems on the job
- Next most recent job (same information as most recent job)

Current adjustment
- Diagnoses: Psychiatric disorder(s), substance use disorder(s)
- Early warning signs of relapse
- Symptoms and coping strategies
- Medication management
- Pattern of substance use
- Physical health, endurance, grooming
- Interpersonal skills

Work skills
- Job-seeking skills and specific vocational skills
- Aptitude and interests (vocational and nonvocational)
- Motivation
- Work habits: Attendance, dependability, stress tolerance

Other work-related factors
- Transportation
- Social support network (family, friends)
- Living situation
- Criminal record
- Disclosure of disorders
- Expectations for work (personal, financial, social)
- Money management skills
- Income and benefits
- Daily activities and routines, regular contacts

Networking contacts for job search
- Family and friends
- Previous employers

let clients work for a few hours a week to see how they do. Often an employer finds that a client is a likable person and a good worker, so the individual's hours are increased. Then the employer is sometimes willing to hire another client.

The key to successful job development in IPS is the job match. Simply put, the job should fit the client. For example, in the old train–place model, vocational counselors spent considerable time trying to teach clients how to comb their hair, dress nicely, and bathe before they were considered ready for job placement and work. In the IPS model, clients who do not bathe, change their clothes, or comb their hair, and who smell terrible, are perfectly acceptable. Such a person may be helped to find a job in a recycling center where everything smells, and he or she fits in perfectly. For another example, imagine a man with schizophrenia who screams at his voices all day long. This man will not fit in well in an office setting. So where can he fit in? In a sawmill! The sawmill is buzzing all day long and this fellow may be screaming, but nobody can hear him, and he can do the job.

CASE EXAMPLE

Sharon was a woman with borderline personality disorder and alcohol abuse who often cut herself with razor blades. She had not benefited from several psychotherapy experiences, although she expressed a desire to work. Sharon began meeting with an employment specialist from an IPS program, who explored possible job interests with her. The employment specialist finally helped her to find a job doing autopsies on animals at a medical research laboratory. She enjoyed doing these autopsies and was able to stop cutting herself when she focused on her work. Sharon also liked the fact that her work involved evening and nighttime hours, since these were especially difficult times for her to be alone and were when most of her abusive drinking occurred. Over time, Sharon met some other people at the laboratory who also worked late into the night, who became her friends. Her alcohol use gradually decreased as she spent more time with others, often in the evening, and felt less of an urge to drink.

Employment specialists interview clients about their job preferences when they first enter an IPS program. Although clients sometimes have unrealistic expectations about the kinds of jobs they would like to do, most clients immediately express job preferences that are fairly realistic. For the others, the employment specialists work with them to identify more realistic job possibilities related to their interests. For example, a client may express a desire to be a doctor, but careful exploration of this ambition reveals that the primary attraction is to the clothing doctors wear. There are many jobs other than being a doctor in which people get to wear white coats, and the employment specialist can help the client get one of these jobs.

Clients sometimes express ambitious but quite genuine vocational goals that may be attainable in the long run; for instance, someone who did not complete high school may want to become a mental health professional. The employment specialist explores such interests with the client and works to develop a long-range plan for achieving the goal. Steps toward that goal may involve obtaining further education or training, and less skilled work in related jobs or professions. For most clients, some type of current work experience is useful for making progress toward longer-term goals.

For a client with persistent symptoms, the goal is to find a job that not only matches who the person is, but also helps him or her to control symptoms. Clients use a variety of strategies to manage their symptoms. For example, some clients have learned that they need to be in a quiet place, and others need to be in a noisy place where there is music or other continuous sound. Some people need to be alone, while others need to be around people. Some clients like to sit and work with their hands on assembly tasks or a computer, and others like talking to the public. The job-matching process is very idiosyncratic. An optimal job is one that fits with a client's natural strategies for controlling his or her symptoms so that it enhances overall coping effectiveness.

The typical client in an IPS program starts at a few hours a week at an entry-level job and ends up working from 18 to 22 hours a week. Some clients begin working as few as 2 hours a week. Most clients begin by earning minimum wage and, when their jobs are consistent with their preferences, stay on these jobs for about 6 months. Although 6 months is not very long, people without psychiatric disabilities stay in entry-level jobs for about the same amount of time, and for many clients this work may be their first paid employment in years. Most clients go on to find several more jobs over time.

CASE EXAMPLE

Nancy liked painting, and the store that really fascinated her was a local picture-framing shop. The employment specialist talked with the owner of the frame shop, who agreed to give Nancy a job helping to clean up for 2 hours a week. Nancy liked being at the shop, and the job grew. Over the next several months, her hours gradually increased to 20 per week. She also began painting, and she was given two raises in her hourly wage. After 8 months at this job, Nancy decided to pursue a job with a painting company; she successfully secured this job with the help of her employment specialist, and held it for several years.

IPS Strategies

There are several characteristic strategies of the IPS model, summarized in Table 18.2 and described below.

Integration of Treatment and Rehabilitation

The provision of vocational services in the IPS model is fully integrated with all aspects of psychiatric treatment, including case management, symptom monitoring, and medication. In fact, IPS conceptualizes rehabilitation *as* treatment. Work is not something peripheral to treatment, such as getting clients jobs because they have lots of time on their hands, or because they are now doing well and want to work. Rehabilitation is at the very center of treatment. Rehabilitation involves taking the healthiest, most functional part of a person and helping that part to expand into normal role functioning. Through working, people develop self-esteem, friends, a structured activity, personal meaning, and motivation for managing their disorders and symptoms.

The integration of vocational rehabilitation and clinical treatment is accomplished in IPS programs by having an employment specialist, who provides supported employment services, and functions as a member of a client's multidisciplinary treatment team. The employment specialist attends all team meetings (usually several times per week); provides updates concerning the client's progress toward employment goals; problem-solves with team members about possible obstacles to employment; and receives information from other team members concerning job leads, clinical issues relevant to the client's work performance, and other clients who may benefit from supported employment.

Team Approach to Vocational Rehabilitation

IPS uses a team approach to improving work outcomes for clients. As mentioned above, the employment specialist functions as a member of a multidisciplinary team (including the psychiatrist, case managers, nurse, etc.). In addition, the employment specialist works collaboratively with extended members of the client's treatment team, such as residential care providers, family members, friends, landlords, and probation or parole officers. Collaboration with everyone involved in treatment ensures that everybody on the team can support the focus on work, and can view it as central to treatment and to the recovery process.

One of the problems with providing vocational services that are not integrated with other aspects of psychiatric treatment, such as medication and monitoring symptoms, is that clients often give (and receive) contradictory messages to (and from) different providers. For example, a client may go to a vocational program, express readiness to work, and receive help from the employment specialist in finding a job. The client then goes back to the mental health program and expresses the other half of his or her ambivalence by saying, "Gee, I don't think I'm ready to work yet. I'm really too anxious right now, and maybe I should put this off for a while." This common scenario can lead to conflict between members of the vocational program and the treatment team as to who really understands the client.

The bottom line is this: Just as psychiatric and substance abuse services need to be integrated to improve the outcomes of clients with dual disorders, vocational services also need to be integrated with dual-disorder treatment in order to improve work outcomes. When

TABLE 18.2. Strategies of the Individual Placement and Support (IPS) Model

Strategy	Description
Integration of treatment and rehabilitation	Vocational services are provided by an employment specialist who functions as a member of the client's treatment team.
Team approach to vocational rehabilitation	Employment specialists work with other team members collaboratively to help clients find and keep desired jobs.
Emphasis on competitive work	The focus is on helping clients get competitive jobs paying competitive wages in community settings.
Rapid job search	Prevocational assessment and training are deemphasized in favor of rapid individualized job search and attainment.
Provision of follow-along supports	On-site and/or off-site support is provided to each client after obtaining a job, to ensure success or smooth transition to a new job.
Attention to client preferences	A client's preferences determine the type of job sought, the disclosure (or not) of the client's disability to employers, and the nature of job support provided.
Provision of services in the community	Most vocational services are provided in natural settings in the community, such as in a restaurant, park, the client's home, or the workplace, rather than the mental health center.

clients go to work, it is common for them to experience momentary periods of increased anxiety, depression, substance abuse, and other problems, which can be frightening or destabilizing. When this occurs, it is not helpful to say, "You shouldn't be working yet. It looks like your disorders are acting up, so why don't you take a week off, calm down, and think about it?" Rather, clients need support for sticking to and following through on their vocational plans, and help in dealing with substance abuse, disruptive symptoms, and stressors that threaten to derail these plans. Interventions such as medication dosing can be more precisely tailored to clients' needs when there is feedback from vocational services.

Emphasis on Competitive Work

IPS focuses on helping clients find and hold competitive jobs—not sheltered work, volunteer jobs, or transitional jobs. The reason for emphasizing competitive work is that clients with severe mental illness are capable of it and value it. Traditionally, clients have rarely been given the opportunity to work competitively because of all the "preparation" deemed necessary, such as extensive prevocational assessment or skills training. If clients are placed in prevocational programs that involve very low expectations on their performance, such as sheltered workshops, skills training groups, or transitional jobs, they tend to become stalled and never move on to competitive employment positions.

Rapid Job Search

Collaborative work with clients focuses on rapid job searches. Rather than conducting extensive assessments or job training activities, IPS prescribes helping clients look for jobs as soon as possible. An employment specialist actively helps a client to find a job. Assessment is done along the way, but does not slow the process. The best way to learn about what a client likes to do, what the person can do, and what troubles the person is likely to encounter on the job is to help that individual find a job and see how it goes. This is especially the case for persons who have not worked in a long time. An example of the rapid and individual approach to job placement is provided below.

CASE EXAMPLE

Selma was a 26-year-old woman with major depression and polysubstance abuse who had recently been discharged from the hospital following alcohol detoxification. Soon after her discharge, a member of her treatment team began talking with her about her job interests, and a part-time job was found for her sorting mail at a local insurance company. However, after only an hour Selma walked off the job. She came in to an appointment, and a team member said to her, "Well, congratulations! That's terrific. You worked an hour, and I bet you learned a lot about what you like and what you don't like about work. So tell me all about it, and then we can find another job that is more consistent with what you want." The IPS counselor contacted the employer to help explain Selma's difficulty tolerating the job, and to maintain a positive rapport with the employer. All the team members treated Selma's effort at working as a great success, even though she was on the job for only 1 hour.

Provision of Follow-Along Supports

Providing clients with follow-along supports after they have found work is crucial to ensuring success on the job or a smooth transition to another job. The nature of follow-along supports can take many different forms and depends on both a client's needs and preferences, including whether the psychiatric disability has been disclosed to the employer. The client may be visited on the job, picked up after working, or helped to learn part of the job. The employment specialist may talk with the client's employer about the job; arrange for reasonable accommodations for the psychiatric disorder (e.g., brief scheduled breaks each hour for attention problems, decreased hours during a symptom exacerbation, wearing headphones to cope with persistent auditory hallucinations); practice a social skill with the client that may facilitate interactions with coworkers; teach strategies for improving attention (e.g., writing things down) or managing problematic symptoms; or just provide empathic listening and emotional support. In other words, clients are provided the assistance they need in order to make their efforts to join the workforce rewarding and successful.

Attention to Client Preferences

In line with the role of shared decision making in the integrated dual-disorder treatment approach (see Chapter 2), IPS gives priority to clients' preferences—including preferences regarding disclosure to employers about the psychiatric illness, the type of job sought, the job setting, and the provision of follow-along supports. About half the time, clients do not want their employers to know that they have a mental illness. However, there are advantages if an employer knows that a person has a disability, because the team can work with the employer from the beginning. Team members can intervene when problems emerge, and the employee has certain rights and protections under the Americans with Disabilities Act legislation (Fabian, Waterworth, &

Ripke, 1993; Furlong-Norman, 1997; Kaufmann, 1993; Mancuso, 1990).

Nevertheless, there is a long history of discrimination against people with psychiatric disorders in obtaining work and at the workplace (Farina, 1998). For this reason and others, many clients feel stigmatized by their mental illness and prefer to get jobs on their own, without disclosing their disability to employers. Although this often does not work out, it is important to respect each client's choice. If a job is not successful and a client moves on to another job, in the second or third job the client may change his or her mind and be willing to disclose the mental illness. Or, with the off-site support of the employment specialist, the client may experience success on the job without disclosing his or her disability to the employer.

When the client permits disclosure, it is preferable for the employment specialist to talk to the employer in advance to explain that the person has a disability and is interested in getting back to work. More specific information about the client, such as diagnosis and history of hospitalization, is not necessary. It can be helpful for the employment specialist to advise the employer about certain behaviors peculiar to the client, such as talking to him- or herself. If the employer notices any problems, the employment specialist can be contacted, and someone can come over and determine whether the client needs help. Employers value the backup provided by the team. Many employees in entry-level jobs have problems, whether or not they have disabilities, and it is common for people to walk off the job and disappear without even informing their employers about what the trouble was. Employers like the reassurance that a job counselor provides, and they are often willing and eager to hire clients when they know that this type of support is available.

Employment specialists strive to achieve a balance between providing as little information as necessary about the nature of clients' disorders to their employers, and giving enough information to prepare the employers for possible difficulties on the job. In general, employers do not like to be surprised by unexpected problems in employees, and preparing employers in advance may help to avoid "burning bridges" with them. At the same time, providing too much information may discourage a prospective employer from hiring a client, or may create negative expectations and thus inadvertently stigmatize the client.

Client preferences for the kind of work they want to do are also important. Before beginning the job search, the employment specialist spends time with clients exploring the types of work they would like to do, the preferred work setting, and so forth. Research shows that client preferences for type of work are re-

lated to job tenure. Clients in IPS programs whose jobs match their preferences remain on those jobs about twice as long as clients whose jobs do not match their preferences, and they report higher satisfaction with their jobs as well (Becker, Bebout, & Drake, 1998; Becker, Drake, Farabaugh, & Bond, 1996; Mueser, Becker, & Wolfe, 2001). Thus client preferences are important in determining both the nature of the support provided and the types of jobs sought.

CASE EXAMPLE

Marcus had bipolar disorder, as well as drug dependence on marijuana and sedatives. He spent most of his time alone using drugs, and he had not worked in many years. In exploring the prospect of work with his employment specialist, Marcus expressed ambivalence: Although he wanted to work, he did not feel he was capable of it, and doubted that he could meet the expectations of paid employment. Marcus also was not sure what he wanted to do, but he noted that he always loved animals. The employment specialist was not able to convince Marcus that he would be able to meet the demands of a paid job. To help Marcus explore what it was like to work, but in a situation with low expectations, the employment specialist suggested that he try a volunteer position. Marcus agreed to this, and a volunteer job walking dogs for the local animal shelter was found. Marcus enjoyed the job, and he showed he could be reliable. With this success, Marcus's confidence increased, and the employment specialist helped him find a paid job working at a local pet store. While Marcus continued to walk dogs for the animal shelter as a volunteer, he decreased his time doing this in order to spend more time working at the pet store.

Provision of Services in the Community

The employment specialist tries to build a relationship with the client in the real world. Both searching for jobs and providing job support are community-based activities; thus most vocational services are provided in the community and not the office. In fact, many employment specialists do not even have their own private offices; instead, they share space with each other or with case managers to facilitate collaboration, and have access to a private meeting area where they can occasionally get together with clients. When employment specialists share space, it is helpful to plot and prominently display on a blackboard the current jobs held by clients. This can facilitate the specialists' sharing of job leads, and can also make it clear when specialists are having difficulty getting their clients employed.

When employment specialists work with clients who have never worked and have no idea what they would like to do, they get out of the office and into the city or town. They spend their time walking around together, looking in stores, visiting restaurants or coffee shops, and trying to think about what it might be like to work in these different places. They get to know their clients by interacting with them in the community rather than the mental health center.

CASE EXAMPLE

Juan was a 36-year-old man who had moved to the United States from Mexico at the age of 4. He had been involved in the mental health system since he was 8 years old, when he demonstrated significant conduct problems (lying, petty theft, frequent fights) and borderline intellectual functioning. Juan began drinking alcohol at the age of 10, and experimenting with a wide variety of drugs by the time he was 12. Juan dropped out of high school in his first year, and had his first psychotic episode soon afterward at the age of 15. After several psychiatric hospitalizations, Juan was diagnosed with schizophrenia. His substance use problems continued unabated throughout his adolescence, and for most of his adult life Juan met criteria for polysubstance dependence. His most recent drug problems were related to heroin, amphetamines, and marijuana. Juan had been in jail or prison on several occasions for such charges as public intoxication, theft, setting fires, and assault.

Since the onset of his illness, Juan had experienced persistent symptoms of his schizophrenia, including auditory hallucinations. He sometimes had delusions (e.g., believing that others could read his mind), which tended to worsen with acute alcohol and drug abuse. When Juan was referred to the IPS program, he was using marijuana daily, injecting amphetamines once every day or two, and either snorting or injecting heroin once or twice per week. Juan's alcohol use was limited to episodes of abusive drinking every several weeks, usually when drugs were not available. Much of Juan's drug use occurred with friends; he supported his addiction by allowing his apartment to be used for dealing drugs, which provided him with free access to the substances. Juan acknowledged some of the problems he had experienced because of his substance abuse, but expressed limited interest in working on it.

Despite moving to the United States at a relatively young age, Juan's language skills in English were not strong. He was able to communicate fairly effectively, but he spoke ungrammatically and with a limited vocabulary. When Juan began meeting with his employment specialist, his job history revealed that his work experience was limited to working in a state-sponsored janitorial program, and doing a limited amount of piecework

while in prison. Although Juan's level of education was low and he had limited work experience, he also had several notable strengths. First, he was artistically inclined: He had good drawing and painting skills, he enjoyed listening to music, and he had taught himself how to play the guitar. Juan was also interested in working, with his major motivation being to purchase art supplies. Last, although Juan appeared rather unkempt, he had relatively good personal hygiene, including regular bathing, toothbrushing, and use of deodorant.

Juan's job preferences centered mainly on work that had some connection to the arts. The employment specialist explored a variety of options with Juan, such as working in an art or music store. Eventually they were able to find a job for Juan working as an usher at a local theater company. The job started out at 4 hours per week. Juan and his employment specialist worked out an agreement that the specialist would manage the additional income Juan earned on the job, and that the money could be spent on art supplies and (eventually) a new guitar.

Juan enjoyed interacting with the stage performers and set designers, who were not put off by his disability. They reached out to him and liked him as a person. Over time, the theater managers recognized Juan's artistic skills, and they began to give him other tasks to do. They increased his hours at the theater. They also asked Juan to design some of the brochures and advertisements for upcoming performances, and to help paint sets and design other props for plays. Juan's working hours were increased to between 16 and 24 hours per week, with a variable schedule depending on whether a play was being performed.

Over the first 6 months on this job, Juan experienced a number of setbacks related to his substance abuse. On several occasions he did not show up for work because of substance use, and he was informed by his employer that his job was in jeopardy if he could not be counted on. At first, Juan responded to these concerns by trying not to use substances in the afternoon, when it interfered with his ability to go to work. However, he found that once he started using substances it was hard to stop, and he made an agreement with his employment specialist not to use on the same days that he had to work. As Juan's working hours increased and he began to make friends with people at the theater company, his interest in using substances declined. He enlisted the help of his case manager in meeting and talking with his drug-using friends, in order to get them out of his apartment. This effort was partially successful, but Juan and his case manager agreed that moving to another apartment would make it easier to break his connection with these friends. One year after starting the job, Juan was continuing to work and had not used amphetamines or heroin for the past 2 months. He continued to have occasional problems related to marijuana and alcohol use, which had decreased but not stopped altogether. Juan felt good about his job and his decreased substance use, and began to talk about wanting to stop using marijuana and alcohol.

SUMMARY

Work plays an important role in the recovery process for people with dual disorders. Competitive employment helps clients structure their lives by giving them something positive and respected to do with their time. Work also provides many real-life opportunities for clients to experience the natural consequences of substance abuse, and to develop motivation for addressing their substance use problems in order to achieve desired changes in their lives.

The most effective approach to vocational rehabilitation for persons with severe mental illness, including those with dual disorders, is supported employment. One widely used supported employment program is the IPS model. The principles of this model include deemphasis on prevocational training and assessment; rapid job search and attainment; provision of follow-along supports; attention to client preferences in type of job and nature of support provided; and integration of vocational rehabilitation with treatment at the level of the treatment team. Clients at any stage of dual-diagnosis treatment can participate in and benefit from supported employment, regardless of the extent of their current substance use problems. Employment specialists can use a variety of strategies to address common issues related to providing vocational rehabilitation to clients with dual disorders, such as handling additional money from paid employment, disclosing the disorders to employers, and dealing with job losses due to substance abuse. Through perseverance and collaboration, supported employment programs can help clients develop meaning in their lives, and motivate them to address their substance abuse problems in order to pursue their personal goals.

19

Psychopharmacology

Although physicians and other prescribers have long administered *psychopharmacological* treatments to clients with severe mental illness, there has been only limited recognition of the high prevalence of co-occurring substance use disorders. Research indicates that clients with persistent psychiatric syndromes do respond to medications, although their substance abuse does not automatically improve (Nunes & Quitkin, 1997). Few guidelines exist for psychopharmacological treatment for clients with dual disorders, despite the numerous potential complications. The most serious concerns relate to medication nonadherence, substance–medication interactions, and the potential of some medicines for abuse.

In this chapter, we review the principles of pharmacology for clients with dual disorders. The emphasis is on more general issues, although we also discuss specific medications, describe our clinical experiences, and review pertinent research literature. For further information about medications for different psychiatric disorders, readers should review three educational handouts in Appendix B of this book (see Handouts B.7, B.8, and B.9); for even more detailed information, they should consult a recent textbook on psychopharmacology (e.g., Buckley & Waddington, 2000; Schatzberg & Nemeroff, 2001). Because most standard texts omit the topic of co-occurring substance use disorders, we suggest ways in which standard pharmacological treatment must be modified when dual disorders are present. Clearly, the scope of this chapter is wide, as is the intended audience. Due to the chapter's broad coverage, program directors, physicians and other prescribers, case managers, counselors, clients, and family members may all find reading it useful.

We begin with a discussion of the role of psycho-

pharmacology in dual-disorder treatment, followed by general guidelines and a review of central issues in treatment, such as diagnosis and the optimum times to initiate pharmacotherapy. We next consider medications for specific comorbid psychiatric syndromes, including psychosis, bipolar disorder, depression, and anxiety; this discussion is followed by a description of medications for comorbid substance use disorders. We next discuss pharmacological treatment for detoxification, and conclude by considering strategies for monitoring treatment and outcomes of clients with dual disorders.

THE ROLE OF PSYCHOPHARMACOLOGY IN DUAL-DISORDER TREATMENT

Psychopharmacological treatment is the mainstay of treatment for severe mental illnesses, such as schizophrenia, bipolar disorder, and treatment-refractory major depression. Furthermore, there is a growing literature testifying to the beneficial effects of specific medications for substance abuse. However, despite the importance of medication, nonadherence to prescribed medication is common, and comorbid substance abuse often worsens adherence further. Even when clients take their medication, the presence of substance use disorders can mask the clinical effects of medication, making it difficult to optimize treatment. These problems are compounded by the fact that in many settings clinical personnel are confused about potential interactions between substances of abuse and prescribed medications; this confusion often results in contradictory messages to clients and undertreatment of psychiatric disorders. In the absence of competent psychopharmacological treatment, the psychosocial components of integrated treatment are compromised, and in some cases may be rendered altogether ineffective.

Psychopharmacology has two major roles in the treatment of dual disorders. First, pharmacological treatment is necessary to stabilize the major symptoms of severe mental illness in a substantial majority of clients, and to avert or reduce the likelihood of subsequent symptom relapses. The need for such stabilization should be apparent during the assessment of a client's psychiatric diagnosis and symptoms, and by a thorough review of the client's treatment history (Chapter 4).

Symptom stabilization is an important tool at every stage of treatment. At the engagement stage, when a client lacks a working alliance with a clinician, pharmacological treatment can reduce acute symptoms and produce rapid subjective relief, which can facilitate the formation of a therapeutic relationship. At the persuasion stage, when clients have a working alliance with clinicians but lack the motivation to work on their substance abuse, pharmacological symptom stabilization can be critical to decreasing distracting symptoms, improving cognitive functioning, and enhancing insight—thereby creating the psychological foundation necessary for the clients to understand the effects of substance abuse on their psychiatric disorder and their lives. At the active treatment stage, when clients have begun to reduce their substance use or have recently achieved abstinence, pharmacological treatment can alleviate symptoms that might otherwise contribute to substance use and abuse. In the relapse prevention stage, when clients have not recently experienced problems related to substance use, pharmacological treatment of their psychiatric disorders serves primarily to reduce risk of symptom relapses, enabling the clients to remain focused on their personal recovery goals and the avoidance of substance abuse relapses.

Second, psychopharmacological treatment has a more circumscribed role to play in the direct treatment of substance abuse. Several effective medications have been shown to improve the outcome of substance abuse, and judicious use of these medications in clients with dual disorders may produce similar effects. At the same time, awareness of a client's stage of treatment and the appropriate timing of pharmacological interventions, and the coordination of such treatments for substance abuse with psychosocial interventions, can make the difference between a good and a bad outcome.

Thus psychopharmacology is a critical intervention in the treatment of dual disorders. It is important at all stages of treatment, and its implementation needs to be closely coordinated with the psychosocial treatment components.

GENERAL GUIDELINES

Clients with dual disorders are often warned that their medications may interact dangerously with their use of alcohol and drugs. Clients may also find that their medications interfere with the "high" or "buzz" they expect from using substances. They often resolve these conflicts by skipping their medications when using substances, which may contribute to their high relapse and rehospitalization rates (Drake & Brunette, 1998). Another problem is that physicians sometimes withhold medications from clients with dual disorders because of fears regarding safety or liability. Probably the most common difficulty is that physicians fail to identify and appreciate comorbid substance use disorders and the related nonadherence to medications. As a result, they may attribute continued or recurrent symptoms to lack of medication efficacy rather than to medication nonadherence and substance abuse. To avoid these pitfalls and to optimize a therapeutic response to medications, a physician should carefully consider both the severe mental illness and substance use disorder when prescribing for such a client, and should follow the guidelines described below.

Ciraulo and Renner (1991) have articulated the following guidelines for the use of medications with alcoholic clients, which have general applicability to the broader population of persons with dual disorders:

- Determine the diagnosis, so that medications are not used to treat substance-induced symptoms.
- Use medications that have low abuse potential, to avoid creating another addiction and making the situation worse.
- Use medications that have low lethality in overdose, since clients with substance use disorders are prone to overdoses and suicide attempts.
- Dispense limited amounts of medication, and follow clients closely.
- Use random urine or plasma toxicology when they might help to identify misuse.

To these recommendations, we add two more:

- When selecting a medication to treat psychiatric symptoms, include evidence of potential to reduce craving for substances of abuse in the selection process.
- Consider prescribing medications specific for the treatment of addiction.

These principles are useful for all clients with dual disorders, and we consider these issues below in regard to the specific comorbid conditions that are most common.

ISSUES IN PSYCHOPHARMACOLOGICAL TREATMENT OF DUAL DISORDERS

Several issues are central to all pharmacological treatment of co-occurring disorders, including establishing a diagnosis and initiating treatment; education, shared decision making, and informed consent; and drug interactions and safety.

Establishing a Diagnosis and Initiating Treatment

In Chapters 4 and 5, we have discussed the assessment of substance use disorders in clients with severe mental illness. Because substance use or withdrawal can mimic the symptoms of psychiatric disorders, as well as exacerbate a preexisting psychiatric disorder, distinguishing the effects of substances from psychiatric illness can be difficult or impossible. Determining the independence of a psychiatric disorder from substance abuse is especially difficult in work with a new client, due to the lack of information about the course and interactions between the disorders.

Family history, the temporal onset of the two disorders, persistence of symptoms, and the presence or absence of symptoms during substance-free periods (e.g., during inpatient hospitalization) may help to clarify the relationship. However, the situation often remains ambiguous. For example, consider a young man who presents at the emergency room with a history of hallucinations and delusions dating back several months, a 3-year history of heavy cannabis use, long-term psychosocial problems, and vague symptoms of disordered thinking for an unclear period of time. There is no family history of psychosis or substance abuse, and there has been no time over the past 3 years during which he has been free of substances for a month or more. Typically, this client would be hospitalized and quickly treated with an antipsychotic medication. Regardless of the degree and timing of his clinical response, it would usually not be possible to observe him for an extended period (e.g., a month) without substances or medications.

For the clinician, the critical issue is not so much the independence of the psychiatric and substance abuse syndromes (which often cannot be determined without longitudinal observation), but rather the best time to treat psychiatric symptoms. The general principle we recommend is that clients with severe or persistent psychiatric symptoms, such as psychosis, mania, or depression, require pharmacological treatment for those symptoms, regardless of the presumed cause. Clinical experience suggests several rules for treating symptoms in the absence of sustained periods without substance use.

Substance-induced symptoms of psychosis or ma-nia usually remit within several days of stopping substance use, making it easier to diagnose schizophrenia or mania than depression. However, in practice most physicians treat psychotic or manic symptoms immediately, without waiting to determine whether symptoms will spontaneously remit after cessation of substance use, unless there is compelling evidence that the onset of the symptoms recently coincided with substance abuse. Although 2–3 weeks of abstinence are usually recommended before treatment of depressive symptoms (Brady & Roberts, 1995), physicians often treat severe and unremitting depression soon after detoxification, particularly if there is a family history of mood disorders or a past history of depression without a substance use disorder. Two studies of tricyclic antidepressants (Mason et al., 1996; McGrath et al., 1996) and another of fluoxetine (Cornelius et al., 1997) support this practice. These studies found that treating depression immediately following detoxification decreases depression and is associated with longer periods of abstinence, regardless of whether the depression's onset came before or after the alcohol abuse.

In many cases, the psychiatric diagnosis is necessarily tentative and must be confirmed or changed over time. Most guidelines suggest slow tapering of psychiatric medication after 6–24 months of sustained remission of symptoms, with careful monitoring and observation. If a client is unable to achieve full remission of psychiatric symptoms despite integrated dual-disorder treatment, the presence of a chronic mental disorder is supported, and attempts to discontinue medication are not recommended. Medication is generally discontinued only when a client has experienced a sustained remission of symptoms, and when psychosocial functioning is no longer impaired, usually in the context of a sustained remission of substance abuse. In our experience, this rarely occurs; when it does, it tends to be in individuals with fairly recent onset of a psychiatric disorder, apparently precipitated by or complicated by substance abuse.

We place greater emphasis on the importance of careful assessment to support safe, informed treatment than on the avoidance of treating substance-induced symptoms. For example, although treating cocaine-induced anxiety or paranoia could enable ongoing use, identifying the precise cause of symptoms is frequently impossible because the psychiatric and substance use disorders are intertwined, and untreated psychiatric symptoms often interfere with successful treatment of the substance abuse. In general, elaborate attempts to distinguish which disorders are causing which symptoms consume a great deal of time and resources, are rarely fruitful, and may lead to the undertreatment of psychiatric disorders. Furthermore, psychopharmacology informed by careful assessment of substance use may enhance treatment outcomes in several ways. Assessment can focus attention on the potential for substance use to interfere with treatment efficacy and contribute to medication nonadherence, can reduce the risk of dangerous substance–medication interactions, can help physicians avoid prescribing medications with high abuse potential, and can lead to the consideration of agents that may reduce craving for alcohol or drugs.

Education, Shared Decision Making, and Informed Consent

When a physician has determined that a client's psychiatric symptoms are severe and persistent, consistent with an independent diagnosis (or at least a tentative diagnosis) of severe mental illness, medications should be considered in accordance with standard psychopharmacology practice. Current medication guidelines, treatment algorithms, educational materials for clients and family members (see the appropriate handouts in Appendix B), and methods for engaging in shared decision making and monitoring response in routine mental health settings are being developed by several groups and projects, such as the Texas Medication Algorithm Project (Chiles et al., 1999; Rush et al., 1999). However, these materials often neglect the issue of co-occurring substance use disorders. We outline modifications for working with clients with a dual disorder.

As always, clients (and usually family members or other support persons) need to be engaged in a discussion about diagnoses, treatment options, and the risks and benefits of different treatments. Clients and families should be educated about the complexities of making an accurate psychiatric diagnosis in the context of substance abuse, to create appropriate expectations about the evolutionary process of longitudinal assessment (see Chapters 4 and 5). They also need to be made aware that pharmacological treatments alone have little chance of success. Discussion of treatment options should include a review of the evidence that psychosocial interventions—for instance, social skills training (Chapter 11), family interventions (Chapters 13–15), and vocational rehabilitation (Chapter 18)—enhance treatment outcomes when used in combination with medications. Moreover, clients and their families need specific information about the advantages of integrating treatment for comorbid substance use disorders with psychiatric treatment. The discussion of the risks and benefits of recommended medication options should include information about the potential impact of psychiatric medications on the substance use disorder (Table 19.1), as well as the risk of interactions with commonly abused

substances (Table 19.2; see also "Drug Interactions and Safety," below).

As discussed in Chapter 2, shared decision making is the process of laying out all treatment options, describing the advantages and disadvantages of each, identifying a clinician's recommendations and rationale for reaching them, and then trusting a client to chose his or her treatment as an informed consumer (Noordsy et al., 2000). Shared decision making is more than informed consent. It involves exposing the subtle coercion and dependency inherent in doctor–patient relationships—factors that are expedient in the short term, but hinder the client's development of responsibility and self-control in the long run. It means investing in the client's education and development of decision-making abilities, rather than relying on compliance as the primary means of ensuring good outcomes.

When a client's judgment is impaired, shared decision making is threatened. However, even the most impaired clients, who may have guardians making their ultimate treatment decisions, can be encouraged to understand and participate in treatment decisions to the best of their ability. Finding areas in which to give clients control (e.g., choosing the time of administration or frequency of dosing), and helping clients learn about their diagnoses, medications, and rehabilitation, give them a greater sense of responsibility for the outcome of their treatment. The more clients understand their treatment options and are responsible for making their own treatment decisions, the more invested they will be in the chosen treatment.

Drug Interactions and Safety

Medications may interact with alcohol and drugs. Physicians should be aware of specific interactions and avoid those that are clinically significant whenever possible. They should also be aware of safety issues in a population that is prone to overdose and suicide. Table 19.2 presents an overview of such interactions.

Although drug interactions are among the most dramatic and frightening complications of prescribing psychiatric medications for clients with dual disorders, we have found that following a few basic guidelines can eliminate most concerns about these interactions in day-to-day care. First, the newer antidepressant and antipsychotic medications (except clozapine) are safer than older compounds, and generally pose lower risks in overdose or in combination with substances of abuse.

Second, it is best whenever possible to avoid prescribing medications with high potential for abuse, such as benzodiazepines, amphetamines, and acetylcholine-blocking antiparkinsonian agents. These agents have

TABLE 19.1. Psychotropic Medications: Potential Impact on Substance Use Disorders

Medication	Potential impact on substance use disorders
Antipsychotic medications	
Conventional	• Theoretically, could dampen mesolimbic responsiveness and increase drive to use substances • May interfere with cocaine high
Novel	• Clozapine and olanzapine associated with improved substance use disorders in uncontrolled trials and case reports • Risperidone associated with reduced alcohol preference in animals
Antidepressant medications	
Tricyclic antidepressants	• Desipramine associated with reduced craving for cocaine in some studies, not in others • Imipramine and desipramine associated with reduced relapse rates in abstinent, depressed clients with alcoholism
MAOIs	• No known effects
SSRIs	• No consistent effects on substance use disorders • Fluoxetine associated with reduced relapse rates in abstinent, depressed clients with alcoholism
Other compounds	• Bupropion reduces craving for nicotine • No other known effects
Mood stabilizers	
Lithium	• Associated with reduced alcohol use in some studies, not in others
Valproic acid	• No known effects
Carbamazepine	• Effective for detoxification from alcohol
Anxiolytics	
Benzodiazapines	• Effective for detoxification from alcohol • May stimulate craving for sedatives and alcohol
Buspirone	• May reduce craving
Stimulants	• Theoretically, could produce craving for stimulants
Antidipsomanic medications	
Disulfiram	• Facilitates reductions in drinking when administered under supervision
Naltrexone	• Reduces craving for alcohol, leading to fewer days of drinking • Blocks high from opiates • Some clients report anxiolytic effect
Acamprosate	• Reduces craving for alcohol, leading to fewer days of drinking
Ondansetron	• Reduces days of drinking for early-onset alcoholism
Nalmefene	• Reduces relapses of alcohol abuse
Medications for herion dependence	
Methodone	• Facilitates reductions in opiate abuse when administered under supervision
Buprenorphine	• Facilitates reductions in opiate abuse when administered under supervision

Note. Data from Anton et al., 1999; Barnett, Rogers, & Bloch, 2001; Brewer, 1992; Carroll et al., 1994; Chambers et al., 2001; Ciraulo et al., 1988; Clark & Fawcett, 1989; Cornelius et al., 1997; de la Fuente et al., 1989; Dorus et al., 1989; Drake & Brunette, 1998; Drake et al., 2000; Garbutt et al., 1999; Johnson et al., 2000; Kranzler et al., 1994; Littrell et al., 2001; Malcolm et al., 1989; Mason et al., 1996, 1999; McGrath et al., 1996; Merry et al., 1976; Noordsy et al., 2001; Pani et al., 1997; Panocka et al., 1993; Sullivan et al., 1989; Volpicelli et al., 1992; Wilkins, 1997; Ziedonis et al., 1992; Zimmet et al., 2000.

TABLE 19.2. Psychotropic Medications: Potential Risks and Interactions in Clients with Dual Disorders

Medication	Potential risk/interaction
Antipsychotic medications	
Conventional	• Possible increased risk of dystonia, akathisia, and tardive dyskinesia • Risk for hyperpyrexia in combination with stimulants • Cigarette smoking lowers blood levels (also true for clozapine) • Prolongation of QTc interval, which predisposes to cardiac arrhythmia, could interact with cardiac effects of cocaine and other stimulants (thioridazine, mesoridazine)
Novel	• Risk of respiratory arrest with combination of clozapine and benzodiazapines • Alcohol may synergistically increase sedative effects of clozapine • Clozapine lowers seizure threshold substantially • Prolongation of QTc interval, which predisposes to cardiac arrhythmia, could interact with cardiac effects of cocaine and other stimulants (ziprasidone)
Mood stabilizers	
Lithium	• Specific interactions not documented
Valproic acid	• Potential for liver toxicity
Carbamazepine	• Potential for liver toxicity
Antidepressant medications	
Tricyclic antidepressants	• Chronic alcohol use may induce metabolism and decrease levels • Additive cardiotoxicity with cocaine
MAOIs	• Tyramine present in alcoholic beverages may produce elevated blood pressure or hypertensive crisis • Potentiation of sympathomimetic effects of stimulants—hypertension/hyperpyrexia • Toxic interaction with meperidine (hypertensive crisis)
SSRIs	• May lower seizure threshold
Other compounds	• Alcohol or benzodiazepines increase cognitive and motor side effects of mirtazapine • Venlafaxine elevates blood pressure, as does alcohol use and withdrawal • Bupropion lowers seizure threshold, which could increase risk of seizure with cocaine use or alcohol withdrawal
Anxiolytics	
Benzodiazapines	• Considerable abuse potential
Buspirone	• Specific interactions not documented
Stimulants	• Possible abuse potential
Antiparkinsonian medications	• Possible abuse potential
Antidipsomanic medications	
Disulfiram	• At high doses, may stimulate psychosis in clients not on antipsychotic medication • Potential for liver toxicity
Naltrexone	• Potential for liver toxicity
Nalmefene	• Minimal potential for liver toxicity
Acamprosate	• Specific interactions not yet known
Ondansetron	• Specific interactions not yet known

Note. Data from Soyka (1996), Poulsen et al. (1992), Glassman and Salzman (1987), Steffens et al. (1997), Krystal et al. (1999), and Brady and Roberts (1995).

significant potential for drug interactions, as they share mechanisms of action with commonly abused substances. Also, it is preferable to avoid medications with high potential for interactions with substances of abuse, such as monoamine oxidase inhibitors (MAOIs).

Third, it is useful to help clients learn how to manage their mental illness better by teaching them about the benefits of taking their medications regularly, and the risks of relapse and rehospitalization associated with substance use. We encourage clients to make careful adherence to their medication regimens a priority, and avoid actively discouraging them from taking their medications when they are using substances. (See the "Coordinating Medication Treatment" section of Chapter 6, and Table 6.4, for strategies on improving adherence to prescribed medications.) The provision of information to clients about the benefits of medication, the negative effects of alcohol and drugs, and the interactions between medications and substances of abuse (when present) should be clearly documented in their charts, and this information should be periodically reviewed in clients with active substance abuse. This ensures that decisions to use substances with medications are clearly the clients' informed responsibility.

Withholding medications from clients who are actively abusing substances may undermine their clinical stability and their commitment to treatment. At most, a physician may hold or reduce the dose of a specific medication with high potential for interaction when a client presents intoxicated for medication monitoring. In addition, it is useful to have information about the extent of a client's substance abuse. For example, a client who is depressed and drinking heavily may not be an appropriate person to treat with a tricyclic antidepressant, for reasons of safety. Keeping a focus on the client's responsibility for deciding to use substances is consistent with the motivational development process described throughout this book (see especially Chapter 7). The advantage of integrating psychiatric and substance abuse treatments is that clients' symptoms can be stabilized while simultaneously developing their motivation to work on substance abuse, promoting progress toward recovery and decreased risk over time.

CASE EXAMPLE

Jay's treatment team began monitoring his medication adherence daily after he experienced a relapse of symptoms (e.g., auditory hallucinations, delusions of reference) associated with low blood levels of his medication. One day, his case manager found Jay obviously intoxicated when he went to his apartment for medication monitoring. Jay was slurring his words and unsteady on his feet. He initially de-

nied substance use, but eventually acknowledged drinking "a few beers" when empty cans lying around his apartment were pointed out to him. The odor of marijuana was also present in the apartment. Jay's case manager called the team psychiatrist and described the situation. The psychiatrist ordered that Jay's clozapine dose be reduced by half that evening to reduce risk for synergistic sedative effects, but approved proceeding with the full doses of sertraline and thyroxine. Jay was advised to contact the treatment team or seek emergency medical attention if he had any difficulties, and to resume the full dose of his medications the following day. His case manager called his father and described the team's concerns. Jay's father agreed to stop by in a few hours to check on him.

Jay's case manager followed up with him the next morning. They discussed the risk that Jay's substance use would interfere with his medications' effectiveness and prevent him from regaining psychiatric stability, which would jeopardize his visitation rights with his daughter and his ability to work. Work was important to Jay, as he was trying to save money for a car.

MEDICATIONS FOR SPECIFIC COMORBID PSYCHIATRIC SYNDROMES

In this section, we address pharmacological treatment of four specific psychiatric syndromes comorbid with substance abuse: psychosis, bipolar disorder, depression, and anxiety.

Medications for Comorbid Psychosis

The effects of substance abuse on responses to antipsychotic medications are unclear. Clinical experience suggests that many clients with dual disorders respond to antipsychotic medications even in the context of active substance use, and that serious side effects are uncommon. Some reports, however, suggest poor response and increased incidence of *tardive dyskinesia* among clients with schizophrenia and substance abuse (Dixon et al., 1992; Olivera, Kiefer, & Manley, 1990). Other reports have failed to find an association between substance abuse and tardive dyskinesia, but have reported that clients with schizophrenia and alcohol use disorder have more severe *akathisia* (Duke et al., 1994; Salyers & Mueser, 2001). Many other concerns have been raised about side effects among clients with dual disorders (as outlined in Table 19.2), such as seizures, orthostatic hypotension, sedation, and respiratory depression. The actual incidence and clinical significance of these side effects are poorly understood.

Research on medication response is sparse. One

study suggested that history of substance abuse in clients with schizophrenia predicted poorer response to conventional antipsychotic medications (Bowers, Mazure, Nelson, & Jatlow, 1990). A subsequent study found that clients with treatment-resistant schizophrenia responded equally well to the novel antipsychotic clozapine, regardless of their substance abuse history (Buckley, Thompson, Way, & Meltzer, 1994). There is little evidence that substance abuse interferes with clinical response to antipsychotic medications, although numerous studies demonstrate that substance abuse, even in relatively small quantities, can contribute to significant deterioration in symptom control despite pharmacological treatment (e.g., Drake, Mueser, et al., 1996).

Clients and families frequently ask whether alcohol or drug use will interfere with or interact with medication treatment. To respond to this, we educate clients and their relatives about the stress–vulnerability model of psychiatric disorders (see Appendix B, Handout B.10). This model posits that biological vulnerability to mental illness increases a person's sensitivity to a variety of stressors, including the effects of alcohol and drugs on the brain; the results may be relapses and rehospitalizations. Whereas medications reduce symptoms and sensitivity to stress, substance use tends to worsen the mental illness, undermining the benefits of medication. In fact, it may take higher doses of medication to control symptoms even tenuously when an individual is using substances, and higher doses may compound problems with side effects.

Clozapine may be unique in the treatment of clients with schizophrenia, because it has a greater efficacy for the symptoms of schizophrenia *and* it may also have a positive effect on substance use disorders. Two recent uncontrolled studies found rapid and dramatic reductions in substance use disorders for clients with comorbid schizophrenia who were started on clozapine (Drake et al., 2000; Zimmet, Strous, Burgess, Kohnstamm, & Green, 2000). The primary concern with the use of clozapine compared to other antipsychotics is its risk of causing *agranulocytosis* (a significant reduction in the white blood cell count that if unchecked can lead to vulnerability to serious infection and even death). However, if clients' white blood cells are routinely monitored, clozapine can be safely prescribed (Wahlbeck, Cheine, Essali, & Adams, 1999), especially compared to the well-documented risks of serious infection and early mortality related to substance use disorders.

An open-label report found reductions in substance abuse and craving among clients with treatment-refractory schizophrenia and substance abuse in response to olanzapine treatment (Conley, Kelly, & Gale, 1998). Two uncontrolled studies have also found reductions in substance use disorders for clients with dual

disorders who were started on olanzapine (Littrell, Petty, Hilligoss, Peabody, & Johnson, 2001; Noordsy et al., 2001). Olanzapine has been associated with reduced cocaine use, and risperidone with reduced alcohol preference in rodents (Meil & Schter, 1997; Panocka, Pomeei, & Massi, 1993). Open-label risperidone treatment was associated with reduced symptoms and improved functioning in 14 clients with dual disorders, but substance use outcomes were not reported (Albanese, 2001). There are no reports to date of research with quetiapine or ziprasidone. It has been hypothesized that the dibenzodiazepine and thienobenzodiazepine classes of novel antipsychotics have unique effects on dopaminergic transmission in the mesocorticolimbic system, and that these effects lead to reduced substance abuse (Chambers et al., 2001; Green et al., 1999).

In addition to abusing alcohol and drugs, clients with substance use disorders are more likely than other clients to abuse prescribed medications. Antipsychotic medications themselves appear to be rarely abused. We have occasionally seen clients overuse low-potency, sedating antipsychotic medications to achieve nonspecific oversedation; this abuse is rarely sustained. However, medications for side effects, particularly benzodiazepines (see below) and antiparkinsonian medications such as benztropine (Buhrich, Weller, & Kevans, 2000), are more commonly abused. The abuse of these medications in our studies of clients with dual disorders is quite low, however. This may be due in part to physician awareness, close monitoring, and limited access to these medications. Physicians should be aware of the risk and should monitor prescriptions and potential abuse carefully. In practice, this means small prescriptions, close follow-up by case managers in the community and with significant others, and frequent review of medications.

The *novel* (or *atypical*) antipsychotic medications have rapidly become accepted as first-line treatments for clients with psychotic disorders. The use of these medications is associated with a substantially lower need for medications to treat side effects. Therefore, the use of novel antipsychotics for clients with dual disorders can reduce the need to prescribe side effect medications that have some abuse potential. In addition to their abuse potential, benzodiazepines and anticholinergic medications have side effects that can include substantial cognitive impairment, which may interfere with rehabilitation efforts. When a client is switched from a conventional to a novel antipsychotic medication, the physician should carefully review any adjunctive medications and gradually taper off those that may be unnecessary and/or may contribute to abuse liability and overall side effect burden.

Because of the more benign side effects and better

clinical efficacy of novel antipsychotics, clients with schizophrenia and substance abuse should be tried on these medications for their psychiatric disorder first. There are no documented differences in the impact of available first-line novel antipsychotic agents (i.e., risperidone, olanzapine, quetiapine, ziprasidone, or aripiprazole) on the outcome of comorbid substance use disorders. Therefore, the choice of medication is based on an assessment of a client's symptom profile (i.e., the prominence of positive, disorganization, negative, cognitive, and mood symptom clusters) and tolerability of potential side effects using a shared decision-making approach with the client and family. For clients with unremitting substance abuse, a clozapine or olanzapine trial should be considered. Clozapine should also be considered for refractory psychosis as usual.

The older, *conventional* antipsychotic medications should be reserved for third-line use in situations where clients' symptoms are refractory to medication, or where clients do not adhere to novel antipsychotic medications. Although these agents can improve positive and disorganization symptoms in clients with psychotic disorders, they tend to be less effective for negative and cognitive symptoms, and may contribute to dysphoria. Negative and cognitive symptoms have been shown to be more strongly related than psychotic symptoms to functional outcomes (Breier, Schreiber, Dyer, & Pickar, 1991; Brekke, Debonis, & Graham, 1994; Trumbetta & Mueser, 2001), and to have a greater impact on response to rehabilitation (Green, 1996; Kopelowicz, Liberman, Mintz, & Zarate, 1997). The impact of conventional antipsychotics on dysphoria and/or on dopaminergic transmission in the mesolimbic system may actually worsen substance use disorders (Littrell et al., 2001) (see the discussion of comorbidity theories in Chapter 1). However, long-acting, depot preparations are only available for conventional antipsychotics at this writing. Medication monitoring is commonly used by dual-diagnosis treatment teams to assure medication adherence without resorting to depot medication. Even when depot preparations are required, the dose can be kept low by combining with a novel antipsychotic agent. Once newer routes of delivery are developed for the novel agents, conventional antipsychotics will be reserved for trials in clients whose disorder has remained refractory to novel antipsychotics, similar to how newer antidepressant medications replaced tricyclic antidepressants in the 1990s.

Combinations of two antipsychotic medications have become increasingly common in clinical practice, as more varied agents with unique mechanisms of activity have become available (Meltzer & Kostakoglu, 2000). However, there is a lack of controlled trials examining the efficacy of such combinations for either clients with psychosis alone or clients with dual disorders. Until data are available, combinations of antipsychotic medications should only be used after at least two adequate trials of single-antipsychotic treatment. Some practice guidelines recommend a trial of clozapine prior to combination therapy (Chiles et al., 1999). Treatment targets for combination therapy should be clearly defined prior to a trial, with careful follow-up assessment of the benefits and side effects. Typically one agent is used at full therapeutic dosage, with a second augmenting agent prescribed in low to moderate dosage. Alternatively, the dosage of an effective single agent (e.g., clozapine or haloperidol decanoate) might be lowered from full to moderate to reduce bothersome side effects, and then augmented with a moderate dosage of a second agent with fewer side effects to maintain antipsychotic effect. Outcomes of treatment targets should be evaluated at regular intervals, and the combination treatment should be terminated if improvements are not observed.

Medications for Comorbid Bipolar Disorder

Bipolar disorder (or bipolar I disorder, as it is now formally known; see American Psychiatric Association, 1994) along with schizophrenia, has the highest rate of comorbid substance abuse of all mental illnesses (Regier et al., 1990; see Chapter 1). Several studies have found that disinhibition during episodes of mania creates particular vulnerability to substance abuse (Hensel, Dunner, & Fieve, 1979; Mayfield & Coleman, 1968; Reich, Davies, & Himmelhoch, 1974; Zisook & Schuckit, 1987), although others report that depressive episodes may more often trigger substance abuse (Bernadt & Murray, 1986; Minski, 1938). Some research indicates that comorbid substance abuse in clients with bipolar disorder decreases the efficacy of lithium (Himmelhoch, Mulla, Neil, Detre, & Kupfer, 1976; Himmelhoch, Neil, May, Fuchs, & Licata, 1980; Prien, Caffey, & Klett, 1974), although it is unclear whether medication nonadherence mediates the poorer outcomes (Goodwin & Jamison, 1990). Despite this, little is firmly established about the effects of substance use disorders on medication treatment response in bipolar disorder. Clinical experience suggests that many clients with dual disorders respond to mood-stabilizing medications even in the context of active substance abuse, and that serious side effects are uncommon.

Substance abuse is often observed to worsen the course of bipolar disorder, although disentangling effects of substances from phasic changes in the illness is difficult (Bernadt & Murray, 1986; Strakowski & DelBello, 2000). Substance use can compound problems with poor discretion, agitation, and excessive spending. Stimulants directly mimic symptoms of mania and may be particularly destabilizing for clients with bipolar disorder (Post & Kopanda, 1976). In line with the stress–vulnerability model of severe mental illness, we advise clients and families that substance use can destabilize bipolar disorder by creating an intermittent variation in the already delicate balance of brain chemistry. Although no clear evidence on the impact of substance use on medication treatment is available, it is reasonable to assume that the alteration of brain chemistry resulting from the use of most substances makes medication response less reliable.

As indicated in Table 19.1, some research has suggested that lithium treatment can have beneficial effects on the outcome of alcohol use disorders (Clark & Fawcett, 1989; de la Fuente, Morse, Niven, & Ilstrup, 1989; Merry, Reynolds, Bailey, & Coppen, 1976), although the largest and most rigorous controlled trial did not support this (Dorus et al., 1989). The major recent advances in the pharmacological treatment of bipolar disorder include the study of novel antipsychotic agents and a number of newer anticonvulsant agents as mood stabilizers. As of this writing, this work has led to the approval of olanzapine as a treatment for acute mania in the United States, although its effects on substance use disorders have not been systematically evaluated. Clozapine has been demonstrated to be effective for clients with bipolar disorder as well (Green et al., 2000; McElroy et al., 1991; Suppes et al., 1999). Naturalistic data suggest that clozapine is associated with improvement in alcohol use disorders in clients with schizophrenia (Drake et al., 2000), but its effects on alcohol abuse in clients with comorbid bipolar disorder have not been explored. Anticonvulsant medications, though effective in the management of bipolar disorder, have not been shown to have a significant impact on the outcome of co-occurring substance use disorders.

The core pharmacological treatments for bipolar disorder (i.e., lithium, anticonvulsants, antipsychotics) do not have addictive potential. However, benzodiazepines are commonly prescribed for the management of agitation and insomnia associated with bipolar disorder. When benzodiazepines are used for clients with bipolar and substance use disorders, the duration of treatment should be carefully considered, and the medications should be tapered when clinically appropriate to reduce exposure to side effects and abuse potential. Outpatient physicians should carefully monitor the need for ongoing benzodiazepine treatment that is started during an inpatient stay. Inpatient physicians should consider alternative medications, such as sedating antipsychotic medications, for agitated clients who have a history of benzodiazepine abuse.

Because there is no clear evidence of a differential

impact on substance use disorders, the choice of a first-line pharmacological treatment for clients with bipolar disorder and substance abuse is based on the clinical characteristics of the bipolar illness. One pilot study suggested that clients with bipolar disorder and substance abuse responded less well to lithium than clients with only bipolar disorder, but that clients with a dual disorder responded equally well to valproate (Brady et al., 1996); however, this has not been replicated. Olanzapine has recently been approved by the U.S. Food and Drug Administration (FDA) for the treatment of bipolar disorder. There is strong evidence for the efficacy of carbamazepine in bipolar disorder as well, but it has not gone through regulatory review for this indication. If a client does not respond well to an adequate trial of one of these agents, switching to another is recommended. Clozapine, which does not have formal FDA approval for the treatment of bipolar disorder and which has mostly open-label evidence for its efficacy, should be considered if other agents have not been successful in stabilizing the disorder. Clozapine may be considered earlier in clients with comorbid refractory alcohol use disorders, given its association with improved recovery rates in schizophrenia (Drake et al., 2000).

Combination treatment with two medications for bipolar disorder is widely recommended in practice guidelines when clients are refractory to monotherapy, and in our experience is also helpful in clients with comorbid substance abuse. Combinations of agents with different mechanisms of action (e.g., lithium and an antipsychotic) are recommended to enhance complementary effects. The combination of carbamazapine and valproate should be avoided, however, due to an elevated risk of hepatotoxicity.

Medications for Comorbid Depression

The capacity for alcohol use disorders to cause symptoms indistinguishable from major depression is the most widely recognized interaction between a substance use disorder and a mental illness. It is generally accepted that continued alcohol use interferes with recovery from depression. As a result, many physicians have been trained not to treat depression until a client has been sober for an extended period of time, to ensure that it is so-called "primary" depression (i.e., endogenous in origin, and therefore likely to respond to antidepressant medications). However, as reviewed previously in this chapter (see "Establishing a Diagnosis and Initiating Treatment"), several studies have challenged these assumptions by demonstrating that antidepressant treatment for depression in alcohol-abusing clients immediately following detoxification improves mood problems and is associated with longer periods of abstinence, regardless of whether the depression began before ("primary" depression) or after ("secondary" depression) the alcohol use disorder.

This work represents the clearest evidence to date that a substance-induced mental syndrome may respond to medications, and that the treatment of psychiatric symptoms improves the outcome of a substance use disorder. Abuse of sedative/hypnotic medications and withdrawal from cocaine and other stimulants can also produce symptoms of depression; however, there is no clear evidence that the pharmacological treatment of depression influences the course of these other types of substance abuse. As we do for clients with schizophrenia and bipolar disorder, we advise clients with depression (and their relatives) that substance use is likely to interfere with the treatment of depression, resulting in higher medication doses and increasing the chances of not responding.

Since the mid-1990s, a new class of antidepressants, the selective serotonin reuptake inhibitors (SSRIs), has become the first line of antidepressant treatment. This shift has occurred not because of greater efficacy, but because of greater tolerability and safety (Schatzberg, Cole, & DeBattista, 1997). Medication interactions do occur with SSRIs, but alcohol and drugs are not mentioned as concerns in most textbooks. The SSRIs are also relatively safe when taken in overdose and have low abuse potential.

Specific interactions are concerns with some of the other novel antidepressants. These compounds, like the SSRIs, have good tolerability and low abuse potential. However, alcohol and benzodiazepines increase the motor and cognitive side effects of mirtazapine (Steffens, Krishnan, & Doraiswamy, 1997). Venlafaxine may elevate blood pressure, as do alcohol use and withdrawal. Bupropion is another novel antidepressant agent with good tolerability and low abuse potential. Its dopaminergic properties suggest that it may benefit clients with negative symptoms of a psychotic disorder and comorbid depression. However, the primary side effect of bupropion is lowered seizure threshold; it thus increases risk for people who may be predisposed to seizures, including those who abuse cocaine and those in alcohol withdrawal (Steffens et al., 1997).

Tricyclic antidepressants are still used in the treatment of depression and have low abuse potential, but greater concerns about side effects and safety make them less useful in clients with dual disorders. Barbiturates or alcohol may induce hepatic metabolism and decrease the clinical effect of tricyclic antidepressants at usual dosages (Glassman & Salzman, 1987). Blood levels of these antidepressants should be monitored (Ciraulo & Renner, 1991). Although alcohol increases the sedative effects of tricyclic antidepressants, this interaction tends not to be clinically significant (Glassman & Salzman, 1987). These medications are cardiotoxic in overdose and therefore are contraindicated in clients who are prone to overdoses.

There is mixed evidence that adding tricyclic antidepressants may be helpful for clients with substance abuse and depression. In a small, uncontrolled study of 11 clients, Siris, Bermanzohn, Mason, and Shuwell (1991) reported that some clients with schizophrenia or schizoaffective disorder, clinical depression, and substance use disorders benefited from adjunctive imipramine treatment. In a controlled, double-blind study of adjunctive desipramine treatment over 12 weeks for 27 clients with schizophrenia and cocaine use disorders, Ziedonis, Richardson, Lee, Petrakis, and Kosten (1992) found lower rates of cocaine use. Wilkins (1997) studied the long-term effects of 12 weeks of adjunctive desipramine on 80 clients with schizophrenia or schizoaffective disorder and cocaine dependence. Interestingly, lower rates of cocaine use for clients receiving desipramine were reported in weeks 10–26 (medication was given in weeks 1–12), but not for the remaining period of the 15-month study. Last, in a 12-week study of desipramine for clients with cocaine abuse and depression, no beneficial effect of medication on cocaine use was found (Carroll et al., 1994). Thus tricyclic antidepressants may reduce substance abuse in clients with comorbid depression, although the available data are not strong.

Even greater concerns are raised about using MAOIs for clients with dual disorders. These drugs specifically interact with beer and red wine, as well as other common foods such as sausage and bananas, to cause hypertensive crises. Stimulants are also dangerous in combination with MAOIs. Furthermore, MAOIs have been associated with higher dropout rates than those for desipramine in at least one controlled study of clients with schizophrenia and cocaine use disorders (Ziedonis et al., 1996). It is best to avoid prescribing the MAOIs for clients with active substance use disorders. In rare situations where an MAOI is the treatment of choice for a client's disorder, the clinician can point out the medication's risks and benefits as a way of helping the client develop motivation for sobriety.

When a client with depression has a very severe substance use disorder, such as heavy alcohol dependence, it can be helpful to get to know the client and his or her pattern of substance use before attempting to treat the depression pharmacologically. Nevertheless, we generally offer pharmacological treatment of depression to clients with dual disorders in any stage of treatment, even when substance abuse is ongoing, to enhance their capacity to engage in treatment. Clients need to be clearly advised that ongoing substance use may interfere with their response to treatment. It is best to start with safer agents such as SSRIs or bupropion, and advance to other agents as needed to achieve a satisfactory clinical response. If a client responds poorly, treatment adherence and ongoing substance use should be evaluated and addressed. Clients whose depression remains refractory despite good treatment adherence and abstinence from substance use should be managed according to standard treatment algorithms—including consideration of a combination of two antidepressant medications with different mechanisms of action (e.g., an SSRI and bupropion), tricyclic antidepressants, MAOIs, or electroconvulsive therapy if necessary.

Medications for Comorbid Anxiety

Anxiety is extremely common among clients with dual disorders. Clients frequently cite the need to manage anxiety as compelling them to continue substance use (e.g., Mueser, Nishith, et al., 1995; Noordsy et al., 1991). Anxiety and substance use often have a circular relationship: Active use of many substances temporarily relieves anxiety, but then increases anxiety beyond its original intensity during the withdrawal phase (i.e., *rebound anxiety*). Symptoms of anxiety emanating from the mental illness and the substance abuse become rapidly intertwined and indistinguishable. Given the temporal relationships of substance use and its consequences, most clients are only able to recognize that they feel better when they use substances.

We are aware of no research that addresses the effects of substance use on medication response in the treatment of anxiety. Two studies have failed to find beneficial effects of buspirone on alcohol abuse in clients with comorbid anxiety disorders (Kranzler et al., 1994; Malcolm et al., 1992), and the impact of other anxiolytics has not been established. It should be noted, however, that antidepressant medications have potent anxiolytic effects. Therefore, the studies cited above demonstrating improved outcomes associated with antidepressant treatment could involve anxiolytic mechanisms of action as well.

Modern treatment of anxiety disorders has evolved dramatically in recent years. Whereas tricyclic antidepressants and MAOIs have long been recognized to have anxiolytic properties, a flurry of research activity and FDA approval of many SSRIs and other compounds as first-line treatments for various anxiety disorders has shifted prescribing practices and reduced the prominence of benzodiazepines in their management. As described above, newer antidepressants are generally safe and well tolerated, and have low abuse potential. (It is important to distinguish that bupropion does *not* have anxiolytic properties, and may in fact worsen anxiety.)

Concerns about safety and abuse potential are frequently raised when benzodiazepines are considered for the treatment of anxiety in clients with dual disorders. Because alcohol increases the sedating effects of benzodiazepines, the risks of severe respiratory depression and death are heightened when the two are combined (Glassman & Salzman, 1987). Overdoses involving both are particularly dangerous. Benzodiazepines also potentiate the respiratory depression produced by clozapine and may produce dangerous interactions if used in high doses. Therefore, any benzodiazepine use in clients with dual disorders should be monitored carefully.

There is cross-tolerance between alcohol and benzodiazepines, which raises concerns about the abuse potential of prescribed benzodiazepines (Ciraulo et al., 1988). The actual risk of benzodiazepine abuse in persons with alcoholism is unclear, although it is probably higher than in the general population (Ciraulo et al., 1988). The potential for abuse varies across different benzodiazepines and is greater for the rapid-onset, short-acting medications such as diazepam and alprazolam than for the long-acting medications such as clonazepam (Griffiths & Wolf, 1990). A recent review of research on prescription of benzodiazepines for persons with addictive disorders concluded that abuse potential was overestimated (Posternak & Mueller, 2001).

Benzodiazepine use in clients with dual disorders is a complicated topic that is frequently a source of clinical controversy. Some physicians advocate complete avoidance; others frequently prescribe long-acting benzodiazepines such as clonazepam. Few data address the effects of prescribing benzodiazepines to clients with dual disorders. In a long-term follow-up of approximately 200 clients with dual disorders, about 20% reported benzodiazepine use at each 6-month follow-up, but only a small number of these reported abuse of prescribed medications (Brunette, Noordsy, & Drake, 2002). In this cohort, clients who were prescribed benzodiazepines were just as likely to become abstinent from alcohol and drugs as those who were not prescribed benzodiazepines. However, there was no evidence that benzodiazepine use was associated with improvement in symptoms, or that benzodiazepine discontinuation was associated with worsening of anxiety.

In the absence of research-based guidelines, we recommend a cautious, stepwise approach to treating anxiety in clients with dual disorders. Consideration should be given to the possibility that clients presenting with anxiety complaints may be engaging in medication-seeking behavior, and may be prone to anxiolytic abuse. In clients taking conventional antipsychotic medications, anxiety may be due to the side effect of akathisia, which should be evaluated and treated first when present. If anxiety remains, a careful analysis of the relationships between substance use and anxiety should be performed with the client.

Amphetamines and cocaine cause relatively immediate, and therefore fairly obvious, increases in anxiety. However, the anxiety-precipitating effects of alcohol and other sedative/hypnotics occur remotely, often many hours after substance use. It typically takes work with a client over an extended period of time to help him or her understand the impact of substance use on anxiety. When multiple periods of substance use and abstinence are contrasted, the connection between substance abuse and anxiety often becomes clear and helps to motivate the client for change. Use of any substance may also destabilize psychotic and mood disorders, indirectly increasing anxiety.

We usually begin psychopharmacological treatment of anxiety in clients with dual disorders at any of the four stages of substance abuse treatment: engagement, persuasion, active treatment, or relapse prevention (see Chapter 2 for a review of these stages). This includes providing pharmacological treatment for anxiety to clients who are in the engagement stage of treatment, when their connection with treatment providers is tenuous and a strong therapeutic relationship has not been established. Pharmacological treatment of anxiety at this early stage can facilitate clients' engagement in dual-disorder treatment and instill hope that positive change is possible.

Although pharmacological intervention can be effective for anxiety disorders, cognitive-behavioral treatments should be the first step in the treatment of anxiety for clients with a dual disorder when possible. Standardized, empirically validated cognitive-behavioral treatment protocols have been developed for all the major anxiety disorders, including posttraumatic stress disorder (Foa & Rothbaum, 1998; Resick & Schnicke, 1992), panic disorder (Barlow & Craske, 2000; Craske, Barlow, & Meadows, 2000; Zuercher-White, 1999a, 1999b), obsessive–compulsive disorder (Foa & Kozak, 1997; Kozak & Foa, 1997; Steketee, 1999a, 1999b), social phobia (Bourne, 1998a, 1998b; Craske, Antony, & Barlow, 1997; Heimberg & Becker, 2002), generalized anxiety disorder (Craske, Barlow, & O'Leary, 1992; White, 1999a, 1999b; Zinbarg, Craske, & Barlow, 1993), and specific phobia (Antony, Craske, & Barlow, 1995; Bourne, 1998a, 1998b; Craske et al., 1997). In line with the principles of integrated treatment, we recommend that members of the client's dual-disorder treatment team deliver cognitive-behavioral treatment for an anxiety disorder directly, rather than referring the individual to another clinician. Considering the ubiquitous nature of anxiety in dual disorders, training team members

in the principles of cognitive-behavioral anxiety management has great practical value.

If pharmacological treatment of anxiety appears to be necessary, either alone or in addition to cognitive-behavioral treatment, serotonergic agents such as SSRIs or buspirone should be used as first-line agents. Management of anxiety disorders may require doses in the upper therapeutic range for SSRIs. In our experience, high doses of buspirone are required to achieve therapeutic effects as well. Other antidepressant compounds may also be effective for anxiety management. If a client fails to respond clinically, treatment adherence (to both medication and cognitive-behavioral interventions) and ongoing substance use should be evaluated and addressed. Clients with persistent anxiety despite good treatment adherence and abstinence from substance use may require further intervention. SSRIs and buspirone enhance serotonergic activity through different mechanisms, and some research indicates that they may be combined to achieve greater effect (Joffe & Schuller, 1993). However, physicians must be careful to monitor for the *serotonin syndrome* (Sternbach, 1991)—a rare complication of excessive serotonergic activation that leads to malaise and autonomic instability.

If a client presents a convincing picture of a primary anxiety disorder that is refractory despite good adherence to first-line anxiolytic medications and abstinence from substances, a trial of a benzodiazapine may be considered, especially in clients who do not have a history of benzodiazepine abuse. It is best to avoid "as-needed" (p.r.n.) dosing, as this can inadvertently heighten clients' sensitivity to signs of anxiety, resulting in escalating use. A trial should proceed with careful monitoring and attention to treatment outcomes. Benzodiazepines also have street value, and clients may sell their medication or exchange it with others. Particular attention to any signs of overuse, such as running out of medication early or frequently reporting that medication was lost or stolen, should lead a physician to question the safety and appropriateness of ongoing treatment with a benzodiazepine.

MEDICATIONS FOR
SUBSTANCE USE DISORDERS

Several different types of medication have been shown to be effective for the treatment of substance use disorders, including disulfiram, opiate antagonists (naltrexone, nalmefene), acamprosate, ondansetron, and methadone. However, no controlled studies examining the efficacy of these agents for clients with dual disorders have been published. We recommend using these medications with such clients in a stage-specific fashion, after they have failed to respond to standard integrated treatment approaches (see below). We discuss here the use of specific medications for treating substance abuse in clients with dual disorders; the preponderance of space is devoted to disulfiram and naltrexone, with which we have the most clinical experience.

Disulfiram

Disulfiram is an approved agent for the treatment of alcohol use disorders in the United States (Carroll, Nich, Ball, McCance, & Rounsaville, 1998; Chick et al., 1992). Disulfiram inhibits the metabolism of alcohol, causing acetaldehyde to accumulate. Acetaldehyde produces the toxic aftereffects of alcohol consumption commonly known as a "hangover." When it accumulates, these toxic effects are magnified, producing headache, flushing, malaise, nausea, and vomiting. If excessive, blood pressure can rise to dangerous levels. Clients experiencing a disulfiram–alcohol reaction require emergency medical evaluation. In the early years of disulfiram use, when dosage levels between 1000 and 2000 mg/day were prescribed, some deaths due to interactions with alcohol were reported (e.g., Becker & Sugarman, 1952; Jacobsen, 1952). No deaths due to such interactions have been reported in recent years, presumably because of lower prescribed dosages (Chick, 1999). Current guidelines recommend prescription of 125–500 mg of disulfiram daily.

Disulfiram does not have any known abuse potential, but it does carry some risk of hepatotoxicity. In clients with substantial liver damage due to alcohol abuse or hepatitis C infection, the risk–benefit ratio of disulfiram must be considered carefully, and liver enzyme levels must be closely monitored. Interactions between disulfiram and substances of abuse, other than the obvious alcohol–disulfiram reaction, have not been established.

In order for disulfiram to be effective, it must be administered under supervision (Brewer, 1992). Clinicians may directly supervise adherence to disulfiram 2–5 days per week. As an alternative, family members can provide even more frequent supervision (Azrin et al., 1982; Brewer, 1992; Chick et al., 1992).

Disulfiram is intended to create a barrier to drinking alcohol for a period of 7–14 days following the last dose of the medication. This is the period of time required for normal alcohol dehydrogenase activity to resume. The desired effect is a psychological barrier to drinking, causing clients to postpone the impulse to drink and giving them time to change their minds. However, many clients will drink within less than 7 days of disulfiram treatment. When they experience a disulfiram–alcohol reaction, it may decrease their motivation to drink further. Some reports have suggested that experiencing a disulfiram–alcohol reaction will increase the success of disulfiram treatment through aversive conditioning, although the primary effect on reducing alcohol use and abuse is through deterrence (Brewer, 1992).

Actual response to disulfiram is quite variable, probably due to individual variation in alcohol dehydrogenase activity. Some clients have no reaction to alcohol despite treatment with 500 mg/day of disulfiram, while others react to minute quantities of alcohol in vinegar or cologne. Optimal dosing of disulfiram may vary widely, and dosing should be based on an individual client's clinical response. Some clinicians would advocate raising the dose of disulfiram as high as needed to achieve a clinical response. However, lethal alcohol–disulfiram reactions have been associated with high-dose therapy (over 1000 mg/day), as noted above. Current regulatory approval of disulfiram for treatment of alcoholism in the United States is for doses up to 500 mg/day.

The use of disulfiram in clients with dual disorders, especially those with psychotic disorders, has been a topic of some clinical controversy. There are a few case reports of disulfiram being associated with the development or worsening of psychotic symptoms in individuals who were not taking an antipsychotic medication (Liddon & Satran, 1967; Martensen-Larsen, 1951; Nasrallah, 1979), especially at the high dosages of 1000–2000 mg/day (Larson, Olincy, Rummans, & Morse, 1992). Disulfiram inhibits dopamine-beta-hydroxylase, which converts dopamine to norepinephrine. This could cause dopamine to accumulate in the brain. Therefore, some physicians believe that disulfiram is contraindicated for clients with schizophrenia.

On the other hand, there are reports of disulfiram being used safely for clients with schizophrenia who are stable, nonpsychotic, adherent to medication, and actively trying to maintain abstinence (Kingsbury & Salzman, 1990). Our experience with disulfiram (and that of others; see Kofoed, Kania, Walsh, & Atkinson, 1986; Larson et al., 1992) is that it can be used safely and effectively for clients with active dual disorders. In a series of uncontrolled case studies including 33 clients with alcoholism and severe mental illness (70% with schizophrenia or schizoaffective disorder) treated for an average of almost 2 years and followed up for 3 years, we found that 64% achieved a remission of their alcoholism for at least 1 year, and 30% achieved a remission for at least 2 years (Mueser, Noordsy, Fox, & Wolfe, in press). Like Kofoed and colleagues (1986), we also found little evidence for exacerbation of psychosis or other symptoms associated with disulfiram use, or for problematic alcohol–disulfiram interactions.

It is appropriate to consider disulfiram for alcohol-abusing clients who are in the active treatment stage and have had at least several days of abstinence to clear the substance from their system and avoid dangerous drug interactions. Given concerns about disulfiram's capacity to raise central dopamine levels, disulfiram within the 500-mg dosage limit is prudent for clients with psychotic disorders. Prescription of disulfiram above 500 mg/day may be justified in some clinical situations where the risks of unremitting alcohol use are very high, but this should be considered only with careful informed consent.

When we treat clients with disulfiram, we start with very careful education about the nature of the treatment and the risks associated with it, to ensure informed consent. If a client is motivated to maintain abstinence but has been unable to do so despite multiple attempts, disulfiram may be started with monitoring of medication doses. We ask the client to notify us of any alcohol use. If reactions are reported after use of alcohol while the client is on disulfiram, emergency medical evaluation is conducted. The decision to continue disulfiram therapy is reassessed after each relapse, with client motivation for abstinence being the critical determining factor. Once a client achieves the relapse prevention stage, especially when the alcoholism has been in remission for 1–2 years, ongoing treatment with disulfiram may no longer be necessary and should be reconsidered.

CASE EXAMPLE

Abdul was a 31-year-old man with diagnoses of bipolar disorder and alcohol dependence. His alcohol use had precipitated numerous symptom relapses and rehospitalizations—and, in combination with manic episodes, involvement in the criminal justice system for disorderly conduct and getting into fights. In most discussions with his outpatient treatment team, Abdul expressed ambivalence about his alcohol abuse. He recognized the troubles that alcohol often caused, but he frequently gave in to cravings after only a few days of abstinence. During one of Abdul's hospitalizations for treatment of a manic episode, his inpatient psychiatrist discussed with him the potential benefits of disulfiram in helping him achieve abstinence from alcohol. Abdul expressed an interest in trying disulfiram, and he was started while in the hospital at a dosage of 250 mg/day, which was subsequently increased to 500 mg/day after 3 days.

Abdul was discharged from the hospital and remained on the dosage of 500 mg/day. Early during disulfiram therapy, Abdul's case manager closely monitored his taking of the medication (usually daily). After 3 months on disulfiram, Abdul experienced some overwhelming cravings and tried drinking alcohol. The next day Abdul told his case manager about his slip into alcohol use, which he said

caused a flushed face and made him feel very nauseated. A meeting was arranged between Abdul and his psychiatrist, who determined that medical treatment was not needed, as the alcohol–disulfiram interaction had ended. Abdul still endorsed abstinence as a goal, and his disulfiram was continued at the same dosage. After 6 months of abstinence, the monitoring of Abdul's taking disulfiram was tapered to three times per week. Approximately 10 months after achieving abstinence (16 months after initiating disulfiram), Abdul stopped taking disulfiram over a weekend and had a 2-day drinking binge. Inpatient hospitalization was not required. After a meeting between Abdul and his treatment team (during which it became clear that Abdul was still committed to abstinence), his disulfiram was resumed at the same dosage, and the frequency of monitoring was temporarily increased. Four months later, Abdul stopped taking disulfiram again and had another brief relapse, after which the medication was resumed.

Abdul eventually developed a strong commitment to abstinence, due to the sobriety that disulfiram enabled him to achieve. He began working for the first time since his mental illness began, and started to reconnect with and make amends to family members whom he had alienated during his manic and drinking episodes. Abdul also found social support by attending Alcoholics Anonymous, which he began 4 months after initiating disulfiram therapy. Three years after Abdul began taking disulfiram, following 16 months of continuous abstinence from alcohol, Abdul felt that he was ready to stop the medication. Abdul remained abstinent without disulfiram, and a 2-year follow-up indicated no slips or relapses.

Opiate Antagonists

In addition to disulfiram, naltrexone (Anton et al., 1999; O'Malley et al., 1992; Volpicelli, Alterman, Hayashida, & O'Brien, 1992; Volpicelli et al., 1997) is an approved agent for the treatment of alcohol use disorders in the United States. Also similar to disulfiram, naltrexone does not have abuse potential, but it does carry some risk of hepatotoxicity; thus its use in clients with liver damage must be considered carefully, and liver enzyme levels must be monitored closely. Like naltrexone, nalmefene (another opiate antagonist) has been shown to be effective for the treatment of alcoholism (Mason, Salvato, Williams, Ritvo, & Cutler, 1999), but it has a lower risk of hepatotoxicity. However, nalmefene is not available in an oral route of administration at this writing, and there are no reports available about its use with clients with dual disorders.

It is appropriate to discuss naltrexone for suppression of craving for alcohol in the late persuasion and active treatment stages, as clients are attempting to reduce their alcohol use and beginning abstinence. There is no danger to clients if they use alcohol while on naltrexone, so this medication is appropriate for clients who have not yet developed a strong commitment to sobriety. On the other hand, there is no evidence that unmotivated clients will change their alcohol-using behaviors with prescription of naltrexone alone, so it is difficult to justify the risks of exposure for unmotivated clients. In our clinical experience, roughly half of clients with dual disorders taking naltrexone in the late persuasion and active treatment stages have reported some benefits, in terms of reduced craving for alcohol and enhanced capacity to avoid alcohol use. Some clients also report feeling calmer on naltrexone.

For the treatment of opiate addiction, naltrexone therapy must be delayed until a client is free from opiates, to avoid precipitating an acute opiate withdrawal syndrome. Once initiated, naltrexone will block the euphoric effects of opiate use, but is not associated with adverse reactions when opiates are used. If naltrexone therapy is uninterrupted, it may continue despite slips into opiate use. As with disulfiram, naltrexone therapy for opiate addiction is most likely to be successful if supervised, and motivation for maintaining abstinence should be reassessed after episodes of relapse.

Acamprosate and Ondansetron

Two other compounds have been recently demonstrated to be effective in reducing cravings and alcohol relapses: acamprosate (Garbutt, West, Carey, Lohr, & Crews, 1999) and ondansetron (Johnson et al., 2000). Neither of these compounds has any known abuse potential, and problematic interactions with commonly abused substances are not established. Although the limited research on these medications for alcoholism is promising, their effects in clients with dual disorders are not known.

Methadone and Buprenorphine

Methadone maintenance therapy is used in many states for the treatment of refractory opiate addiction. There are few systematically collected data concerning the effects of methadone maintenance on clients with dual disorders, but clinical lore suggests beneficial effects (e.g., Feinberg & Hartman, 1991). Although the severity of psychiatric comorbidity is correlated with the severity of opiate abuse problems in clients maintained on methadone (Mason et al., 1998), treatment response to methadone appears to be comparable between clients with dual disorders and clients with opiate addiction alone (Pani, Trogu, Contu, Agus, & Gessa, 1997). There are no well-established contraindications to methadone maintenance treatment for clients with dual disorders.

The little available research on use of methadone in schizophrenia has yielded mixed results. One small controlled trial suggested that single doses of methadone for clients with schizophrenia produced a mild worsening in negative symptoms and dysphoria, but had no effect on psychosis (Judd, Janowsky, Segal, Parker, & Huey, 1981). However, another small controlled trial found beneficial effects on severity of psychosis when methadone was administered to clients with schizophrenia for a 3-week period (Brizer, Hartman, Sweeney, & Millman, 1985). The use of methadone in combination with integrated dual-diagnosis treatment appears to be a reasonable treatment approach for some clients.

Buprenorphine was approved by the FDA in 2002 as an alternative to methadone for treatment of people with opiate addiction (Comer & Collins, 2002; DiPaula, Schwartz, Montoya, Barrett, & Tang, 2002; Lintzeris, Bell, Bammer, Jolley, & Rushworth, 2002). There are no data currently available on buprenorphine treatment among clients with comorbid mental illness. Buprenorphine has the potential to be more readily available to clients with severe mental illness, however. In the United States its use will not be restricted to specialized clinics, so that a psychiatrist on an integrated dual-disorder treatment team could prescribe it directly after completing a required training session. This has the potential to substantially expand available treatment alternatives for clients with dual disorders who abuse opiates.

DETOXIFICATION

Pharmacological treatment is also used to *detoxify* clients—that is, to wean them from physical dependence on substances. Detoxification approaches for both outpatient and inpatient settings have been described in the literature (Galanter & Kleber, 1999). For clients with dual disorders, detoxification is appropriate in the late persuasion and early active treatment stages, as the clients attempt to achieve sobriety after a period of sustained use. Research evidence is lacking on detoxification of clients with dual disorders. In clinical practice, we have followed routine detoxification protocols with minor modification for such clients. Often detoxification can be successfully conducted on an outpatient basis. However, in circumstances where abstinence from abused substances is unlikely on an outpatient basis, or where detoxification involves significant medical risks (see below), inpatient detoxification is justified. We describe the steps for detoxification below; they are summarized in Table 19.3.

First, the treatment team should carefully consider whether detoxification is necessary. Clients with dual

TABLE 19.3. Guidelines for Detoxification of Clients with Dual Disorders

- Evaluate whether detoxification is necessary, based on signs of physical dependence on substance.

- During detoxification, monitor clients closely for signs of a relapse of the psychiatric disorder, and treat vigorously if early warning signs are detected.

- Attend to the interactions between different medications and substance withdrawal, and increased risk of side effects, including:
  - Excessive respiratory depression and sedation when clozapine is combined with high doses of benzodiazepines.
  - Lower seizure threshold for clients on antipsychotics or bupropion.
  - Lower seizure threshold during acute withdrawal from alcohol or sedative/hypnotics.

- Monitor metabolic status of clients during detoxification, and treat if abnormalities are detected (if necessary, in the hospital).

disorders may develop negative consequences of substance use, despite intermittent or moderate use that may not be sufficient to cause symptoms of physiological dependence (nausea, headache, tremors, delirium tremens, etc.). Such clients may be able to discontinue substance use safely without medication detoxification. Close monitoring and social support are important to maintaining motivation and identifying clients who may require more intensive treatment.

Second, each client should be monitored closely for signs of relapse of the mental illness during detoxification. Depression, insomnia, anxiety, activation, and agitation that emerge as part of withdrawal may destabilize the mental illness, and the result can be an episode of active mental illness. Symptoms should be closely monitored and vigorously treated to prevent full-blown psychiatric relapse.

Third, attention must be paid to issues of drug interactions and increased risks of side effects associated with psychotropic medications. The most prominent concerns are the risk of excessive respiratory depression and sedation with high doses of benzodiazepines in combination with clozapine, and the lower threshold for developing seizures associated with antipsychotics (particularly clozapine) and bupropion. Because the acute withdrawal period from alcohol and sedative/hypnotics is associated with an elevated seizure risk, close monitoring of clients on these agents is required, and prophylaxis should be considered for those with a history of seizures. A detoxification protocol using carbamazepine may be preferable in this situation (Malcolm, Ballenger, Sturgis, & Anton, 1989). When benzodiazepines are used, doses should be kept moderate for clients who are

already being treated with highly sedating psychotropic medication. Ideally, benzodiazepine doses should be based only on objective signs of withdrawal, according to a standardized scale such as the Revised Clinical Institute Withdrawal Assessment for Alcohol Scale (Sullivan, Sykora, Schneiderman, Naranjo, & Sellers, 1989). Respiration should also be monitored, particularly at night. A lower threshold for referral to a hospital setting for detoxification should be used with clients at risk for these interactions.

Finally, the metabolic status of clients with dual disorders should be carefully assessed during detoxification. Clients with severe mental illness are prone to poor nutrition, heavy smoking, and inactivity. Some clients with schizophrenia develop polydipsia (excessive fluid intake), which produces hyponatremia (low sodium) (Leadbetter, Shutty, Higgins, & Pavalonis, 1994; Tracy et al., 1997). Hyponatremia may predispose them to medical complications during withdrawal, such as seizure or cardiac complications. If laboratory testing reveals metabolic abnormalities, detoxification should take place in a hospital setting.

MONITORING TREATMENT RESPONSE

Effective strategies for monitoring treatment response are critical to pharmacological treatment of clients with dual disorders. Monitoring treatment includes both tracking medication blood levels and monitoring treatment response in the community.

Medication Blood Levels

The measurement of medication blood levels should be considered for any client with a poorly controlled psychiatric illness or severe side effects, in addition to routine monitoring for such medications as lithium, carbamazapine, and valproate. Blood levels, which are useful primarily in knowing whether clients are taking their medications, are available for most psychiatric medications. For some, such as clozapine, lithium, carbamazapine, valproate, and tricyclic antidepressants, there is a clearly defined therapeutic range; in these cases, certain medication levels have been associated with optimal clinical response. Levels below the therapeutic range are associated with poor clinical response, while levels above the therapeutic range may be associated with poor clinical response or with high risk for side effects.

It is important to be mindful that reference or therapeutic ranges are based on averages, and that each client is an individual for whom optimal pharmacological treatment may fall outside the established therapeutic range. The pharmacologist's mantra is "Treat the client, not the blood level." When a client has a good therapeutic response, the dosage should not be adjusted simply because the blood level is outside of population norms. However, blood levels can provide valuable information for solving clinical problems in dual-disorder treatment, as well as for identifying drug interactions and other areas of risk.

If a blood level is low, a client may not be taking medication, may be prescribed an inadequate dose, or may be rapidly metabolizing the medication. As failure to adhere to a medication regimen is common in the dual-disorder population, the first step when a low blood level is discovered is to present the result to the client and inquire about the individual's pattern of taking medication. If the client has missed many doses, a problem-solving approach is used to address the reasons underlying the nonadherence. Questions for detecting problems related to not taking medication are provided in Table 19.4. After possible reasons for poor medication adherence are identified, a plan is developed with the client and family to address these concerns (see the Problem-Solving or Goal-Setting Sheet—Appendix C, Form C.20), and the blood level is rechecked after several weeks (see also Chapter 6 for discussion of methods for improving adherence to medications). It is usually helpful to simplify the dosing schedule to once daily whenever possible.

If the blood level remains low, it is useful to observe the client taking each dose to determine whether adherence is truly a problem. This may be done by treatment team members, family members, or other support network members (see Chapters 6 and 17 for more on close monitoring). If medication adherence is assured, blood levels remain low, and clinical response is not satisfactory, increases in the dosage should be

considered. Once clients have achieved an adequate blood level of medication associated with a good response, periodic random blood levels may be checked to monitor their adherence to medication after they have resumed responsibility for self-monitoring doses.

Occasionally clients go to great lengths to avoid taking medication; for example, they may hide tablets in their mouth and spit them out or vomit after observation has ended. If such behavior is suspected, it is best to renew efforts to educate clients about their illness and the role of medication as a tool to serve them in their recovery process. Helping clients identify personal reasons why taking medication is in their own best interest can instill motivation in clients who have limited or no insight into their psychiatric disorder (i.e., motivational interviewing; see Kemp et al., 1998; see also Chapter 7). Clients with cognitive deficits are more prone to problems with adherence to medication (Robinson et al., 2002). *Behavioral tailoring*, or helping clients fit the taking of medication into their daily routines, can facilitate medication adherence (Mueser, Corrigan, et al., 2002). Alternate routes for delivery of medication can also be considered, such as crushed tablets in soft food, liquid medication, or intramuscular injection. If vomiting is suspected, staying with a client for 30 minutes after each dose may ensure absorption of a reasonable proportion of the dose. Scheduling case management functions or family events after medication dosing makes this task more efficient.

Rarely, a client's liver may metabolize medications unusually rapidly, and thus the client may achieve only a very low blood level despite good adherence to a usual dose. When other, more common explanations for low blood levels have been addressed, rapid metabolism should be considered. One can be more confident in accepting rapid metabolism as an explanation for low blood levels of a medication when other prescribed medications yield expected blood levels. In this case, the medication dosage may be raised and the blood level rechecked in several weeks. Usual guidelines for dosing can generally be surpassed with informed consent, as the blood level gives a more accurate reflection of the client's actual exposure to the medication.

However, oral medications must pass through the liver before entering the bloodstream and making their way to the brain, where they have their action. A client who metabolizes a medication unusually rapidly has high levels of activity of enzymes in the liver that break down the medication in question. Therefore, substantial increases in a dose of oral medication may result in only small increases in blood levels. If an adequate therapeutic response is not achieved despite progressive dose increases, the physician should consider using another medication that has a different route of metabolism or a

TABLE 19.4. Questions for Assessing Reasons for Medication Nonadherence

- Does the client understand the benefits of taking medication?
- Does the client believe that taking medication will help him or her make progress toward achieving personally desired goals?
- Are there bothersome side effects that need to be addressed?
- Does the client misattribute certain problems or symptoms to the medication that may be due to other causes?
- Is the client afraid of specific interactions between medication and substances of abuse? If so, is this fear leading to nonadherence when the client is using substances?
- Does the client need a helpful prompt to overcome forgetfulness or disorganization?
- Can taking medication regularly be fitted into the client's daily routine?
- Is the medication regimen unnecessarily complicated?

different route of administration. Intramuscular injection allows absorption of medication into the bloodstream and then to the brain prior to passing through the liver, and may be useful in delivering more of the medication to a rapidly metabolizing client.

If the blood level is within the expected reference or therapeutic range, one can be relatively confident that the client is getting a reasonable trial of the medication. It is important not to assume that any level within the therapeutic range will be optimally effective. Some clients respond better to a level at the upper end of the range than to one at the lower end. The level informs the physician about whether there is room to increase the dose of medication and remain within the expected range.

Nonadherent clients may sometimes take a dose just prior to the blood draw and achieve a reasonable blood level to conceal their nonadherence. An unannounced blood level check may be useful in sorting this out. If a client remains poorly responsive despite good blood levels for an adequate duration of time and careful consideration of medication adherence, it usually makes sense to move on to a different medication. Although the treatment team cannot be entirely confident that the client is unresponsive to a particular medication as long as there is active substance abuse, there is more to be gained pragmatically from trying a new medication regimen than sticking with a regimen known to be minimally effective or ineffective. If a better response is achieved, it may assist the client in progressing through the stages of dual-disorder treatment. If a pattern of repeated poor responsiveness to adequate trials of medication develops in association with ongoing substance use, this information is used as part of the process of developing motivation for change in substance use behaviors (see Chapter 7).

If the blood level of a medication is higher than the expected reference or therapeutic range, this may indicate that the client is receiving too much medication. However, some individuals will respond best at levels higher than population norms. The key question when one is reviewing a high blood level with a client is how well the medication is tolerated. If the client is doing well on the medication with few side effects, he or she should be educated carefully about any known risks associated with high levels (e.g., increased risk for seizures with clozapine), and a shared decision should be made on how to proceed. If lower doses have been associated with poorer response, it may be reasonable to continue medication at a high blood level. If substantial side effects are present, the high blood level indicates the need to lower even modest doses of medication. Elderly individuals, women, and people who do not smoke are generally at higher risk for metabolizing medica-

tions more slowly and building up higher levels. Some clients with particular sensitivity to side effects may not be able to tolerate medication even within expected ranges. Gradual dose reductions with close observation or a change in medications may be warranted.

Altered blood levels may also indicate an interaction between different medications or between a medication and a substance of abuse. For example, fluvoxamine can impede the metabolism of clozapine, resulting in high blood levels of clozapine when the two are combined. Ibuprofen can interfere with lithium clearance, leading to perplexing variation in lithium levels as a client intermittently uses over-the-counter ibuprofen. Alcohol and cigarettes can both increase liver metabolism, which may generally reduce blood levels of prescribed medications.

Community Monitoring

Physicians should consider carefully the specific benefits and risks associated with particular medications in the context of particular substances of abuse. The great majority of clients are able to use medications to reduce or control symptoms of their psychiatric illness while residing in the community, even when they are actively using alcohol or drugs. Most available evidence indicates that abuse of prescribed medications is rare, and that medication–substance interactions are very rare. Moreover, the risks of active substance abuse, including disease and death, are substantial; they are probably of a much higher magnitude than the risks posed by interactions between medication and commonly abused substances. Finally, symptom control is probably a necessary first step in the process of pursuing recovery from substance use disorder. Nevertheless, caution is warranted, and the key to safe and effective use of medications in clients with dual disorders is careful monitoring.

Careful monitoring means that medications are prescribed with clear and accurate information about risks as well as benefits; that potentially dangerous medications are prescribed in relatively small doses or not at all; and that the family and the clinical team, not just the physician, are committed to following the client carefully and monitoring symptom response and warning signs of misuse. For example, the case manager may notice that the client is disinhibited or overly sedated while on benzodiazepines, even though he or she does not present for a medication check in this state. As always, medications that are not clearly producing a desired effect should be tapered and withdrawn, so that the client does not suffer the cumulative effects of an increasingly complicated regimen of possibly helpful medications. Through ongoing collaboration among the client, the treatment providers, and the social support network, pharmacological treatment for dual disorders can be effectively provided and monitored in the community. When these efforts are integrated with other components of dual-disorder treatment, optimal outcomes can be achieved.

SUMMARY

Psychopharmacological treatment is the mainstay in the treatment of severe mental illness, and it has an equally important role to play in the management of dual disorders. The presence of substance abuse in persons with severe mental illness complicates the process of pharmacological treatment, because of the inherent difficulties in distinguishing the two disorders. Nevertheless, it is critical to initiate pharmacological treatment based on the best diagnostic information available, with the expectation that ongoing assessment over time will resolve many of the diagnostic dilemmas. In the vast majority of cases, this can be done safely because of the minimal interactions between prescribed medications and commonly abused substances. Educating clients and their families about the nature of dual disorders and pharmacological treatment, including medication–substance interactions, creates a context of shared decision making that is necessary for clients to be fully informed about treatment and consent to it.

Physicians have a vast armamentarium for the pharmacological treatment of dual disorders. Medications can be broadly divided into those that target the mental illness and those that focus on the substance abuse. Among medications for psychiatric disorders, various effective compounds exist for psychosis, bipolar disorder, depression, and anxiety disorders. In addition, several medications have been shown to be effective in preventing relapses of substance use disorders, mainly alcoholism. Medications are also used in the detoxification of clients with dual disorders, which can often be safely conducted on an outpatient basis. Effective pharmacological treatment requires close monitoring of both medication blood levels and clinical response. Involving a client and his or her natural support system, along with the treatment team, in monitoring the dual disorders and the effects of pharmacological treatment optimizes the outcomes of both disorders.

VII

Research

20

Research on Integrated Dual-Disorder Treatment

A substantial body of research has accumulated in recent years supporting the effectiveness of integrated treatment programs for dual disorders. In this chapter, we provide a brief synthesis of research on the treatment of these disorders. Almost all of the research on outpatient dual-disorder treatment has been conducted within mental health programs, because of the greater feasibility of adding substance abuse treatment to existing community support services (Mercer-McFadden, Drake, Brown, & Fox, 1997). Research on dual-disorder treatment in general can be divided into four different types of studies: (1) traditional substance abuse treatments in mental health settings; (2) early studies of integrated treatment programs; (3) controlled studies of long-term outpatient integrated treatment; and (4) controlled studies of integrated residential or intensive day treatment programs. We summarize the findings of these studies below, emphasizing the controlled research on integrated treatment programs. We conclude with a brief discussion of future directions for this body of research.

TRADITIONAL SUBSTANCE ABUSE TREATMENT IN MENTAL HEALTH SETTINGS

Early studies of dual-disorder treatment, most conducted in the 1980s, examined the effects of providing traditional substance abuse treatment in addition to ongoing psychiatric care in mental health settings—for example, incorporating group or inpatient programs based on Twelve-Step principles. Some of these studies were conducted with randomized designs (Hellerstein et al., 1995; Herman et al., 1997; Lehman et al., 1993; Mowbray et al., 1995), but none demonstrated strong positive

effects on substance abuse outcomes. One possible explanation for the poor outcomes of these studies is that these programs failed to adhere to the basic values and the core components of integrated treatment outlined in this book. For example, none of the programs was based on the concept of stages of change (Prochaska, DiClemente, & Norcross, 1992) or the stages of treatment (see Chapter 2). Consequently, these programs focused on abstinence as the primary goal from the beginning of treatment, rather than on engaging clients, reducing the negative consequences of substance abuse, and gradually reducing substance use. Furthermore, most programs were time-limited and short-term, and were not comprehensive.

EARLY STUDIES OF INTEGRATED TREATMENT PROGRAMS

Coincident with research documenting the failures of simply incorporating substance abuse treatment into mental health services, other programs utilizing the principles of integrated treatment were being developed, with pilot findings suggesting better outcomes (Mercer-McFadden et al., 1997). Based on the success of these efforts, further exploratory studies were conducted that adhered to many of the principles of integrated treatment outlined in this book, such as reduction of substance abuse's negative consequences; comprehensive, long-term treatment; outreach for difficult-to-engage clients (see Chapter 2); the use of varied psychotherapeutic treatment strategies (e.g., individual, group, family; see Parts III, IV, and V); and incorporation of motivational (Chapter 7) and cognitive-behavioral (Chapter 8) treatment strategies. The results of these latter studies were that clients generally showed substantial rates of substance abuse remission, accompanied by other positive outcomes (Detrick & Stiepock, 1992; Drake, Bartels, et al., 1993; Durell, Lechtenberg, Corse, & Frances, 1993; Meisler & Williams, 1998). The encouraging results of these uncontrolled studies served as an impetus for conducting more rigorous research to evaluate the benefits of integrated dual-disorder treatment.

Controlled Studies of Long-Term Outpatient Integrated Treatment

With the success of these early studies, subsequent controlled research was conducted to evaluate the benefits of integrated treatment programs more rigorously, and to compare different outpatient approaches to such treatment. As summarized in Table 20.1, six controlled studies of long-term outpatient integrated treatment have been conducted to date. Four of these studies compared integrated with nonintegrated treatment programs (Barrowclough et al., 2001; Carmichael et al., 1998; Drake et al., 1997; Godley, Hoewing-Roberson, & Godley, 1994); the other two compared different types of long-term integrated treatment (Drake, McHugo, et al., 1998; Jerrell & Ridgely, 1995a).

Among the four studies comparing long-term outpatient integrated treatment with nonintegrated programs, several patterns emerge. All four studies reported more improvement in substance abuse outcomes for clients who received the long-term integrated treatment. Three of the studies found no differences between the integrated and nonintegrated treatment groups in psychiatric outcomes (Carmichael et al., 1998; Drake et al., 1997; Godley et al., 1994), whereas the fourth study found that integrated treatment resulted in fewer relapses and hospitalizations, as well as less severe symptoms (Barrowclough et al., 2001). It is notable that this fourth study was the only one in which the integrated treatment included a family intervention component for all participating clients (Barrowclough et al., 2001). Family treatment for dual disorders may serve to improve the monitoring of clients' psychiatric disorders, resulting in fewer relapses and rehospitalizations (Mueser & Fox, 2002), as it does in the primary population of clients with severe mental illness (Dixon et al., 2001; Pitschel-Walz, Leucht, Bäuml, Kissling, & Engel, 2001).

The two studies comparing different models of long-term integrated dual-disorder treatment addressed rather different questions (Drake, McHugo, et al., 1998; Jerrell & Ridgely, 1995a). The study by Drake, McHugo, and colleagues (1998) compared two different case management approaches for integrated treatment: assertive community treatment (ACT) and standard case management. Outcomes tended to favor ACT over standard case management, and clients in both treatment groups improved considerably, but the magnitude of the differences between the groups was not great. This study suggests that the ACT model of case management may be beneficial to some clients with a dual disorder (e.g., clients prone to frequent crises, relapses and rehospitalizations, legal problems), and thus merits inclusion as a component of integrated treatment. However, as discussed in Chapter 3, ACT-level case management is not required for all clients with dual disorders.

The Jerrell and Ridgely study (Jerrell, Hu, & Ridgely, 1994; Jerrell & Ridgely, 1995a, 1995b) compared behavioral skills training, intensive case management, and a Twelve-Step approach. Overall, substance abuse and psychiatric outcomes favored the skills training approach the most and the Twelve-Step approach the least. It is noteworthy that one short-term (1-month) quasi-experimental study (not included in Table 20.1) comparing cognitive-behavioral group counseling to a Twelve-Step group approach for dual disorders also reported better substance abuse outcomes at 6 months posttreatment for the cognitive-behavioral treatment group (Fisher & Bentley, 1996). These studies support the importance of cognitive-behavioral counseling (see Chapter 8) as one important component of integrated dual-disorder treatment.

CONTROLLED STUDIES OF INTEGRATED RESIDENTIAL OR INTENSIVE DAY TREATMENT PROGRAMS

Five studies examining the effectiveness of integrated residential or intensive day treatment programs have been completed to date (Blankertz & Cnaan, 1994; Brunette et al., 2001; Burnam et al., 1995; Penn & Brooks, 1999; Rehav et al., 1995). Four of these programs examined relatively short-term intensive treatments (e.g., 3–6 months), and all suffered from rates of client dropout exceeding 50% (Blankertz & Cnaan, 1994; Burnam et al., 1995; Penn & Brooks, 1999; Rehav et al., 1995). The fifth study (Brunette et al., 2001) employed a quasi-experimental design to compare the effects of a short-term residential program (3–4 months; see Bartels & Drake, 1996) with a long-term program (2 years), the Gemini House program (see Chapter 16 for an in-depth description of this program). In addition to its longer-term nature, Gemini House provided a gradual transition for all clients from the residence back into the community. The results indicated that more clients in the long-term program (Gemini House) were successfully engaged in treatment, and they had better substance abuse outcomes as well. Clients in the long-term and

TABLE 20.1. Controlled Studies of Outpatient Integrated Treatment Programs

Study characteristics	Godley et al. (1994)	Jerrell & Ridgely (1995a)	Drake et al. (1997)	Drake et al. (1998)	Carmichael et al. (1998)	Barrowclough et al. (2001)
Sample size	38	132	217	203	208	36
Mental illness	44% schizophrenia 39% affective psychosis	—	50% schizophrenia 47% mood disorders	77% schizophrenia 23% bipolar disorder	31% schizophrenia 21% bipolar disorder 39% major depression	Schizophrenia
Substance use disorder	58% AUD ≥42% DUD	40% AUD 19% DUD	55% AUD 61% DUD	73% AUD 42% DUD	47% AUD[a] 53% SUD	64% AUD 69% DUD
Other features	None	30% minority groups	89% African American Homeless	None	15% African American 14% Hispanic 26% homeless	—
Interventions	ICM + IT vs. SS	BST vs. ICM vs. Twelve-Step	IT vs. SS	ACT + IT vs. SCM + IT	IT vs. SS	IT[b] vs. SS
Research design	Experimental Integrated vs. nonintegrated	Quasi-experimental[b] Integrated vs. integrated	Quasi-experimental Integrated vs. nonintegrated	Experimental Integrated vs. integrated	Experimental/quasi-experimental[c] Integrated vs. nonintegrated	Experimental Integrated vs. nonintegrated
Follow-up period	2 years	18 months	18 months	3 years	1 year	1 year
Research attrition[d]	21%	31%	14%	9%	45%	84%
Substance abuse outcomes	ICM > SS on days of drug use	BST > Twelve-Step ICM = Twelve-Step	IT >SS for treatment progress and decreased alcohol use severity	ACT > SCM on treatment progress and decreased alcohol use severity	IT > SS (alcohol) IT SS (drug)	IT > SS on days abstinent
Hospital use outcomes	ICM = SS for days of hospitalization	—	IT = SS for reduced days in hospital	ACT = SCM	IT = SS	IT > SS
Symptom outcomes	ICM = SS	BST > Twelve-Step ICM > Twelve-Step	IT = SS	ACT = SCM	IT = SS	IT > SS
Other outcomes	—	No difference for social functioning and role performance	IT = SS for QOL; legal, medical, and work status; and homeless days	ACT = SCM on QOL	IT > SS in medication compliance, suicidal thoughts, income, arrests, and consumer satisfaction IT = SS in community functioning	No differences for social functioning

Note. Dashes, no data; >, better than; ACT, assertive community treatment; AUD, alcohol use disorder; BST, behavioral skills training; CM, case management; DUD, drug use disorder; ICM, intensive case management; IT, integrated dual-disorder treatment; QOL, quality of life; SCM, standard case management; SS, standard services; SUD, substance use disorder.

[a]Some clients were randomly assigned to treatment groups, but not others.

[b]IT = family intervention, motivational interviewing, and cognitive-behavioral counseling.

[c]Random assignment to IT or SS at two sites (n = 144), but not the third site (n = 64).

[d]*Research attrition* refers to percentage of clients lost to research follow-up.

short-term programs did not differ in symptom and hospitalization outcomes.

The results of these five studies indicate that short-term programs tended to have very high dropout rates, due to both the brevity of the interventions and their lack of outreach. Clients who were retained in intensive programs did well while they were in these programs, mainly because of the restricted access to substances. However, once they were discharged, their relapse rates were high. In contrast, the study of the one long-term program, Gemini House (Brunette et al., 2001), indicated higher rates of engagement and better substance abuse outcomes—perhaps in part because it facilitated the transition of clients from the residence into the community. Thus research suggests a possible role for longer-term integrated dual-disorder treatment, but not for short-term, intensive programs.

SUMMARY OF THE RESEARCH ON INTEGRATED TREATMENT

There is substantial research supporting the effectiveness of integrated treatment programs for clients with dual disorders. The strongest evidence comes from the six controlled studies of outpatient integrated treatment (Table 20.1). Four of these studies showed that comprehensive, motivation-based, long-term integrated treatment programs resulted in significantly better substance abuse outcomes than those of standard, nonintegrated care (Barrowclough et al., 2001; Carmichael et al., 1998; Drake et al., 1997; Godley et al., 1994). Two studies compared different approaches to integrated dual-disorder treatment, with one study (Drake, McHugo, et al., 1998) reporting beneficial effects of ACT for some clients, and the other study (Jerrell & Ridgely, 1995a) reporting better outcomes with behavioral skills training compared to intensive case management, which in turn was better than a Twelve-Step approach.

In general, the effects of integrated short-term residential or intensive day treatment programs were not positive. Such programs had difficulty engaging and retaining clients, and relapse rates tended to be high following discharge into the community. One study (Brunette et al., 2001) found that Gemini House—a long-term residential program for dual disorders, with a gradual process for helping clients move back into the community—had good retention rates and better substance abuse outcomes following discharge than a short-term residential program did. These findings suggest that brief, intensive treatments for dual disorders are not helpful, and that treatment other than detoxification or stabilization should usually occur in the community

(Drake & Noordsy, 1995; Greenfield, Weiss, & Tohen, 1995). However, some clients with dual disorders may benefit from longer-term residential programs.

FUTURE DIRECTIONS FOR RESEARCH

Given the magnitude of the dual-disorder problem, more controlled research is needed to examine the effectiveness of integrated treatment models, and to understand the critical components of treatment. Prior research in this area suggests several minimal standards for conducting research on integrated dual-disorder treatment. Programs need to be comprehensive—including assertive outreach and case management, as well as stage-wise, motivational interventions for substance abuse. Treatment interventions need to be guided by program manuals, and implementation should be assessed carefully with fidelity measures. Studies should have controls and enough clients to achieve statistical validity. Since substance use disorders, like severe mental disorders, are chronic and relapsing, programs and services need to span a time period of at least 2 years (Drake, Mueser, et al., 1996).

Another methodological issue in conducting research on dual disorder programs concerns the measurement of substance abuse. Research shows that reliance on self-report of substance abuse alone, especially single self-report measures, yields inadequate information (Corse et al., 1995; Drake et al., 1990; Galletly et al., 1993; Goldfinger et al., 1996; Shaner et al., 1993; Stone et al., 1993; Wolford et al., 1999). Self-report therefore needs to be supplemented by at least one other source of data about substance abuse, such as multiple instruments, clinical ratings, or laboratory tests (see Chapter 4). Furthermore, since most clients with dual disorders make progress and recover from substance use disorders in stages, assessment needs to measure clients' stages of treatment (McHugo et al., 1995; Mueser, Drake, et al., 1995; see Chapter 5).

Programs' fidelity to the integrated dual-diagnosis treatment model is also an important issue in need of further attention. Two studies indicate that across different program sites, fidelity to a specific integrated model is related to better substance abuse outcomes (Jerrell & Ridgely, 1999; McHugo, Drake, Teague, & Xie, 1999). In order to ensure proper implementation of an integrated treatment model, and to compare implementation fidelity across programs, standardized fidelity measures need to be employed, such as the fidelity scale included in Appendix A. In addition to verifying program implementation or identifying needs for further training or administrative support, the measurement of program fidelity may lead to a better understanding of which treatment components are most crucial to improving dual-disorder outcomes.

Yet another critical issue is the heterogeneity of the dual-disorder population. More research is needed on various types of heterogeneity among clients: motivated versus unmotivated clients; men versus women; clients with diagnoses of substance dependence versus substance abuse; those with polysubstance use versus those with alcohol use alone; those with trauma histories versus those with none; and those with antisocial behavior versus those with none. The individual differences in clients' treatment needs have only recently begun to be documented. For example, the treatment needs of women with dual disorders differ substantially from those of men (Alexander, 1996; Brunette & Drake, 1997, 1998).

Greater understanding of the organization and costs of these treatment systems is another important research need. The few existing data at this point suggest that community-based care for individuals with dual disorders is expensive (Bartels et al., 1993; Jerrell, 1996) and places burdens on families (Clark, 1994; Clark & Drake, 1994). Integrated dual-disorder treatment has the potential to reduce costs substantially (Jerrell et al., 1994), but this potential needs to be evaluated in controlled studies. Since clients with dual disorders consume extensive resources outside the mental health system, cost studies should also include a societal perspective (Clark, 2001; Clark & Fox, 1993).

A final area in need of more research concerns the specific components of integrated dual-disorder treatment, and the timing of the delivery of those components. Various psychotherapeutic strategies are employed in dual-disorder programs, including individual, group, and family interventions; however, the specific impact of different interventions remains unclear, because most studies have compared multiple interventions provided in integrated treatment programs with standard, nonintegrated care. As convincing evidence supporting integrated dual-disorder treatment has accumulated (Drake et al., 2001), there is a need for research that goes beyond the simple comparison of integrated versus nonintegrated programs to evaluating and comparing the specific components of integrated treatment programs, including individual, group, and family psychotherapeutic modalities.

SUMMARY

Research provides support for the effectiveness of integrated treatment programs for dual disorders. Six controlled studies have been conducted to date of long-term integrated outpatient programs, and these provide solid evidence supporting the integration of services. Research on short-term residential or intensive day treatment programs has been less encouraging, with problems due to poor retention and high dropout rates following discharge. Evidence from one study suggests that long-term residential treatment may be beneficial for severely ill clients with dual disorders, provided that the transition back to community living is very gradual.

Considerable progress has occurred in understanding the core components of integrated dual disorder treatment. Research provides encouragement for the effectiveness of long-term, stage-wise, motivational treatment. Clients, their families, and clinicians have reason to be optimistic over the long term concerning the potential for recovery from substance use disorders.

Epilogue: Avoiding Burnout and Demoralization

Working with clients with a dual disorder is often diffi-cult, challenging, and sometimes downright exasperat-ing. Although a clinician sometimes experiences short-term rewards when beginning work with a new client, such as intervening to resolve a crisis or establishing good rapport, more often the rewards are few and far between; they also tend to be long-term, accumulating over months or even years. In this book, we have de-scribed both a philosophy and various strategies for helping dually diagnosed clients. However, clinicians will be able to use and adapt these methods creatively and effectively only if they are able to remain invested in, optimistic about, and energized about their clients' prospects for recovery. This epilogue focuses on helping clinicians remain spirited and upbeat in working with their clients, and avoid demoralization and burnout.

AVOIDING BLAME OF CLIENTS

An easy temptation when treating a challenging client is to blame the person for his or her problems. Clients of-ten do not seem to appreciate their clinicians' efforts to help them. They appear unmotivated, insincere, avoid-ant, or belligerent in responding to offers of assistance. For many clients, there is a frustrating disconnection between what they say and what they do. Such clients may *say* they want treatment, but then they fail to ap-pear for scheduled appointments. They may swear in all earnestness that they endorse abstinence, but within hours they can be found drinking or using drugs again. Some clients steadfastly deny using substances even though the effects on their behavior are clearly evident to everyone else, and they may even test positive for al-cohol or drug use during routine screens for substances.

Many clients just don't seem to want help with either their psychiatric or their substance use problems.

Clients who reject help often seem rational, de-spite the apparent chaos of their lives. Assuming that a client's judgment is intact and that the responsibility for getting better is the client's, not the clinician's, is a natu-ral response when treatment appears to have reached an impasse. However, this reaction is tantamount to blam-ing the client or giving up efforts to engage the client in the recovery process.

There are several problems with blaming a client that may ultimately undermine treatment success. First, blaming the client for not getting better can interfere with the clinician's continuing efforts to help. The clini-cian may reason, "If Tom doesn't want to get better, why should I keep trying to help him?" Second, blam-ing the client can pollute the working alliance by inject-ing a degree of clinician distrust or skepticism concern-ing the client's motives. Third, clients who are blamed for their problems may internalize this blame, thereby further damaging their self-esteem and increasing feel-ings of guilt. Most clients with a dual disorder usually have experienced ample recrimination for their mis-deeds, and feel much doubt about their ability to over-come their problems. Increasing their self-doubt by blaming them for their problems is countertherapeutic; it only increases the shame clients already feel. There are several useful alternatives to blaming clients for their problems.

Recognizing That Both Disorders Are "Primary"

Psychiatric and substance use disorders are both best conceptualized as "primary" disorders with more simi-larities than differences. Both disorders are biologically based illnesses that are partly hereditary and often have a chronic course. Denial is an important symptom of both disorders. Clients are no more personally responsible for their substance use behavior than they are for their psychiatric symptoms. By maintaining awareness that these disorders are true illnesses, clinicians can understand difficult client behaviors as one or both illnesses' "speaking," rather than as a genuine desire to remain ill.

Remembering That Challenging Clients Need the Most Help

Most clinicians enjoy treating clients who are verbal, motivated, earnest, and dependable. Fortunately, many clients with a dual diagnosis with these attributes either get better on their own, or improve rapidly over short periods of time with professional help. Unfortunately for clinicians, these articulate and invested clients need few dual-disorder services. Clients with persistent dual disorders often have numerous other handicaps that make their treatment more difficult, such as cognitive deficits, lack of social supports, trauma history, poverty, and poor motivation. Yet these are the same clients who need the most help, and for whom motivational and rehabilitation-based dual-diagnosis treatment are essential. Recognizing the multiple challenges these clients face makes it easier to avoid blaming them for their predicament.

Acknowledging That Clients Are Doing the Best They Can

When clinicians are working with challenging individuals—especially those whose progress does not appear to measure up to hopes and expectations, or who seem to engage in blatantly destructive or self-destructive behavior—it is helpful to remember the adage that "people cope the best they can." Individuals' ability to manage their affairs, to achieve goals, and to deal with the day-to-day stresses of life is a function of the dynamic interplay among their biological vulnerabilities, their coping skills, and the resources available to them. Poor adjustment and problem behaviors are less reflections of clients' desire to "be that way" than they are of their coping skills and supports. An insufficient repertoire of coping skills may interfere with reducing substance abuse, which itself can be a coping skill used in response to other life challenges. Recognizing that clients' behaviors represent efforts at maintaining a homeostatic adaptation (however tenuous this adaptation may be) appreciates the fact that clients are invested in managing their lives as effectively as possible, despite the apparent destructiveness of some of their coping efforts.

AVOIDING FRUSTRATION

If a client is not to blame, and things do not seem to be going well, then whom is the clinician to blame? All too often the answer is him- or herself. Even when the clinician is successful in avoiding self-blame, the struggle against treatment-refractory dual disorders can lead to frustration—and ultimately burnout and demoralization—if the clinician does not perceive the benefits of his or her work. Avoiding such frustration is critical for clinicians to remain energized, hopeful, and creative in their work with clients. Several ways of doing this are available.

Taking a Long-Term Perspective

Some clients with a dual disorder respond quickly to integrated treatment, and achieve stable remission of their substance use disorders within a year of beginning treatment. Many clients, however, respond to integrated care over a much longer period of time—from 2 to 4 years or even longer. Therefore, it is important to remember that although improvements in some clients may not be evident early in the course of treatment, in the long run integrated dual-diagnosis care works, and most clients get better. In addition, the longer a client is engaged in treatment, the more likely it is that he or she will make progress toward substance use reduction and abstinence.

Assuming That the "Best" Solution Is Not Obvious

The problems presented by clients with a dual diagnosis are often complex and multifaceted. Treatment providers often cling to the belief that if their clinical acumen is sufficiently strong, the proper solution to a problem will be readily apparent. Conversely, if a clinician tries a strategy and it fails, the clinician may interpret this as a negative reflection on his or her clinical skill.

Despite the belief that the "best" solution to a thorny problem should be knowable in advance, often it is not, and a process of trial and error is required to find effective solutions. In fact, more "promising" solutions often have to be eliminated before a suitable solution can be identified and tried. Therefore, rather than assuming that the optimal solution to a problem should be apparent from the outset, and then blaming oneself when the first attempt to solve the problem is not successful, it is preferable to adopt a collaborative/empirical approach to solving problems. It is also important not to cling doggedly to a single "one size fits all" treatment, but to have a range of approaches available to meet individual client needs.

A collaborative/empirical approach to dual-disorder treatment recognizes that multiple efforts are usually necessary to solve difficult problems, and that only through trial and error can effective solutions be found. When using this approach, clinicians collaborate with clients and other stakeholders (e.g., relatives) to identify a "best" solution to a problem. That solution is implemented, and a follow-up is conducted to evaluate whether the problem was solved or improved. If the problem remains, information is gleaned from the unsuccessful attempt, and a new solution is identified and implemented. Through this iterative process, unsuccessful efforts to solve a problem are construed as "learning experiences" that provide valuable information about the nature of the problem and possible strategies for resolving it.

Remembering the Importance of a Functional Analysis

Dual-disorder work often involves responding to, and attempting to resolve, crisis situations related to substance abuse. Common crises that absorb clinicians' time include the loss of stable housing, psychiatric relapses, and conflict with social network members. Dealing with crises effectively is stressful work, because by their very nature they are difficult to anticipate, and their outcome is uncertain. Clinicians who spend most of their time waiting for and responding to crises are vulnerable to burnout, due to the high cost of vigilance and their limited control over the clients' situations.

Clinicians who spend most of their time dealing with crises operate primarily in a *reactive* mode, in which their main function is to respond to emergent situations that threaten their clients' stability. The solution to stress associated with operating in a reactive mode is to become more *proactive* in work with clients. Proactive work involves setting and working toward specific goals identified for specific clients, with at least some of these goals aimed at reducing the chances of future crises.

The functional analysis, as described in Chapter 5, is a vital assessment tool in which specific factors believed to maintain a client's substance abuse are identified. The identification of factors that maintain substance abuse, as well as of obstacles to changing substance use behavior, can lead to interventions addressing those areas and thereby (ideally) reducing substance use. For example, addressing common motives for using substances (e.g., social facilitation, coping with symptoms, and recreation) may lower clients' reliance on using substances to get their needs met in these areas.

In the midst of multiple crises, documentation requirements, team meetings, and other seemingly more pressing professional responsibilities, it is easy for a clinician to neglect to conduct a functional analysis, or to fail to update the analysis on a regular basis. However, developing a functional analysis is crucial because it lays the groundwork for working proactively with a client toward achieving specific goals, rather than reactively responding to an endless series of crises. Clinicians who work proactively with their clients are usually able to make progress toward such goals, which is satisfying to both clinicians and clients. In addition, by taking steps toward desired goals, clinicians and clients may feel less susceptible to the unpredictable nature of the clients' illnesses. Focusing on proactive changes based on the functional analysis is usually the most effective strategy in the long run for reducing substance abuse and the crises associated with it.

CONCLUSIONS

Motivating clients with dual disorders to begin working on their problems, and helping them regain control over their lives, are challenging but rewarding enterprises. In order to be effective and remain invested, clinicians need to form collaborative relationships with clients and other stakeholders, and to broaden their focus from simply eliminating substance abuse to creating positive changes in the clients' lives. When all concerned parties work together and look toward the future, integrated treatment can improve the long-term course of clients with a dual disorder.

References

Addington, J., & Addington, D. (1998). Effect of substance misuse in early psychosis. *British Journal of Psychiatry, 172*(Suppl. 33), 134–136.

Addington, J., & Duchak, V. (1997). Reasons for substance use in schizophrenia. *Acta Psychiatrica Scandinavica, 96,* 329–333.

Addington, J., el-Guebaly, N., Duchak, V., & Hodgins, D. (1999). Using measures of readiness to change in individuals with schizophrenia. *American Journal of Drug and Alcohol Abuse, 25,* 151–161.

Albanese, M. J. (2001). Safety and efficacy of risperidone in substance abusers with psychosis. *American Journal on Addictions, 10,* 190–191.

Alcoholics Anonymous (AA). (1953). *Twelve Steps and Twelve Traditions.* New York: Author.

Alcoholics Anonymous (AA). (1990). *The AA Group: Where It All Begins* (rev. ed.). New York: Author.

Alexander, M. J. (1996). Women with co-occurring addictive and mental disorders: An emerging profile of vulnerability. *American Journal of Orthopsychiatry, 66,* 61–70.

Alfs, D. S., & McClellan, T. A. (1992). A day hospital program for dual diagnosis patients in a VA medical center. *Hospital and Community Psychiatry, 43,* 241–244.

Allness, D. J., & Knoedler, W. H. (1998). *The PACT Model of Community-Based Treatment for Persons with Severe and Persistent Mental Illness: A Manual for PACT Start-Up.* Arlington, VA: National Alliance for the Mentally Ill.

Alterman, A. I., & Cacciola, J. S. (1991). The antisocial personality disorder diagnosis in substance abusers: Problems and issues. *Journal of Nervous and Mental Disease, 179,* 167–175.

Alverson, H., Alverson, M., & Drake, R. E. (2001). Social patterns of substance-use among people with dual diagnoses. *Mental Health Services Research, 3,* 3–14.

Alverson, M., Becker, D. R., & Drake, R. E. (1995). An ethnographic study of coping strategies used by people with severe mental illness participating in supported employment. *Psychosocial Rehabilitation Journal, 18*(4), 115–128.

American Psychiatric Association. (1994). *Diagnostic and Statistical Manual of Mental Disorders* (4th ed.). Washington, DC: Author.

Americans with Disabilities Act of 1990, P. L. 101-336, 104 Stat. 327 (1991).

Ananth, J., Vandewater, S., Kamal, M., Brodsky, A., Gamal, R., & Miller, M. (1989). Missed diagnosis of substance abuse in psychiatric patients. *Hospital and Community Psychiatry, 40,* 297–299.

Anderson, C. M., Reiss, D. J., & Hogarty, G. E. (1986). *Schizophrenia and the Family.* New York: Guilford Press.

Andreasen, N. C. (1984). *Modified Scale for the Assessment of Negative Symptoms.* Bethesda, MD: U.S. Department of Health and Human Services.

Andrews, D. A., & Bonta, J. L. (1994). *The Psychology of Criminal Conduct.* Cincinnati, OH: Anderson.

Andrews, D. A., Zinger, I., Hoge, R. D., Bonta, J., Gendreau, P., & Cullen, F. T. (1990). Does correctional treatment work? A clinically relevant and psychologically informed meta-analysis. *Criminology, 28,* 369–404.

Anthenelli, R. M., & Schuckit, M. A. (1992). Genetics. In J. H. Lowinson, P. Ruiz, R. B. Millman, & J. G. Langrod (Eds.), *Substance Abuse: A Comprehensive Textbook* (2nd ed., pp. 39–50). Baltimore: Williams & Wilkins.

Anthony, J. C., & Helzer, J. E. (1991). Syndromes of drug abuse and dependence. In L. N. Robins & D. A. Regier (Eds.), *Psychiatric Disorders in America: The Epidemiologic Catchment Area Study* (pp. 116–154). New York: Free Press.

Anthony, W. A. (1993). Recovery from mental illness: The guiding vision of the mental health service system in the 1990s. *Psychosocial Rehabilitation Journal, 16,* 11–23.

Anton, R. F., Moak, D. H., Waid, L. R., Latham, P. K., Malcolm, R. J., & Dias, J. K. (1999). Naltrexone and cognitive behavioral therapy for the treatment of outpatient alcoholics: Results of a placebo-controlled trial. *American Journal of Psychiatry, 156*, 1758–1764.

Antony, M. M., Craske, M. G., & Barlow, D. H. (1995). *Mastery of Your Specific Phobia: Client Workbook*. San Antonio, TX: Psychological Corporation.

Applebaum, P. S. (1994). *Almost a Revolution: Mental Health Law and the Limits of Change*. New York: Oxford University Press.

Arndt, S., Tyrrell, G., Flaum, M., & Andreasen, N. C. (1992). Comorbidity of substance abuse and schizophrenia: The role of pre-morbid adjustment. *Psychological Medicine, 22*, 379–388.

Ascher-Svanum, H., & Krause, A. A. (1991). *Psychoeducational Groups for Patients with Schizophrenia: A Guide for Practitioners*. Gaithersburg, MD: Aspen.

Atkinson, J. M., & Coia, D. A. (1995). *Families Coping with Schizophrenia*. New York: Wiley.

Azrin, N. H., Sissons, R., Meyers, S. R., & Godley, M. (1982). Alcoholism treatment by disulfiram and community reinforcement therapy. *Journal of Behavioral Therapy and Experimental Psychiatry, 13*, 105–112.

Backer, T., Liberman, R., & Kuehnel, T. (1986). Dissemination and adoption of innovative psychosocial interventions. *Journal of Consulting and Clinical Psychology, 54*, 111–118.

Baigent, M., Holme, G., & Hafner, R. J. (1995). Self reports of the interaction between substance abuse and schizophrenia. *Australian and New Zealand Journal of Psychiatry, 29*, 69–74.

Barbee, J. G., Clark, P. D., Craqanzano, M. S., Heintz, G. C., & Kehoe, C. E. (1989). Alcohol and substance abuse among schizophrenic patients presenting to an emergency service. *Journal of Nervous and Mental Disease, 177*, 400–407.

Barlow, D. H. (2002). *Anxiety and Its Disorders: The Nature and Treatment of Anxiety and Panic* (2nd ed.). New York: Guilford Press.

Barlow, D. H., & Craske, M., G. (2000). *Mastery of Your Anxiety and Panic: Client Workbook for Anxiety and Panic MAP-3* (3rd ed.). San Antonio, TX: Psychological Corporation.

Barnett, P. G., Rogers, J. H., & Bloch, D. A. (2001). A meta-analysis comparing buprenorphine to methadone for treatment of opiate dependence. *Addiction, 96*, 683–690.

Barrowclough, C., Haddock, G., Tarrier, N., Lewis, S., Moring, J., O'Brien, R., Schofield, N., & McGovern, J. (2001). Randomized controlled trial of motivational interviewing, cognitive behavior therapy, and family intervention for patients with comorbid schizophrenia and substance use disorders. *American Journal of Psychiatry, 158*, 1706–1713.

Bartels, S. J., & Drake, R. E. (1996). A pilot study of residential treatment for dual diagnoses. *Journal of Nervous and Mental Disease, 184*, 379–381.

Bartels, S. J., Drake, R. E., & McHugo, G. (1992). Alcohol use, depression, and suicidal behavior in schizophrenia. *American Journal of Psychiatry, 149*, 394–395.

Bartels, S. J., Drake, R. E., & Wallach, M. A. (1995). Long-term course of substance use disorders in severe mental illness. *Psychiatric Services, 46*, 248–251.

Bartels, S. J., Teague, G. B., Drake, R. E., Clark, R. E., Bush, P. W., & Noordsy, D. L. (1993). Substance abuse in schizophrenia: Service utilization and costs. *Journal of Nervous and Mental Disease, 181*, 227–232.

Beale, V., & Lambric, T. (1995). *The Recovery Concept: Implementation in the Mental Health System: A Report by the Community Support Program Advisory Committee*. Columbus: Ohio State Department of Mental Health, Office of Consumer Services.

Beck, A. T., & Emery, G., with Greenberg, R. L. (1985). *Anxiety Disorders and Phobias: A Cognitive Perspective*. New York: Basic Books.

Beck, A. T., Rush, A. J., Shaw, B. F., & Emery, G. (1979). *Cognitive Therapy of Depression*. New York: Guilford Press.

Beck, A. T., & Steer, R. A. (1990). *Manual for the Beck Anxiety Inventory*. San Antonio, TX: Psychological Corporation.

Beck, A. T., Steer, R. A., & Garbin, M. G. (1988). Psychometric properties of the Beck Depression Inventory: Twenty-five years of evaluation. *Clinical Psychology Review, 8*, 77–100.

Beck, A. T., Wright, F. D., Newman, C. F., & Liese, B. S. (1993). *Cognitive Therapy of Substance Abuse*. New York: Guilford Press.

Becker, D. R., Bebout, R. R., & Drake, R. E. (1998). Job preferences of people with severe mental illness: A replication. *Psychiatric Rehabilitation Journal, 22*, 46–50.

Becker, D. R., & Drake, R. E. (1993). *A Working Life: The Individual Placement and Support (IPS) Program*. Concord: New Hampshire-Dartmouth Psychiatric Research Center.

Becker, D. R., Drake, R. E., Farabaugh, A., & Bond, G. R. (1996). Job preferences of clients with severe psychiatric disorders participating in supported employment programs. *Psychiatric Services, 47*, 1223–1226.

Becker, D. R., Torrey, W. C., Toscano, R., Wyzik, P. F., & Fox, T. S. (1998). Building recovery-oriented services: Lessons from implementing IPS in community mental health centers. *Psychiatric Rehabilitation Journal, 22*, 51–54.

Becker, H. S. (1953). Becoming a marijuana user. *American Journal of Sociology, 59*, 235–242.

Becker, M. C., & Sugarman, G. (1952). Death following a test drink of alcohol in patients receiving Antabuse. *Journal of the American Medical Association, 149*, 568–569.

Becker, R. E., Meisler, N., Stormer, G., & Brondino, M. J. (1999). Employment outcomes for clients with severe mental illness in a PACT model replication. *Psychiatric Services, 50*, 104–106.

Belenko, S. (1998). Research on drug courts: A critical review. *National Drug Court Institute Review, 1*, 1–42.

Bell, M., Greig, T., Gill, P., Whelahan, H., & Bryson, G. (2002). Work rehabilitation and patterns of substance use among persons with schizophrenia. *Psychiatric Services, 53*, 63–69.

Bellack, A. S., & DiClemente, C. C. (1999). Treating substance abuse among patients with schizophrenia. *Psychiatric Services, 50*, 75–79.

Bellack, A. S., Morrison, R. L., Wixted, J. T., & Mueser, K. T. (1990). An analysis of social competence in schizophrenia. *British Journal of Psychiatry, 156*, 809–818.

Bellack, A. S., Mueser, K. T., Gingerich, S., & Agresta, J. (1997). *Social Skills Training for Schizophrenia: A Step-by-Step Guide.* New York: Guilford Press.

Bellack, A. S., Mueser, K. T., Wade, J. H., Sayers, S. L., & Morrison, R. L. (1992). The ability of schizophrenics to perceive and cope with negative affect. *British Journal of Psychiatry, 160*, 473–480.

Bellack, A. S., Sayers, M., Mueser, K. T., & Bennett, M. (1994). An evaluation of social problem solving in schizophrenia. *Journal of Abnormal Psychology, 103*, 371–378.

Bennett, N. S., Lidz, C. W., Monahan, J., Mulvey, E., Hoge, S. K., Roth, L. H., & Gardner, W. (1993). Inclusion, motivation, and good faith: The morality of coercion in mental hospital admission. *Behavioral Sciences and the Law, 11*, 295–306.

Berman, S. M., & Noble, E. P. (1993). Childhood antecedents of substance misuse. *Current Opinion in Psychiatry, 6*, 382–387.

Bermanzohn, P. C., & Siris, S. G. (1992). Akinesia: A syndrome common to parkinsonism, retarded depression, and negative symptoms of schizophrenia. *Comprehensive Psychiatry, 33*, 221–232.

Bernadt, M. W., & Murray, R. M. (1986). Psychiatric disorder, drinking and alcoholism: What are the links? *British Journal of Psychiatry, 148*, 393–400.

Bernheim, K. F., & Lehman, A. F. (1985). *Working with Families of the Mentally Ill.* New York: Norton.

Bidaut-Russell, M., Bradford, S. E., & Smith, E. M. (1994). Prevalence of mental illnesses in adult offspring of alcoholic mothers. *Drug and Alcohol Dependence, 35*, 81–90.

Bijou, S. W., & Peterson, R. F. (1971). Functional analysis in the assessment of children. In P. McReynolds (Ed.), *Advances in Psychological Assessment* (Vol. 2, pp. 63–78). Palo Alto, CA: Science & Behavior Books.

Birmaher, B., Ryan, N. D., Williamson, D. E., Brent, D. A., Kaufman, J., Dahl, R. E., Perel, J., & Nelson, B. (1996). Childhood and adolescent depression: A review of the past 10 years. Part I. *Journal of the American Academy of Child and Adolescent Psychiatry, 35*, 1427–1439.

Blanchard, E. P., Jones-Alexander, J., Buckley, T. C., & Forneris, C. A. (1996). Psychometric properties of the PTSD Checklist. *Behavior Therapy, 34*, 669–673.

Blanchard, J. J., Bellack, A. S., & Mueser, K. T. (1994). Affective and social-behavioral correlates of physical and social anhedonia in schizophrenia. *Journal of Abnormal Psychology, 103*, 719–728.

Blanchard, J. J., Brown, S. A., Horan, W. P., & Sherwood, A. R. (2000). Substance use disorders in schizophrenia: Review, integration, and a proposed model. *Clinical Psychology Review, 20*, 207–234.

Blanchard, J. J., Mueser, K. T., & Bellack, A. S. (1998). Anhedonia, positive and negative affect, and social functioning in schizophrenia. *Schizophrenia Bulletin, 24*, 413–424.

Blanchard, J. J., Squires, D., Henry, T., Horan, W. P., Bogenschutz, M., Lauriello, J., & Bustillo, J. (1999). Examining an affect regulation model of substance abuse in schizophrenia: The role of traits and coping. *Journal of Nervous and Mental Disease, 187*, 72–79.

Bland, R. C., Newman, S. C., & Orn, H. (1987). Schizophrenia: Lifetime comorbidity in a community sample. *Acta Psychiatrica Scandinavica, 75*, 383–395.

Blankertz, L. E., & Cnaan, R. A. (1994). Assessing the impact of two residential programs for dually diagnosed homeless individuals. *Social Service Review, 68*, 536–560.

Bond, G. R., Becker, D. R., Drake, R. E., Rapp, C. A., Meisler, N., Lehman, A. F., Bell, M. D., & Blyler, C. R. (2001). Implementing supported employment as an evidence-based practice. *Psychiatric Services, 52*, 313–322.

Bond, G. R., Drake, R. E., Mueser, K. T., & Becker, D. R. (1997). An update on supported employment for people with severe mental illness. *Psychiatric Services, 48*, 335–346.

Bond, G. R., Drake, R. E., Mueser, K. T., & Latimer, E. (2001). Assertive community treatment for people with severe mental illness: Critical ingredients and impact on clients. *Disease Management and Health Outcomes, 9*, 141–159.

Bond, G. R., McDonel, E. C., Miller, L. D., & Pensec, M. (1991). Assertive community treatment and reference groups: An evaluation of their effectiveness for young adults with serious mental illness and substance abuse problems. *Psychosocial Rehabilitation Journal, 15*(2), 31–43.

Bordin, E. S. (1976). The generalizability of the psychoanalytic concept of the working alliance. *Psychotherapy: Theory, Research and Practice, 16*, 252–260.

Bourne, E. J. (1998a). *Overcoming Specific Phobia: A Hierarchy and Exposure-Based Protocol for the Treatment of All Specific Phobias—Client Manual.* Oakland, CA: New Harbinger.

Bourne, E. J. (1998b). *Overcoming Specific Phobia: A Hierarchy and Exposure-Based Protocol for the Treatment of All Specific Phobias—Therapist Protocol.* Oakland, CA: New Harbinger.

Bowers, M. B., Mazure, C. M., Nelson, C. J., & Jatlow, P. I. (1990). Psychotogenic drug use and neuroleptic response. *Schizophrenia Bulletin, 16*, 81–85.

Brady, K. T., & Roberts, J. M. (1995). The pharmacotherapy of dual diagnosis. *Psychiatric Annals, 25*, 344–352.

Brady, S., Hiam, C. M., Saemann, R., Humbert, L., Fleming, M. Z., & Dawkins-Brickhouse, K. (1996). Dual diagnosis: A treatment model for substance abuse and major mental illness. *Community Mental Health Journal, 32*, 573–578.

Breakey, W. R., Goodell, H., Lorenz, P. C., & McHugh, P. R. (1974). Hallucinogenic drugs as precipitants of schizophrenia. *Psychological Medicine, 4*, 255–261.

Brehm, J. W. (1966). *A Theory of Psychological Reactance.* New York: Academic Press.

Breier, A., Schreiber, J., Dyer, J., & Pickar, D. (1991). National Institute of Mental Health longitudinal study of chronic schizophrenia. *Archives of General Psychiatry, 48*, 239–246.

Brekke, J. S., Debonis, J. A., & Graham, J. W. (1994). A latent structure analysis of the positive and negative symptoms in schizophrenia. *Comprehensive Psychiatry, 35,* 252–259.

Brewer, C. (1992). Controlled trials of Antabuse in alcoholism: The importance of supervision and adequate dosage. *Acta Psychiatrica Scandinavica, 86,* 51–58.

Briere, J., Woo, R., McRae, B., Foltz, J., & Sitzman, R. (1997). Lifetime victimization history, demographics, and clinical status in female psychiatric emergency room patients. *Journal of Nervous and Mental Disease, 185,* 95–101.

Brizer, D. A., Hartman, N., Sweeney, J., & Millman, R. B. (1985). Effect of methadone plus neuroleptics on treatment-resistant chronic paranoid schizophrenia. *American Journal of Psychiatry, 142,* 1106–1107.

Bruce, M. L., Takeuchi, D. T., & Leaf, P. J. (1991). Poverty and psychiatric status: Longitudinal evidence from the New Haven Epidemiologic Catchment Area Study. *Archives of General Psychiatry, 48,* 470–474.

Brunette, M. F., & Dean, W. (2002). Community mental health care of women with severe mental illness who are parents. *Community Mental Health Journal, 38,* 153–165.

Brunette, M. F., & Drake, R. E. (1997). Gender differences in patients with schizophrenia and substance abuse. *Comprehensive Psychiatry, 38,* 109–116.

Brunette, M. F., & Drake, R. E. (1998). Gender differences in homeless persons with schizophrenia and substance abuse. *Community Mental Health Journal, 34,* 627–642.

Brunette, M. F., Drake, R. E., Woods, M., & Hartnett, T. (2001). A comparison of long-term and short-term residential treatment programs for dual diagnosis patients. *Psychiatric Services, 52,* 526–528.

Brunette, M. F., Mueser, K. T., Xie, H., & Drake, R. E. (1997). Relationships between symptoms of schizophrenia and substance abuse. *Journal of Nervous and Mental Disease, 185,* 13–20.

Brunette, M. F., Noordsy, D., & Drake, R. E. (2002). *Benzodiazepine use and abuse by clients with severe mental illness and substance use disorders.* Manuscript submitted for publication.

Buckley, P. F., Thompson, P., Way, L., & Meltzer, H. Y. (1994). Substance abuse among patients with treatment-resistant schizophrenia: Characteristics and implications for clozapine therapy. *American Journal of Psychiatry, 151,* 385–389.

Buckley, P. F., & Waddington, J. L. (Eds.). (2000). *Schizophrenia and Mood Disorders: The New Drug Therapies in Clinical Practice.* Woburn, MA: Butterworth-Heinemann.

Bühler, B., Hambrecht, M., Löffler, W., An der Heiden, W., & Häfner, H. (2002). Precipitation and determination of the onset and course of schizophrenia by substance abuse: A retrospective and prospective study of 232 population-based first illness episodes. *Schizophrenia Research, 54,* 243–251.

Buhrich, N., Weller, A., & Kevans, P. (2000). Misuse of anticholinergic drugs by people with severe mental illness. *Psychiatric Services, 51,* 928–929.

Burnam, M. A., Morton, S. C., McGlynn, E. A., Peterson, L. P., Stecher, B. M., Hayes, C., & Vaccaro, J. V. (1995). An experimental evaluation of residential and nonresidential treatment for dually diagnosed homeless adults. *Journal of Addictive Diseases, 14,* 111–134.

Butzlaff, R. L., & Hooley, J. M. (1998). Expressed emotion and psychiatric relapse. *Archives of General Psychiatry, 55,* 547–552.

Caballo, V. E. (Ed.). (1998). *International Handbook of Cognitive-Behavioral Treatments for Psychological Disorders.* Oxford: Elsevier Science.

Campbell, J. (1997). How consumers/survivors are evaluating the quality of psychiatric care. *Evaluation Review, 21,* 357–363.

Cannon, T. D., Mednick, S. A., Parnas, J., Schulsinger, F., Praestholm, J., & Vestergaard, A. (1993). Developmental brain abnormalities in the offspring of schizophrenic mothers. *Archives of General Psychiatry, 50,* 551–564.

Cantor-Graae, E., Nordström, L. G., & McNeil, T. F. (2001). Substance abuse in schizophrenia: A review of the literature and study of correlates in Sweden. *Schizophrenia Research, 48,* 69–82.

Carey, K. B. (1996). Substance use reduction in the context of outpatient psychiatric treatment: A collaborative, motivational, harm reduction approach. *Community Mental Health Journal, 32,* 291–306.

Carey, K. B., & Carey, M. P. (1995). Reasons for drinking among psychiatric outpatients: Relationship to drinking patterns. *Psychology of Addictive Behaviors, 9,* 251–257.

Carey, K. B., & Correia, C. J. (1998). Severe mental illness and addictions: Assessment considerations. *Addictive Behaviors, 23,* 735–748.

Carey, K. B., Purnine, D. M., Maisto, S. A., Carey, M. P., & Barnes, K. L. (1999). Decisional balance regarding substance use among persons with schizophrenia. *Community Mental Health Journal, 35,* 289–299.

Carey, M. P., Carey, K. B., Maisto, S. A., Gleason, J. R., Gordon, C. M., & Brewer, K. K. (1999). HIV-risk behavior among outpatients at a state psychiatric hospital: Prevalence and risk modeling. *Behavior Therapy, 30,* 389–406.

Carey, M. P., Weinhardt, L. S., & Carey, K. B. (1995). Prevalence of infection with HIV among the seriously mentally ill: Review of research and implications for practice. *Professional Psychology: Research and Practice, 26,* 262–268.

Carling, P. J. (1995). *Return to Community: Building Support Systems for People with Psychiatric Disabilities.* New York: Guilford Press.

Carmen, E., Rieker, P. P., & Mills, T. (1984). Victims of violence and psychiatric illness. *American Journal of Psychiatry, 141,* 378–383.

Carmichael, D., Tackett-Gibson, M., O'Dell, L., Jayasuria, B., Jordan, J., & Menon, R. (1998). *Texas Dual Diagnosis Project Evaluation Report 1997–1998.* College Station: Public Policy Research Institute/Texas A&M University.

Carroll, K. M., Nich, C., Ball, S. A., McCance, E., & Rounsaville, B. J. (1998). Treatment of cocaine and alcohol dependence with psychotherapy and disulfiram. *Addiction, 93,* 713–728.

Carroll, K. M., Rounsaville, B. J., Nich, C., Gordon, L. T., Wirtz, P. W., & Gawin, F. (1994). One-year follow-up of psychotherapy and pharmacotherapy for cocaine dependence: Delayed emergence of psychotherapy effects. *Archives of General Psychiatry, 51*, 989–997.

Carter, B., & McGoldrick, M. (1988). *The Changing Family Life Cycle: A Framework for Family Therapy* (2nd ed.). New York: Gardner Press.

Cascardi, M., Mueser, K. T., DeGiralomo, J., & Murrin, M. (1996). Physical aggression against psychiatric inpatients by family members and partners: A descriptive study. *Psychiatric Services, 47*, 531–533.

Catalano, E. (1990). *Getting to Sleep.* Oakland, CA: New Harbinger.

Caton, C. L., Shrout, P. E., Dominguez, B., Eagle, P. F., Opler, L. A., & Cournos, F. (1995). Risk factors for homelessness among women with schizophrenia. *American Journal of Public Health, 85*, 1153–1156.

Caton, C. L., Shrout, P. E., Eagle, P. F., Opler, L. A., Felix, A. F., & Dominguez, B. (1994). Risk factors for homelessness among schizophrenic men: A case–control study. *American Journal of Public Health, 84*, 265–270.

Center for Mental Health Services. (1994). *Making a Difference: Interim Status Report of the McKinney Research Demonstration Program for Homeless Mentally Ill Adults.* Rockville, MD: Substance Abuse and Mental Health Services Administration.

Chamberlin, J., & Rogers, J. A. (1990). Planning a community-based mental health system: Perspectives of service recipients. *American Psychologist, 45*, 1241–1244.

Chambers, R. A., Krystal, J. H., & Self, D. W. (2001). A neurobiological basis for substance abuse comorbidity in schizophrenia. *Biological Psychiatry, 50*, 71–83.

Chick, J. (1999). Safety issues concerning the use of disulfiram in treating alcohol dependence. *Drug Safety, 20*, 427–435.

Chick, J., Gough, K., Falkowski, W., Kershaw, P., Hore, B., Mehta, B., Ritson, B., Ropner, R., & Torley, D. (1992). Disulfiram treatment of alcoholism. *British Journal of Psychiatry, 161*, 84–89.

Chilcoat, H. D., & Breslau, N. (1998). Posttraumatic stress disorder and drug disorders: Testing causal pathways. *Archives of General Psychiatry, 55*, 913–917.

Chiles, J. A., Miller, A. L., Crismon, M. L., Rush, A. J., Krasof, A. S., & Shon, S. S. (1999). The Texas Medication Algorithm Project: Development and implementation of the schizophrenia algorithm. *Psychiatric Services, 50*, 69–74.

Chouljian, T. L., Shumway, M., Balancio, E., Dwyer, E. V., Surber, R., & Jacobs, M. (1995). Substance use among schizophrenic outpatients: Prevalence, course, and relation to functional status. *Annals of Clinical Psychiatry, 7*, 19–24.

Ciraulo, D. A., Barnhill, J. G., Greenblatt, D. J., Shader, R. I., Ciraulo, A. M., Tarmey, M. F., Molloy, M. A., & Foti, M. E. (1988). Abuse liability and clinical pharmacokinetics of alprazolam in alcoholic men. *Journal of Clinical Psychiatry, 49*, 333–337.

Ciraulo, D. A., & Renner, J. A. (1991). Alcoholism. In D. A. Ciraulo & R. I. Shader (Eds.), *Clinical Manual of Chemical Dependence* (pp. 1–93). Washington, DC: American Psychiatric Press.

Clark, D. C., & Fawcett, J. (1989). Does lithium carbonate therapy for alcoholism deter relapse drinking? In M. Galanter (Ed.), *Recent Developments in Alcoholism: Vol. 7. Treatment Research* (pp. 315–328). New York: Plenum Press.

Clark, R. E. (1994). Family costs associated with severe mental illness and substance use: A comparison of families with and without dual disorders. *Hospital and Community Psychiatry, 45*, 808–813.

Clark, R. E. (1996). Family support for persons with dual disorders. In R. E. Drake & K. T. Mueser (Eds.), *New Directions for Mental Health Services: Vol. 70. Dual Diagnosis of Major Mental Illness and Substance Abuse Disorder, Volume 2: Recent Research and Clinical Implications* (pp. 65–78). San Francisco: Jossey-Bass.

Clark, R. E. (2001). Family support and substance use outcomes for persons with mental illness and substance use disorders. *Schizophrenia Bulletin, 27*, 93–101.

Clark, R. E., & Drake, R. E. (1994). Expenditures of time and money by families of people with severe mental illness and substance use disorders. *Community Mental Health Journal, 30*, 145–163.

Clark, R. E., Drake, R. E., McHugo, G. J., & Ackerson, T. H. (1995). Incentives for community treatment mental illness management services. *Medical Care, 33*, 729–738.

Clark, R. E., & Fox, T. (1993). A framework for evaluating the economic impact of case management. *Hospital and Community Psychiatry, 44*, 469–473.

Cohen, M., & Klein, D. F. (1970). Drug abuse in a young psychiatric population. *American Journal of Orthopsychiatry, 40*, 448–455.

Coldham, E. L., Addington, J., & Addington, D. (2002). Medication adherence of individuals with a first episode of psychosis. *Acta Psychiatrica Scandinavica, 106*, 286–290.

Comas-Díaz, L. (1981). Puerto Rican espiritismo and psychotherapy. *American Journal of Orthopsychiatry, 51*, 636–645.

Comer, S. D., & Collins, E. D. (2002). Self-administration of intravenous buprenorphine and the buprenorphine/naloxone combination by recently detoxified herion abusers. *Journal of Pharmacology and Experimental Therapeutics, 303*, 695–703.

Conley, R. R., Kelly, D. L., & Gale, E. A. (1998). Olanzapine response in treatment-refractory schizophrenic patients with a history of substance abuse. *Schizophrenia Research, 33*, 95–101.

Connors, G. J., Donovan, D. M., & DiClemente, C. C. (2001). *Substance Abuse Treatment and the Stages of Change.* New York: Guilford Press.

Cooper, C. S., & Trotter, J. A., Jr. (1994). Recent developments in drug case management: Reengineering the judicial process. *Justice System Journal, 17*, 83–98.

Copeland, M. E. (1994). *Living without Depression and Manic Depression.* Oakland, CA: New Harbinger.

Copeland, M. E. (1997). *Wellness Recovery Action Plan.* Brattleboro, VT: Peach Press.

Cornelius, J. R., Salloum, I. M., Ehler, J. G., Jarret, P. J., Cornelius, M. D., Perel, J. M., Thase, M. E., & Black, A. (1997). Fluoxetine in depressed alcoholics: A double-blind placebo-controlled trial. *Archives of General Psychiatry, 54,* 700–705.

Corrigan, P. W. (1995). Wanted: Champions of rehabilitation for psychiatric hospitals. *American Psychologist, 50,* 514–521.

Corrigan, P. W., Liberman, R. P., & Wong, S. E. (1993). Recreational therapy and behavior management on inpatient units: Is recreational therapy therapeutic? *Journal of Nervous and Mental Disease, 181,* 644–646.

Corrigan, P. W., McCracken, S. G., & Holmes, E. P. (2001). Motivational interviews as goal assessment for persons with psychiatric disability. *Community Mental Health Journal, 37,* 113–122.

Corrigan, P. W., & Penn, D. L. (1999). Lessons from social psychology on discrediting psychiatric stigma. *American Psychologist, 54,* 765–776.

Corrigan, P. W., River, L. P., Lundin, R. K., Penn, D. L., & Kubiak, M. A. (2001). Three strategies for changing attributions about severe mental illness. *Schizophrenia Bulletin, 27,* 187–196.

Corse, S. J., Hirschinger, N. B., & Zanis, D. (1995). The use of the Addiction Severity Index with people with severe mental illness. *Psychiatric Rehabilitation Journal, 19,* 9–18.

Cournos, F., Empfield, M., Horwath, E., McKinnon, K., Meyer, I., Schrage, H., Currie, C., & Agosin, B. (1991). HIV prevalence among patients admitted to two psychiatric hospitals. *American Journal of Psychiatry, 148,* 1225–1229.

Cournos, F., & McKinnon, K. (1997). HIV seroprevalence among people with severe mental illness in the United States: A critical review. *Clinical Psychology Review, 17,* 159–169.

Craine, L. S., Henson, C. E., Colliver, J. A., & MacLean, D. G. (1988). Prevalence of a history of sexual abuse among female psychiatric patients in a state hospital system. *Hospital and Community Psychiatry, 39,* 300–304.

Craske, M. G., Antony, M. M., & Barlow, D. H. (1997). *Mastery of Your Specific Phobia: Therapist Guide.* San Antonio, TX: Psychological Corporation.

Craske, M. G., Barlow, D. H., & Meadows, E. A. (2000). *Mastery of Your Anxiety and Panic: Therapist Guide for Anxiety, Panic, and Agoraphobia MAP-3* (3rd ed.). San Antonio, TX: Psychological Corporation.

Craske, M. G., Barlow, D. H., & O'Leary, T. A. (1992). *Mastery of Your Anxiety and Worry: Client Workbook.* San Antonio, TX: Psychological Corporation.

Crowley, T. J., Chesluck, D., Dilts, S., & Hart, R. (1974). Drug and alcohol abuse among psychiatric admissions. *Archives of General Psychiatry, 30,* 13–20.

Cuffel, B. J. (1996). Comorbid substance use disorder: Prevalence, patterns of use, and course. In R. E. Drake & K. T. Mueser (Eds.), *New Directions for Mental Health Services: Vol. 70. Dual Diagnosis of Major Mental Illness and Substance Abuse Volume 2: Recent Research and Clinical Implications* (pp. 93–105). San Francisco: Jossey-Bass.

Cuffel, B., & Chase, P. (1994). Remission and relapse of substance use disorders in schizophrenia: Results from a one year prospective study. *Journal of Nervous and Mental Disease, 182,* 704–708.

Culver, C. M., & Gert, B. (1982). *Philosophy in Medicine: Conceptual and Ethical issues in Medicine and Psychiatry.* New York: Oxford University Press.

Dansky, B. S., Saladin, M. E., Brady, K. T., Kilpatrick, D. G., & Resnick, H. S. (1995). Prevalence of victimization and posttraumatic stress disorder among women with substance use disorders: Comparison of telephone and in-person assessment samples. *International Journal of the Addictions, 30,* 1079–1099.

Deegan, P. E. (1988). Recovery: The lived experience of rehabilitation. *Psychosocial Rehabilitation Journal, 11,* 11–19.

Deegan, P. E. (1990). Spirit breaking: When the helping professionals hurt. *The Humanistic Psychologist, 18,* 301–313.

Deegan, P. E. (1992). The independent living movement and people with psychiatric disabilities: Taking back control over our own lives. *Psychosocial Rehabilitation Journal, 15,* 3–19.

de la Fuente, J. R., Morse, R. M., Niven, R. G., & Ilstrup, D. M. (1989). A controlled study of lithium carbonate in the treatment of alcoholism. *Mayo Clinic Proceedings, 64,* 177–180.

DelBello, M. P., Strakowski, S. M., Sax, K. W., McElroy, S. L., Keck, P. E. J., West, S. A., & Kmetz, G. F. (1999). Effects of familial rates of affective illness and substance abuse on rates of substance abuse in patients with first-episode mania. *Journal of Affective Disorders, 56,* 55–60.

de Leon, J., Dadvand, M., Canuso, C., White, A. O., Stanilla, J. K., & Simpson, G. M. (1995). Schizophrenia and smoking: An epidemiological survey at a state hospital. *American Journal of Psychiatry, 152,* 453–455.

Denning, P. (2000). *Practicing Harm Reduction Psychotherapy: An Alternative Approach to Addictions.* New York: Guilford Press.

Derogatis, L. R. (1993). *Brief Symptom Inventory (BSI): Administration, Scoring, and Procedures Manual* (3rd ed.). Minneapolis, MN: National Computer Systems.

Des Jarlais, D. C. (1995). Harm reduction: A framework for incorporating science into drug policy [Editorial]. *American Journal of Public Health, 85,* 10–12.

Deschenes, E., & Greenwood, P. (1995). Drug court or probation?: An experimental evaluation of Maricopa County's drug court. *Justice System Journal, 18,* 55–73.

Detrick, A., & Stiepock, V. (1992). Treating persons with mental illness, substance abuse, and legal problems: The Rhode Island experience. In L. I. Stein (Ed.), *New Directions for Mental Health Services: Vol. 56. Innovative Community Mental Health Programs* (pp. 65–77). San Francisco: Jossey-Bass.

Deykin, E. Y., & Buka, S. L. (1997). Prevalence and risk factors for posttraumatic stress disorder among chemically dependent adolescents. *American Journal of Psychiatry, 154,* 752–757.

Dickey, B., & Azeni, H. (1996). Persons with dual diagnoses of substance abuse and major mental illness: Their excess costs of psychiatric care. *American Journal of Public Health, 86,* 973–977.

DiClemente, C. C., & Prochaska, J. O. (1998). Toward a comprehensive, transtheoretical model of change: Stages of change and addictive behaviors. In W. R. Miller & N. Heather (Eds.), *Treating Addictive Behaviors* (2nd ed., pp. 3–24). New York: Plenum Press.

Dilk, M. N., & Bond, G. R. (1996). Meta-analytic evaluation of skills training research for individuals with severe mental illness. *Journal of Consulting and Clinical Psychology, 64,* 1337–1346.

DiPaula, B. A., Schwartz, R., Montoya, I. D., Barrett, D., & Tang, C. (2002). Heroin detoxification with buprenorphine on an inpatient psychiatric unit. *Journal of Substance Abuse Treatment, 23,* 163–169.

Dixon, L., Adams, C., & Lucksted, A. (2000). Update on family psychoeducation for schizophrenia. *Schizophrenia Bulletin, 26,* 5–20.

Dixon, L., Haas, G., Weiden, P., Sweeney, J., & Frances, A. J. (1990). Acute effects of drug abuse in schizophrenic patients: Clinical observation and patients' self-reports. *Schizophrenia Bulletin, 16,* 69–70.

Dixon, L., Haas, G., Weiden, P. J., Sweeney, J., & Frances, A. J. (1991). Drug abuse in schizophrenic patients: Clinical correlates and reasons for use. *American Journal of Psychiatry, 148,* 224–230.

Dixon, L., McFarlane, W., Lefley, H., Lucksted, A., Cohen, C., Falloon, I., Mueser, K. T., Miklowitz, D., Solomon, P., & Sondheimer, D. (2001). The state of evidence based practices for services to family members of people with psychiatric disabilities. *Psychiatric Services, 52,* 903–910.

Dixon, L., McNary, S., & Lehman, A. (1995). Substance abuse and family relationships of persons with severe mental illness. *American Journal of Psychiatry, 152,* 456–458.

Dixon, L., Weiden, P. J., Haas, G., Sweeney, J., & Frances, A. J. (1992). Increased tardive dyskinesia in alcohol-abusing schizophrenic patients. *Comprehensive Psychiatry, 33,* 121–122.

Dorus, W., Ostrow, D. G., Anton, R., Cushman, P., Collins, J. F., Schaefer, M., Charles, H. L., Desai, P., Hayashida, M., Malkerneker, U., Willenbring, M., Fiscella, R., & Sather, M. R. (1989). Lithium treatment of depressed and nondepressed alcoholics. *Journal of the American Medical Association, 262,* 1646–1652.

Drake, R. E., Antosca, L. M., Noordsy, D. L., Bartels, S. J., & Osher, F. C. (1991). New Hampshire's specialized services for the dually diagnosed. In K. Minkoff & R. E. Drake (Eds.), *New Directions for Mental Health Services: Vol. 50. Dual Diagnosis of Major Mental Illness and Substance Disorder* (pp. 57–67). San Francisco: Jossey-Bass.

Drake, R. E., Bartels, S. J., Teague, G. B., Noordsy, D. L., & Clark, R. E. (1993). Treatment of substance abuse in severely mentally ill patients. *Journal of Nervous and Mental Diseases, 181,* 606–611.

Drake, R. E., Becker, D. R., Clark, R. E., & Mueser, K. T. (1999). Research on the Individual Placement and Support model of supported employment. *Psychiatric Quarterly, 70,* 627–633.

Drake, R. E., & Brunette, M. F. (1998). Complications of severe mental illness related to alcohol and other drug use disorders. In M. Galanter (Ed.), *Recent Developments in Alcoholism: Vol. 14. Consequences of Alcoholism* (pp. 285–299). New York: Plenum Press.

Drake, R. E., Brunette, M. F., & Mueser, K. T. (1998). Substance use disorder and social functioning in schizophrenia. In K. T. Mueser & N. Tarrier (Eds.), *Handbook of Social Functioning in Schizophrenia* (pp. 280–289). Boston: Allyn & Bacon.

Drake, R. E., Essock, S. M., Shaner, A., Carey, K. B., Minkoff, K., Kola, L., Lynde, D., Osher, F. C., Clark, R. E., & Rickards, L. (2001). Implementing dual diagnosis services for clients with severe mental illness. *Psychiatric Services, 52,* 469–476.

Drake, R. E., Gates, C., Whitaker, A., & Cotton, P. G. (1985). Suicide among schizophrenics: A review. *Comprehensive Psychiatry, 26,* 90–100.

Drake, R. E., McHugo, G., & Noordsy, D. L. (1993). Treatment of alcoholism among schizophrenic outpatients: Four-year outcomes. *American Journal of Psychiatry, 150,* 328–329.

Drake, R. E., McHugo, G. J., Clark, R. E., Teague, G. B., Xie, H., Miles, K., & Ackerson, T. H. (1998). Assertive community treatment for patients with co-occurring severe mental illness and substance use disorder: A clinical trial. *American Journal of Orthopsychiatry, 68,* 201–215.

Drake, R. E., Mercer-McFadden, C., Mueser, K. T., McHugo, G. J., & Bond, G. R. (1998). Review of integrated mental health and substance abuse treatment for patients with dual disorders. *Schizophrenia Bulletin, 24,* 589–608.

Drake, R. E., Mueser, K. T., Clark, R. E., & Wallach, M. A. (1996). The course, treatment, and outcome of substance disorder in persons with severe mental illness. *American Journal of Orthopsychiatry, 66,* 42–51.

Drake, R. E., & Noordsy, D. L. (1994). Case management for people with coexisting severe mental disorder and substance use disorder. *Psychiatric Annals, 24,* 427–431.

Drake, R. E., & Noordsy, D. L. (1995). The role of inpatient care for patients with co-occurring severe mental disorder and substance use disorder. *Community Mental Health Journal, 31,* 279–282.

Drake, R. E., Osher, F. C., Noordsy, D. L., Hurlbut, S. C., Teague, G. B., & Beaudett, M. S. (1990). Diagnosis of alcohol use disorders in schizophrenia. *Schizophrenia Bulletin, 16,* 57–67.

Drake, R. E., Osher, F. C., & Wallach, M. A. (1989). Alcohol use and abuse in schizophrenia: A prospective community study. *Journal of Nervous and Mental Disease, 177,* 408–414.

Drake, R. E., Rosenberg, S. D., & Mueser, K. T. (1996). Assessing substance use disorder in persons with severe mental illness. In R. E. Drake & K. T. Mueser (Eds.), *New Directions for Mental Health Services: Vol. 70. Dual Diagnosis of Major Mental Illness and Substance Abuse Volume 2: Recent Research and Clinical Implications* (pp. 3–17). San Francisco: Jossey-Bass.

Drake, R. E., & Wallach, M. A. (1988). Mental patients' attitudes toward hospitalization: A neglected aspect of hospital tenure. *American Journal of Psychiatry, 145,* 29–34.

Drake, R. E., & Wallach, M. A. (1993). Moderate drinking

among people with severe mental illness. *Hospital and Community Psychiatry, 44*, 780–782.

Drake, R. E., Wallach, M. A., & Hoffman, J. S. (1989). Housing instability and homelessness among aftercare patients of an urban state hospital. *Hospital and Community Psychiatry, 40*, 46–51.

Drake, R. E., Xie, H., McHugo, G. J., & Green, A. I. (2000). The effects of clozapine on alcohol and drug use disorders among schizophrenic patients. *Schizophrenia Bulletin, 26*, 441–449.

Drake, R. E., Yovetich, N. A., Bebout, R. R., Harris, M., & McHugo, G. J. (1997). Integrated treatment for dually diagnosed homeless adults. *Journal of Nervous and Mental Disease, 185*, 298–305.

Duke, P. J., Pantelis, C., & Barnes, T. R. E. (1994). South Westminster schizophrenia survey: Alcohol use and its relationship to symptoms, tardive dyskinesia and illness onset. *British Journal of Psychiatry, 164*, 630–636.

Durell, J., Lechtenberg, B., Corse, S., & Frances, R. (1993). Intensive case management of persons with chronic mental illness who abuse substances. *Hospital and Community Psychiatry, 44*, 415–416.

Dusenbury, L., Botvin, G. J., & James-Ortiz, S. (1989). The primary prevention of adolescent substance abuse through the promotion of personal and social competence. *Prevention in Human Services, 7*, 201–224.

Dyson, V., Appleby, L., Altman, E., Doot, M., Luchins, D. J., & Delehant, M. (1998). Efficiency and validity of commonly used substance abuse screening instruments in public psychiatric patients. *Journal of Addictive Diseases, 17*, 57–76.

D'Zurilla, T. J., & Nezu, A. M. (1999). *Problem-Solving Therapy: A Social Competence Approach to Clinical Intervention* (2nd ed.). New York: Springer.

Edens, J. F., Peters, R. H., & Hills, H. A. (1997). Treating prison inmates with co-occurring disorders: An integrative review of existing programs. *Behavioral Sciences and the Law, 15*, 439–457.

El-Guebaly, N. (1990). Substance abuse and mental disorders: The dual diagnoses concept. *Canadian Journal of Psychiaty, 35*, 261–341.

Ellis, A., & Harper, R. A. (1975). *A New Guide to Rational Living*. North Hollywood, CA: Wilshire.

Emrick, C. D., Tonigan, J. S., Montgomery, H., & Little, L. (1993). Alcoholics Anonymous: What is currently known. In B. S. McCrady & W. R. Miller (Eds.), *Research on Alcoholics Anonymous* (pp. 41–76). New Brunswick, NJ: Rutgers Center of Alcohol Studies.

Equal Employment Opportunity Commission. (1997). *Enforcement Guidance on the Americans with Disabilities Act and Psychiatric Disabilities* (915.002). Washington, DC: Americans with Disabilities Act Division, Office of Legal Counsel.

Estroff, S. (1981). *Making It Crazy: An Ethnography of Psychiatric Clients in an American Community*. Berkeley: University of California Press.

Fabian, E. S., Waterworth, A., & Ripke, B. (1993). Reasonable accommodation for workers with serious mental illness: Type, frequency, and associated outcomes. *Psychosocial Rehabilitation Journal, 17*(2), 163–172.

Falloon, I. R. H., Boyd, J. L., & McGill, C. W. (1984). *Family Care of Schizophrenia: A Problem-Solving Approach to the Treatment of Mental Illness*. New York: Guilford Press.

Falloon, I. R. H., Boyd, J. L., McGill, C. W., Williamson, M., Razani, J., Moss, H. B., Gilderman, A. M., & Simpson, G. M. (1985). Family management in the prevention of morbidity of schizophrenia: Clinical outcome of a two year longitudinal study. *Archives of General Psychiatry, 42*, 887–896.

Fals-Stewart, W., Birchler, G. R., & O'Farrell, T. J. (1996). Behavioral couples therapy for male substance-abusing patients: Effects on relationship adjustment and drug using behavior. *Journal of Consulting and Clinical Psychology, 64*, 959–972.

Fals-Stewart, W., O'Farrell, T. J., Freitas, T. T., McFarlin, S. K., & Rutigliano, P. (2000). The Timeline Followback reports of psychoactive substance use by drug-abusing patients: Psychometric properties. *Journal of Consulting and Clinical Psychology, 68*, 134–144.

Farina, A. (1998). Stigma. In K. T. Mueser & N. Tarrier (Eds.), *Handbook of Social Functioning in Schizophrenia* (pp. 247–279). Boston: Allyn & Bacon.

Feinberg, D. T., & Hartman, N. (1991). Methadone and schizophrenia. *American Journal of Psychiatry, 148*, 1750–1751.

Fernandez, G., & Nygard, S. (1990). Impact of involuntary outpatient commitment on the revolving-door syndrome in North Carolina. *Hospital and Community Psychiatry, 41*, 1001–1004.

Ferster, C. B. (1965). Classification of behavioral pathology. In L. Krasner & L. P. Ullman (Eds.), *Research in Behavior Modification* (pp. 2–26). New York: Holt, Rinehart & Winston.

Fichter, M. M., Glynn, S. M., Weyer, S., Liberman, R. P., & Frick, U. (1997). Family climate and expressed emotion in the course of alcoholism. *Family Process, 36*, 203–221.

Fisher, D. B. (1992). Humanizing the recovery process. *Resources, 4*, 5–6.

Fisher, M. S., & Bentley, K. J. (1996). Two group therapy models for clients with a dual diagnosis of substance abuse and personality disorder. *Psychiatric Services, 47*, 1244–1250.

Foa, E. B., & Kozak, M. J. (1997). *Mastery of Obsessive–Compulsive Disorder: Client Workbook*. San Antonio, TX: Psychological Corporation.

Foa, E. B., & Rothbaum, B. O. (1998). *Treating the Trauma of Rape: Cognitive-Behavioral Therapy for PTSD*. New York: Guilford Press.

Fogarty, J. S. (1997). Reactance theory and patient noncompliance. *Social Science and Medicine, 45*, 1277–1288.

Foote, J., DeLuca, A., Magura, S., Warner, A., Grand, A., Rosenblum, A., & Stahl, S. (1999). A group motivational treatment for chemical dependency. *Journal of Substance Abuse Treatment, 17*, 181–192.

Fowler, D., Garety, P., & Kuipers, E. (1995). *Cognitive Behaviour Therapy for Psychosis: Theory and Practice. Chichester, England: Wiley.

Fowler, I. L., Carr, V. J., Carter, N. T., & Lewin, T. J. (1998). Patterns of current and lifetime substance use in schizophrenia. *Schizophrenia Bulletin, 24,* 443–455.

Fox, L. (1999). Missing out on motherhood. *Psychiatric Services, 50,* 193–194.

Frese, F. J., & Davis, W. W. (1997). The consumer-survivor movement, recovery, and consumer professionals. *Professional Psychology: Research and Practice, 28,* 243–245.

Furlong-Norman, K. (Ed.). (1997). ADA and reasonable accommodations [Special issue]. *Community Support Network News, 12*(1).

Galanter, M., Castaneda, R., & Ferman, J. (1988). Substance abuse among general psychiatric patients: Place of presentation, diagnosis and treatment. *American Journal of Drug and Alcohol Abuse, 14,* 211–235.

Galanter, M., & Kleber, H. D. (Eds.). (1999). *Textbook of Substance Abuse Treatment* (2nd ed.). Washington, DC: American Psychiatric Press.

Galletly, C., Field, C., & Prior, M. (1993). Urine drug screening of patients admitted to a state psychiatric hospital. *Hospital and Community Psychiatry, 44,* 587–589.

Garbutt, J. C., West, S. L., Carey, T. S., Lohr, K. N., & Crews, F. T. (1999). Pharmacological treatment of alcohol dependence: A review of the evidence. *Journal of the American Medical Association, 28,* 1318–1325.

Garety, P. A., Fowler, D., & Kuipers, E. (2000). Cognitive-behavioral therapy for medication-resistant symptoms. *Schizophrenia Bulletin, 26,* 73–86.

Gartner, A., & Riessman, F. (1977). *Self-Help in the Human Services.* San Francisco: Jossey-Bass.

Gendreau, P. (1996). Offender rehabilitation: What we know and what needs to be done. *Criminal Justice and Behavior, 23,* 144–161.

Gershon, E. S., DeLisi, L. E., Hamovit, J., Nurnberger, J. I., Maxwell, M. E., Schreiber, J., Dauphinais, D., Dingman, C. W., & Guroff, J. J. (1988). A controlled family study of chronic psychoses: Schizophrenia and schizoaffective disorder. *Archives of General Psychiatry, 45,* 328–336.

Glassman, R., & Salzman, C. (1987). Interactions between psychotropic and other drugs: An update. *Hospital and Community Psychiatry, 34,* 897–902.

Godley, S. H., Hoewing-Roberson, R., & Godley, M. D. (1994). *Final MISA Report.* Bloomington, IL: Lighthouse Institute.

Goldfinger, S. M., Schutt, R. K., Seidman, L. J., Turner, W. M., Penk, W. E., & Tolomiczenko, G. S. (1996). Self-report and observer measures of substance abuse among homeless mentally ill persons in cross-section and over time. *Journal of Nervous and Mental Disease, 184,* 667–672.

Goldfinger, S. M., Schutt, R. K., Tolomiczenko, G. S., Seidman, L., Penk, W. E., Turner, W., & Caplan, B. (1999). Housing placement and subsequent days homeless among formerly homeless adults with mental illness. *Psychiatric Services, 50,* 674–679.

Goldfried, M. R., & Pomeranz, D. M. (1968). The role of assessment in behavior modification. *Psychological Reports, 23,* 75–87.

Goldiamond, I. (1974). Toward a constructional approach to social problems: Ethical and constitutional problems raised by applied behavioral analysis. *Behaviorism, 2,* 1–85.

Goldman, C. R., & Quinn, F. L. (1988). Effects of a patient education program in the treatment of schizophrenia. *Hospital and Community Psychiatry, 39,* 282–286.

Goodman, L. A., Salyers, M. P., Mueser, K. T., Rosenberg, S. D., Swartz, M., Essock, S. M., Osher, F. C., & Butterfield, M. I. (2001). Recent victimization in women and men with severe mental illness: Prevalence and correlates. *Journal of Traumatic Stress, 14,* 615–632.

Goodman, L. A., Thompson, K. M., Weinfurt, K., Corl, S., Acker, P., Mueser, K. T., & Rosenberg, S. D. (1999). Reliability of reports of violent victimization and PTSD among men and women with SMI. *Journal of Traumatic Stress, 12,* 587–599.

Goodwin, F. K., & Jamison, K. R. (1990). *Manic Depressive Illness.* New York: Oxford University Press.

Gould, R. A., Mueser, K. T., Bolton, E., Mays, V., & Goff, D. (2001). Cognitive therapy for psychosis in schizophrenia: A preliminary meta-analysis. *Schizophrenia Research, 48,* 335–342.

Graham, H. L. (1998). The role of dysfunctional beliefs in individual who experience psychosis and use substances: Implications for cognitive therapy and medication adherence. *Behavioural and Cognitive Psychotherapy, 26,* 193–207.

Graham, H. L., & Maslin, J. (2002). Problematic cannabis use amongst those with severe mental health problems in an inner city area of the UK. *Addictive Behaviors, 27,* 261–273.

Graham, H. L., Maslin, J., Copello, A., Birchwood, M., Mueser, K., McGovern, D., & Georgiou, G. (2001). Drug and alcohol problems amonst individuals with severe mental health problems in an inner city area of the UK. *Social Psychiatry and Psychiatric Epidemiology, 36,* 448–455.

Grassi, L., Pavanati, M., Cardelli, R., Ferri, S., & Peron, L. (1999). HIV-risk behaviour and knowledge about HIV/AIDS among patients with schizophrenia. *Psychological Medicine, 29,* 171–179.

Green, A. I., Tohen, M., Patel, J. K., Banov, M., DuRand, C., Berman, I., Chang, H., Zarate, C., Jr., Posener, J., Lee, H., Dawson, R., Richards, C., Cole, J. O., & Schatzberg, A. F. (2000). Clozapine in the treatment of refractory psychotic mania. *American Journal of Psychiatry, 157,* 982–986.

Green, A. I., Zimmet, S. V., Strous, R. D., & Schildkraut, J. J. (1999). Clozapine for comorbid substance use disorder and schizophrenia: Do patients with schizophrenia have a reward-deficiency syndrome that can be ameliorated by clozapine? *Harvard Review of Psychiatry, 6,* 287–296.

Green, M. F. (1996). What are the functional consequences of neurocognitive deficits in schizophrenia? *American Journal of Psychiatry, 153,* 321–330.

Green, M. F. (2001). *Schizophrenia Revealed*. New York: Norton.

Greenfield, S. F., Strakowski, S. M., Tohen, M., Batson, S. C., & Kolbrener, M. L. (1994). Childhood abuse in first-episode psychosis. *British Journal of Psychiatry, 164*, 831–834.

Greenfield, S. F., Weiss, R. D., & Tohen, M. (1995). Substance abuse and the chronically mentally ill: A description of dual diagnosis treatment services in a psychiatric hospital. *Community Mental Health Journal, 31*, 265–277.

Greenman, M., & McClellan, T. A. (1985). The impact of a more stringent commitment code in Minnsota. *Hospital and Community Psychiatry, 36*, 990–992.

Griffiths, R. R., & Wolf, B. (1990). Relative abuse liability of different benzodiazepines in drug abusers. *Journal of Clinical Psychopharmacology, 10*, 237–243.

Group for the Advancement of Psychiatry. (1994). *Forced into Treatment: The Role of Coercion in Clinical Practice*. Washington, DC: American Psychiatric Press.

Hall, R. C. W., Popkin, M. K., & DeVaul, R. (1977). The effect of unrecognized drug abuse on diagnosis and therapeutic outcome. *American Journal of Drug and Alcohol Abuse, 4*, 455–465.

Hall, R. G., Duhamel, M., McClanahan, R., Miles, G., Nason, C., Rosen, S., Schiller, P., Tao-Yonenaga, L., & Hall, S. M. (1995). Level of functioning, severity of illness, and smoking status among chronic psychiatric patients. *Journal of Nervous and Mental Disease, 183*, 468–471.

Hamera, E., Schneider, J. K., & Deviney, S. (1995). Alcohol, cannabis, nicotine, and caffeine use and symptom distress in schizophrenia. *Journal of Nervous and Mental Disease, 183*, 559–565.

Hamilton, T., & Sample, P. (1994). *The Twelve Steps and Dual Recovery: A Framework of Recovery for Those of Us with Addiction and an Emotional or Psychiatric Illness*. Center City, MN: Hazelden.

Harris, M., & Bergman, H. C. (1987). Case management with the chronically mentally ill: A clinical perspective. *American Journal of Orthopsychiatry, 57*, 296–302.

Hartman, D. P., Roper, B. L., & Bradford, D. C. (1979). Some relationships between behavioral and traditional assessment. *Journal of Behavioral Assessment, 1*, 3–21.

Hatfield, A. B., & Lefley, H. P. (1987). *Families of the Mentally Ill: Coping and Adaptation*. New York: Guilford Press.

Hatfield, A. B., & Lefley, H. P. (1993). *Surviving Mental Illness: Stress, Coping, and Adaptation*. New York: Guilford Press.

Hauri, P., & Linde, S. (1996). *No More Sleepless Nights* (rev. ed.). New York: Wiley.

Havassy, B. E., Shopshire, M. S., & Quigley, L. A. (2000). Effects of substance dependence on outcomes of patients in a randomized trial of two case management models. *Psychiatric Services, 51*, 639–644.

Hawkins, D. J., Catalano, R. F., & Miller, J. Y. (1992). Risk and protective factors for alcohol and other drug problems in adolescence and early adulthood: Implications for substance abuse prevention. *Psychological Bulletin, 112*, 64–105.

Hawkins, R. P. (1986). Selection of target behaviors. In R. O. Nelson & S. C. Hayes (Eds.), *Conceptual Foundations of Behavioral Assessment* (pp. 331–385). New York: Guilford Press.

Hayes, S. C., & Nelson, R. O. (1986). Assessing the effects of therapeutic interventions. In R. O. Nelson & S. C. Hayes (Eds.), *Conceptual Foundations of Behavioral Assessment* (pp. 430–460). New York: Guilford Press.

Hayes, S. C., Strosahl, K. D., & Wilson, K. G. (1999). *Acceptance and Commitment Therapy: An Experiential Approach to Behavior Change*. New York: Guilford Press.

Healey, A., Knapp, M., Astin, J., Beecham, J., Kemp, R., Kirov, G., & David, A. (1998). Cost-effectiveness evaluation of compliance therapy for people with psychosis. *British Journal of Psychiatry, 172*, 420–424.

Heather, N., Peters, T. J., & Stockwell, T. R. (Eds.). (2001). *Handbook of Alcohol Dependence and Related Problems*. Chichester, England: Wiley.

Heimberg, R. G., & Becker, R. E. (2002). *Cognitive Behavioral Group Therapy for Social Phobia*. New York: Guilford Press.

Heinssen, R. K., Liberman, R. P., & Kopelowicz, A. (2000). Psychosocial skills training for schizophrenia: Lessons from the laboratory. *Schizophrenia Bulletin, 26*, 21–46.

Hellerstein, D. J., & Meehan, B. (1987). Outpatient group therapy for schizophrenic substance abusers. *American Journal of Psychiatry, 144*, 1337–1339.

Hellerstein, D. J., Rosenthal, R. N., & Miner, C. R. (1995). A prospective study of integrated outpatient treatment for substance-abusing schizophrenic outpatients. *American Journal on Addictions, 4*, 33–42.

Hensel, B., Dunner, D. L., & Fieve, R. R. (1979). The relationship of family history of alcoholism to primary affective disorder. *Journal of Affective Disorders, 1*, 105–113.

Herman, S. E., Boots-Miller, B., Jordan, L., Mowbray, C. T., Brown, W. G., Deiz, N., Bandla, H., Solomon, M., & Green, P. (1997). Immediate outcomes of substance use treatment within a state psychiatric hospital. *Journal of Mental Health Administration, 24*, 126–138.

Herz, M. I., Lamberti, J. S., Mintz, J., Scott, R., O'Dell, S. P., McCartan, L., & Nix, G. (2000). A program for relapse prevention in schizophrenia: A controlled study. *Archives of General Psychiatry, 57*, 277–283.

Hester, R. K., & Miller, W. R. (Eds.). (1995). *Handbook of Alcoholism Treatment Approaches: Effective Alternatives* (2nd ed.). Boston: Allyn & Bacon.

Hiday, V. A. (1992). Coercion in civil commitment: Process, preferences and outcome. *International Journal of Law and Psychiatry, 15*, 359–377.

Hiday, V. A. (1996). Involuntary commitment as a psychiatric technology. *International Journal of Technology Assessment in Health Care, 12*, 585–603.

Hiday, V. A., & Scheid-Cook, T. L. (1987). The North Carolina experience with outpatient commitment: A critical appraisal. *International Journal of Law and Psychiatry, 10*, 215–232.

Hiday, V. A., & Scheid-Cook, T. L. (1989). A follow-up of chronic patients committed to outpatient treatment. *Hospital and Community Psychiatry, 40*, 52–58.

Hiday, V. A., & Scheid-Cook, T. L. (1990). Outpatient commitment for revolving door patients: Treatment and compliance. *Journal of Nervous and Mental Disease, 179,* 85–90.

Hiday, V. A., Swartz, M. S., Swanson, J. W., Borum, R., & Wagner, H. R. (1999). Criminal victimization of persons with severe mental illness. *Psychiatric Services, 50,* 62–68.

Hiday, V. A., Swartz, M. S., Swanson, J. W., Borum, R., & Wagner, H. R. (2002). Impact of outpatient commitment on victimization of people with severe mental illness. *American Journal of Psychiatry, 159,* 1403–1411.

Hiday, V. A., Swartz, M. S., Swanson, J. W., & Wagner, H. R. (1997). Patient perceptions of coercion in mental hospital admission. *International Journal of Law and Psychiatry, 20,* 227–241.

Higgins, S. T., Budney, A. J., Bickel, W. K., Foerg, F. E., Donham, R., & Badger, G. J. (1994). Incentives improve outcome in outpatient behavioral treatment of cocaine dependence. *Archives of General Psychiatry, 51,* 568–576.

Himmelhoch, J. M., Mulla, D., Neil, J. F., Detre, T. P., & Kupfer, D. J. (1976). Incidence and significance of mixed affective states in a bipolar population. *Archives of General Psychiatry, 33,* 1062–1066.

Himmelhoch, J. M., Neil, J. F., May, S. J., Fuchs, C. Z., & Licata, S. M. (1980). Age, dementia, dyskinesias, and lithium response. *American Journal of Psychiatry, 137,* 941–945.

Hodgins, S., & Côté, G. (1993). The criminality of mentally disordered offenders. *Criminal Justice and Behavior, 28,* 115–129.

Hodgins, S., Toupin, J., & Côté, G. (1996). Schizophrenia and antisocial personality disorder: A criminal combination. In L. B. Schlesinger (Ed.), *Explorations in Criminal Psychopathology: Clinical Syndromes with Forensic Implications* (pp. 217–237). Springfield, IL: Thomas.

Hser, Y.-I., Hoffman, V., Grella, C. E., & Anglin, D. (2001). A 33–year follow-up of narcotics addicts. *Archives of General Psychiatry, 58,* 503–508.

Hser, Y. I., Anglin, D., & Powers, K. (1993). A 24–year follow-up of California narcotics addicts. *Archives of General Psychiatry, 50,* 577–584.

Hughes, J. R., Hatsukami, D. K., Mitchell, J. E., & Dahlgren, L. A. (1986). Prevalence of smoking among psychiatric outpatients. *American Journal of Psychiatry, 143,* 993–997.

Hughes, J. R., & Howard, T. S. (1997). Nicotine and caffeine use as confounds in psychiatric studies. *Biological Psychiatry, 42,* 1184–1185.

Hunt, G. E., Bergen, J., & Bashir, M. (2002). Medication compliance and comorbid substance abuse in schizophrenia: Impact on community survival 4 years after a relapse. *Schizophrenia Research, 54,* 253–264.

Hutchings, P. S., & Dutton, M. A. (1993). Sexual assault history in a community mental health center clinical population. *Community Mental Health Journal, 29,* 59–63.

Inciardi, J. A., McBride, D. C., & Rivers, J. E. (1996). *Drug Control and the Courts.* Thousand Oaks, CA: Sage.

Intagliata, J. (1982). Improving the quality of community care for the chronically mentally disabled: The role of case management. *Schizophrenia Bulletin, 8,* 655–674.

Jackson, H. J., Whiteside, H. L., Bates, G. W., Rudd, R. P., & Edwards, J. (1991). Diagnosing personality disorders in psychiatric inpatients. *Acta Psychiatrica Scandinavica, 83,* 206–213.

Jacobsen, E. (1952). Deaths of alcoholic patients treated with disulfiram. *Quarterly Journal of Studies on Alcohol, 13,* 16–26.

Jacobson, A. (1989). Physical and sexual assault histories among psychiatric outpatients. *American Journal of Psychiatry, 146,* 755–758.

Jacobson, A., & Herald, C. (1990). The relevance of childhood sexual abuse to adult psychiatric inpatient care. *Hospital and Community Psychiatry, 41,* 154–158.

Janowsky, D. S., & Davis, J. M. (1976). Methylphenidate, dextroamphetamine, and levamphetamine. *Archives of General Psychiatry, 33,* 304–308.

Jerrell, J. M. (1996). Cost-effective treatment for persons with dual disorder. In R. E. Drake & K. T. Mueser (Eds.), *New Directions for Mental Health Services: Vol. 70. Dual Diagnosis of Major Mental Illness and Substance Abuse Volume 2: Recent Research and Clinical Implications* (pp. 79–91). San Francisco: Jossey-Bass.

Jerrell, J. M., Hu, T., & Ridgely, M. S. (1994). Cost-effectiveness of substance abuse treatments for the SMI. *Journal of Mental Health Administration, 21,* 281–295.

Jerrell, J. M., & Ridgely, M. S. (1995a). Comparative effectiveness of three approaches to serving people with severe mental illness and substance use disorders. *Journal of Nervous and Mental Disease, 183,* 566–576.

Jerrell, J. M., & Ridgely, M. (1995b). Evaluating changes in symptoms and functioning of dually diagnosed clients in specialized treatment. *Psychiatric Services, 46,* 233–238.

Jerrell, J. M., & Ridgely, M. S. (1999). Impact of robustness of program implementation on outcomes of clients in dual diagnosis programs. *Psychiatric Services, 50,* 109–112.

Joffe, R. T., & Schuller, D. R. (1993). An open study of buspirone augmentation of serotonin reuptake inhibitors in refractory depression. *Journal of Clinical Psychiatry, 54,* 269–271.

Johnson, B. A., Roache, J. D., Javors, M. A., DiClemente, C. C., Cloninger, C. R., Prihoda, T. J., Bordnick, P. S., Ait-Daoud, N., & Hensler, J. (2000). Ondansetron for reduction of drinking among biologically predisposed alcoholic patients: A randomized controlled trial. *Journal of the American Medical Association, 284,* 963–971.

Johnson, R. E., Chutuape, M. A., Strain, E. C., Walsh, S. L., Stitzer, M. L., & Bigelow, G. E. (2000). A comparison of levomethadyl acetate, buprenorphine and methadone for opioid dependence. *New England Journal of Medicine, 343,* 1290–1297.

Jones, P., Guth, C., Lewis, S., & Murray, R. (1994). Low intelligence and poor educational achievement precede early onset schizophrenic psychosis. In A. S. David & J. C. Cutting (Eds.), *The Neuropsychology of Schizophrenia* (pp. 131–144). Brighton, England: Erlbaum.

Judd, L. L., Janowsky, D. S., Segal, D. S., Parker, D. C., &

Huey, L. Y. (1981). Behavioral effects of methodone in schizophrenic patients. *American Journal of Psychiatry, 138,* 243–245.

Kanfer, F. H., & Saslow, G. (1969). Behavioral diagnosis. In C. M. Franks (Ed.), *Behavior Therapy: Appraisal and Status* (pp. 417–444). New York: McGraw-Hill.

Kanter, J. (1989). Clinical case management: Definitions, principles, components. *Hospital and Community Psychiatry, 40,* 361–368.

Kashner, M., Rader, L., Rodell, D., Beck, C., Rodell, L., & Muller, K. (1991). Family characteristics, substance abuse, and hospitalization patterns of patients with schizophrenia. *Hospital and Community Psychiatry, 42,* 195–197.

Kaufmann, C. (1993). Reasonable accommodation to mental health disabilities at work: Legal constructs and practical applications. *International Journal of Psychiatry and Law, 21,* 153–174.

Kavanagh, D. J. (1995). An intervention for substance abuse in schizophrenia. *Behaviour Change, 12,* 20–30.

Kavanagh, D. J., Greenway, L., Jenner, L., Saunders, J. B., White, A., Sorban, J., & Hamilton, G. (2000). Contrasting views and experiences of health professionals on the management of comorbid substance misuse and mental disorders. *Australian and New Zealand Journal of Psychiatry, 34,* 279–289.

Kay, S. R., Opler, L. A., & Fiszbein, A. (1987). The Positive and Negative Syndrome Scale (PANSS) for schizophrenia. *Schizophrenia Bulletin, 13,* 261–276.

Keith, S. J., Regier, D. A., & Rae, D. S. (1991). Schizophrenic disorders. In L. N. Robins & D. A. Regier (Eds.), *Psychiatric Disorders in America: The Epidemiologic Catchment Area Study* (pp. 33–52). New York: Free Press.

Kemp, R., Hayward, P., Applewhaite, G., Everitt, B., & David, A. (1996). Compliance therapy in psychotic patients: Randomised controlled trial. *British Medical Journal, 312,* 345–349.

Kemp, R., Kirov, G., Everitt, B., Hayward, P., & David, A. (1998). Randomised controlled trial of compliance therapy: 18-month follow-up. *British Journal of Psychiatry, 173,* 271–272.

Kessler, R. C., Crum, R. M., Warner, L. A., Nelson, C. B., Schulenberg, J., & Anthony, J. C. (1997). Lifetime co-occurrence of DSM-III-R alcohol abuse and dependence with other psychiatric disorders in the National Comorbidity Survey. *Archives of General Psychiatry, 54,* 313–321.

Kessler, R. C., Nelson, C. B., McGonagle, K. A., Edlund, M. J., Frank, R. G., & Leaf, P. J. (1996). The epidemiology of co-occurring addictive and mental disorders: Implications for prevention and service utilization. *American Journal of Orthopsychiatry, 66,* 17–31.

Khantzian, E. J. (1985). The self-medication hypothesis of addictive disorders: Focus on heroin and cocaine dependence. *American Journal of Psychiatry, 142,* 1259–1264.

Khantzian, E. J. (1997). The self-medication hypothesis of substance use disorders: A reconsideration and recent applications. *Harvard Review of Psychiatry, 4,* 231–244.

Kilpatrick, D. G., Acierno, R., Resnick, H. S., Saunders, B. E., & Best, C. L. (1997). A 2-year longitudinal analysis of the relationships between violent assault and substance use in women. *Journal of Consulting and Clinical Psychology, 65,* 834–847.

Kingsbury, S. J., & Salzman, C. (1990). Disulfiram in the treatment of alcoholic patients with schizophrenia. *Hospital and Community Psychiatry, 41,* 133–134.

Kline, J., Harris, M., Bebout, R. R., & Drake, R. E. (1991). Contrasting integrated and linkage models of treatment for homeless, dually diagnosed adults. In K. Minkoff & R. Drake (Eds.), *New Directions for Mental Health Services: Vol. 50. Dual Diagnosis of Major Mental Illness and Substance Disorder* (pp. 95–106). San Francisco: Jossey-Bass.

Kloos, B., Zimmerman, S. O., Scrimenti, K., & Crusto, C. (2002). Landlords as partners for promoting success in supported housing: "It takes more than a lease and a key." *Psychiatric Rehabilitation Journal, 25,* 235–244.

Kofoed, L., Kania, J., Walsh, T., & Atkinson, R. (1986). Outpatient treatment of patients with substance abuse and coexisting psychiatric disorders. *American Journal of Psychiatry, 143,* 867–872.

Kofoed, L., & Keys, A. (1988). Using group therapy to persuade dual-diagnosis patients to seek substance abuse treatment. *Hospital and Community Psychiatry, 39,* 1209–1211.

Kopelowicz, A., Liberman, R. P., Mintz, J., & Zarate, R. (1997). Comparison of efficacy of social skills training for deficit and nondeficit negative symptoms in schizophrenia. *American Journal of Psychiatry, 154,* 424–425.

Kozak, M. J., & Foa, E. B. (1997). *Mastery of Obsessive–Compulsive Disorder: Therapist Guide.* San Antonio, TX: Psychological Corporation.

Kranzler, H., Burleson, J., DelBoca, F., Babor, T., Korner, P., Brown, J., & Bohn, M. (1994). Buspirone treatment of anxious alcoholics. *Archives of General Psychiatry, 51,* 720–731.

Krystal, J. H., D'Souza, D. C., Madonick, S., & Petrakis, I. L. (1999). Toward a rational pharmacotherapy of comorbid substance abuse in schizophrenic patients. *Schizophrenia Research, 35,* S35–S49.

Kuipers, L., Leff, J., & Lam, D. (1992). *Family Work for Schizophrenia: A Practical Guide.* London: Gaskell.

Kurtz, L., Garvin, C., Hill, E., Pollio, D., McPherson, S., & Powell, T. (1995). Involvement in Alcoholics Anonymous by persons with dual disorders. *Alcoholism Treatment Quarterly, 12,* 1–17.

Kushner, M. G., Abrams, K., & Borchardt, C. (2000). The relationship between anxiety disorders and alcohol use disorders: A review of major perspectives and findings. *Clinical Psychology Review, 20,* 149–171.

Kushner, M. G., & Mueser, K. T. (1993). Psychiatric co-morbidity with alcohol use disorders. In *Eighth Special Report to the U.S. Congress on Alcohol and Health* (NIH Publication No. 94-3699, pp. 37–59). Rockville, MD: U.S. Department of Health and Human Services.

Lam, J. A., & Rosenheck, R. (1998). The effect of victimization on clinical outcomes of homeless persons with serious mental illness. *Psychiatric Services, 49,* 678–683.

Lamb, H. R., & Weinberger, L. E. (1993). Therapeutic use of conservatorship in the treatment of gravely disabled psychiatric patients. *Hospital and Community Psychiatry, 44,* 147–150.

Langer, E. J. (1989). *Mindfulness.* Reading, MA: Addison-Wesley.

Larson, E. W., Olincy, A., Rummans, T. A., & Morse, R. M. (1992). Disulfiram treatment of patients with both alcohol dependence and other psychiatric disorders: A review. *Alcoholism: Clinical and Experimental Research, 16,* 125–130.

Laudet, A. B., Magura, S., Vogel, H. S., & Knight, E. (2000). Addiction services: Support, mutual aid and recovery from dual diagnosis. *Community Mental Health Journal, 36,* 457–476.

Leadbetter, R. A., Shutty, M. S. J., Higgins, P. B., & Pavalonis, D. (1994). Multidisciplinary approach to psychosis, intermittent hyponatremia, and polydipsia. *Schizophrenia Bulletin, 20,* 375–385.

Leete, E. (1989). How I perceive and manage my illness. *Schizophrenia Bulletin, 15,* 197–200.

Lefley, H. P. (1996). *Family Caregiving in Mental Illness.* Thousand Oaks, CA: Sage.

Lehman, A. F., Goldberg, R., Dixon, L. B., McNary, S., Postrado, L., Hackman, A., & McDonnell, K. (2002). Improving employment outcomes for persons with severe mental illnesses. *Archives of General Psychiatry, 59,* 165–172.

Lehman, A. F., Herron, J., Schwartz, R., & Myers, C. (1993). Rehabilitation for adults with severe mental illness and substance use disorders: A clinical trial. *Journal of Nervous and Mental Disease, 181,* 86–90.

Lehman, A. F., Myers, C., Corty, E., & Thompson, J. (1994). Severity of substance-use disorders among psychiatric inpatients. *Journal of Nervous and Mental Disease, 182,* 164–167.

Liberman, R. P. (Ed.). (1992). *Handbook of Psychiatric Rehabilitation.* Boston: Allyn & Bacon.

Liberman, R. P., DeRisi, W. J., & Mueser, K. T. (1989). *Social Skills Training for Psychiatric Patients.* Needham Heights, MA: Allyn & Bacon.

Liberman, R. P., Mueser, K. T., Wallace, C. J., Jacobs, H. E., Eckman, T., & Massel, H. K. (1986). Training skills in the psychiatrically disabled: Learning coping and competence. *Schizophrenia Bulletin, 12,* 631–647.

Liberman, R. P., Wallace, C. J., Blackwell, G., Kopelowicz, A., Vaccaro, J. V., & Mintz, J. (1998). Skills training versus psychosocial occupational therapy for persons with persistent schizophrenia. *American Journal of Psychiatry, 155,* 1087–1091.

Liddon, S. C., & Satran, R. (1967). Disulfiram (Antabuse) psychosis. *American Journal of Psychiatry, 123,* 1284–1289.

Lidz, C. W., Mulvey, E. P., Arnold, R. P., Bennett, N. S., & Kirsch, B. L. (1993). Coercive interactions in a psychiatric emergency room. *Behavioral Sciences and the Law, 11,* 269–280.

Lieberman, J. A., Kinon, B. J., & Loebel, A. D. (1990). Dopaminergic mechanisms in idiopathic and drug-induced psychoses. *Schizophrenia Bulletin, 16,* 97–110.

Lindsley, O. R. (1964). Direct measurement and prosthesis of retarded behavior. *Journal of Education, 147,* 304–312.

Linehan, M. M. (1993). *Cognitive-Behavioral Treatment of Borderline Personality Disorder.* New York: Guilford Press.

Linszen, D., Dingemans, P., Van der Does, A. J. W., Scholte, P., Lenior, R., & Goldstein, M. J. (1996). Treatment, expressed emotion and relapse in recent onset schizophrenic disorders. *Psychological Medicine, 26,* 333–342.

Lintzeris, N., Bell, J., Bammer, G., Jolley, D. J., & Rushworth, L. (2002). A randomized controlled trial of buprenorphine in the management of short-term ambulatory heroin withdrawal. *Addiction, 97,* 1395–1404.

Lipsey, M. W. (1995). What do we learn from 400 research studies on the effectiveness of treatment with juvenile delinquents? In J. McGuire (Ed.), *What Works: Reducing Reoffending* (pp. 63–78). Chichester, England: Wiley.

Littrell, K. H., Petty, R. G., Hilligoss, N. M., Peabody, C. D., & Johnson, C. G. (2001). Olanzapine treatment for patients with schizophrenia and substance abuse. *Journal of Substance Abuse Treatment, 21,* 217–221.

Lösel, F. (1995). The efficacy of correctional treatment: A review and synthesis of meta-evaluations. In J. McGuire (Ed.), *What Works: Reducing Reoffending* (pp. 79–111). Chichester, England: Wiley.

Lucksted, A., & Coursey, R. D. (1995). Therapeutic use of conservatorship in the treatment of gravely disabled psychiatric patients. *Psychiatric Services, 46,* 146–152.

Lukoff, D., Nuechterlein, K. H., & Ventura, J. (1986). Manual for the Expanded Brief Psychiatric Rating Scale (BPRS). *Schizophrenia Bulletin, 12,* 594–602.

Madera, E. J. (1988, May). Seven principles in self help: Understanding how self-help groups help. *New Program Initiatives in Mental Health* [Newsletter published by the New Jersey State Division of Mental Health and Hospitals], pp. 3–4.

Mahoney, M. J. (1991). *Human Change Processes: The Scientific Foundations of Psychotherapy.* New York: Basic Books.

Maier, W., Lichtermann, D., Minges, J., Delmo, C., & Heun, R. (1995). The relationship between bipolar disorder and alcoholism: A controlled family study. *Psychological Medicine, 25,* 787–796.

Maisto, S. A., Carey, M. P., Carey, K. B., Gordon, C. M., & Gleason, J. R. (2000). Use of the AUDIT and the DAST-10 to identify alcohol and drug use disorders among adults with a severe and persistent mental illness. *Psychological Assessment, 12,* 186–192.

Malcolm, R., Anton, R. F., Randall, C. L., Johnston, A., Brady, K., & Thevos, A. (1992). A placebo controlled trial of buspirone in anxious inpatient alcoholics. *Alcoholism: Clinical and Experimental Research, 16,* 1007–1013.

Malcolm, R., Ballenger, J. C., Sturgis, E. T., & Anton, R. (1989). Double-blind controlled trial comparing carbamazepine to oxazepam treatment of alcohol withdrawal. *American Journal of Psychiatry, 146,* 617–621.

Mancuso, L. L. (1990). Reasonable accommodation for workers with psychiatric disabilities. *Psychosocial Rehabilitation Journal, 14*(2), 3–19.

Mansour, A., Meador-Woodruff, J. H., López, J. F., & Watson, S. J. (1998). Biochemical anatomy: Insights into the cell biology and pharmacology of the dopamine and serotonin systems in the brain. In A. F. Schatzberg & C. B. Nemeroff (Eds.), *The American Psychiatric Press Textbook of Psychopharmacology* (2nd ed., pp. 55–73). Washington, DC: American Psychiatric Press.

Marder, S. R., Wirshing, W. C., Mintz, J., McKenzie, J., Johnston, K., Eckman, T. A., & Johnston-Cronk, K. (1996). Two-year outcome for social skills training and group psychotherapy for outpatients with schizophrenia. *American Journal of Psychiatry, 153*, 1585–1592.

Marlatt, G. A. (Ed.). (1998). *Harm Reduction: Pragmatic Strategies for Managing High-Risk Behaviors*. New York: Guilford Press.

Marlatt, G. A., & Gordon, J. R. (Eds.). (1985). *Relapse Prevention: Maintenance Strategies in the Treatment of Addictive Behaviors*. New York: Guilford Press.

Marlatt, G. A., & Witkiewitz, K. (2002). Harm reduction approaches to alcohol use: Health promotion, prevention, and treatment. *Addictive Behaviors, 27*, 867–886.

Marlin, E. (1989). *Genograms: The New Tool for Exploring the Personality, Career, and Love Patterns You Inherit*. Chicago: Contemporary Books.

Martensen-Larsen, O. (1951). Psychotic phenomena provoked by tetra-ethylthiuram disulfide. *Quarterly Journal of Studies on Alcohol, 12*, 206–216.

Maslin, J., Graham, H. L., Cawley, M., A, C., Birchwood, M., Georgiou, G., McGovern, D., Mueser, K., & Orford, J. (2001). Combined severe mental health and substance use problems: What are the training and support needs of staff working with this client group? *Journal of Mental Health, 10*, 131–140.

Mason, B. J., Kocsis, J. H., Melia, D., Khuri, E. T., Sweeney, J., Wells, A., Borg, L., Millman, R. B., & Kreek, M. J. (1998). Psychiatric comorbidity in methadone maintained patients. *Journal of Addictive Diseases, 17*, 75–89.

Mason, B. J., Kocsis, J. H., Ritvo, E. C., & Cutler, R. B. (1996). A double-blind, placebo controlled trial of desipramine for primary alcohol dependence stratified on the presence or absence of major depression. *Journal of the American Medical Association, 275*, 761–767.

Mason, B. J., Salvato, F. R., Williams, L. D., Ritvo, E. C., & Cutler, R. B. (1999). A double-blind, placebo-controlled study of oral nalmefene for alcohol dependence. *Archives of General Psychiatry, 56*, 719–724.

Matousek, N., Edwards, J., Jackson, H. J., Rudd, R. P., & McMurry, N. E. (1992). Social skills training and negative symptoms. *Behavior Modification, 16*, 39–63.

Mayfield, D., McCleod, G., & Hall, P. (1974). The CAGE questionnaire: Validation of a new alcoholism screening questionnaire. *American Journal of Psychiatry, 131*, 1121–1123.

Mayfield, D. G., & Coleman, L. L. (1968). Alcohol use and affective disorder. *Diseases of the Nervous System, 29*, 467–474.

McDowell, D., Galanter, M., Goldfarb, L., & Lifshutz, H.

(1996). Spirituality and the treatment of the dually-diagnosed: An investigation of patient and staff attitudes. *Journal of Addictive Diseases, 15*, 55–68.

McElroy, S. L., Dessain, E. C., Pope, H. G., Jr., Cole, J. O., Keck, P. E., Jr., Frankenburg, F. R., Aizley, H. G., & O'Brien, S. (1991). Clozapine in the treatment of psychotic mood disorders, schizoaffective disorder, and schizophrenia. *Journal of Clinical Psychiatry, 52*, 411–414.

McFarlane, A. C. (1998). Epidemiologic evidence about the relationship between PTSD and alcohol abuse: The nature of the association. *Addictive Behaviors, 6*, 813–825.

McFarlane, A. C., Bookless, C., & Air, T. (2001). Posttraumatic stress disorder in a general psychiatric inpatient population. *Journal of Traumatic Stress, 14*, 633–645.

McFarlane, W. R. (1990). Multiple family groups and the treatment of schizophrenia. In M. I. Herz, S. J. Keith, & J. P. Docherty (Eds.), *Handbook of Schizophrenia: Vol. 4. Psychosocial Treatment of Schizophrenia* (pp. 167–189). Amsterdam: Elsevier.

McFarlane, W. R. (2002). *Multifamily Groups in the Treatment of Severe Psychiatric Disorders*. New York: Guilford Press.

McGrath, P. J., Nunes, E. V., Stewart, J. W., Goldman, D., Agosti, V., Ocepek-Welikson, K., & Quitkin, F. M. (1996). Imipramine treatment of alcoholics with primary depression. *Archives of General Psychiatry, 53*, 232–240.

McHugo, G. J., Drake, R. E., Burton, H. L., & Ackerson, T. H. (1995). A scale for assessing the stage of substance abuse treatment in persons with severe mental illness. *Journal of Nervous and Mental Disease, 183*, 762–767.

McHugo, G. J., Drake, R. E., Teague, G. B., & Xie, H. (1999). Fidelity to assertive community treatment and client outcomes in the New Hampshire dual disorders study. *Psychiatric Services, 50*, 818–824.

McLellan, A. T., Alterman, A. I., Metzger, D. S., Grisson, G. R., Woody, G. E., Luborsky, L., & O'Brien, C. P. (1994). Similarity of outcome predictors across opiate, cocaine, and alcohol treatment services. *Journal of Consulting and Clinical Psychology, 62*, 1141–1158.

McPhillips, M. A., Kelly, F. J., Barnes, T. R. E., Kuke, P. J., Gene-Cos, N., & Clark, K. (1997). Detecting comorbid substance misuse among people with schizophrenia in the community: A study comparing the results of questionnaires with analysis of hair and urine. *Schizophrenia Research, 25*, 141–148.

Meil, W. M., & Schter, M. D. (1997). Olanzapine attenuates the reinforcing effects of cocaine. *European Journal of Pharmacology, 340*, 17–26.

Meisler, N., & Williams, O. (1998). Replicating effective supported employment models for adults with psychiatric disabilities. *Psychiatric Services, 49*, 1419–1421.

Meissen, G., Powell, T. J., Wituk, S. A., Girrens, K., & Arteaga, S. (1999). Attitudes of AA contact persons toward group participation by persons with a mental illness. *Psychiatric Services, 50*, 1079–1081.

Meltzer, H. Y., & Kostakoglu, A. E. (2000). Combining antipsychotics: Is there evidences for efficacy? *Psychiatric Times, 17*(9), 25–34.

Mercer-McFadden, C., Drake, R. E., Brown, N. B., & Fox, R. S. (1997). The community support program demonstrations of services for young adults with severe mental illness and substance use disorders 1987–1991. *Psychiatric Rehabilitation Journal, 20*(3), 13–24.

Mercer-McFadden, C., Drake, R. E., Clark, R. E., Verven, N., Noordsy, D. L., & Fox, T. S. (1998). *Substance Abuse Treatment for People with Severe Mental Disorders: A Program Manager's Guide.* Concord: New Hampshire–Dartmouth Psychiatric Research Center.

Merry, J., Reynolds, C. M., Bailey, J., & Coppen, A. (1976). Prophylactic treatment of alcoholism by lithium carbonate. *Lancet, i,* 481–482.

Meyer, R., Babor, T., & Hesselbrock, V. (1988). An alcohol research center in concept and practice: Interdisciplinary collaboration at the UConn ARC. *British Journal of Addiction, 83,* 245–252.

Meyers, R. J., & Smith, J. E. (1995). *Clinical Guide to Alcohol Treatment: The Community Reinforcement Approach.* New York: Guilford Press.

Miklowitz, D. J., Simoneau, T. L., George, E. L., Richards, J. A., Kalbag, A., Sachs-Sricsson, N., & Suddath, R. (2000). Family-focused treatment of bipolar disorder: 1–year effects of a psychoeducational program in conjunction with pharmacotherapy. *Biological Psychiatry, 48,* 582–592.

Miller, B. A., Downs, W. R., & Testa, M. (1993). Interrelationships between victimization experiences and women's alcohol use. *Journal of Studies on Alcohol, 54*(Suppl. 11), 109–117.

Miller, L. J., & Finnerty, M. (1996). Sexuality, pregnancy, and childrearing among women with schizophrenia-spectrum disorders. *Psychiatric Services, 4,* 502–506.

Miller, W. R. (1995). Increasing motivation to change. In R. K. Hester & W. R. Miller (Eds.), *Handbook of Alcoholism Treatment Approaches: Effective Alternatives* (2nd ed., pp. 89–104). Boston: Allyn & Bacon.

Miller, W. R., Brown, J. M., Simpson, T. L., Handmaker, N. S., Bien, T. H., Luckie, L. F., Montgomery, H. A., Hester, R. K., & Tonigan, J. S. (1995). What works?: A methodological analysis of the alcohol treatment outcome literature. In R. K. Hester & W. R. Miller (Eds.), *Handbook of Alcoholism Treatment Approaches: Effective Alternatives* (2nd ed., pp. 12–44). Boston: Allyn & Bacon.

Miller, W. R., & Rollnick, S. (2002). *Motivational Interviewing (2nd ed.): Preparing People for Change.* New York: Guilford Press.

Millett, K. (1991). *The Loony Bin Trip.* London: Virago Press.

Milton, F., Patwa, V. K., & Hafner, R. J. (1978). Confrontation vs. belief modification in persistently deluded patients. *British Journal of Medical Psychology, 51,* 127–130.

Miner, C. R., Rosenthal, R. N., Hellerstein, D. J., & Muenz, L. R. (1997). Prediction of compliance with outpatient referral in patients with schizophrenia and psychoactive substance use disorders. *Archives of General Psychiatry, 54,* 706–712.

Minkoff, K. (1989). An integrated treatment model for dual diagnosis of psychosis and addiction. *Hospital and Community Psychiatry, 40,* 1031–1036.

Minkoff, K., Rossi, A., Ajilore, C., & Cahill, C. (1997). *Center for Mental Health Services Managed Care Initiative: Clinical Standards and Workforce Competencies Project. Annotated Bibliography.* Rockville, MD: Center for Mental Health Services.

Minski, L. (1938). Psychopathology and psychoses associated with alcohol. *Journal of Mental Science, 84,* 985–990.

Mischel, W. (1968). *Personality and Assessment.* New York: Wiley.

Monahan, J., Hoge, S. K., Lidz, C., Roth, L. H., Bennett, N., Gardner, W., & Mulvey, E. (1995). Coercion and commitment: Understanding involuntary mental hospital admission. *International Journal of Law and Psychiatry, 18,* 249–263.

Monahan, J., Hoge, S. K., Lidz, C. W., Eisenberg, M. M., Bennett, N. S., Gardner, W. P., Mulvey, E. P., & Roth, L. H. (1996). Coercion to inpatient treatment: Initial results and implications for assertive treatment in the community. In D. L. Dennis & J. Monahan (Eds.), *Coercion and Aggressive Community Treatment* (pp. 13–28). New York: Plenum Press.

Monti, P. M., Abrams, D. B., Kadden, R. M., & Cooney, N. L. (2002). *Treating Alcohol Dependence* (2nd ed.). New York: Guilford Press.

Morales-Dorta, J. (1976). *Puerto Rican Espiritismo: Religion and Psychotherapy.* New York: Vantage.

Morgenstern, J., Labouvie, E., McCrady, B. S., Kahler, C. W., & Frey, R. M. (1997). Affiliation with Alcoholics Anonymous after treatment: A study of its therapeutic effects and mechanisms of action. *Journal of Consulting and Clinical Psychology, 65,* 768–777.

Mowbray, C. T., Solomon, M., Ribisl, K. M., Ebejer, M. A., Deiz, N., Brown, W., Banla, H., Luke, D. A., Davidson, W. S., & Herman, S. (1995). Treatment for mental illness and substance abuse in a public psychiatric hospital. *Journal of Substance Abuse Treatment, 12,* 129–139.

Mowrer, O. H. (1950). *Learning Theory and Personality Dynamics.* New York: Ronald Press.

Mueser, K. T. (1998). Social skill and problem solving. In A. S. Bellack & M. Hersen (Eds.), *Comprehensive Clinical Psychology* (Vol. 6, pp. 183–201). New York: Pergamon Press.

Mueser, K. T., Becker, D. R., & Wolfe, R. (2001). Supported employment, job preferences, and job tenure and satisfaction. *Journal of Mental Health, 10,* 411–417.

Mueser, K. T., & Bellack, A. S. (1998). Social skills and social functioning. In K. T. Mueser & N. Tarrier (Eds.), *Handbook of Social Functioning in Schizophrenia* (pp. 79–96). Needham Heights, MA: Allyn & Bacon.

Mueser, K. T., Bellack, A. S., Douglas, M. S., & Morrison, R. L. (1991). Prevalence and stability of social skill deficits in schizophrenia. *Schizophrenia Research, 5,* 167–176.

Mueser, K. T., Bellack, A. S., Wade, J. H., Sayers, S. L., & Rosenthal, C. K. (1992). Educational needs assessment of chronic psychiatric patients and their relatives. *British Journal of Psychiatry, 160,* 674–680.

Mueser, K. T., Bennett, M., & Kushner, M. G. (1995). Epidemiology of substance abuse among persons with chronic mental disorders. In A. F. Lehman & L. Dixon (Eds.),

Double Jeopardy: Chronic Mental Illness and Substance Abuse (pp. 9–25). New York: Harwood Academic.

Mueser, K. T., Bond, G. R., Drake, R. E., & Resick, S. G. (1998). Models of community care for severe mental illness: A review of research on case management. *Schizophrenia Bulletin, 24*, 37–74.

Mueser, K. T., Corrigan, P. W., Hilton, D., Tanzman, B., Schaub, A., Gingerich, S., Essock, S. M., Tarrier, N., Morey, B., Vogel-Scibilia, S., & Herz, M. I. (2002). Illness management and recovery for severe mental illness: A review of the research. *Psychiatric Services, 53*, 1272–1284.

Mueser, K. T., Drake, R. E., Ackerson, T. H., Alterman, A. I., Miles, K. M., & Noordsy, D. L. (1997). Antisocial personality disorder, conduct disorder, and substance abuse in schizophrenia. *Journal of Abnormal Psychology, 106*, 473–477.

Mueser, K. T., Drake, R. E., Clark, R. E., McHugo, G. J., Mercer-McFadden, C., & Ackerson, T. (1995). *Toolkit for Evaluating Substance Abuse in Persons with Severe Mental Illness*. Cambridge, MA: Evaluation Center at Human Services Research Institute.

Mueser, K. T., Drake, R. E., & Noordsy, D. L. (1998). Integrated mental health and substance abuse treatment for severe psychiatric disorders. *Journal of Practical Psychiatry and Behavioral Health, 4*, 129–139.

Mueser, K. T., Drake, R. E., & Wallach, M. A. (1998). Dual diagnosis: A review of etiological theories. *Addictive Behaviors, 23*, 717–734.

Mueser, K. T., Essock, S. M., Drake, R. E., Wolfe, R. S., & Frisman, L. (2001). Rural and urban differences in dually diagnosed patients: Implications for service needs. *Schizophrenia Research, 48*, 93–107.

Mueser, K. T., & Fox, L. (2000). Family-friendly services: A modest proposal [Letter to the editor]. *Psychiatric Services, 51*, 1452.

Mueser, K. T., & Fox, L. (2002). A family intervention program for dual disorders. *Community Mental Health Journal, 38*, 253–270.

Mueser, K. T., Fox, M., Kenison, L. B., & Geltz, B. L. (1995). *The Better Living Skills Group*. Concord, NH: New Hampshire–Dartmouth Psychiatric Research Center.

Mueser, K. T., & Gingerich, S. L. (1994). *Coping with Schizophrenia: A Guide for Families*. Oakland, CA: New Harbinger.

Mueser, K. T., & Glynn, S. M. (1999). *Behavioral Family Therapy for Psychiatric Disorders* (2nd ed.). Oakland, CA: New Harbinger.

Mueser, K. T., Glynn, S. M., Corrigan, P. W., & Baber, W. (1996). A survey of preferred terms for users of mental health services. *Psychiatric Services, 47*, 760–761.

Mueser, K. T., Goodman, L. B., Trumbetta, S. L., Rosenberg, S. D., Osher, F. C., Vidaver, R., Auciello, P., & Foy, D. W. (1998). Trauma and posttraumatic stress disorder in severe mental illness. *Journal of Consulting and Clinical Psychology, 66*, 493–499.

Mueser, K. T., Nishith, P., Tracy, J. I., DeGirolamo, J., & Molinaro, M. (1995). Expectations and motives for substance use in schizophrenia. *Schizophrenia Bulletin, 21*, 367–378.

Mueser, K. T., & Noordsy, D. L. (1996). Group treatment for dually diagnosed clients. In R. E. Drake & K. T. Mueser (Eds.), *New Directions for Mental Health Services: Vol. 70. Dual Diagnosis of Major Mental Illness and Substance Abuse Volume 2: Recent Research and Clinical Implications* (pp. 33–51). San Francisco: Jossey-Bass.

Mueser, K. T., Noordsy, D. L., Fox, L., & Wolfe, R. (in press). Disulfiram treatment for alcoholism in severe mental illness. *American Journal on Addictions*.

Mueser, K. T., Rosenberg, S. D., Drake, R. E., Miles, K. M., Wolford, G., Vidaver, R., & Carrieri, K. (1999). Conduct disorder, antisocial personality disorder, and substance use disorders in schizophrenia and major affective disorders. *Journal of Studies on Alcohol, 60*, 278–284.

Mueser, K. T., Rosenberg, S. D., Goodman, L. A., & Trumbetta, S. L. (2002). Trauma, PTSD, and the course of schizophrenia: An interactive model. *Schizophrenia Research, 53*, 123–143.

Mueser, K. T., Salyers, M. P., & Mueser, P. R. (2001). A prospective analysis of work in schizophrenia. *Schizophrenia Bulletin, 27*, 281–296.

Mueser, K. T., Salyers, M. P., Rosenberg, S. D., Ford, J. D., Fox, L., & Cardy, P. (2001). A psychometric evaluation of trauma and PTSD assessments in persons with severe mental illness. *Psychological Assessment, 13*, 110–117.

Mueser, K. T., Sayers, S. L., Schooler, N. R., Mance, R. M., & Haas, G. L. (1994). A multisite investigation of the reliability of the Scale for the Assessment of Negative Symptoms. *American Journal of Psychiatry, 151*, 1453–1462.

Mueser, K. T., Sengupta, A., Schooler, N. R., Bellack, A. S., Xie, H., Glick, I. D., & Keith, S. J. (2001). Family treatment and medication dosage reduction in schizophrenia: Effects on patient social functioning, family attitudes, and burden. *Journal of Consulting and Clinical Psychology, 69*, 3–12.

Mueser, K. T., Valentiner, D. P., & Agresta, J. (1997). Coping with negative symptoms of schizophrenia: Patient and family perspectives. *Schizophrenia Bulletin, 23*, 329–339.

Mueser, K. T., Yarnold, P. R., & Bellack, A. S. (1992). Diagnostic and demographic correlates of substance abuse in schizophrenia and major affective disorder. *Acta Psychiatrica Scandinavica, 85*, 48–55.

Mueser, K. T., Yarnold, P. R., Levinson, D. F., Singh, H., Bellack, A. S., Kee, K., Morrison, R. L., & Yadalam, K. G. (1990). Prevalence of substance abuse in schizophrenia: Demographic and clinical correlates. *Schizophrenia Bulletin, 16*, 31–56.

Mueser, K. T., Yarnold, P. R., Rosenberg, S. D., Swett, C., Miles, K. M., & Hill, D. (2000). Substance use disorder in hospitalized severely mentally ill psychiatric patients: Prevalence, correlates, and subgroups. *Schizophrenia Bulletin, 26*, 179–192.

Munetz, M. R. (Ed.). (1997). *Can mandatory treatment be therapeutic?* (New Directions for Mental Health Services, Vol. 75). San Francisco: Jossey-Bass.

Munsey, D. F., Galanter, M., Lifshutz, H., & Franco, H.

(1992). Antecedents, severity of abuse, and response to treatment in substance-abusing schizophrenic individuals. *American Journal on Addictions, 1*, 210–216.

Nasrallah, H. A. (1979). Vulnerability to disulfiram psychosis. *Western Journal of Medicine, 130*, 575–577.

Nelson, R. O., & Hayes, S. C. (1986). The nature of behavioral assessment. In R. O. Nelson & S. C. Hayes (Eds.), *Conceptual Foundations of Behavioral Assessment* (pp. 3–41). New York: Guilford Press.

Neria, Y., Bromet, E. J., Sievers, S., Lavelle, J., & Fochtmann, L. J. (2002). Trauma exposure and posttraumatic stress disorder in psychosis: Findings from a first-admission cohort. *Journal of Consulting and Clinical Psychology, 70*, 246–251.

Nezu, A. M., & Nezu, C. M. (Eds.). (1989). *Clinical Decision Making in Behavior Therapy: A Problem-Solving Perspective*. Champaign, IL: Research Press.

Nezu, A. M., Nezu, C. M., & Perri, M. G. (1989). *Problem-Solving Therapy for Depression: Therapy, Research, and Clinical Guidelines*. New York: Wiley.

Nishith, P., Mueser, K. T., Srsic, C. S., & Beck, A. T. (1997). Expectations and motives for alcohol use in a psychiatric outpatient population. *Journal of Nervous and Mental Disease, 185*, 622–626.

Nishith, P., Resick, P. A., & Mueser, K. T. (2001). Sleep disturbances and alcohol use motives in female rape victims with posttraumatic stress disorder. *Journal of Traumatic Stress, 14*, 469–479.

Noordsy, D. L., & Drake, R. E. (1994). Case management. In N. Miller (Ed.), *Treating Coexisting Psychiatric and Addictive Disorders: A Practical Guide* (pp. 231–244). Center City, MN: Hazelden.

Noordsy, D. L., Drake, R. E., Biesanz, J. C., & McHugo, G. J. (1994). Family history of alcoholism in schizophrenia. *Journal of Nervous and Mental Disease, 186*, 651–655.

Noordsy, D. L., Drake, R. E., Teague, G. B., Osher, F. C., Hurlbut, S. C., Beaudett, M. S., & Paskus, T. S. (1991). Subjective experiences related to alcohol abuse among schizophrenics. *Journal of Nervous and Mental Disease, 179*, 410–414.

Noordsy, D. L., & O'Keefe, C. (1999). Effectiveness of combining atypical antipsychotics and psychosocial rehabilitation in a CMHC setting. *Journal of Clinical Psychiatry, 60*(Suppl. 19), 47–51.

Noordsy, D. L., O'Keefe, C., Mueser, K. T., & Xie, H. (2001). Six month outcomes for patients switched to olanzapine treatment in community psychiatric care. *Psychiatric Services, 52*, 501–507.

Noordsy, D. L., Schwab, B., Fox, L., & Drake, R. E. (1996). The role of self-help programs in the rehabilitation of persons with severe mental illness and substance use disorders. *Community Mental Health Journal, 32*, 71–81.

Noordsy, D. L., Torrey, W. C., Mead, S., Brunette, M., Potenza, D., & Copeland, M. E. (2000). Recovery-oriented pharmacology: Redefining the goals of antipsychotic treatment. *Journal of Clinical Psychiatry, 61* (Suppl. 3), 22–29.

Nuechterlein, K. H., & Dawson, M. E. (1984). A heuristic vulnerability/stress model of schizophrenic episodes. *Schizophrenia Bulletin, 10*, 300–312.

Nunes, E. V., & Quitkin, F. M. (1997). Treatment of depression in drug-dependent patients: Effects on mood and drug use. In L. S. Onken, J. D. Blaine, S. Genser, & A. M. Horton (Eds.), *Treatment of Drug-Dependent Individuals with Comorbid Mental Disorders* (NIDA Research Monograph No. 172, pp. 61–85). Rockville, MD: National Institute on Drug Abuse.

O'Farrell, T. J., Cutter, H. S., & Floyd, F. J. (1985). Evaluating behavioral marital therapy for male alcoholics: Effects on marital adjustment and communication from before to after treatment. *Behavior Therapy, 16*, 147–167.

O'Farrell, T. J., Cutter, H. S. G., Chouquette, K. S., Floyd, F. J., & Bayog, R. D. (1992). Behavioral marital therapy for male alcoholics: Marital and drinking adjustment during the two years after treatment. *Behavior Therapy, 23*, 529–549.

O'Keefe, C., Potenza, D. P., & Mueser, K. T. (1997). Treatment outcomes for severely mentally ill patients on conditional discharge to community-based treatment. *Journal of Nervous and Mental Disease, 185*, 409–411.

O'Leary, K. D., & Wilson, G. T. (1975). *Behavior Therapy: Application and Outcome*. Englewood Cliffs, NJ: Prentice-Hall.

Olfson, M., Mechanic, D., Hansell, S., Boyer, C. A., & Walkup, J. (1999). Prediction of homelessness within three months of discharge among inpatients with schizophrenia. *Psychiatric Services, 50*, 667–673.

Olivera, A. A., Kiefer, M. W., & Manley, N. K. (1990). Tardive dyskinesia in psychiatric patients with substance use disorders. *American Journal of Drug and Alcohol Abuse, 16*, 57–66.

O'Malley, S. S., Jaffe, A. J., Chang, G., Schottenfeld, R. S., Meyer, R. E., & Rounsaville, B. (1992). Naltrexone and coping skills therapy for alcohol dependence: A controlled study. *Archives of General Psychiatry, 49*, 881–887.

Osher, F. C., & Dixon, L. B. (1996). Housing for persons with co-occurring mental and addictive disorders. In R. E. Drake & K. T. Mueser (Eds.), *New Directions for Mental Health Services: Vol. 70. Dual Diagnosis of Major Mental Illness and Substance Abuse Volume 2: Recent Research and Clinical Implications* (pp. 53–64). San Francisco: Jossey-Bass.

Osher, F. C., & Drake, R. E. (1996). Reversing a history of unmet needs: Approaches to care for persons with co-occurring addictive and mental disorders. *American Journal of Orthopsychiatry, 66*, 4–11.

Osher, F. C., Drake, R. E., Noordsy, D. L., Teague, G. B., Hurlbut, S. C., & Paskus, T. J. (1994). Correlates and outcomes of alcohol use disorder among rural schizophrenic outpatients. *Journal of Clinical Psychiatry, 55*, 109–113.

Osher, F. C., & Kofoed, L. L. (1989). Treatment of patients with psychiatric and psychoactive substance use disorders. *Hospital and Community Psychiatry, 40*, 1025–1030.

Pandina, R. J., Labouvie, E. W., Johnson, V., & White, H. R. (1990). The relationship between alcohol and marijuana use and competence in adolescence. *Journal of Health and Social Policy, 1,* 89–108.

Pani, P. P., Trogu, E., Contu, P., Agus, A., & Gessa, G. L. (1997). Psychiatric severity and treatment response in a comprehensive methadone maintainance treatment program. *Drug and Alcohol Dependence, 48,* 119–126.

Panocka, I., Pomeei, P., & Massi, M. (1993). Suppression of alcohol preference in rats induced by risperidone, a serotonin 5–HT2 and dopamine D2 antagonist. *Brain Research Bulletin, 31,* 595–599.

Parks, G. A., Anderson, B. K., & Marlatt, G. A. (2001). Relapse prevention therapy. In N. Heather, T. J. Peters, & T. Stockwell (Eds.), *Handbook of Alcohol Dependence and Problems* (pp. 575–592). Chichester, England: Wiley.

Paul, G. L., & Lentz, R. J. (1977). *Psychosocial Treatment of Chronic Mental Patients: Milieu versus Social-Learning Programs.* Cambridge, MA: Harvard University Press.

Paulman, R., Devous, M., Gregory, R., Herman, J., Jennings, L., Bonte, F., Nasrallah, H., & Raese, J. (1990). Hypofrontality and cognitive impairment in schizophrenia: Dynamic single-photon tomography and neuropsychological assessment of schizophrenic brain function. *Biological Psychiatry, 27,* 377–399.

Penn, P. E., & Brooks, A. J. (1999). *Comparing Substance Abuse Treatments for Dual Diagnosis. Final Report.* Tucson, AZ: La Frontera Center.

Perry, A., Tarrier, N., Morriss, R., McCarthy, E., & Limb, K. (1999). Randomised controlled trial of efficacy of teaching patients with bipolar disorder to identify early symptoms of relapse and obtain treatment. *British Medical Journal, 318,* 149–153.

Peters, R. H., & Bartoi, M. G. (1997). *Screening and Assessment of Co-Occurring Disorders in the Justice System.* Delmar, NY: National GAINS Center.

Peters, R. H., Greenbaum, P. E., Edens, J. F., Carter, C. R., & Ortiz, M. M. (1998). Prevalence of DSM-IV substance abuse and dependence disorders among prison inmates. *American Journal of Drug and Alcohol Abuse, 24,* 573–587.

Peters, R. H., & Hills, H. A. (1999). Community treatment and supervision strategies for offenders with co-occurring disorders: What works? In E. Latessa (Ed.), *Strategic Solutions: The International Community Corrections Association Examines Substance Abuse* (pp. 81–137). Lanham, MD: American Correctional Association.

Peters, R. H., Kearns, W. D., Murrin, M. R., & Dolente, A. S. (1992). Psychopathology and mental health needs among drug-involved inmates. *Journal of Prison and Jail Health, 111,* 3–25.

Peters, R. H., & Murrin, M. R. (2000). Effectiveness of treatment-based drug courts in reducing criminal recidivism. *Criminal Justice and Behavior, 27,* 72–96.

Phillips, P., & Johnson, S. (2001). How does drug and alcohol misuse develop among people with psychotic illness?: A literature review. *Social Psychiatry and Psychiatric Epidemiology, 36,* 269–276.

Pitschel-Walz, G., Leucht, S., Bäuml, J., Kissling, W., & Engel, R. R. (2001). The effect of family interventions on relapse and rehospitalization in schizophrenia: A meta-analysis. *Schizophrenia Bulletin, 27,* 73–92.

Polcin, D. L. (1992). Issues in the treatment of dual diagnosis clients who have chronic mental illness. *Professional Psychology: Research and Practice, 23,* 30–37.

Policy Research Associates. (1998). *Final Report: Research Study of the New York City Involuntary Outpatient Commitment Program.* New York: New York City Department of Mental Health, Mental Retardation, and Alcoholism Services.

Popper, K. R. (1959). *The Logic of Scientific Discovery.* New York: Harper & Row.

Post, R. M., & Kopanda, R. T. (1976). Cocaine, kindling, and psychosis. *American Journal of Psychiatry, 133,* 627–634.

Posternak, M. A., & Mueller, T. I. (2001). Assessing the risks and benefits of benzodiazepines for anxiety disorders in patients with a history of substance abuse or dependence. *American Journal on Addictions, 10,* 48–68.

Poulsen, E., Loft, S., Anderson, J. R., & Andersen, M. (1992). Disulfiram therapy: Adverse drug reactions and interactions. *Acta Psychiatrica Scandinavica, 86,* 59–66.

Prien, R. F., Caffey, E. M., Jr., & Klett, J. (1974). Factors associated with treatment success in lithium carbonate prophylaxis: Report of the Veterans Administration and National Institute of Mental Health Collaborative Study Group. *Archives of General Psychiatry, 31,* 189–192.

Prochaska, J. O. (1984). *Systems of Psychotherapy: A Transtheoretical Analysis.* Homewood, IL: Dorsey Press.

Prochaska, J. O., & DiClemente, C. C. (1984). *The Transtheoretical Approach: Crossing the Traditional Boundaries of Therapy.* Homewood, IL: Dow-Jones/Irwin.

Prochaska, J. O., DiClemente, C. C., & Norcross, J. C. (1992). In search of how people change: Applications to addictive behaviors. *American Psychologist, 47,* 1102–1114.

Prochaska, J. O., Norcross, J. C., & DiClemente, C. C. (1994). *Changing for Good.* New York: Avon Books.

Project Link. (1999). Prevention of jail and hospital recidivism among persons with severe mental illness. *Psychiatric Services, 50,* 1477–1480.

Project MATCH Research Group. (1997). Matching alcohol treatment to client heterogeneity: Project MATCH posttreatment drinking outcomes. *Journal of Studies on Alcohol, 58,* 7–29.

Pulver, A. E., Wolyniec, P. S., Wagner, M. G., Moorman, C. C., & McGrath, J. A. (1989). An epidemiologic investigation of alcohol-dependent schizophrenics. *Acta Psychiatrica Scandinavica, 79,* 603–612.

RachBeisel, J., Scott, J., & Dixon, L. (1999). Co-occurring severe mental illness and substance abuse disorders: A review of recent research. *Psychiatric Services, 50,* 1427–1434.

Rajkumar, S., & Thara, R. (1989). Factors affecting relapse in schizophrenia. *Schizophrenia Research, 2,* 403–409.

Randolph, E. T., Glynn, S. M., Eth, S., Paz, G. G., Leong, G. B., & Shaner, A. L. (1995). *Family therapy for schizophrenia: Two year outcome.* Paper presented at the annual meeting of the American Psychiatric Association, Miami, FL.

Rapp, C. A. (1993). Theory, principles, and methods of the strengths model of case management. In M. Harris & H. C. Bergman (Eds.), *Case Management: Theory and Practice* (pp. 143–164). New York: Harwood Academic.

Rapp, C. A. (1998a). The active ingredients of effective case management: A research synthesis. *Community Mental Health Journal, 34,* 363–380.

Rapp, C. A. (1998b). *The Strengths Model: Case Management with People Suffering from Severe and Persistent Mental Illness.* New York: Oxford University Press.

Räsänen, P., Tiihonen, J., Isohanni, M., Rantakallio, P., Lehtonen, J., & Moring, J. (1998). Schizophrenia, alcohol abuse, and violent behavior: A 26-year followup study of an unselected birth cohort. *Schizophrenia Bulletin, 24,* 437–441.

Raskin, D. E. (1972). Akathisia: A side effect to be remembered. *American Journal of Psychiatry, 129,* 121–123.

Regier, D. A., Farmer, M. E., Rae, D. S., Locke, B. Z., Keith, S. J., Judd, L. L., & Goodwin, F. K. (1990). Comorbidity of mental disorders with alcohol and other drug abuse: Results from the Epidemiologic Catchment Area (ECA) study. *Journal of the American Medical Association, 264,* 2511–2518.

Rehabilitation Act Amendments of 1998: Title IV of the Workforce Investment Act of 1998, Pub. Law 105-220, 112 Stat. 936.

Rehav, M., Rivera, J. J., Nuttbrock, L., Ng-Mak, D., Sturz, E. L., Link, B. G., Struening, E. L., Pepper, B., & Gross, B. (1995). Characteristics and treatment of homeless, mentally ill, chemical-abusing men. *Journal of Psychoactive Drugs, 27,* 93–103.

Reich, L. H., Davies, R. K., & Himmelhoch, J. M. (1974). Excessive alcohol use in manic–depressive illness. *American Journal of Psychiatry, 131,* 83–86.

Resick, P. A., & Schnicke, M. K. (1992). Cognitive processing therapy for sexual assault victims. *Journal of Consulting and Clinical Psychology, 60,* 748–756.

Ridgely, M. S., Goldman, H. H., & Willenbring, M. (1990). Barriers to the care of persons with dual diagnoses: Organizational and financing issues. *Schizophrenia Bulletin, 16,* 123–132.

Rimmer, J., & Jacobsen, B. (1977). Alcoholism in schizophrenics and their relatives. *Journal of Studies on Alcohol, 38,* 1781–1784.

Roberts, L. J., Shaner, A., & Eckman, T. A. (1999). *Overcoming Addictions: Skills Training for People with Schizophrenia.* New York: Norton.

Robins, L. N. (1966). *Deviant Children Grown Up.* Huntington, NY: Krieger.

Robinson, D. G., Woerner, M. G., Alvir, J. M. J., Bilder, R. M., Hinrichsen, G. A., & Lieberman, J. A. (2002). Predictors of medication discontinuation by patients with first-episode schizophrenia and schizoaffective disorder. *Schizophrenia Research, 57,* 209–219.

Rogers, E. S., Walsh, D., Masotta, L., & Danley, K. (1991). *Massachusetts Survey of Client Preferences for Community Support Services (Final Report).* Boston: Center for Psychiatric Rehabilitation.

Room, R. (1993). Alcoholics Anonymous as a social movement.

In B. S. McCrady & W. R. Miller (Eds.), *Research on Alcoholics Anonymous* (pp. 167–189). New Brunswick, NJ: Rutgers Center of Alcohol Studies.

Rose, S. M., Peabody, C. G., & Stratigeas, B. (1991). Undetected abuse among intensive case management clients. *Hospital and Community Psychiatry, 42,* 499–503.

Rosen, A. J., Sussman, S., Mueser, K. T., Lyons, J. S., & Davis, J. M. (1981). Behavioral assessment of psychiatric inpatients and normal controls across different environmental contexts. *Journal of Behavioral Assessment, 3,* 25–36.

Rosen, M. I., Rosenheck, R. A., Shaner, A., Eckman, T., Gamache, G., & Krebs, C. (2002). Veterans who may need a payee to prevent misuse of funds for drugs. *Psychiatric Services, 53,* 995–1000.

Rosenberg, S. D., Drake, R. E., Wolford, G. L., Mueser, K. T., Oxman, T. E., Vidaver, R. M., Carrieri, K. L., & Luckoor, R. (1998). The Dartmouth Assessment of Lifestyle Instrument (DALI): A substance use disorder screen for people with severe mental illness. *American Journal of Psychiatry, 155,* 232–238.

Rosenberg, S. D., Goodman, L. A., Osher, F. C., Swartz, M., Essock, S. M., Butterfield, M. I., Constantine, N. T., Wolford, G. L., & Salyers, M. P. (2001). Prevalence of HIV, hepatitis B and hepatitis C in people with severe mental illness. *American Journal of Public Health, 91,* 31–37.

Rosenberg, S. D., Trumbetta, S. L., Mueser, K. T., Goodman, L. A., Osher, F. C., Vidaver, R. M., & Metzger, D. S. (2001). Determinants of risk behavior for HIV/AIDS in people with severe and persistent mental illness. *Comprehensive Psychiatry, 42,* 263–271.

Rosenthal, R. N., Hellerstein, D. J., & Miner, C. R. (1992). Integrated services for treatment of schizophrenic substance abusers: Demographics, symptoms, and substance abuse patterns. *Psychiatric Quarterly, 63,* 3–26.

Ross, C. A., Anderson, G., & Clark, P. (1994). Childhood abuse and the positive symptoms of schizophrenia. *Hospital and Community Psychiatry, 45,* 489–491.

Ross, H. E., Glaser, F. B., & Germanson, T. (1988). The prevalence of psychiatric disorders in patients with alcohol and other drug problems. *Archives of General Psychiatry, 45,* 1023–1031.

Roy, A. (Ed.). (1986). *Suicide in Schizophrenia.* Baltimore: Williams & Wilkins.

Rudgley, R. (1998). *The Encyclopedia of Psychoactive Substances.* New York: Dunn.

Rush, A. J., Rago, W. V., Crismon, M. L., Toprac, M. G., Shon, S. P., Suppes, T., Miller, A. L., Trivedi, M. H., Swann, A. C., Biggs, M. M., Shores-Wilson, K., Kashner, T. M., Pigott, T., Chiles, J. A., Gilbert, D. A., & Altshuler, K. Z. (1999). Medication treatment for the severely and persistently mentally ill: The Texas Medication Algorithm Project. *Journal of Clinical Psychiatry, 60,* 284–291.

Russell, M., Martier, S. S., Sokol, R. J., Mudar, P., Bottoms, S., Jacobson, S., & Jacobson, J. (1994). Screening for pregnancy risk-drinking. *Alcoholism: Clinical and Experimental Research, 18,* 1156–1161.

Safer, D. (1987). Substance abuse by young adult chronic patients. *Hospital and Community Psychiatry, 38,* 511–514.

Salyers, M. P., & Mueser, K. T. (2001). Social functioning, psychopathology, and medication side effects in relation to substance use and abuse in schizophrenia. *Schizophrenia Research, 48*, 109–123.

Saunders, J. B., Aasland, O. G., Babor, T. F., De La Fuente, J. R., & Grant, M. (1993). Development of the Alcohol Use Disorders Identification Test (AUDIT): WHO Collaborative Project on Early Detection of Persons with Harmful Alcohol Consumption II. *Addiction, 88*, 791–804.

Schatzberg, A. F., Cole, J. O., & DeBattista, C. (1997). *Manual of Clinical Psychopharmacology* (3rd ed.). Washington, DC: American Psychiatric Press.

Schatzberg, A. F., & Nemeroff, C. B. (Eds.). (1998). *The American Psychiatric Press Textbook of Psychopharmacology* (2nd ed.). Washington, DC: American Psychiatric Press.

Schatzberg, A. F., & Nemeroff, C. B. (Eds.). (2001). *Essentials of Clinical Psychopharmacology*. Washington, DC: American Psychiatric Press.

Scheller-Gilkey, G., Thomas, S. M., Woolwine, B. J., & Miller, A. J. (2002). Increased early life stress and depressive symptoms in patients with comorbid substance abuse and schizophrenia. *Schizophrenia Bulletin, 28*, 223–231.

Schneier, F. R., & Siris, S. G. (1987). A review of psychoactive substance use and abuse in schizophrenia. *Journal of Nervous and Mental Disease, 175*, 641–652.

Schooler, N. R., Keith, S. J., Severe, J. B., Matthews, S. M., Bellack, A. S., Glick, I. D., Hargreaves, W. A., Kane, J. M., Ninan, P. T., Frances, A., Jacobs, M., Lieberman, J. A., Mance, R., Simpson, G. M., & Woerner, M. G. (1997). Relapse and rehospitalization during maintenance treatment of schizophrenia: The effects of dose reduction and family treatment. *Archives of General Psychiatry, 54*, 453–463.

Schuckit, M. (1983). Alcoholism and other psychiatric disorders. *Hospital and Community Psychiatry, 34*, 1022–1027.

Schuckit, M. A., Zisook, S., & Mortola, J. (1985). Clinical implications of DSM-III diagnoses of alcohol abuse and alcohol dependence. *American Journal of Psychiatry, 142*, 1403–1408.

Schwab, B., Clark, R. E., & Drake, R. E. (1991). An ethnographic note on clients as parents. *Psychiatric Rehabilitation Journal, 15*, 95–99.

Schwartz, A., & Goldiamond, I. (1975). *Social Casework: A Behavioral Approach*. New York: Columbia University Press.

Segal, Z. V., Williams, J. M. G., & Teasdale, J. D. (2002). *Mindfulness-Based Cognitive Therapy for Depression*. New York: Guilford Press.

Seidman, L. J., Kremen, W. S., Koren, D., Farone, S. V., Goldstein, J. M., & Tsuang, M. T. (2002). A comparative profile analysis of neuropsychological functioning in patients with schizophrenia and bipolar psychosis. *Schizophrenia Research, 53*, 31–44.

Seinen, A., Dawe, S., Kavanagh, D. J., & Bahr, M. (2000). An examination of the utility of the AUDIT in people diagnosed with schizophrenia. *Journal of Studies on Alcohol, 61*, 744–750.

Selzer, M. L. (1971). The Michigan Alcoholism Screening Test: The quest for a new diagnostic instrument. *American Journal of Psychiatry, 127*, 1653–1658.

Sengupta, A., Drake, R. E., & McHugo, G. J. (1998). The relationship between substance use disorder and vocational functioning among persons with severe mental illness. *Psychiatric Rehabilitation Journal, 22*, 41–45.

Sensky, T., Turkington, D., Kingdon, D., Scott, J. L., Scott, J., Siddle, R., O'Carroll, M., & Barnes, T. R. E. (2000). A randomized controlled trial of cognitive-behavioral therapy for persistent symptoms in schizophrenia resistant to medication. *Archives of General Psychiatry, 57*, 165–172.

Serper, M. R., Alpert, M., Richardson, N. A., Dickson, S., Allen, M. H., & Werner, A. (1995). Clinical effects of recent cocaine use on patients with acute schizophrenia. *American Journal of Psychiatry, 152*, 1464–1469.

Shaner, A., Khalsa, M. A., Roberts, L., Wilkins, J., Anglin, D., & Hsieh, S. C. (1993). Unrecognized cocaine use among schizophrenic patients. *American Journal of Psychiatry, 150*, 758–762.

Shaner, A., Roberts, L. J., Eckman, T. A., Racenstein, J. M., Tucker, D. E., Tsuang, J. W., & Mintz, J. (1998). Sources of diagnostic uncertainty for chronically psychotic cocaine abusers. *Psychiatric Services, 49*, 684–690.

Silverman, K., Higgins, S. T., Brooner, R. K., Montoya, I. D., Cone, E. J., Schuster, C. R., & Preston, K. L. (1996). Sustained cocaine abstinence in methadone maintenance patients through voucher-based reinforcement therapy. *Archives of General Psychiatry, 53*, 409–415.

Simpson, D. D., Joe, G. W., Lehman, W. E. K., & Sells, S. B. (1986). Addiction careers: Etiology, treatment, and 12 year follow-up procedures. *Journal of Drug Issues, 16*, 107–121.

Siris, S. G., Bermanzohn, P. C., Mason, S. E., & Shuwell, M. A. (1991). Antidepressant for substance-abusing schizophrenic patients: A minireview. *Progress in Neuropsychopharmacology and Biological Psychiatry, 15*, 1–13.

Sitharthan, T., Singh, S., Kranitis, P., Currie, J., Freeman, P., Murugesan, G., & Ludowici, J. (1999). Integrated drug and alcohol intervention: Development of an opportunistic intervention program to reduce alcohol and other substance use among psychiatric patients. *Australian and New Zealand Journal of Psychiatry, 33*, 676–683.

Skinner, H. A. (1982). The Drug Abuse Screening Test. *Addictive Behaviors, 7*, 363–371.

Smith, G. R., & Burns, B. J. (1994). Recommendations of the Little Rock Working Group on mental health and substance abuse disorders in health-care reform. *Journal of Mental Health Administration, 20*, 247–253.

Sobell, M. B., Maisto, S. A., Sobell, L. C., Copper, A. M., & Sanders, B. (1980). Developing a prototype for evaluating alcohol treatment effectiveness. In L. C. Sobell, M. B. Sobell, & E. Ward (Eds.), *Evaluating Alcohol and Drug Abuse Treatment Effectiveness* (pp. 129–150). New York: Pergamon Press.

Sobell, M. B., & Sobell, L. C. (1993). *Problem Drinkers: Guided Self-Change Treatment*. New York: Guilford Press.

Sonne, S. C., Brady, K. T., & Morton, W. A. (1994). Substance abuse and bipolar affective disorder. *Journal of Nervous and Mental Disease, 182*, 349–352.

Soyka, M. (1996). Dual diagnosis in patients with schizophrenia: Issues in pharmacological treatment. *CNS Drugs, 6,* 414–425.

Spaniol, L., Zipple, A., & Cohen, B. (1991). Managing innovation and change in psychosocial rehabilitation: Key principles and guidelines. *Psychosocial Rehabilitation Journal, 14,* 27–38.

Spencer, C., Castle, D., & Michie, P. T. (2002). Motivations that maintain substance use among individuals with psychotic disorders. *Schizophrenia Bulletin, 28,* 233–247.

Stahl, S. M. (1996). *Essential Psychopharmacology: Neuroscientific Basis and Clinical Applications.* Cambridge, England: Cambridge University Press.

Stanovich, K. E. (2001). *How to Think Straight about Psychology* (6th ed.). Needham Heights, MA: Allyn & Bacon.

Stanton, M. D., & Shadish, W. R. (1997). Outcome, attrition, and family–couples treatment for drug abuse: A meta-analysis and review of the controlled, comparative studies. *Psychological Bulletin, 122,* 170–191.

Steadman, H. J., Mulvey, E. P., Monahan, J., Robbins, P. C., Appelbaum, P. S., Grisso, T., Roth, L. H., & Silver, E. (1998). Violence by people discharged from acute psychiatric inpatient facilities and by others in the same neighborhoods. *Archives of General Psychiatry, 55,* 393–401.

Steadman, H. J., Stainbrook, K. A., Griffin, P., Draine, J., Dupont, R., & Horey, C. (2001). A specialized crisis response site as a core element of police-diversion programs. *Psychiatric Services, 52,* 219–222.

Steffens, D. C., Krishnan, K. R. R., & Doraiswamy, P. M. (1997). Psychotropic drug interactions. *Primary Psychiatry, 4,* 24–53.

Stein, L. I., & Santos, A. B. (1998). *Assertive Community Treatment of Persons with Severe Mental Illness.* New York: Norton.

Stein, L. I., & Test, M. A. (1980). Alternatives to mental hospital treatment: Conceptual, model, treatment program and clinical evaluation. *Archives of General Psychiatry, 37,* 392–397.

Steketee, G. (1999a). *Overcoming Obsessive–Compulsive Disorder: A Behavioral and Cognitive Protocol for the Treatment of OCD—Client Manual.* Oakland, CA: New Harbinger.

Steketee, G. (1999b). *Overcoming Obsessive-Compulsive Disorder: A Behavioral and Cognitive Protocol for the Treatment of OCD-Therapist Protocol.* Oakland, CA: New Harbinger.

Sternbach, H. (1991). The serotonin syndrome. *American Journal of Psychiatry, 148,* 705–713.

Stewart, S. H. (1996). Alcohol abuse in individuals exposed to trauma: A critical review. *Psychological Bulletin, 120,* 83–112.

Stone, A. A. (1975). *Mental Health and the Law: A System of Transition.* Washington, DC: Department of Health, Education, and Welfare.

Stone, A. A. (1984). *Law, Psychiatry, and Morality.* Washington, DC: American Psychiatric Press.

Stone, A. M., Greenstein, R. A., Gamble, G., & McLellan, A. T. (1993). Cocaine use by schizophrenic outpatients who

receive depot neuroleptic medication. *Hospital and Community Psychiatry, 44,* 176–177.

Strakowski, S. M., & DelBello, M. P. (2000). The co-occurrence of bipolar and substance use disorders. *Clinical Psychology Review, 20,* 191–206.

Strakowski, S. M., DelBello, M. P., Fleck, D. E., & Arndt, S. (2000). The impact of substance abuse on the course of bipolar disorder. *Biological Psychiatry, 48,* 477–485.

Strakowski, S. M., McElroy, S. L., Keck, P. E. J., & West, S. A. (1996). The effects of antecedent substance abuse on the development of first-episode mania. *Journal of Psychiatric Research, 30,* 59–68.

Strakowski, S. M., Sax, K. W., Setters, M. J., & Keck, P. E. J. (1996). Enhanced response to repeated *d*-amphetamine challenge: Evidence for behavioral sensitization in humans. *Biological Psychiatry, 40,* 872–880.

Strauss, J. S., & Carpenter, W. T. (1977). Prediction of outcome in schizophrenia: III. Five-year outcome and its predictors. *Archives of General Psychiatry, 34,* 159–163.

Sullivan, J. T., Sykora, K., Schneiderman, J., Naranjo, C. A., & Sellers, E. M. (1989). Assessment of alcohol withdrawal: The Revised Clinical Institute Withdrawal Assessment for Alcohol Scale. *British Journal of Addictions, 84,* 1353–1357.

Sullivan, W. P. (1992). Reclaiming the community: The strengths perspective and deinstitutionalization. *Social Work, 37,* 204–209.

Suppes, T., Webb, A., Paul, B., Carmody, T., Kraemer, H., & Rush, A. J. (1999). Clinical outcome in a randomized 1–year trial of clozapine versus treatment as usual for patients with treatment-resistant illness and a history of mania. *American Journal of Psychiatry, 156,* 1164–1169.

Swanson, A. J., Pantalon, M. V., & Cohen, K. R. (1999). Motivational interviewing and treatment adherence among psychiatric and dually diagnosed patients. *Journal of Nervous and Mental Disease, 187,* 630–635.

Swanson, J. W., Swartz, M. S., Borum, R., Hiday, V. A., Wagner, H. R., & Burns, B. J. (2000). Involuntary out-patient commitment and reduction of violent behavior in persons with severe mental illness. *British Journal of Psychiatry, 176,* 324–331.

Swartz, M. S., Swanson, J., W., Wagner, H. R., Burns, B. J., Hiday, V. A., & Borum, R. (1999). Can voluntary outpatient commitment reduce hospital recidivism?: Findings from a randomized trial with severely mentally ill individuals. *American Journal of Psychiatry, 156,* 1968–1975.

Swartz, M. S., Swanson, J. W., Hiday, V. A., Borum, R., Wagner, H. R., & Burns, B. J. (1998a). Taking the wrong drugs: The role of substance abuse and medication noncompliance in violence among severely mentally ill individuals. *Social Psychiatry and Psychiatric Epidemiology, 33,* S75–S80.

Swartz, M. S., Swanson, J. W., Hiday, V. A., Borum, R., Wagner, H. R., & Burns, B. J. (1998b). Violence and mental illness: The effects of substance abuse and nonadherence to medication. *American Journal of Psychiatry, 155,* 226–231.

Swartz, M. S., Swanson, J. W., Wagner, H. R., Burns, B. J., & Hiday, V. A. (2001). Effects of involuntary outpatient commitment and depot antipsychotics on treatment adherence in persons with severe mental illness. *Journal of Nervous and Mental Disease, 189,* 583–592.

Swendsen, J. D., & Merikangas, K. R. (2000). The comorbidity of depression and substance use disorders. *Clinical Psychology Review, 20,* 173–189.

Switzer, G. E., Dew, M. A., Thompson, K., Goycoolea, J. M., Derricott, T., & Mullins, S. D. (1999). Posttraumatic stress disorder and service utilization among urban mental health center clients. *Journal of Traumatic Stress, 12,* 25–39.

Swofford, C. D., Kasckow, J. W., Scheller-Gilkey, G., & Inderbitzin, L. B. (1996). Substance use: A powerful predictor of relapse in schizophrenia. *Schizophrenia Research, 20,* 145–151.

Tarasoff v. Regents of the University of California, 551 P.2d 334 (Cal. 1976).

Tarrier, N., Wittkowski, A., Kinney, C., McCarthy, E., Morris, J., & Humphreys, L. (1999). Durability of the effects of cognitive-behavioural therapy in the treatment of chronic schizophrenia: 12–month follow-up. *British Journal of Psychiatry, 174,* 500–504.

Tauber, R., Wallace, C. J., & Lecomte, T. (2000). Enlisting indigenous community supporters in skills training programs for persons with severe mental illness. *Psychiatric Services, 51,* 1428–1432.

Teeson, M., Hall, W., Lynskey, M., & Degenhardt, L. (2000). Alcohol and drug use disorders in Australia: Implications of the National Survey of Mental Health and Wellbeing. *Australian and New Zealand Journal of Psychiatry, 34,* 206–213.

Teplin, L. A. (1983). The criminalization of the mentally ill: Speculation in search of data. *Psychological Bulletin, 94,* 54–67.

Teplin, L. A. (1985). The criminality of the mentally ill: A dangerous misconception. *American Journal of Psychiatry, 142,* 593–598.

Terkelsen, K. G. (1983). Schizophrenia and the family: II. Adverse effects of family therapy. *Family Process, 22,* 191–200.

Test, M. A., Allness, D. J., & Knoedler, W. H. (1995, October). *Impact of Seven Years of Assertive Community Treatment.* Paper presented at the American Psychiatric Association Institute on Psychiatric Services, Boston.

Test, M. A., & Stein, L. I. (1980). Alternative to mental hospital treatment: III. Social cost. *Archives of General Psychiatry, 37,* 409–412.

Test, M. A., Wallish, L. S., Allness, D. G., & Ripp, K. (1989). Substance use in young adults with schizophrenic disorders. *Schizophrenia Bulletin, 15,* 465–476.

Thurstin, A. H., Alfano, A. M., & Nerviano, V. J. (1987). The efficacy of Alcoholics Anonymous attendance for aftercare of inpatient alcoholics: Some follow-up data. *International Journal of the Addictions, 22,* 1083–1090.

Torrey, E. F., & Kaplan, R. J. (1995). A national survey of the use of outpatient commitment. *Psychiatric Services, 46,* 778–784.

Torrey, W. C., Drake, R. E., & Bartels, S. J. (1996). Suicide and persistent mental illness: A continual clinical and risk-management challenge. In S. M. Soreff (Ed.), *Handbook for the Treqatment of the Seriously Mentally Ill* (pp. 295–313). Seattle, WA: Hogrefe & Huber.

Torrey, W. C., Drake, R. E., Dixon, L., Burns, B. J., Flynn, L., Rush, A. J., Clark, R. E., & Klatzker, D. (2001). Implementing evidence-based practices for persons with severe mental illnesses. *Psychiatric Services, 52,* 45–55.

Torrey, W. C., & Wyzik, P. F. (2000). The recovery vision as a service improvement guide for community mental health center providers. *Community Mental Health Journal, 36,* 209–216.

Tracy, J. I., Nematbakhsh, A., de Leon, J., McCann, E. M., McGrory, A., Quereshi, G., & Josiassen, R. C. (1997). A comparison of polydipsia prevalence among chronic psychiatric patients using three measurement approaches. *Biological Psychiatry, 42,* 1097–1104.

Treffert, D. A. (1978). Marijuana use in schizophrenia: A clear hazard. *American Journal of Psychiatry, 135,* 1213–1215.

Triffleman, E. G., Marmar, C. R., Delucchi, K. L., & Ronfeldt, H. (1995). Childhood trauma and posttraumatic stress disorder in substance abuse inpatients. *Journal of Nervous and Mental Disease, 183,* 172–176.

Trimpey, J. (1992). *The Small Book: A Revolutionary Alternative for Overcoming Alcohol and Drug Dependence.* New York: Dell.

Trimpey, J. (1996). *Rational Recovery: The New Cure for Substance Addiction.* New York: Pocket Books.

Trull, T. J., Sher, K. J., Minks-Brown, C., Durbin, J., & Burr, R. (2000). Borderline personality disorder and substance use disorders: A review and integration. *Clinical Psychology Review, 20,* 235–253.

Trumbetta, S. L., & Mueser, K. T. (2001). Social functioning and its relationship to cognitive deficits. In R. Keefe & J. McEvoy (Eds.), *The Assessment of Negative Symptoms and Cognitive Deficit Response* (pp. 33–67). Washington, DC: American Psychiatric Press.

Trumbetta, S. L., Mueser, K. T., Quimby, E., Bebout, R., & Teague, G. B. (1999). Social networks and clinical outcomes of dually diagnosed homeless persons. *Behavior Therapy, 30,* 407–430.

Tsuang, M. T., Simpson, J. C., & Kronfol, Z. (1982). Subtypes of drug abuse with psychosis. *Archives of General Psychiatry, 39,* 141–147.

Vaillant, G. E. (1983). Natural history of male alcoholism: V. Is alcoholism the cart or the horse to sociopathy? *British Journal of Addiction, 78,* 317–326.

Vaillant, G. E. (1988). What can long term follow-up teach us about relapse and prevention of relapse in addiction? *British Journal of Addiction, 83,* 1147–1157.

Vaillant, G. E. (1995). *Natural History of Alcoholism Revisited.* Cambridge, MA: Harvard University Press.

Vardy, M. M., & Kay, S. R. (1983). LSD psychosis or LSD-induced schizophrenia?: A multimethod inquiry. *Archives of General Psychiatry, 40,* 877–883.

Vogel, H. S., Knight, E., Laudet, A. B., & Magura, S. (1998). Double Trouble in Recovery: Self-help for the dually diagnosed. *Psychiatric Rehabilitation Journal, 21,* 356–364.

Volpicelli, J. R., Alterman, A. I., Hayashida, M., & O'Brien, C.

P. (1992). Naltrexone in the treatment of alcohol dependence. *Archives of General Psychiatry, 49,* 876–880.

Volpicelli, J. R., Rhines, K. C., Rhines, J. S., Volpicelli, L. A., Alterman, A. I., & O'Brien, C. P. (1997). Naltrexone and alcohol dependence: Role of subject compliance. *Archives of General Psychiatry, 54,* 737–742.

Voruganti, L. N. P., Heslegrave, R. J., & Awad, A. G. (1997). Neuroleptic dysphoria may be the missing link between schizophrenia and substance abuse. *Journal of Nervous and Mental Disease, 185,* 463–465.

Wahlbeck, K., Cheine, M., Essali, A., & Adams, C. (1999). Evidence of clozapine's effectiveness in schizophrenia: A systematic review and meta-analysis of randomized trials. *American Journal of Psychiatry, 156,* 990–999.

Wallace, C. J., Tauber, R., & Wilde, J. (1999). Teaching fundamental workplace skills to persons with serious mental illness. *Psychiatric Services, 50,* 1147–1153.

Wallen, M. C., & Weiner, H. D. (1989). Impediments to effective treatment of the dually diagnosed patient. *Journal of Psychoactive Drugs, 21,* 161–168.

Warner, R., Taylor, D., Wright, J., Sloat, A., Springett, G., Amold, S., & Weinberg, H. (1994). Substance use among the mentally ill: Prevalence, reasons for use and effects on illness. *American Journal of Orthopsychiatry, 64,* 30–39.

Wasserman, D. A., Havassy, B. E., & Boles, S. M. (1997). Traumatic events and post-traumatic stress disorder in cocaine users entering private treatment. *Drug and Alcohol Dependence, 46,* 1–8.

Watson, A., Hanrahan, P., Luchins, D., & Lurigio, A. (2001). Mental health courts and the complex issue of mentally ill offenders. *Psychiatric Services, 52,* 477–481.

Wehman, P. (1981). *Competitive Employment: New Horizons for Severely Disabled Individuals.* Baltimore: Brookes.

Wehman, P. (1986). Supported competitive employment for persons with severe disabilities. *Journal of Applied Rehabilitation Counseling, 17,* 24–29.

Weiden, P. J. (Ed.). (1999). *TeamCare Solutions.* Trenton, NJ: Eli Lilly.

Weiden, P. J., Mott, T., & Curcio, N. (1995). Recognition and management of neuroleptic noncompliance. In C. L. Shriqui & H. A. Nasrallah (Eds.), *Contemporary Issues in the Treatment of Schizophrenia* (pp. 411–433). Washington, DC: American Psychiatric Press.

Weiss, K. A., Smith, T. E., Hull, J. W., Piper, A. C., & Hubbert, J. D. (2002). Predictors of risk of nonadherence in outpatients with schizophrenia and other psychotic disorders. *Schizophrenia Bulletin, 28,* 341–349.

Wennberg, J. E. (1991). Outcomes research, patient preference, and the primary care physician. *Journal of the American Board of Family Practice, 4,* 365–367.

Westermeyer, J., Myott, S., Aarts, R., & Thuras, P. (2001). Self-help strategies among patients with substance use disorders. *American Journal on Addictions, 10,* 249–257.

White, J. (1999a). *Overcoming Generalized Anxiety Disorder: A Relaxation, Cognitive Restructuring, and Exposure-Based Protocol for the Treatment of GAD—Client Manual.* Oakland, CA: New Harbinger.

White, J. (1999b). *Overcoming Generalized Anxiety Disorder: A Relaxation, Cognitive Restructuring, and Exposure-Based Protocol for the Treatment of GAD—Therapist Protocol.* Oakland, CA: New Harbinger.

Whitlock, F. A., & Lowrey, J. M. (1967). Drug dependence in psychiatric patients. *Medical Journal of Australia, 1,* 1157–1166.

Wilkins, J. N. (1997). Pharmacotherapy of schizophrenia patients with comorbid substance abuse. *Schizophrenia Bulletin, 23,* 215–228.

Winick, B. J. (1997). *The Right to Refuse Mental Health Treatment.* Washington, DC: American Psychological Association.

Winokur, G., Coryell, W., Akiskal, H. S., Endicott, J., Keller, M., & Mueller, T. (1994). Manic–depressive (bipolar) disorder: The course in light of a prospective ten-year follow-up of 131 patients. *Acta Psychiatrica Scandinavica, 152,* 365–372.

Winokur, G., Coryell, W., Akiskal, H. S., Maser, J. D., Keller, M. B., Endicott, J., & Mueller, T. (1995). Alcoholism in manic–depressive (bipolar) illness: Familial illness, course of illness, and the primary–secondary distinction. *American Journal of Psychiatry, 152,* 365–372.

Wolford, G. L., Rosenberg, S. D., Drake, R. E., Mueser, K. T., Oxman, T. E., Hoffman, D., Vidaver, R. M., Luckoor, R., & Carrieri, K. L. (1999). Evaluation of methods for detecting substance use disorder in persons with severe mental illness. *Psychology of Addictive Behaviors, 13,* 313–326.

Wong, S. E., Terranova, M. D., Bowen, L., Zarate, R., Massel, H. K., & Liberman, R. P. (1987). Providing independent recreational activities to reduce stereotypic vocalizations in chronic schizophrenics. *Journal of Applied Behavior Analysis, 20,* 77–81.

Woody, G. (1996). The challenge of dual diagnosis. *Alcohol Health and Research World, 20,* 76–80.

Xiong, W., Phillips, M. R., Hu, X., Ruiwen, W., Dai, Q., Kleinman, J., & Kleinman, A. (1994). Family-based intervention for schizophrenic patients in China: A randomised controlled trial. *British Journal of Psychiatry, 165,* 239–247.

Yandow, V. (1989). Alcoholism in women. *Psychiatric Annals, 19,* 243–247.

Yesavage, J. A., & Zarcone, V. (1983). History of drug abuse and dangerous behavior in inpatient schizophrenics. *Journal of Clinical Psychiatry, 44,* 259–261.

Ziedonis, D. M., & Fisher, W. (1996). Motivation-based assessment and treatment of substance abuse in patients with schizophrenia. *Directions in Psychiatry, 16,* 1–7.

Ziedonis, D. M., Fisher, W., Harris, P., Trudeau, K., Rao, S., & Kosten, T. R. (1996). Adjunctive selegiline in the treatment of cocaine-abusing schizophrenics. In L. S. Harris (Ed.), *Problems of Drug Dependence, 1995: Proceedings of the 57th Annual Scientific Meeting* (p. 325). Rockville, MD: National Institute on Drug Abuse.

Ziedonis, D. M., Richardson, T., Lee, E., Petrakis, I., & Kosten, T. (1992). Adjunctive desipramine in the treatment of cocaine abusing schizophrenics. *Psychopharmacology Bulletin, 28,* 309–314.

Ziedonis, D. M., & Trudeau, K. (1997). Motivation to quit using substances among individuals with schizophrenia: Implications for a motivation-based treatment model. *Schizophrenia Bulletin, 23,* 229–238.

Zigler, E., & Glick, M. (1986). *A Developmental Approach to Adult Psychopathology.* New York: Wiley.

Zimmerman, M., & Mattia, J. I. (2001). A self-report scale to help make psychiatric diagnoses: The Psychiatric Diagnostic Screening Questionnaire. *Archives of General Psychiatry, 58,* 787–794.

Zimmet, S., Strous, R., Burgess, E. S., Kohnstamm, S., & Green, A. I. (2000). Effects of Clozapine on substance use in patients with schizophrenia and schizoaffective disorder: A retrospective survey. *Journal of Clinical Psychopharmacology, 20,* 94–98.

Zinbarg, R. E., Craske, M. G., & Barlow, D. H. (1993). *Mastery of Your Anxiety and Worry: Therapist Guide.* San Antonio, TX: Psychological Corporation.

Zisook, S., Heaton, R., Moranville, J., Kuck, J., Jernigan, T., & Braff, D. (1992). Past substance abuse and clinical course of schizophrenia. *American Journal of Psychiatry, 149,* 552–553.

Zisook, S., & Schuckit, M. A. (1987). Male primary alcoholics with and without family histories of affective disorder. *Journal of Studies on Alcohol, 48,* 337–344.

Zubin, J., & Spring, B. (1977). Vulnerability: A new view of schizophrenia. *Journal of Abnormal Psychology, 86,* 103–126.

Zuercher-White, E. (1999a). *Overcoming Panic Disorder and Agoraphobia: A Cognitive-Restructuring and Exposure-Based Protocol for the Treatment of Panic and Agoraphobia—Client Manual.* Oakland, CA: New Harbinger.

Zuercher-White, E. (1999b). *Overcoming Panic Disorder and Agoraphobia: A Cognitive-Restructuring and Exposure-Based Protocol for the Treatment of Panic and Agoraphobia—Therapist Protocol.* Oakland, CA: New Harbinger.

Appendices

Dual-Disorder Treatment Fidelity Scale

KIM T. MUESER
LINDY FOX
GARY R. BOND
MICHELLE SALYERS
KIKUKO YAMAMOTO
JANE WILLIAMS

This appendix is intended to help guide you in administering the Dual-Disorder Treatment Fidelity Scale. In this appendix, you will find the following:

1. *Introduction*. This gives an overview of the "who, what, and how" of the scale.
2. *Fidelity assessor checklist*. This is a checklist of suggestions for before, during, and after the fidelity assessment site visit; it should lead to the collection of higher-quality data, more positive interactions with respondents, and a more efficient data collection process.
3. *Protocol*. The protocol explains how to rate each item. In particular, it contains the following:
    a. A *definition* and *rationale* for each fidelity item. These items have been derived from a comprehensive evidence-based literature.
    b. A list of *data sources* (e.g., clinician, chart review, program director) that are most appropriate for each fidelity item.
    c. A set of *probe questions* to help you elicit critical information from respondents for scoring the fidelity items. These probe questions were specifically generated to help you collect information that is free from bias, such as social desirability factors.
    d. *Decision rules* that will help you correctly score each item. As you collect information from various sources, these rules will help you determine the specific rating you give for each item.
4. *Cover Sheet*. This form is used to record background information on the study site. These data are not used in determining fidelity, but provide important information for classifying programs, such as size and duration of program and type of parent organization.
5. *Score Sheet*. This sheet provides instructions for scoring (including how to handle missing data, plus cutoff scores for full, moderate, and inadequate implementation).
6. *Anchor points*. This chart contains anchor points for the fidelity ratings, which are recorded on the Score Sheet.

INTRODUCTION TO THE SCALE

The Dual-Disorder Treatment Fidelity Scale is a 20-item scale assessing the adequacy of implementation of evidence-based practices for treatment of individuals with dual disorders. By definition, clients with dual disorders are diagnosed with both severe mental illness (e.g., schizophrenia) and substance use disorders. The Dual-Disorder

(continued)

Treatment Fidelity Scale is organized around seven principles: *integration* (i.e., provision of mental health and substance abuse assessment and treatment by a single team); *comprehensiveness* (i.e., services across the full range of client needs, including symptom management, housing, finances, and employment); *assertiveness* (e.g., home visits and persistent follow-up); *reduction of negative consequences* (e.g., needle exchange programs, securing stable housing); *long-term perspective* (i.e., no arbitrary time limits or mandatory graduation for service recipients); *motivation-based treatment* (i.e., a stages-of-treatment approach); and *multiple psychotherapeutic modalities* (i.e., individual, group, and family therapy).

How Items Are Rated

Each item on the scale is rated on a 5-point rating scale ranging from 1 ("Not Implemented") to 5 ("Fully Implemented"). The standards used for establishing the anchors for the "Fully Implemented" ratings were determined through a variety of expert sources, as well as empirically based research.

What Is Rated

The scale is rated on current behavior and activities, not planned or intended behavior. For example, if there is a vacancy for a substance abuse counselor, the fact that the clinic is currently interviewing candidates is not sufficient to get full credit for that item.

Who Is Rated

This scale is appropriate for organizations serving clients with severe mental illness, and for assessing fidelity to evidence-based practices *at the clinic level*, rather than at the level of a specific clinician or team. However, separate ratings may be completed for a specialty team in addition to the agency or clinic level.

How the Rating Is Done

We believe that a truly valid fidelity assessment must be done in person (i.e., through a site visit). The fidelity assessment requires a minimum of 3 hours to complete, although a longer period will offer more opportunity to collect information and hence should result in a more valid assessment. The data collection procedures include semistructured interviews, chart reviews, and direct observation of treatment and team meetings.

The site visit should include interviews with key personnel. Our recommendation is that these interviews be done in a group format; the presumed advantage is that the team collectively may provide more balanced and more valid consensus responses than any single individual can. Preliminary experience with group interviews suggests that a group of five or more interviewees works well.

Who Does the Ratings

The Dual-Disorder Treatment Fidelity Scale can be administered internally by an agency or treatment team, or by an external review group. If it is administered internally, it is obviously important for the ratings to be made objectively, based on hard evidence, rather than made to make an agency or its personnel "look good." Circumstances will dictate decisions in this area, but we encourage agencies to choose a review process that fosters objectivity in ratings (e.g., involving one or more staff members who are not centrally involved in providing services). With regard to external reviews, there is a distinct advantage in using assessors who are familiar with the agency, but at the same time are independent. The goal in either case is the selection of objective and competent assessors.

Fidelity assessments should be administered by individuals who have experience and training in interviewing and data collection procedures (including chart reviews). In addition, the interviewers need to have an understanding of the nature and ingredients of integrated dual-disorder treatment, and should be versed in both mental illness and substance abuse treatment principles. We recommend that all fidelity assessments be conducted by at least two assessors.

(continued)

Who Is Interviewed

Roles and titles will vary across agencies; however, the fidelity assessment should include interviews with the program director, the dual-disorder treatment coordinator, and at least one clinician (e.g., case manager or nurse). If there is no one who fills the role of a treatment coordinator, then we suggest including two clinicians with different educational backgrounds (e.g., nurse and case manager). Optimally, psychiatrists, nurses, substance abuse counselors, and consumers should all be interviewed.

Missing Data

The Dual-Disorder Treatment Fidelity Scale is designed to be completely filled out, with no missing data on any items. Therefore, it is essential that assessors obtain the required information for every item. If information cannot be obtained at the time of the site visit, it will be important to be able to collect it at a later date.

FIDELITY ASSESSOR CHECKLIST

Before the Site Visit

1. *Review the sample cover sheet.* This sheet is useful for organizing your fidelity assessment, identifying where the specific fidelity assessment was completed, and recording general descriptive information about the site. You may need to tailor this sheet for your specific needs (e.g., unique data sources, purposes of the fidelity assessment).

2. *Create a time line for the fidelity assessment.* Fidelity assessments require careful coordination of efforts and good communication, particularly if there are multiple assessors. For instance, the time line might include a note to make reminder calls to the program site to confirm interview dates and times.

3. *Establish a contact person at the program.* You should have one key person who arranges your visits and communicates beforehand the purpose and scope of your assessment. Typically, this will be the dual-disorder treatment team leader or the director of community support program services. Exercise common courtesy in scheduling well in advance, respecting the competing time demands on clinical staff members, and so forth.

4. *Establish a shared understanding with personnel at the site being assessed.* We need to go no further than a *Dilbert* cartoon to know how often workers in organizations are subjected to processes that come out of the clear blue sky. It is *essential* that the fidelity assessment team communicate to the program site personnel what the goals of the fidelity assessment are, who will see the report, whether the program site will receive this information, and exactly what information will be provided. The most successful fidelity assessments are those in which the assessors and the program site personnel share the goal of determining how the program is progressing according to evidence-based principles. If administrators or front-line staff members at the study site fear that they will lose funding or look bad if they don't score well, then the accuracy of the data may be compromised. The best agreement is one in which all parties are interested in getting at the truth.

5. *Indicate what you will need from respondents during your fidelity visit.* In addition to the purpose of the assessment, you will need to describe briefly what information you will need, what information the source will need to collect prior to your visit, with whom you will need to speak, and how long each interview or visit will take to complete. Examples will include caseload lists (to determine caseload ratios), schedules of team meetings, schedules and curricula for therapy groups, agency mission statements, tools used to assess substance use, charts, and sample treatment plans.

6. *Alert your contact person that you will need to sample clients' charts.* To score some items, the scale calls for at least 10 charts (20 charts are preferred) to be reviewed by the assessors. Ideally, these charts should be chosen randomly from those clients whom the agency believes qualify for a dual diagnosis. Although there are several ways this can be done, it is preferable from a time efficiency standpoint that these charts be randomly drawn beforehand. Obviously, this is an area where an agency can "game the system" by hand-picking charts and/or updating them right before the visit. If there is a shared understanding that the goal is a better understanding of how a program is implementing services, this is less likely to occur.

7. *Provide clear information to all respondents about the purpose of the assessment.* The quality of your interview will be improved if all sources feel comfortable about providing accurate information. Therefore, it is important

(continued)

to communicate clearly the reason for your visit and your questions. This will serve to reduce any defensiveness or apprehension due to the evaluation process.

During the Site Visit

1. *Tailor the terminology used in the interview to the terminology used at the site.* For example, if the site uses the term *member* for *client*, use that term. If *case managers* are referred to as *clinicians*, use that terminology. Every agency has specific job titles for particular staff roles. By adopting the local terminology, the assessor will improve communication.

2. *Record relevant numbers and titles.* During the interview, record the titles of all relevant programs; the total number of clients with severe mental illness; and the total number of clinicians (excluding psychiatrists) and their titles.

3. *Review at least 10 charts.* We suggest that you ask the agency to select 20 charts for clients with dual disorders, and then that the fidelity assessment team randomly select and review 10 of those charts. This suggestion is made with the assumption that the agency personnel are fully behind the measurement process and that they are not purposely choosing the 10 or 20 "best" charts. When you are coding the items that require chart review, full implementation of a particular practice (i.e., a 5 on the scale) would be given if 7 of the 10 charts displayed evidence that the practice was being implemented.

4. *Before you leave, check for missing data.* As noted earlier, completion of the scale requires information to be obtained for every item.

After the Site Visit

1. *If necessary, follow up on any missing data.* For example, make phone calls to the program site.

2. *Have assessors reach a consensus.* If there are two assessors, both should independently rate the fidelity scale. The assessors should then compare their ratings, resolve any disagreements, and come up with a consensus rating.

3. *Complete the scale itself.* Tally the item scores and determine which level of implementation was achieved (see score sheet).

4. *Send a follow-up letter to the site.* In most cases, this letter will include a *fidelity report,* explaining to the program its scores on the Dual-Disorder Treatment Fidelity Scale and providing some interpretation of the assessment, highlighting both strengths and weaknesses. The report should be informative, factual, and constructive. The recipients of this report will vary according to the purposes, but typically include the key administrators involved in the assessment.

5. *If the scale is administered often, provide a graph.* If the fidelity assessment is given repeatedly, it is often useful to create a graph of a program's progress over time by graphing the total scores obtained on the scale. This graph may be included in the fidelity report.

FIDELITY SCALE PROTOCOL: ITEM DEFINITIONS AND SCORING

1. Identification of Clients with Dual Disorders

Definition: At admission for services, all clients are assessed for substance use (both drugs and alcohol) with standardized instruments (i.e., published instruments). The assessment is included in each client's chart.

Rationale: Substance use disorders are common in persons with severe mental illness, but they are frequently undetected in routine mental health treatment settings. Accurate identification of substance use disorders requires routine screening of all clients with standardized instruments.

Sources of Information: Chart review.

Item Response Coding: If 7 of the 10 charts reviewed provide evidence that a substance abuse screen has been used, the item would be coded as a 5.

Probe Questions: Not applicable.

(continued)

2. Integrated Assessment of Clients with Dual Disorders

Definition: Two factors are taken into account in this rating: the specificity and the integration of the assessment. *Specificity* refers in this context to the behavioral details of the assessment that form the basis for treatment recommendations (see the definition of item 1 above for details). *Integration* refers in this context to the evaluation of how one disorder influences the other disorder, suggesting possible avenues of treatment (e.g., a client with poor social skills uses substances in social situations to meet interpersonal needs; a client with schizophrenia smokes cannabis to relax, but it worsens his or her paranoia and risk of relapses).

Rationale: Specificity is critical in order to identify suitable potential targets of interventions, to measure them, and to know how to modify them. Integration is critical because it addresses how one disorder is influencing the other (contributing to it, worsening it, etc.). Information about the interactions between disorders can help pinpoint areas of integrated dual-disorder treatment that are most important and that have the most promise for affecting the outcomes of both disorders.

Sources of Information: Chart review.

Item Response Coding: If 7 of the 10 charts reviewed provide evidence that an integrated assessment has been conducted, the item would be coded as a 5.

Probe Questions: Not applicable.

3. Comprehensive Mental Health Assessment

Definition: Clients' mental health needs are comprehensively assessed and updated at least yearly. Comprehensive mental health assessment involves a systematic review of the following:
- Psychosocial history
- Symptoms
- Psychiatric hospitalization and use of other emergency/crisis services
- Social and vocational functioning
- Leisure and recreational activities
- Family contacts and other social support contacts
- Housing
- Safety
- Independent living skills
- Medical needs
- Insight into and understanding of mental illness

Rationale: Substance abuse is often an effort to get basic needs met, albeit at a high cost. Effective treatment includes helping clients develop healthy, rewarding lifestyles not dependent on alcohol and drugs. Comprehensive assessment of mental health needs identifies domains of functioning that may need to be improved in order to achieve sustained sobriety.

Sources of Information: Chart review.

Item Response Coding: Calculate the number of factors needed on each chart and calculate the mean per chart. Compare the mean with the level for each alternative. For example, if the mean is 9.0 or higher, this item would be coded as a 5.

Probe Questions: Not applicable.

4. Comprehensive Substance Abuse Assessment

Definition: Clients' substance use behaviors and patterns are comprehensively assessed and updated at least yearly. Comprehensive assessment of substance use includes an assessment of the following:
- History of substance use and abuse
- Treatment history
- Current/recent use of alcohol and specific drugs (including patterns and amounts of use)
- Social context of substance use

(continued)

341

- Motives for substance use
- Consequences of substance use
- Insight
- Motivation to address substance abuse

Rationale: Specific information about substance use habits is important in order to understand the functions of substance use in clients' lives (e.g., social, coping, or recreational), the severity of its effects on their lives, and their motivation to work on the problem.

Sources of Information: Chart review.

Item Response Coding: Calculate the number of factors recorded on each chart and calculate the mean per chart. Compare the mean with the level for each alternative. For example, if the mean is 7.0 or higher, this item would be coded as a 5.

Probe Questions: Not applicable.

5. Integrated Treatment Plan

Definition: Treatment plans for clients with dual disorders address both mental health and substance abuse treatment needs, with both specificity and integration of treatment recommendations. *Specificity* refers in this context to treatment recommendations that identify both the target of the intervention (e.g., specific symptoms, social problems, substance abuse behaviors) and an intervention designed to address that problem and how it will bring about changes. *Integration* refers in this context to treatment recommendations that address the interactions between substance abuse and mental illness. One example of such integration is helping clients to cope with psychiatric symptoms that appear to contribute to their substance use. Another example is providing psychoeducation to clients to help them understand how substance abuse worsens their psychiatric illness.

Rationale: Addressing the areas in which the disorders interact has the most promise for improving the outcome of both disorders.

Sources of Information: Clinical records of clients with active substance use disorders.

Item Response Coding: If 7 of the 10 charts reviewed provide evidence that an integrated treatment plan has been developed, the item would be coded as a 5.

Probe Questions: Not applicable.

6. Integrated Crisis Plan

Definition: Written crisis plans address both mental-health-related and substance-abuse-related crises.

Rationale: Clients with dual disorders are at higher risk for crises (e.g., relapses in disorders, homelessness, legal problems), and therefore have a higher need for workable crisis plans.

Sources of Information: Chart review.

Item Response Coding: If 7 of the 10 charts reviewed provide evidence that an integrated crisis plan has been developed, the item would be coded as a 5.

Probe Questions: Not applicable.

7. Integration of Services

Definition: Mental health and substance abuse treatment services are provided by the same clinician (or team of clinicians).

Rationale: Receiving treatment for dual disorders from a single team of providers leads to better outcomes. In this way, information and interventions are woven together for a stronger clinical approach. It can help to prevent clients from "falling between the cracks" and not receiving treatment for one or both disorders; it can also avert philosophical conflict between different providers, and can improve the providers' communication.

Sources of Information: Director/clinician reports.

(continued)

Probe Questions:

- "How are mental health and substance abuse treatment services organized in your program?"
- "Who provides mental health services?"
- "Who provides substance abuse services?"
- "Do clinicians providing mental health and substance abuse services work for an agency other than the mental health center?" If yes: "Do the different agencies require separate reporting procedures?"
- "How many clients with a dual disorder are being treated by a clinician who focuses on both disorders?"
- "How many clients with a dual disorder are there in all?"

8. Comprehensiveness of Services

Definition: Five types of services that address the full range of needs of clients with dual disorders are available: residential services, family services, illness self-management, assertive community treatment (ACT) or intensive case management (ICM) teams, and vocational services. (Definitions and probe questions for these five types of services are provided below.) In order for a type of service to be considered available, it must both exist and be accessible by clients with needs in those areas within 2 months of referral.

Rationale: Although a major focus of treatment is the elimination or reduction of substance abuse, this goal is more effectively met when other domains of functioning in which clients are typically impaired are also addressed.

Sources of Information: Director/clinician reports and chart review.

Definitions of services:

Residential Services: An agency has some supervised residential services that accept clients with dual disorders. These include supported housing (i.e., outreach for housing purposes to clients living independently) and residential programs with on-site residential staff. They exclude short-term residential services (i.e., a month or less).

Probe Questions:

- "What residential services are available for clients in your agency? If the agency has supervised or supported housing, are clients with dual disorders eligible? Are there exclusion criteria?"
- "What is the waiting period for clients to obtain these residential services after the referral is made?"

Family Services: Family services are available if clinicians have ongoing contact with more than 50% of the families with whom clients are in regular contact (e.g., weekly). Family includes any blood relative or long-term (over 1 year) conjugal partner.

Probe Questions:

- "Among the clients in regular contact with family members, how many of the families do clinicians have contact with?"
- "How soon after a client's referral does a clinician make contact with the family?"

Illness Self-Management: There is systematic teaching of interpersonal skills (social skills) or illness management skills (psychoeducation, relapse prevention, or coping with persistent symptoms).

Probe Questions:

- "Does your agency provide social skills training?"
- "How is skills training done?" Probe for skills training components, including modeling, role playing, positive and corrective feedback, homework.
- "How soon after referral is this skills training available to clients?"
- "Is your skills training based on a specific written curriculum?" If yes, identify source of curriculum and verify with inspection of materials.
- "Do you conduct psychoeducation about psychiatric illness and its management?" If yes: "Is it a time-limited or time-unlimited course?"
- "Is this course based on a standard, written curriculum?" If yes, identify source of curriculum and verify.

(continued)

ACT or ICM: One or both of these forms of case management, including client-to-clinician ratios of 15:1 or lower, are used. Over 50% of the services provided by the team are in the community.

Probe Questions:
- "Are ACT or ICM services available for clients with high service utilization [e.g., frequent hospitalizations] or severe psychosocial impairment?" If yes, probe to determine client-to-clinician ratios, as well as the primary locus of service for such services.
- "What is the waiting period for a client to receive ACT or ICM services?"

Vocational Services: Supported employment services are available that do not preclude people with active dual disorders within 2 months of referral. Supported employment programs stress competitive employment in integrated community settings and provide ongoing support to clients to promote job tenure.
- "Supported employment programs stress competitive employment in integrated community settings and provide ongoing support to clients to promote job tenure. Do clients have access to supported employment?" Deemphasize prevocational assessment and training, and focus on rapid job seeking and attainment.
- "What is the waiting period to receive vocational rehabilitation services?"
- "Are vocational rehabilitation services available to clients with active substance use disorders?"

9. Time-Unlimited Services

Definition: The provision of dual-disorder services is not limited by time constraints.

Rationale: The evidence suggests that both psychiatric and substance use disorders tend to be chronic and severe. Continuity of treatment—that is, ongoing services by a single treatment team without arbitrary time limits—is believed to be the most effective long-term strategy with the dual-disorder population.

Sources of Information: Director/clinician reports.

Probe Questions:
- "Are there any time limits for the provision of mental health services in your agency?" If yes: "How long may services be provided?"
- "Are there any time limits for the provision of substance abuse treatment services in your agency?" If yes: "How long may services be provided?"
- If the respondent reports that there are time limits for mental health services, substance abuse treatment services, or both, although there are not time limits: "Is there any pressure in your system to limit the amount of time or services devoted to mental health and/or substance abuse treatment?"
- If the answer is "no" for either or both mental health and substance abuse treatment services: "Although there are no time limits, is there any pressure in your system to limit the amount of time or services devoted to mental health and/or substance abuse treatment?"

10. Outreach Capability

Definition: Services are provided outside of the clinic or institutional setting (e.g., in a client's home, in a park, etc.). Outreach includes both engagement of new clients and (re)engagement of clients previously admitted who are not currently participating in agency programs.

Rationale: Because clients with dual disorders tend to have high dropout rates from treatment, lower levels of motivation, and cognitive impairment, keeping them engaged in programs is difficult. Therefore, interventions that reach out to assist such clients can be helpful for developing engagement, as well as for other important therapeutic outcomes.

Sources of information: Director/clinician reports.

Probe Questions:
- "Where are most services for clients provided?" Probe to determine how often services are provided outside the office.
- "Could you tell me what types of services are provided?" Probe for outreach done to provide emergency services, to address housing/clothing/food needs, to engage clients, or to provide *in vivo* skills training.

(continued)

11. Client-to-Clinician Ratio

Definition: The ratio of clients to clinicians within the agency (including all clinicians who provide actual services, but excluding vocational staff members and psychiatrists) is satisfactorily low. If separate dual-disorder teams exist, compute client-to-clinician ratio for those separate teams; otherwise, compute the average ratio for the agency.

Rationale: Effective dual-disorder treatment requires that clinicians engage in many functions (e.g., coordination of treatment, medication supervision, symptom monitoring), and thus such treatment is best implemented with a lower client-to-clinician ratio.

Sources of Information: Director/clinician reports.

Probe Questions:

- "How many clinicians do you have? For each, what is his or her current caseload?" These answers are then used to determine the average client-to-clinician ratio. If teams share caseloads, then simply divide the number of clients with severe mental illness by the number of clinicians (excluding psychiatrists and vocational specialists).

12. Integrated Group Treatment for Clients with Dual Disorders

Definition: The agency provides groups specifically designed to address both mental health and substance abuse problems at the same time.

Rationale: Research indicates that better outcomes are achieved when treatment is integrated to address both disorders. In addition, group settings are often effectively used in the treatment of substance abuse.

Sources of Information: Director/clinician reports.

Probe Questions:

- "Can you tell me about the types of groups that are run in your center?"
- "How many different groups do you run for clients? How do you decide which group each client should be in?"
- "What topics do you cover in the groups?"
- "Do you have groups that address both mental health and substance abuse problems?"
- "Do groups address both types of problems at the same time, or are there separate groups that address these problems?"

13. Group Treatment

Definition: The agency provides different, professionally led group interventions that specifically target clients with dual disorders. Six different types of groups are identified: education, persuasion, active treatment, combined persuasion and active treatment, social skills training, and relapse prevention. Descriptions of these six types of groups are given below.

Rationale: Groups have powerful effects on individuals, both positive and negative. Substance abuse frequently occurs in group settings, as does treatment of substance abuse. Group treatment for dual disorders has several advantages: It is a cost-effective approach to working with individuals; it provides opportunities for social modeling; it furnishes social support; and it makes more sources of feedback available to individuals. Various group interventions for dual disorders have been included in effective treatment programs for this population.

Sources of Information: Director/clinician reports.

Probe Questions:

- "Are there any particular groups, led by professionals, that are specifically oriented toward persons with dual disorders?"
- "Please describe these groups." Probe to determine the availability of the six different types of dual-disorder groups, as mentioned above and described below. For a type of group to be considered available, a client must be able to have access to it within 1 month of referral.

(continued)

345

Types of Groups:

Education groups: These curriculum-driven groups are aimed at teaching clients about substance abuse, mental illness, and their interactions. Note whether these groups are available, and, if so, whether they are time-limited or time-unlimited

Persuasion groups: These groups are aimed at engaging clients in discussion about substance use and mental illness, and motivating them to address substance abuse through personal exploration and avoidance of confrontation. Motivation to address substance abuse is not a prerequisite for participation. Note whether these groups are available.

Active treatment groups: These groups address practical skills aimed at helping clients reduce their use of substances and/or maintain abstinence. Teaching cognitive-behavioral strategies for dealing with high-risk situations for substance abuse may be a common feature of such groups, as well as developing group support for working on substance abuse. Note whether these groups are available.

Combined persuasion and active treatment groups: These groups include a mix of people in persuasion and active treatment. The groups address topics that meet the needs of clients in both stages. Note whether these groups are available.

Social skills training groups: These groups systematically use social learning methods (modeling, role playing, positive and corrective feedback, homework) to teach social skills for dealing with substance use situations and/or for getting social needs met in ways other than using substances. Skills training groups follow a preplanned curriculum. Note whether these groups are available.

Relapse prevention groups: These groups are specifically intended for clients whose substance use disorder is now in remission. Groups may focus on developing relapse prevention/management plans and providing mutual support for maintaining sobriety. Note whether these groups are available.

14. Individual Motivational Interviewing

Definition: The steps involved in motivational interviewing for dual disorders include expressing empathy, identifying personal goals, developing discrepancy, rolling with resistance, and supporting self-efficacy.

Rationale: The premise of motivational interviewing is that clients with substance use disorders can be motivated to work on their substance abuse problems by first helping them identify personal goals, and then developing discrepancy between continued substance abuse and achieving these personal goals.

Sources of Information: Director/clinician reports.

Probe Questions:

- "When a client first starts treatment, what things do you work on? Can you provide an example?"
- "Are the clinicians treating clients with dual disorders familiar with motivational interviewing approaches to substance abuse?" If yes: "Please describe these." Probe to evaluate understanding, including the steps of motivational interviewing. If the respondent is not familiar with motivational interviewing, explain: "Motivational interviewing is a set of strategies used to help clients *first* focus on their personal goals, and *then* explore how substance abuse may interfere with achieving these goals."
- "Do your clinicians use a book or manual to guide their motivational interviewing work?"
- "Do clinicians receive ongoing training or supervision in motivational interviewing?"
- "Is motivational interviewing systematically done with all clients with dual disorders?" If so: "Please elaborate." If not: "What proportion? Are there clients with whom this is *not* done? If so, why?"

15. Individual Cognitive-Behavioral Counseling

Definition: Cognitive-behavioral counseling for substance abuse problems is aimed at teaching new skills for managing urges to use substances, for dealing with situations in which a person is at risk for substance use, and for responding to the early stages of a relapse. Counseling may take several forms, including developing relapse prevention plans, teaching strategies for dealing with cravings, training in problem solving to address high-risk situations, or teaching specific strategies for coping with symptoms or mood states that lead to substance abuse.

(continued)

Rationale: Cognitive-behavioral counseling has been shown to be effective in treating substance abuse and other addictive disorders.

Information Sources: Director/clinician reports.

Probe Questions:

- "Are other types of individual treatment done with clients (other than motivational interviewing)?"
- "Is individual cognitive-behavioral counseling for substance abuse provided to clients with dual disorders?" If yes: "Please explain."
- "How often and to how many clients is counseling provided?"
- If regular counseling is provided, assess which of the following strategies are taught:
  - Managing cravings
  - Relapse prevention training
  - Teaching strategies to deal with high-risk situations
  - Systematically helping clients challenge their beliefs about substances
  - Teaching coping strategies to deal with symptoms or negative mood states related to substance abuse (e.g., relaxation training, sleep hygiene, cognitive therapy for depression or anxiety, coping strategies for hallucinations)

16. Family Interventions

Definition: Family interventions led by professionals are designed to educate family members about dual disorders, to reduce stress in the family, and to promote collaboration with the treatment team.

Rationale: Families provide extensive supports to individuals with dual disorders, and the loss of such supports contributes to housing instability and homelessness. Family interventions are potent treatments for severe mental illness and for addictive disorders, and some research shows that they are effective for dual disorders as well.

Sources of Information: Director/clinician reports and chart reviews.

Probe Questions:

- "How many clients in the program are in contact with family members (or significant others) on a weekly basis?" (Estimates suggest that about 60% of clients with dual disorders have weekly contact with their families.)
- "Of those clients, how many families have received family services?"
- "Do you do outreach to families?"
- "Is there a manual or book you use to guide family treatment?"
- "What family formats are used—single-family, multiple-family groups, or both?"
- Assess what clinicians usually do in their family work:
  - Education about dual disorders
  - Communication skills training
  - Problem-solving training
  - General stress reduction training
  - Relapse prevention planning
  - Collaborative treatment planning
  - Other (ask for details)

17. Pharmacological Treatment of Mental Illness

Definition: Psychotropic medications are prescribed for the treatment of mental illness in clients who also have active substance use disorders.

Rationale: Research indicates that psychotropic medications are effective in the treatment of severe mental illness, even when active substance abuse problems are present. Access to such medications, including antipsychotics, mood stabilizers, and antidepressants, is critical to effective treatment of dual disorders.

Sources of Information: Director/clinician/psychiatrist reports.

(continued)

Probe Questions:
- "Are psychotropic medications prescribed to clients with active substance abuse problems?"
- "Are there certain restrictions, in terms of specific types of substances abused or specific mental illnesses, in which psychotropic medications are not to be prescribed [exclude benzodiazepines]?"
- "How often are psychotropic medications not prescribed because of a concurrent substance use disorder?"

18. Self-Help Liaison

Definition: Clients are connected with consumer-run self-help groups for addiction problems, such as Alcoholics Anonymous (AA), Narcotics Anonymous (NA), Rational Recovery, Double Trouble in Recovery, or Dual Recovery Anonymous.

Rationale: Self-help groups are widely used resources in the treatment of addiction, and enjoy moderate popularity among clients with dual disorders. Participation in self-help is associated with greater improvements in substance abuse.

Sources of Information: Director/clinician reports.

Probe Questions:
- "Are clients with dual disorders referred to self-help groups in the community, such as AA, NA, or Double Trouble in Recovery?" If yes: "How often are clients referred to such groups? How often do clients follow up on these referrals?"
- "Do clinicians ever attend self-help group meetings with clients to help them identify suitable groups?" If yes: "How often does this happen?"
- "Is a self-help group operated out of the agency?" If yes: "How often are clients with dual disorders referred to these groups? How often do clients follow through on these referrals?"
- "Does the agency have a designated individual who is a liaison to self-help groups for clients with dual disorders?"

19. Stage-Wise Treatment

Definition: Specific interventions are based on an evaluation of each client's motivation to address and work on substance abuse. Stages of treatment (or stages of change) are reflected in the understanding that a clinical relationship must be established before attempting to address substance abuse. Once such a relationship is established, attention is paid to helping clients understand the effects of substance use on their lives, and motivating them to address it. Then attention turns to substance use reduction, and finally to relapse prevention.

Rationale: There is a strong research base suggesting that modifications in maladaptive behavior occur most effectively when stage of treatment is taken into account.

Sources of Information: Director/clinician reports.

Probe Questions:

Ask the respondent to identify three clients: one who is relatively new; one who has been in the program for a moderate amount of time (i.e., about 1 year); and one who has been in the program for a longer period of time (i.e., >3 years). Ask the respondent to discuss each individual's treatment and progress. The goal is to see whether the respondent talks about stages and appropriate interventions for that client. The following questions should also be asked:
- "Are you familiar with the concept of stages of change or stages of treatment?" If so, ask respondent to elaborate on specific stages and how stages are used in treatment planning.
- "Do you use confrontation early in treatment?" If so, ask for examples.
- "Do you teach relapse prevention skills?" If yes: "What do you mean by relapse prevention skills? When in the recovery process are they taught? Are they taught when substance abuse is still active?"
- "How do you deal with unmotivated clients?"
- "When in treatment does abstinence become a goal?"
- "Is cutting down on substance use a viable goal for some clients?"

(continued)

20. Reduction of Negative Consequences

Definition: Efforts are made to reduce the negative consequences of substance abuse directly, via methods other than substance use reduction itself. Typical negative consequences of substance abuse that are foci of intervention include physical effects (e.g., disease, triggering of mental illness relapses, prostitution involving unsafe sex); social effects (e.g., loss of family support, victimization); self-care and independent functioning (e.g., housing instability, incarceration, malnutrition); and use of substances in unsafe situations (e.g., driving while intoxicated). Examples of strategies designed to reduce negative consequences include needle exchange programs, teaching safe-sex practices, supporting clients who switch to less harmful substances, providing support to families, helping clients avoid high-risk situations for victimization, securing housing that recognizes clients' ongoing substance abuse problems, and "safe driver" programs.

Rationale: Because substance abuse has such detrimental effects for people with severe mental illness, and treatment is often a lengthy process, it can be helpful to use strategies to reduce negative consequences. These are particularly important early in the course of dual-disorder treatment.

Sources of Information: Director/clinician reports.

Probe Questions:

- "What do you do with individuals who continue to drink or use drugs?"
- "What is your program's policy regarding treatment for individuals who continue to drink or use drugs?"
- "Is there an emphasis on abstinence?"
- "What do you do if an individual engages in risky sexual behavior?"
- "What do you do if an individual reports using dirty needles?"
- "What is your program's philosophy toward reducing the negative consequences of substance abuse in clients who continue to use substances?"

Dual-Disorder Treatment Fidelity Scale: Cover Sheet

Date: _____   Assessor(s): _____

_____

Program Name: _____

Agency Name: _____

Contact Person: _____

Phone Number: _____

E-mail: _____

Sources Used:

___ Interview with: _____

_____

_____

_____

_____ Chart Reviews (number of charts: _____)

Number of Staff Members: _____

Number of Clients Served in Preceding Year: _____

Date Program Was Started: _____

Dual-Disorder Treatment Fidelity Scale: Score Sheet

Center: _____ Date of Visit: _____

Informants—Name(s) and Positions: _____, _____

Number of Records Reviewed: _____ Rater: _____

		Ratings			
1. Identification of Clients with Dual Disorders	1	2	3	4	5
2. Integrated Assessment of Clients with Dual Disorders	1	2	3	4	5
3. Comprehensive Mental Health Assessment	1	2	3	4	5
4. Comprehensive Substance Abuse Assessment	1	2	3	4	5
5. Integrated Treatment Plan	1	2	3	4	5
6. Integrated Crisis Plan	1	2	3	4	5
7. Integration of Services	1	2	3	4	5
8. Comprehensiveness of Services	1	2	3	4	5
9. Time-Unlimited Services	1	2	3	4	5
10. Outreach Capability	1	2	3	4	5
11. Client-to-Clinician Ratio	1	2	3	4	5
12. Integrated Group Treatment for Dual Disorders	1	2	3	4	5
13. Group Treatment	1	2	3	4	5
14. Individual Motivational Interviewing	1	2	3	4	5
15. Individual Cognitive-Behavioral Counseling	1	2	3	4	5
16. Family Interventions	1	2	3	4	5
17. Pharmacological Treatment of Mental Illness	1	2	3	4	5
18. Self-Help Liaison	1	2	3	4	5
19. Stage-Wise Treatment	1	2	3	4	5
20. Reduction of Negative Consequences	1	2	3	4	5

Total Score: _____

Scoring System: 79–105 =   Fully Implemented
                  50–78 =   Moderately Implemented
                  20–49 =   Not Implemented

Anchor Points for Dual-Disorder Treatment Fidelity Scale Ratings

Items	1	2	3	4	5
1. Identification of Dual-Disorder Clients	No systematic method to identify dual-disorder clients.	Clients are screened for dual-disorder problems when substance abuse is suspected, but the screening is inconsistent.	Clients are screened for dual-disorder problems when substance abuse is suspected, and the screening process is standardized.	Every new client admitted to the agency is screened for dual-disorder problems, but the screening is inconsistent.	Every new client admitted to the agency is systematically screened for dual-disorder problems.
2. Integrated Assessment of Dual-Disorder Clients	Neither disorder assessed with specificity.	One disorder assessed with some specificity, and the other disorder not assessed.	Both disorders assessed, with good specificity of one disorder.	Both disorders assessed with good specificity, but no integration.	Both disorders assessed with good specificity, and integration is mentioned.
3. Comprehensive Mental Health Assessment (see protocol for list of areas)	No comprehensive assessment available (fewer than half of the areas assessed).	Comprehensive assessment available (at least half of the areas assessed), but not updated (>1 year old).	Comprehensive and updated assessment covers 5–6 areas.	Comprehensive and updated assessment covers 7–8 areas.	Comprehensive and updated assessment covers at least 9 areas.
4. Comprehensive Substance Abuse Assessment (see protocol for list of areas)	No comprehensive assessment available (fewer than half of the areas assessed).	Comprehensive assessment available (at least half of the areas assessed), but not updated (>1 year old).	Comprehensive and updated assessment covers 3–4 areas.	Comprehensive and updated assessment covers 5–6 areas.	Comprehensive and updated assessment covers 7–8 areas.
5. Integrated Treatment Plan	Both disorders addressed in <25% of treatment plans.	Both disorders addressed in 25–75% of the treatment plans.	Both disorders addressed in >75% of plans, but plans lack specificity and integration.	Both disorders addressed in >75% of plans, plus good specificity.	Both disorders addressed in >75% of plans, plus good specificity and integration.
6. Integrated Crisis Plan	Fewer than 25% of dual-disorder clients have a written crisis plan (for either disorder).	25–79% of dual-disorder clients have a written crisis plan for at least one disorder.	Crisis plan present for 80% of dual-disorder clients, but plans target both substance abuse and mental illness in <25% of the charts.	Crisis plan present for 80% of dual-disorder clients, and plans target both substance abuse and mental illness in 25–75% of the charts.	Crisis plan present for 80% or more of dual-disorder clients, and plans target both substance abuse and mental illness in >75% of the charts.

(continued)

APPENDIX A. Anchor Points for Dual-Disorder Treatment Fidelity Scale Ratings (page 2 of 3)

Items	1	2	3	4	5
7. Integration of Services	Clinicians who treat both disorders see <25% of dual-disorder clients.	Clinicians who treat both disorders see 25–49% of dual-disorder clients.	Clinicians who treat both disorders see 50–69% of dual-disorder clients.	Clinicians who treat both disorders see 70–89% of dual-disorder clients.	Clinicians who treat both disorders see 90% or more of dual-disorder clients.
8. Comprehensiveness of Services (# accessible to dual-disorder clients within 2 months): • Residential Services • Family Services • Illness Self-Management • ACT or ICM Teams • Vocational Services	One or none of listed services are accessible.	Two of these services are accessible.	Three of these services are accessible.	Four of these services are accessible.	Five of these services are accessible.
9. Time-Unlimited Services	Specific time limits of up to a year are placed on dual-disorder services.	Specific time limits of 1–2 years are placed on dual-disorder services.	Specific time limits of more than 2 years are placed on dual-disorder services.	No specific time limits on dual-disorder services, but there is pressure for clients to move out of these services.	No specific time limits on dual-disorder services, and no pressure for clients to move out of these services.
10. Outreach Capability Clients (i.e., home and community visits for clients who need it)	Outreach rarely if ever done.	Outreach done for emergency purposes.	Outreach done for emergency purposes and medication and symptom monitoring.	Outreach done for emergency purposes, medication/symptom monitoring, and attending to basic needs (food, clothing, shelter).	Outreach done to develop and maintain therapeutic alliance, in addition to the other purposes specified.
11. Client-to-Clinician Ratio (excluding psychiatrist)	Over 50 clients per clinician.	41–50 clients per clinician.	31–40 clients per clinician.	21–30 clients per clinician.	20 or fewer clients per clinician.
12. Integrated Group Treatment for Dual Disorders	No groups are offered for dual-disorder clients.	Groups are offered for only one of the two disorders.	Separate groups for each disorder are offered, but no integration of the disorders in the groups.	Separate groups for each disorder, but some discussion of the other disorder does take place.	Integrated groups where both disorders are the focus of the treatment.
13. Group Treatment: • Education • Persuasion • Active Treatment • Combined Persuasion and Active Treatment • Social Skills Training • Relapse Prevention	No groups.	One group type.	Two group types.	Three group types.	Four or more group types.

(continued)

APPENDIX A. Anchor Points for Dual-Disorder Treatment Fidelity Scale Ratings (page 3 of 3)

Items	1	2	3	4	5
14. Individual Motivational Interviewing	Motivational interviewing is done with <20% of dual-disorder clients.	Motivational interviewing is done with 20–39% of dual-disorder clients.	Motivational interviewing is done with 40–59% of dual-disorder clients.	Motivational interviewing is done with 60–79% of dual-disorder clients.	Motivational interviewing is done with 80% of dual-disorder clients.
15. Individual Cognitive-Behavioral Counseling (CBC)	CBC is done with <20% of dual-disorder clients.	CBC is done with 20–39% of dual-disorder clients.	CBC is done with 40–59% of dual-disorder clients.	CBC is done with 60–79% of dual-disorder clients.	CBC is done with 80% of dual-disorder clients.
16. Family Interventions	Fewer than 20% of families in weekly contact with clients are receiving services.	20–39% of families in weekly contact with clients are receiving services.	40–59% of families in weekly contact with clients are receiving services.	60% or more of families in weekly contact with clients are receiving services, but no standard curriculum or manual is used.	60% or more of families in weekly contact with clients are receiving services, and a curriculum or manual is used.
17. Pharmacological Treatment of Mental Illness	Pharmacological treatment provided to <25% of clients with an active substance use disorder.	Pharmacological treatments provided for 25–49% of clients with an active substance use disorder.	Pharmacological treatments provided for 50–79% of clients with an active substance use disorder.	Pharmacological treatments provided for 80–89% of clients with an active substance use disorder.	Pharmacological treatments provided for 90% of clients with an active substance use disorder.
18. Self-Help Liaison	No referral of dual-disorder clients to self-help in the community.	Occasional referral of clients to self-help.	Clients are routinely referred to self-help groups, but clinicians do not attend these groups with clients.	Clients are routinely referred to self-help groups, and clinicians sometimes attend these groups with clients.	Clients are routinely referred to self-help groups, clinicians frequently attend these groups with clients, and agency has liaison.
19. Stage-Wise Treatment	Interventions contrary to stages.	Some (<40%) interventions are consistent with clients' motivational stages.	Many (40–59%) interventions are consistent with motivational stages.	Most (60–79%) interventions are consistent with motivational stages.	Most (80% or more) interventions are consistent with motivational stages and *explicitly* reflect stages of treatment.
20. Reducing Negative Consequences	No awareness of this principle.	Staff shows little awareness of principle, although some interventions are consistent with it.	Agency endorses principle, but staff only occasionally acts on this principle.	Agency endorses principle, but staff does not routinely implement strategies consistent with this philosophy.	Staff routinely implements strategies consistent with this philosophy.

Educational Handouts

Understanding Bipolar Disorder

Bipolar disorder is a major psychiatric illness, also known as *manic–depressive disorder*. People with this illness sometimes experience extremely high moods (*mania*) and sometimes extremely low moods (*depression*). Symptoms of mania and depression usually occur at different times, but they may exist together in what is called a *mixed episode*. A person may also have normal moods.

The cause of bipolar disorder is unknown. Scientists believe the disorder may be caused by an imbalance in brain chemicals, particularly the chemical *norepinephrine*. This imbalance may be due to genetic factors. About 1% of people develop bipolar disorder in their lifetime.

Bipolar disorder usually develops between the ages of 16 and 35, but may develop in a person's 40s or even 50s. Bipolar disorder is a lifelong disorder, but between mood episodes many people can function well. Many famous people have had bipolar disorder and contributed greatly to society, such as the artist Vincent Van Gogh, the writer Edgar Allen Poe, and the actress Patty Duke.

Bipolar disorder is diagnosed with a clinical interview. The interviewer checks to see whether the person has experienced specific symptoms for a period of at least 2 weeks. The clinician must also make sure that the person has no physical problems that could cause symptoms like those of bipolar disorder, such as thyroid gland disease.

Bipolar disorder is a major psychiatric illness that is diagnosed with a clinical interview.

About 1% of people develop bipolar disorder.

SYMPTOMS OF MANIA

The symptoms of mania involve a change in mood states (usually irritability or euphoria), increased self-esteem and confidence, and increased goal-directed activity (for example, the person spends an excessive amount of time and energy on work, school, or other activities). Some of these symptoms will affect how people perform their daily activities. A person does not have to have all of the following symptoms to be diagnosed with mania.

Common symptoms of mania include the following:

- Euphoria
- Irritability
- Reduced need for sleep

(continued)

- Increased talkativeness
- Inflated self-esteem
- Grandiosity
- Increased goal-directed activity
- Racing thoughts
- Distractibility

The term *hypomanic symptoms* refers to manic symptoms that are less severe and less disruptive.

SYMPTOMS OF DEPRESSION

Depressive symptoms are the opposite of manic symptoms, with low mood and inactivity as the major features. A person does not need to have all of the following symptoms to be diagnosed with depression.

Common symptoms of depression include the following:

- Depressed mood or sadness
- Decreased interest or pleasure
- Feeling worthless, hopeless, or helpless
- Guilt
- Suicidality
- Change in appetite and/or weight
- Sleep disturbances
- Lethargy or agitation
- Fatigue
- Problems with attention, concentration, and making decisions

> Common symptoms of bipolar disorder include:
> - Mania (euphoria, irritability, etc.)
> - Depression (low mood, etc.)

FREQUENTLY ASSOCIATED SYMPTOMS

Some people with bipolar disorder may experience other psychiatric symptoms when they have a manic or depressive episode, although these symptoms are not among those used to diagnose the disorder. Such symptoms include *hallucinations* (hearing, seeing, feeling, or smelling things that aren't there) and *delusions* (unusual beliefs that other people don't have—for example, paranoia or fear of being persecuted).

(continued)

SIMILAR PSYCHIATRIC DISORDERS

Bipolar disorder shares some symptoms with other major psychiatric disorders, including schizophrenia and schizoaffective disorder. There are differences between bipolar disorder and these other disorders, however. The primary difference is that when a person with bipolar disorder has a stable mood, he or she usually does not experience hallucinations or delusions, while a person with schizophrenia or schizo- affective disorder may have these symptoms even during periods when his or her mood is stable. People with posttraumatic stress disorder (PTSD) or personality disorders also experience intense mood shifts. The mood shifts in bipolar disorder typically last for weeks to months, while mood shifts among people with PTSD or personality disorder may last only minutes or hours.

> The symptoms of bipolar disorder
> overlap with those of other psychiatric disorders.

TREATMENT

Medications are used to treat the symptoms of bipolar disorder. Lithium, carbamazepine, and valproic acid are effective medications. Antipsychotic medications like olanzapine can also treat the symptoms of bipolar disorder. Antidepressant medications are sometimes used to treat depression in bipolar disorder, but they may increase the frequency of hypomanic or manic episodes.

Many people with bipolar disorder also use supportive counseling and family treatment to help them cope with the disruptive aspects of the disorder.

> Bipolar disorder is treated
> with medication, as well as other services
> (such as counseling and family treatment).

FURTHER READING

Copeland, M. E. (1994). *Living without Depression and Manic Depression: A Workbook for Maintaining Mood Stability*. Oakland, CA: New Harbinger.

Jamison, K. R. (1995). *An Unquiet Mind: A Memoir of Moods and Madness*. New York: Vintage.

Miklowitz, D. (2002). *The Bipolar Disorder Survival Guide: What You and Your Family Need to Know*. New York: Guilford Press.

Mondimore, F. M. (1999). *Bipolar Disorder: A Guide for Patients and Families*. Baltimore: John Hopkins University Press.

Understanding Major Depression

Major depression is a psychiatric disorder in which a person experiences a very low mood, or *depressed mood*. The person may also have a loss of interest in activities and low energy. Depression differs from feeling "blue," in that it causes severe enough problems to interfere with a person's day-to-day functioning.

The cause of major depression is unknown. Theories suggest that there may be more than one cause. Biochemical theories suggest that two chemicals, *norepinephrine* and *serotonin*, play an important role in depression. Imbalances of these chemicals may be caused by genetic factors, early experiences (such as the loss of a parent at an early age), or both. Between 10% and 15% of people experience an episode of depression during their lifetime.

Depression can happen at any point in a person's life. Some people experience depression but then fully recover from the disorder. Other people struggle with depression throughout much of their lives. People struggling with depression can nevertheless lead very useful and successful lives, as President Abraham Lincoln and the writer Ernest Hemingway did.

Major depression is diagnosed with a clinical interview. The interviewer checks to see whether the person has experienced severe symptoms for at least 2 weeks. Less severe symptoms over a more extended period of time may be diagnosed as *dysthymic disorder*.

> Major depression is a psychiatric illness
> that is diagnosed with a clinical interview.
> Major depression occurs in 10–15% of people.

SYMPTOMS OF DEPRESSION

The primary symptoms of depression include low mood, as well as problems with activity level, sleep, appetite, and thinking. A person does not have to have all the symptoms listed below to receive a diagnosis of major depression.

Common symptoms of depression include the following:

- Depressed mood
- Decreased interest or pleasure
- Feeling worthless, hopeless, or helpless
- Guilt
- Suicidality
- Change in appetite and/or weight
- Sleep disturbances (too much or too little)

(continued)

- Lethargy or agitation
- Fatigue
- Problems with attention, concentration, and making decisions

FREQUENTLY ASSOCIATED SYMPTOMS

Some people with depression may experience other psychiatric symptoms, although these symptoms are not among those used to diagnose depression. They may include *hallucinations* (hearing, seeing, feeling, or smelling things that aren't there) or *delusions* (unusual beliefs that other people don't have, such as persecutory delusions), when their mood is depressed. These symptoms usually go away when their mood is normal.

> Common symptoms of depression include:
> - Depressed mood
> - Weight/appetite and sleep changes
> - Changes in energy and activity level
> - Feeling worthless, helpless, hopeless, guilty, suicidal
> - Concentration/attention problems

SIMILAR PSYCHIATRIC DISORDERS

Major depression shares symptoms with other major psychiatric disorders. People with bipolar disorder, schizoaffective disorder, or schizophrenia may experience symptoms of depression, but there are important differences as well. People with bipolar disorder also have manic episodes, whereas people with major depression do not. People with schizophrenia or schizoaffective disorder may experience depression, but when their mood is normal they may continue to experience hallucinations and delusions.

> The symptoms of major depression
> may overlap with those of other psychiatric disorders.

TREATMENT

Special medications called *antidepressants* are often used to treat major depression. For depressions that don't respond to medication, sometimes *electroconvulsive therapy* (*ECT*) can be an effective treatment.

Many people with depression may also benefit from psychotherapy and family treatment to help them deal with the disruptive aspects of the disorder.

> Effective treatments for major depression include
> medication, counseling, and sometimes ECT.

(continued)

FURTHER READING

Burns, D. (1999). *Feeling Good: The New Mood Therapy* (rev. ed.). New York: Bantam.

Copeland, M. E. (1992). *The Depression Workbook: A Guide for Living with Depression and Manic Depression*. Oakland, CA: New Harbinger.

DePaulo, J. R., Jr. (2002). *Understanding Depression: What We Know and What You Can Do about It*. New York: Wiley.

Papolos, D. F., & Papolos, J. (1997). *Overcoming Depression* (3rd ed.). New York: HarperPerennial.

Understanding Obsessive–Compulsive Disorder

Obsessive–compulsive disorder (OCD) is a major psychiatric disorder. People with OCD may have anxiety related to severe *obsessions* (repeated worries that are difficult to stop thinking about) or *compulsions* (recurrent behaviors or thoughts that must be repeated over and over to reduce anxiety). People with OCD often recognize that their obsessions and compulsions are not normal or rational, but they can't seem to stop them.

The cause of OCD is unknown, but there are several theories. One theory is based on learning. A person experiences a minor distressing thought, image, or impulse, which causes anxiety. The person tries to use thoughts or behaviors to dispel the anxiety, and these are temporarily successful. However, over time the anxiety gets worse as the obsessions increase, and the person develops elaborate thinking strategies or compulsions as attempts to lower the anxiety. There are also biological theories of OCD that focus on an imbalance of brain chemicals, particularly the neurotransmitter (brain chemical) *serotonin*.

Between 2% and 3% of people develop OCD in their lifetime. OCD often develops in late adolescence or early adulthood, although it may occur at any time in a person's life. For some people, OCD is a chronic lifelong disorder. Others may achieve complete recovery.

OCD is diagnosed with a clinical interview. The interviewer checks to see whether the person has experienced specific symptoms for a period of time.

> OCD is a major psychiatric illness that is diagnosed with a clinical interview.
> OCD occurs in 2–3% of people.

OBSESSIVE SYMPTOMS

A person with obsessions has disturbing recurrent thoughts, impulses, or images that cause a great deal of anxiety, such as thoughts of hurting a loved one or thoughts of having been exposed to a fatal disease. Sometimes people realize these obsessions aren't real, but other times they do not. These obsessions lead to efforts to avoid, suppress, or neutralize the thoughts.

COMPULSIVE SYMPTOMS

A person with compulsions repeats behaviors or thoughts to reduce the anxiety related to obsessions, or does so because he or she can't resist doing it. The person may spend several hours a day engaging in these compulsions.

(continued)

Common compulsions include the following:

- Checking things, such as making sure doors and windows are locked, lights are turned off, and appliances are turned off
- Washing and cleaning, such as repeated hand washing
- Repeating behaviors over and over, such as dressing and undressing
- Ordering, such as having objects line up
- Hoarding things like old newspapers
- Thinking rituals, such as repeating prayers over and over

FREQUENTLY ASSOCIATED SYMPTOMS

For some people with OCD, the obsessions and compulsions may take over their lives and lead to depression. When a person develops obsessions that are bizarre and strong, the obsessions can become *delusions* (or false beliefs). The diagnosis of OCD is not based on depression or delusions, however.

> Common symptoms of OCD include:
> - Obsessions (recurrent thoughts, etc.)
> - Compulsions (checking, washing, etc.)

SIMILAR PSYCHIATRIC DISORDERS

OCD shares some symptoms with other psychiatric disorders. The pervasive anxiety in OCD can be similar to that in posttraumatic stress disorder, and the depression can be similar to major depression. Obsessions that become delusional may be difficult to distinguish from the delusions that are present in schizophrenia or schizoaffective disorder. A person may have OCD and one of these other disorders, or the symptoms may only be related to the obsessions and compulsions.

> The symptoms of OCD overlap
> with those of other psychiatric disorders.

TREATMENT

Two types of treatment for OCD are effective: *behavior therapy* and *medication*. Behavior therapy works by employing two therapeutic principles: *exposure* and *response generation*. In exposure, people learn to confront their fears rather than escaping from them and over time their anxiety decreases. In response prevention, people are taught to stop compulsions and break the cycle of repeated behaviors. Family treatment can also help to reduce the stress a person with OCD experiences.

Antidepressant medications can help to alleviate the symptoms of OCD as well. These medications are believed to change levels of the neurotransmitter (brain chemical) serotonin, leading to improvements in OCD symptoms.

(continued)

Effective treatments for OCD
are behavior therapy and medication.

FURTHER READING

Foa, E. B., & Wilson, R. (2001). *Stop Obsessing!: How to Overcome Your Obsessions and Compulsions* (rev. ed.). New York: Bantam.

Goodman, W. K., Rudorfer, M. V., & Maser, J. D. (Eds.). (2000). *Obsessive–Compulsive Disorder: Contemporary Issues in Treatment*. Mahwah, NJ: Erlbaum.

Rapoport, J. L. (1989). *The Boy Who Couldn't Stop Washing: The Experience and Treatment of Obsessive–Compulsive Disorder*. New York: Dutton.

Steketee, G., & White, K. (1990). *When Once Is Not Enough: Help for Obsessive Compulsives*. Oakland, CA: New Harbinger.

Understanding Posttraumatic Stress Disorder

Posttraumatic stress disorder (PTSD) is a major psychiatric disorder that may occur when a person experiences or witnesses a traumatic, often life-threatening event. Examples of common traumatic events that may cause PTSD are combat, sexual abuse, assault or rape, accidents, natural disasters, and the sudden, unexpected death of a loved one. People with PTSD experience high levels of anxiety, arousal, and avoidance due to recurrent memories of the traumatic event.

It is not clear why some people develop PTSD after a trauma and others do not. Theories suggest that both learning and biological factors may contribute to the cause of PTSD. The number of traumas a person experiences is also important. The effects of repeated traumas may be cumulative and result in increased severity of symptoms. From 1% to 10% of people develop PTSD at some point in their lives.

PTSD may develop anytime in a person's life, after experiencing a traumatic event. For some people, the symptoms of PTSD gradually disappear over weeks or months, but for other people they may get worse over time. With treatment a person may fully recover from PTSD, although some people may continue to experience symptoms after treatment.

PTSD is diagnosed with a clinical interview. The interviewer checks to see whether the person has experienced specific symptoms for more than a month.

> PTSD is a major psychiatric illness
> that is diagnosed with a clinical interview.
> PTSD occurs in 1–10% of people at some point in their lives.

SYMPTOMS OF PTSD

PTSD is diagnosed based on the presence of three types of symptoms: reexperiencing the trauma, avoidance of stimuli associated with the trauma, and increased arousal. People do not have to have all of the following symptoms to be diagnosed with PTSD, but they need to have at least some of each type of symptom.

Reexperiencing the Trauma

- Recurrent nightmares of the event
- Recurrent and intrusive memories of the event
- Distress at events that are reminders of the trauma
- Suddenly acting or feeling as if the event were recurring

(continued)

Avoidance of the Stimuli Associated with the Trauma

- Efforts to avoid thoughts, feelings, situations, or activities that trigger memories of the trauma
- Feeling detached or estranged from others
- A sense of foreshortened future
- Inability to recall an important aspect of the trauma
- Diminished interest in significant activities

Increased Arousal

- Hypervigilance (e.g., always "looking over one's shoulder")
- Increased arousal in situations that remind the person of the trauma
- Difficulty sleeping
- Difficulty concentrating
- Exaggerated startle response
- Irritability or anger outbursts

Common symptoms of PTSD include:
- Reexperiencing the trauma
- Avoidance of stimuli associated with the trauma
- Feeling emotionally numb
- Overarousal

FREQUENTLY ASSOCIATED SYMPTOMS

People with PTSD often experience other psychiatric symptoms, although these are not among the symptoms used to diagnose PTSD. Depression is a very common problem. Some people may experience *hallucinations* (hearing, seeing, feeling, or smelling things that aren't there) or *delusions* (unusual beliefs that other people don't have—for example, persecutory delusions) related to their traumatic experience.

SIMILAR PSYCHIATRIC DISORDERS

PTSD shares some symptoms with other psychiatric disorders. The anxiety, anger, and overarousal of PTSD may seem like the mania of bipolar disorder. Some of the symptoms of PTSD may overlap with those of schizophrenia or schizoaffective disorder. For example, people with PTSD may reexperience the trauma to the point of hallucinations. Their avoidance of people who remind them of their trauma may lead to social withdrawal, and their emotional numbing may resemble the blunted (or flattened) affect often present in schizophrenia or schizoaffective disorder. People with PTSD may also experience symptoms of major depression or obsessive–compulsive disorder. A person may have PTSD and also one of these other disorders, or the symptoms may only be related to the traumatic event.

(continued)

TREATMENT

Several different treatments are effective for people with PTSD. *Behavior therapy* is a very effective treatment approach for PTSD. Two types of behavior therapy are used to treat PTSD: *exposure therapy* (also called *flooding*) and *cognitive restructuring* (also called *cognitive therapy* or *cognitive processing therapy*). In exposure therapy, the client is helped to confront feared memories and safe situations that remind him or her of the trauma, rather than avoiding them, in order to learn that feared memories and situations cannot hurt him or her. In cognitive restructuring, the client is helped to challenge distorted beliefs about him- or herself and the world that are related to the trauma in order to develop more realistic and cognitive beliefs. Behavior therapy for PTSD may involve exposure therapy, cognitive restructuring, or a combination of the two.

In addition to behavior therapy, medication and supportive counseling may improve the symptoms of PTSD. Antidepressant and antipsychotic medications can decrease symptoms. Supportive counseling, in which the person can talk about feelings and get help resolving problems, can also be helpful.

> There are several treatments for PTSD, which include:
> - Behavior therapy
> - Supportive counseling
> - Medication

FURTHER READING

Foa, E. B., Keane, T. M., & Friedman, M. J. (Eds.). (2000). *Effective Treatments for PTSD*. New York: Guilford Press.

Rosenbloom, D., & Williams, M. B., with Watkins, B. E. (1999). *Life after Trauma: A Workbook for Healing*. New York: Guilford Press.

Schiraldi, G. R. (2000). *The Post-Traumatic Stress Disorder Sourcebook: A Guide to Healing, Recovery, and Growth*. Los Angeles, CA: Lowell House.

Understanding Schizoaffective Disorder

Schizoaffective disorder is a major psychiatric disorder that is similar to schizophrenia. People with this illness may experience *hallucinations* (hearing, seeing, feeling, or smelling things that aren't there) or *delusions* (unusual beliefs that other people don't have, such as paranoid beliefs that others are against them), as well as low motivation and poor attention. Unlike schizophrenia, people with schizoaffective disorder may also experience extremely high moods (*mania*) or extremely low moods (*depression*) for prolonged periods of time.

The cause of schizoaffective disorder is unknown. Scientists believe the disorder may be caused by an imbalance in neurotransmitters (brain chemicals), particularly the neurotransmitter *dopamine*. These imbalances may be due to genetic factors, early effects of the environment on the developing brain (such as when the baby is in the womb or during birth), or both.

About 0.5% of people (1 in 200) develop schizoaffective disorder in their lifetime. Schizoaffective disorder is diagnosed with a clinical interview. The interviewer checks to see whether the person has experienced specific symptoms over a long enough period of time. The clinician must also make sure that the person has no physical problems that could cause symptoms like those of schizoaffective disorder, such as a brain tumor.

> Schizoaffective disorder is a major psychiatric illness
> that is diagnosed with a clinical interview.
> Schizoaffective disorder occurs in 0.5% of people (1 of 200).

SYMPTOMS OF SCHIZOAFFECTIVE DISORDER

Four broad types of symptoms are very common in schizoaffective disorder: *psychotic symptoms*, *negative symptoms*, *mania*, and *depression*. Psychotic symptoms are thoughts, perceptions, and behaviors that are present in people with schizoaffective disorder (and also schizophrenia), but not in other people. These symptoms often reflect difficulties distinguishing between what is real and not real. Negative symptoms are the absence of thoughts, perceptions, and behaviors that are usually present in other people. Manic symptoms reflect heightened mood states (especially euphoria and irritability), increased self-esteem and confidence, and increased goal-directed activity (such as spending an excessive amount of time and energy on work, school, or other activities). Depressive symptoms are the opposite of manic symptoms, with low mood and inactivity as the major features.

A person does not have to have all of these types of symptoms to be diagnosed with schizoaffective disorder.

(continued)

Common Psychotic Symptoms

- Hallucinations
- Delusions
- Bizarre, disorganized, or strange behaviors
- Disorganized speech

Common Negative Symptoms

- Flattened affect
- Apathy and low motivation
- Loss of pleasure
- Lack or low amount of speech, or limited content of speech

Common Symptoms of Mania

- Euphoria
- Irritability
- Reduced need for sleep
- Increased talkativeness
- Inflated self-esteem
- Grandiosity
- Increased goal-directed activity
- Racing thoughts
- Distractibility

Common Symptoms of Depression

- Depressed mood or sadness
- Decreased interest or pleasure
- Feeling worthless, hopeless, or helpless
- Guilt
- Suicidality
- Change in appetite and/or weight
- Sleep disturbances (too much or too little)
- Lethargy or agitation
- Fatigue
- Problems with attention, concentration, and making decisions

> Common symptoms of schizoaffective disorder include:
> - Psychotic symptoms
> - Negative symptoms
> - Mania
> - Depression
> - Disorganization

(continued)

FREQUENTLY ASSOCIATED SYMPTOMS

Some people with schizoaffective disorder may also experience thinking problems, though these are not among the symptoms used in making a schizoaffective diagnosis. These may include difficulties with memory, trouble with abstract reasoning, difficulty planning, and attention problems.

SIMILAR PSYCHIATRIC DISORDERS

Schizoaffective disorder shares some symptoms with other major psychiatric disorders, such as schizophrenia, bipolar disorder, and major depression. However, there are some important differences. People with schizoaffective disorder or schizophrenia often have hallucinations or delusions even when their mood is stable, whereas people with major depression or bipolar disorder do not have these symptoms when their mood is stable. People with schizoaffective disorder often experience mood symptoms such as mania or depression, while people with schizophrenia usually experience less severe mood symptoms.

> The symptoms of schizoaffective disorder overlap
> with those of other psychiatric disorders.

TREATMENT

As in schizophrenia, antipsychotic medications are effective in treating the symptoms of schizoaffective disorder. Mood-stabilizing medications and antidepressant medications are sometimes used to treat the mood symptoms of this disorder. It is very important that medications be taken regularly to decrease symptoms, to prevent relapses, and to make sure that the illness does not become more severe.

Many people with schizoaffective disorder also benefit from social skills training, supported employment, case management, family treatment, and learning illness management techniques (such as how to prevent relapses and cope with symptoms).

> Schizoaffective disorder is treated with medication,
> as well as other services (including family treatment,
> vocational rehabilitation, and skills training approaches).

FURTHER READING

Mueser, K. T., & Gingerich, S. L. (in press). *Coping with Schizophrenia: A Guide for Families* (2nd ed.). New York: Guilford Press.

Schiller, L., & Bennett, A. (1994). *The Quiet Room: A Journey Out of the Torment of Madness.* New York: Warner Books.

Torrey, E. F. (2001). *Surviving Schizophrenia: A Family Manual* (4th ed.). New York: HarperTrade.

Understanding Schizophrenia

Schizophrenia is a major psychiatric illness. People often experience symptoms such as *hallucinations* (hearing, seeing, feeling, or smelling things that aren't there) or *delusions* (unusual beliefs that other people don't have, such as paranoid beliefs that others are against them). They may also have other symptoms, such as low motivation, poor attention, and inability to experience pleasure. Sometimes it is hard for people with schizophrenia to distinguish fantasy from reality.

The cause of schizophrenia is unknown. Scientists believe it may be caused by an imbalance in neurotransmitters (brain chemicals), especially the chemical *dopamine*. Imbalances of these neurotransmitters may be caused by genetic factors, early effects of the environment on the developing brain (such as when the baby is in the womb or during birth), or both.

About 1% of people develop schizophrenia during their lifetime. Schizophrenia usually develops between the ages of 16 and 30, but may develop after that. It is a lifelong disorder.

Schizophrenia is diagnosed with a clinical interview. The interviewer checks to see whether a person has experienced symptoms and, if so, for how long. To be diagnosed with schizophrenia, a person must experience a decrease in social functioning (school, work, social relationships, or self-care) for at least 6 months. The clinician must also make sure that the person has no physical problems that could cause problems like those of schizophrenia, such as a brain tumor.

> Schizophrenia is a major psychiatric illness
> that is diagnosed with a clinical interview.
> Schizophrenia occurs in 1% of people.

SYMPTOMS OF SCHIZOPHRENIA

Two broad types of symptoms are very common in schizophrenia: *psychotic symptoms* and *negative symptoms*. Psychotic symptoms are thoughts, perceptions, and behaviors that are present in people with schizophrenia, but not in other people. These symptoms often reflect difficulties distinguishing between what is real and not real. Negative symptoms are the absence of thoughts, perceptions, and behaviors that are present in other people. A person does not have to have all of the following symptoms to be diagnosed with schizophrenia.

Common Psychotic Symptoms

- Hallucinations
- Delusions
- Bizarre, disorganized, or strange behaviors
- Disorganized speech

(continued)

Common Negative Symptoms

- Flattened affect (diminished expressiveness)
- Apathy and low motivation
- Loss of pleasure
- Lack or low amount of speech, or limited content of speech

> Common symptoms of schizophrenia include:
> - Psychotic symptoms (hallucinations, delusions, etc.)
> - Negative symptoms (apathy and low motivation, loss of pleasure, etc.)
> - Disorganization

FREQUENTLY ASSOCIATED SYMPTOMS

Some people with schizophrenia may also experience cognitive problems and other symptoms, though these are not used in making the diagnosis of schizophrenia. Cognitive problems include difficulties with memory, trouble with abstract reasoning, difficulty planning, and attention problems. Some other associated symptoms are depression, fluctuating mood, anxiety, and anger or hostility.

SIMILAR PSYCHIATRIC DISORDERS

Schizophrenia shares some symptoms with other major psychiatric disorders, such as bipolar disorder, major depression, and schizoaffective disorder. However, there are important differences between schizophrenia and these other disorders. People with bipolar disorder or major depression sometimes experience hallucinations or delusions when their mood is abnormal (depressed or manic). In contrast, people with schizophrenia or schizoaffective disorder often continue to experience hallucinations or delusions even when their mood is normal. People with schizoaffective disorder experience prolonged or frequent problems with their mood (either depression, mania, or both), whereas people with schizophrenia tend to have less severe problems with their mood.

> The symptoms of schizophrenia overlap
> with those of other psychiatric disorders.

TREATMENT

Antipsychotic medications are used to treat schizophrenia. Sometimes antidepressant and mood-stabilizing medications are used as well. It is very important that medications are taken regularly to decrease symptoms, to prevent relapses, and to make sure that the illness does not become more severe.

(continued)

Many people with schizophrenia also benefit from social skills training, supported employment, case management, family treatment, and learning illness management techniques, such as how to prevent relapses and cope with symptoms.

> Schizophrenia is treated with medication,
> as well as other services (including family treatment,
> vocational rehabilitation, and skills training approaches).

FURTHER READING

Mueser, K. T., & Gingerich, S. L. (in press). *Coping with Schizophrenia: A Guide for Families* (2nd ed.). New York: Guilford Press.

Schiller, L., & Bennett, A. (1994). *The Quiet Room: A Journey Out of the Torment of Madness*. New York: Warner Books.

Torrey, E. F. (2001). *Surviving Schizophrenia: A Family Manual* (4th ed.). New York: Harper Trade.

Understanding Antidepressant Medications

Antidepressant medications are primarily used to treat depression, but they may also be used to treat other symptoms, such as anxiety and chronic pain. Antidepressant medications were first discovered in the 1950s, and new ones continue to be developed.

> Antidepressant medications are effective
> in reducing depression and anxiety.

Antidepressant medications are frequently used in the treatment of major depression and some anxiety disorders, such as posttraumatic stress disorder, obsessive–compulsive disorder, panic disorder, and social phobia. Sometimes these medications are also used to treat bipolar disorder.

> Antidepressant medications are used
> in the treatment of major depression
> and other psychiatric disorders.

Antidepressant medications work by affecting neurotransmitters (chemicals in the brain). Two neurotransmitters that are important include *serotonin* and *norepinephrine*. Some antidepressant medications mainly affect serotonin; others mainly affect norepinephrine; and others affect both neurotransmitters.

> Antidepressant medications work
> by altering chemicals in the brain
> called *neurotransmitters*.

FACTS ABOUT ANTIDEPRESSANT MEDICATIONS

- Antidepressant medications are usually taken by mouth.
- They are not addictive.
- The medications may work in a few days, but they usually require 4–6 weeks to become completely effective.

(continued)

- Taking antidepressant medications has two main effects:
  - They reduce the severity of depression and anxiety.
  - They lower the chances of relapses of depression and anxiety in the future.
- If symptom relapses occur, a temporary increase in antidepressant medication dosage may be helpful.

COMMON ANTIDEPRESSANT MEDICATIONS

Following is a table of the most common antidepressants. They are divided into four major groups: *tricyclic antidepressants*, *monoamine oxidase inhibitors (MAOIs)*, *selective serotonin reuptake inhibitors (SSRIs)*, and *other compounds*.

Antidepressant Medications

Type of drug	Brand name	Chemical name
Tricyclics	Anafranil	Clomipramine
	Elavil	Amitriptyline
	Norpramin	Desipramine
	Pamelor, Aventyl	Nortriptyline
	Sinequan, Adapin	Doxepin
	Tofranil	Imipramine
	Vivactil	Protriptyline
MAOIs	Marplan	Isocarboxazid
	Nardil	Phenelzine
	Parnate	Tranylcypromine
SSRIs	Celexa	Citalopram
	Lexapro	Escitalopram
	Luvox	Fluvoxamine
	Paxil	Paroxtine
	Prozac	Fluoxetine
	Zoloft	Sertraline
Other compounds	Desyrel	Trazodone
	Effexor	Venlafaxine
	Ludiomil	Maprotiline
	Remeron	Mirtazapine
	Serzone	Nefazodone
	Wellbutrin, Zyban	Bupropion

There are four major groups of antidepressant medications:
tricyclics, *MAOIs*, *SSRIs*, and *other compounds*.

(continued)

SIDE EFFECTS

Antidepressant medications can have some unpleasant side effects. To reduce these side effects, either the dosages or the medications themselves can be changed.

There are particular risks for people with bipolar disorder taking antidepressants. These medications may cause hypomania or mania. If this occurs, the dosages may need to be reduced or the medications stopped.

Antidepressant medications can also occasionally cause hypomanic or manic symptoms (such as increased irritability or euphoria, decreased need for sleep, inflated self-esteem, or grandiosity) in people with depression who have no prior history of such symptoms. If hypomanic or manic symptoms are observed in someone who is being treated with antidepressant medications for depression, the prescribing physician should be consulted immediately. Again, these symptoms can usually be resolved by stopping the antidepressant medications or adjusting the dosages.

The MAOIs have side effects with the chemical tyramine, which is found in certain foods and drinks. People taking MAOIs should get a complete list of the foods and beverages to be avoided from their doctor.

Following is a table of common side effects.

Side Effects of Antidepressant Medications

Drug group	Side effects
Tricyclics	Dry mouth, dizziness, sedation or agitation, weight gain, constipation, heart palpitations, cardiac abnormalities
MAOIs	Insomnia, dizziness, weight gain, sexual difficulties, confusion, memory problems, overstimulation, hypertensive crisis
SSRIs	Nausea, vomiting, excitement, agitation, headache, sexual problems (delayed ejaculation, not experiencing orgasm)
Other compounds	Same as SSRIs, plus potential to elevate blood pressure, sedation, or agitation

> Antidepressant medications can have some unpleasant side effects.
>
> The dosages can be adjusted or the medications can be changed to relieve these side effects.

Understanding Antipsychotic Medications

Antipsychotic medications (also called *major tranquilizers* or *neuroleptics*) were first discovered in the 1950s. Many antipsychotic medications have been developed since then. Antipsychotic medications are effective in treating *psychotic symptoms*, such as hallucinations, delusions, and disorganized thinking. They can also be helpful in reducing *negative symptoms*, such as apathy and social withdrawal. In addition, antipsychotic medications are useful in controlling mood swings.

> Antipsychotic medications are effective
> in reducing psychotic symptoms and other symptoms.

Antipsychotic medications are frequently used in the treatment of schizophrenia and schizoaffective disorder. They are also often used to treat bipolar disorder. Sometimes these medications are used to treat major depression and other disorders as well.

> Antipsychotics are used to treat
> schizophrenia and other psychiatric disorders.

Antipsychotic medications work by affecting the neurotransmitter (brain chemical) *dopamine*. Some of the newer antipsychotic medications (called *second-generation, atypical,* or *novel antipsychotics*) also affect the neurotransmitter *serotonin*.

> Antipsychotic medications work by altering chemicals
> in the brain called *neurotransmitters*.

FACTS ABOUT ANTIPSYCHOTIC MEDICATIONS

- Antipsychotic medications are usually taken by mouth, but some short-acting and long-acting injectable forms exist.
- They are not addictive.
- The medications may work in a few days, but they usually require several weeks to become completely effective.
- Taking antipsychotic medications has two main effects:
  - They reduce the severity of symptoms.
  - They lower the chances of symptom relapses in the future.
- If symptom relapses occur, a temporary increase in antipsychotic medication dosage may be helpful.

(continued)

NOVEL ANTIPSYCHOTIC MEDICATIONS

The novel antipsychotics, mentioned above, work differently than the conventional antipsychotics do. They appear to affect different neurotransmitters in the brain. The novel antipsychotics include Clozaril, Risperdal, Zyprexa, Seroquel, Geodon, and Abilify. More novel antipsychotics are currently being developed. Some of these medications may be effective when the conventional medications have only been partially effective. Novel antipsychotics may also be more effective in treating the negative and cognitive symptoms than the conventional medications.

COMMON ANTIPSYCHOTIC MEDICATIONS

A table of commonly used antipsychotic medications (both conventional and novel) follows.

Antipsychotic Medications

Type of medication	Chemical name
Conventional	
Haldol[**]	Haloperidol
Loxitane	Loxapine
Mellaril	Thioridazine
Moban	Molindone
Navane	Thiothixene
Prolixin[**]	Fluphenazine
Serentil	Mesoridazine
Stelazine	Trifluoperazine
Thorazine	Chlorpromazine
Trilafon	Perphenazine
Novel	
Abilify	Aripiprazole
Clozaril	Clozapine
Geodon	Ziprasidone
Risperdal	Risperidone
Seroquel	Quetiapine
Zyprexa	Olanzapine

[**]Medications available in long-acting, injectable preparations.

> There are both conventional and novel antipsychotics, with many new medications currently under development.

(continued)

SIDE EFFECTS OF CONVENTIONAL ANTIPSYCHOTIC MEDICATIONS

The conventional antipsychotic medications have a number of side effects, some mild and some serious. These include the following:

- Drowsiness
- Muscle stiffness
- Dizziness
- Dry mouth
- Mild tremors
- Restlessness
- Increased appetite, weight gain
- Blurred vision
- Sexual difficulties
- Heart rhythm abnormalities

Tardive dyskinesia is a serious side effect that occurs in 10–20% of people taking conventional antipsychotics. Higher rates of tardive dyskinesia may occur in people taking these medications over very long periods of time. This is a neurological syndrome that causes involuntary muscle movements, usually in the tongue, the mouth or lips, the trunk, or the extremities (such as hands, fingers, or toes). It is usually mild, but sometimes may be severe and disfiguring. It usually does not go away, but reducing the dose of the conventional antipsychotic or switching to a novel antipsychotic may improve it.

> Antipsychotic medications cause several side effects.
> Tardive dyskinesia is one of the serious side effects.

MEDICATIONS FOR SIDE EFFECTS

Two types of medications (called *anticholinergics* and *dopamine agonists*) are used to treat side effects like muscle stiffness, tremors, and increased salivation. These are called *extrapyramidal side effects*.

Medications for Extrapyramidal Side Effects of Antipsychotics

Type of drug	Brand name	Chemical name
Anticholinergic	Akineton	Biperiden
	Artane	Trihexyphenidyl
	Cogentin	Benztropine
	Kemadrin	Procyclidine
Dopamine agonist	Symmetrel	Amantadine

(continued)

Another side effect of antipsychotics is *akathisia*, which is restlessness, agitation, or trouble sitting still. Medications like *beta-blockers* (such as Inderal, Tenormin, or Corgard) or *benzodiazepines* (such as Ativan or Valium) may help with akathisia. Unfortunately, there are also side effects associated with these medications.

Possible Side Effects of Side Effect Medications

Drug class	Side effects
Anticholinergics	Dry mouth, constipation, blurry vision, drowsiness, urinary retention, memory loss
Dopamine agonists	Increase in psychotic symptoms
Beta-blockers	Fatigue, depression
Benzodiazepines	Drowsiness, psychological or physiological dependence, psychomotor impairment, memory loss

> There are medications to treat side effects of conventional antipsychotics, but they have side effects of their own.

SIDE EFFECTS OF NOVEL ANTIPSYCHOTICS

Common side effects of Clozaril include drowsiness, increased salivation, dizziness, a slight increase in body temperature, changes in blood pressure, constipation, weight gain, *tachycardia* (rapid heart rate), *cataplexy* (sudden loss of muscle tone), and seizures. *Agranulocytosis* is a dangerous drop in a person's white blood cell count. This occurs less than 1% of the time with people taking Clozaril. To detect this problem, weekly blood tests are done so that the medication can be stopped if agranulocytosis occurs. Clozaril is also rarely associated with myocardia, or inflammation of the heart, which can be fatal.

Novel antipsychotic medications can cause some of the same side effects as the conventional antipsychotics, but usually they are much less severe and side effect medications are often not required to treat them. However, novel antipsychotics may cause some other side effects, which are listed below.

- Risperdal: Elevation of the hormone prolactin, sexual side effects, sedation, weight gain
- Zyprexa: Sedation, weight gain
- Seroquel: Dizziness, sedation, increased risk for cataracts
- Geodon: Possible heart rhythm abnormalities, sedation, nausea, constipation, dizziness
- Abilify: Headache, insomnia, nausea, vomiting, lightheadedness

> Novel antipsychotics tend to cause different side effects from conventional antipsychotics.

Understanding Mood-Stabilizing Medications

Mood-stabilizing medications are primarily used to treat the symptoms of bipolar disorder, including mania and depression, but they may also be used to treat other disorders, such as schizoaffective disorder. Several mood-stabilizing medications have been discovered over the past century, including lithium (the 1940s), carbamazepine and valproic acid (1970s and 1980s), and olanzapine (2000).

> Mood-stabilizing medications are effective
> in reducing episodes of mania and depression.
> They are used to treat bipolar disorder
> (and sometimes other disorders).

FACTS ABOUT MOOD-STABILIZING MEDICATIONS

- Mood-stabilizing medications are believed to work by affecting levels of neurotransmitters (chemicals in the brain).
- The medications are taken by mouth.
- They are not addictive.
- The medications may work in a few days, but they usually require several weeks to become completely effective.
- Mood-stabilizing medications can affect other symptoms, such as impulsiveness, agitation, hallucinations, delusions, and anxiety.
- Taking these medications has two main effects:
  - They reduce the severity of symptoms.
  - They lower the chances of symptom relapses in the future.
- If symptom relapses occur, a temporary increase in mood-stabilizing medication dosage may be helpful.

> Mood stabilizers affect certain
> neurotransmitters in the brain.

(continued)

TYPES OF MOOD STABILIZERS

There are three broad categories of mood-stabilizing medications: lithium, anticonvulsants (medications originally used to treat seizure disorders), and antipsychotics. See the following table.

Mood Stabilizers

Type of drug/brand name	Chemical name	Side effects
Lithium Eskalith, Eskalith Controlled Release, Lithobid, Lithonate	*Lithium carbonate*	*Common side effects* Nausea, weight gain, slowed thinking, fatigue, tremor
		Serious side effects Vomiting, diarrhea, slurred speech, confusion
Anticonvulsants Depakote, Depakene Tegretol	Valproic acid Carbamazepine	*Common side effects* Fatigue, weight gain, nausea, headache, decreased sexual desire
		Serious side effects Confusion, vomiting, abdominal pain, vision problems, fever, jaundice or liver damage, abnormal bleeding or bruising, blood cell count abnormalities, swelling lymph glands
Antipsychotics Zyprexa Clozaril	Olanzapine Clozapine	*Side effects* See "Understanding Antipsychotic Medications" handout

> There are three categories of mood stabilizers:
> - Lithium
> - Anticonvulsants
> - Antipsychotics

SPECIAL ISSUES WITH LITHIUM

If any of the serious side effects are experienced, clients should contact their doctor. High doses of lithium can be harmful to the brain; therefore, regular blood levels of lithium are routinely checked when someone is taking lithium. Low-salt diets and diuretic medications should be avoided, as they lower lithium levels. Anti-inflammatory drugs may increase lithium levels.

> Consult a physician if lithium causes side effects.

(continued)

SPECIAL ISSUES WITH ANTICONVULSANTS

Again, if any of the serious side effects are experienced, clients should contact their doctor. Anticonvulsants can be sedating, and alcohol may increase this sedation, so people using these medications should be careful when driving or operating machinery. Routine blood levels are conducted in order to monitor how the medication is affecting blood cells and the liver.

> Consult a physician if anticonvulsant medications cause side effects.

The Stress–Vulnerability Model of Psychiatric Disorders

Psychiatric illnesses tend to fluctuate over time, with their severity increasing and decreasing at different points in time. An episode of an illness (or a relapse) occurs when symptoms are severe and functioning is impaired. Understanding what factors contribute to relapses can help people learn how to manage their illness more effectively, and to prevent relapses or decrease their severity.

> Psychiatric illnesses fluctuate over time in their severity.

The *stress–vulnerability model of psychiatric disorders* provides a useful way of understanding how different factors influence the course of mental illness. According to this model, the course of a psychiatric illness is influenced by several factors: biological vulnerability, stress, medication, drugs and alcohol, coping skills, and social support. Each of these factors is described below, and illustrated in the accompanying diagram.

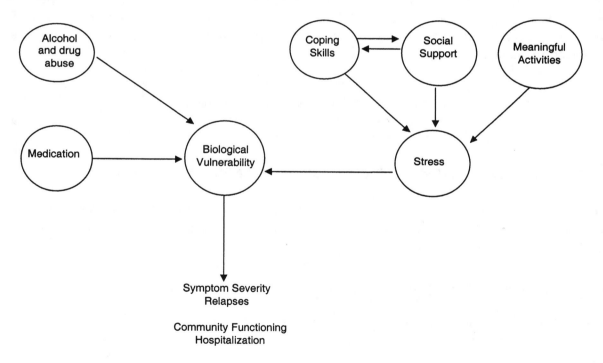

A diagram of the stress–vulnerability model.

(continued)

BIOLOGICAL VULNERABILITY

Each person has *biological vulnerability* to different diseases. This vulnerability is determined by a combination of genetic and other biological factors. For example, some people have a biological vulnerability to cardiac disease; some people have a vulnerability to specific types of cancer; and some people have a vulnerability to specific psychiatric disorders. Common psychiatric disorders to which people are biologically vulnerable include schizophrenia, schizoaffective disorder, bipolar disorder, major depression, and anxiety disorders.

Once a person has a biological vulnerability to a mental illness, that mental illness may either develop spontaneously or be triggered by stress. Even among people who have a psychiatric illness, vulnerability may differ from one person to another. On average, people who have a greater biological vulnerability to an illness experience more severe symptoms and difficulties.

STRESS

Stress refers to something in the environment that forces the person to adjust or adapt in some way. Stress can take the form of specific life events, such as the death of a loved one, a major move, or being a victim of crime. Stress can also be caused by living in difficult conditions, such as living with people who are hostile and critical, living in an unpredictable and dangerous environment, or living in poverty.

People who are biologically vulnerable to a psychiatric disorder and who are exposed to stress are more likely to develop that disorder. Once people have a psychiatric disorder, stress can cause relapses and worsen the course of the illness.

> Stress can affect biological vulnerability,
> leading to symptom relapses.

FACTORS THAT AFFECT BIOLOGICAL VULNERABILITY AND STRESS

Although biological vulnerability and stress influence the course of the psychiatric disorder, they can be affected by several factors. Those factors include medication, drugs and alcohol, coping skills, and social support.

Factors That Affect Biological Vulnerability

Biological vulnerability can be affected both by medications and by drugs and alcohol.

Medications

Medications for psychiatric disorders can decrease biological vulnerability. Medications are effective at both decreasing the severity of symptoms and preventing symptom relapses. People who take medications regularly and do experience relapses tend to have less severe relapses.

(continued)

Alcohol and Drugs

Alcohol and drug use can increase biological vulnerability. Some substances can directly increase biological vulnerability, while other substances can decrease the beneficial effects of medications on vulnerability. People with psychiatric disorders who use alcohol and drugs regularly are prone to more frequent relapses of their symptoms.

> Medications decrease biological vulnerability.
> Alcohol and drugs increase biological vulnerability.

Factors That Affect Stress

Stress can be decreased by coping skills, social support, and engaging in meaningful activity.

Coping Skills

Coping skills are strategies that people use to minimize the effects of stress. Examples of coping skills include relaxation, positive self-talk, problem solving, talking out one's feelings with a friend or support person, exercising, journal writing, and artistic expression. People who have several different coping skills are less susceptible to the negative effects of stress.

> Coping skills decrease
> the negative effects of stress.

Social Support

Social support refers to the help and caring that people feel they can count on from other people. Supportive persons can include family members, friends, members of the treatment team, a clergy member, or anyone else with whom a person has a close relationship. Good social support can decrease the effects of stress. Supportive people can sometimes solve problems with a person and decrease stress. For example, if a man feels criticized by his supervisor at work, a supportive person can help him identify strategies for learning more specifically about his supervisor's concerns. Supportive people can also help a person deal with the negative effects of stress. For example, if a woman has been a victim of crime, she can talk it over with a supportive person, and benefit from that person's concern and empathy.

Social support and coping skills can interact with one another. People with good coping skills can obtain more social support by reaching out and engaging with other people. Supportive people can also improve others' coping skills by helping them develop more effective strategies for dealing with stress. People who have more social support tend to experience fewer and less severe relapses.

> Social support decreases
> the negative effects of stress.

(continued)

Meaningful Activities

Meaningful activities are tasks that provide a strong sense of purpose and gratification to a person. Being involved in meaningful activities helps people to structure their time and gives them something to look forward to every day. Examples of meaningful activities include work, going to school, parenting a child, doing volunteer work, caring for someone else, and being a regular participant at a peer support program. Having meaningful activities to engage in reduces susceptibility to stress, because people are actively pursuing their goals and are less focused on stress.

> Engaging in meaningful activities
> decreases the negative affects of stress.

TREATMENT IMPLICATIONS OF THE STRESS–VULNERABILITY MODEL

The stress–vulnerability model points to five ways people with psychiatric illness (and their families) can improve the course of their illness:

1. Take psychiatric medications as prescribed.
2. Avoid alcohol and drug use.
3. Increase coping skills.
4. Increase social support.
5. Engage in meaningful activities, such as work, school, and parenting.

Taking these steps can help reduce relapses or lessen the severity of relapses, and therefore can help people make progress toward their personal goals.

> The stress–vulnerability model
> points to specific steps
> for reducing relapses and rehospitalizations.

Role of the Family

Family members can play an important role in reducing stress in an ill person's life and helping him or her achieve personal goals. Using good communication and problem-solving skills, creating a role for the ill family member that recognizes the person as the expert on the illness, and helping to monitor symptoms are all ways to enhance the family's role and improve everyone's life.

> Family members can help improve the outcome of a psychiatric disorder by participating in treatment.

EARLY WARNING SIGNS

Relapse is a part of any chronic illness. People with psychiatric disorders often experience small changes in thinking and behavior days or even weeks before a relapse or episode of illness. When family members are able to observe these early warning signs, and then help a client to recognize them and seek an appropriate intervention, it can make a dramatic difference in the outcome of the relapse. Early intervention can often prevent relapses and rehospitalizations, or minimize the severity of a relapse. Here are some examples of common early warning signs:

- Tension or agitation
- Eating problems
- Concentration problems
- Sleeping too little or too much
- Depression
- Social withdrawal
- Irritability
- Decreased compliance with treatment
- Anxiety
- Hallucinations or odd beliefs (delusions)

It is often helpful for the family members to make a list of the early warning signs they have noticed over time with their ill relative. Once they have that list, they should sit down with the client and draw up a list of actions everyone agrees to take once some of the early warning signs occur. This action plan should be agreed upon by client, family, and treatment providers, and signed by all parties.

> Recognizing early warning signs and developing early intervention strategies can help prevent relapse.

(continued)

In developing a plan, everyone should sit down and discuss past relapses, and the early warning signs noticed before. The family should also discuss the types of situations that have been stressful to the ill person in the past, and how to avoid them. A strategy for getting the family members together for a meeting should be put in place. Lastly, actions to be taken should be agreed upon by all family members.

> An action plan needs to include
> recognizing early warning signs,
> avoiding stressful situations,
> and holding a family meeting.

EFFECTS OF MENTAL ILLNESS ON THE FAMILY

Mental illness in a relative can have a major effect on all members of the family. Common reactions to mental illness include anxiety, fear, depression or sadness, guilt, frustration, and anger. In addition, relatives often devote considerable amounts of time and financial help to the ill family member. The net result of these emotional and other consequences of mental illness can be higher levels of stress on family members.

> Common reactions in family members
> to mental illness include:
> - Anxiety
> - Depression
> - Guilt
> - Frustration
> - Anger

When a person has a mental illness, relatives often change their roles to adjust to it. Some family members become very involved in assisting the ill member in meeting his or her day-to-day needs, spending large amounts of time with the person, and devoting much of their lives to helping him or her. Sometimes the level of involvement is so great that although the person appreciates it, he or she finds the attention is more than is truly wanted. Other family members can react to the mental illness by withdrawing from the person and becoming more emotionally distant. These relatives may feel that they don't have anything to offer, may be afraid of mental illness, or may be concerned that they may make matters worse. These changes in family roles are all normal reactions of concerned relatives trying to cope with mental illness.

> Family roles often change
> when relatives try to adjust
> to mental illness in a member.

(continued)

THE FAMILY SYSTEM

When one thing in a system changes, other things shift to accommodate the change. This is a very normal response. The family system is transformed when one member becomes mentally ill. Family members re-define their roles, so that they can maintain a safe environment and continue to get their needs met. Relatives can be supportive of an ill family member and still take care of themselves. Family members can get support for themselves by learning about mental illness, developing a relationship with treatment providers, and participating in support groups for families with a mentally ill member. Family members can also support their ill member in several ways. They can encourage taking medications and attending treatment, can help monitor the illness, can provide a low-stress environment, can help monitor substance use, and can encourage independent living. Providing support and being supported helps families regain their balance.

> Family members can both get support
> for themselves and provide support
> to their mentally ill relative.

FURTHER READING

Marsh, D. T., & Dickens, R. (1997). *How to Cope with Mental Illness in Your Family: A Self-Care Guide for Siblings, Offspring, and Parents.* New York: Tarcher/Putnam.

Neugeboren, J. (1999). *Transforming Madness: New Lives for People Living with Mental Illness.* New York: Morrow.

Secunda, V. (1997). *When Madness Comes Home: Help and Hope for the Children, Siblings, and Partners of the Mentally Ill.* New York: Hyperion.

Woolis, R. (1992). *When Someone You Love Has a Mental Illness: A Handbook for Family, Friends, and Caregivers.* New York: Tarcher/Perigee.

Basic Facts about Alcohol and Drugs

People sometimes use different substances to change the way that they feel, think, or experience the world. Examples of substances commonly used in this way include alcohol, marijuana, and cocaine. These and other substances can have a variety of effects on people. This educational handout reviews the different types of substances commonly used by people and the effects of these substances. In addition, the interactions between substance use and mental illness are discussed.

> This handout reviews the effects
> of different types of commonly used substances.

WHAT ARE PSYCHOACTIVE SUBSTANCES?

Psychoactive substances are substances that have a major effect on the mind. These effects may include the way people feel, how they think, or how they perceive the world around them. Any substance that affects a person's mind this way is a psychoactive substance.

> Psychoactive substances affect
> the way people feel, think, or perceive things.

HISTORY OF PSYCHOACTIVE SUBSTANCE USE

Since earliest civilization, people have used psychoactive substances for a number of different reasons, including medicinal, recreational, and spiritual purposes. For example, the Hittites in central Turkey discovered how to make beer around 7000 B.C., and in the Middle Ages it was a major source of nutrition. Hemp, the plant from which marijuana is derived, has a long history of use in countries in the Far East (such as India). In South America, farmers used to chew leaves of coca, the plant from which cocaine is derived, because of its stimulating properties. Some Indian tribes in Mexico and Central America have used the plant peyote, a powerful substance that can cause hallucinations, as part of religious and spiritual ceremonies.

> Psychoactive substances have been used from earliest civilization for
> medicinal, recreational, and spiritual purposes.

(continued)

DIFFERENT TYPES OF PSYCHOACTIVE SUBSTANCES

There are many different types of psychoactive substances. In order to discuss their effects, it is helpful to consider different types or groups of substances which are commonly used. The table below summarizes broad types of substances, and provides examples of specific substances in each broad category. In addition to describing the specific substances in each broad category, this table also gives examples of slang words for each substance, indicates how each substance is taken ("route of administration"), and describes the effects of the substance.

Different Psychoactive Substances and Their Effects

Substance type	Specific substances	Slang words	Route of administration	Effects
Alcohol	Beer, wine, "hard liquor" (e.g., vodka, Scotch, whiskey, gin, rum, tequila)	Booze; brew (beer)	Oral (drinking)	Relaxation, sedation Slowed reaction time Impaired judgment Loss of inhibition
Cannabis	Marijuana, hashish	Pot, reefer, weed; joint (marijuana cigarette); dope, grass	Smoking (most common), ingestion (eating)	Relaxation Mild euphoria Altered sensory experiences Fatigue Anxiety Panic Increased appetite Paranoia
Stimulants	Cocaine, amphetamines (and related compounds)	Coke, crack, rock (cocaine); crank, speed, crystal meth (amphetamines)	Intranasal (snorting), smoking, injection (cocaine); oral (eating pills), intranasal, injection (amphetamines)	Increased alertness and energy Decreased appetite Positive feelings Anxiety Tension, feeling jittery, heart racing Paranoia
Sedatives	Anxiolytic (anxiety-lowering) medications (e.g., Xanax, Klonopin, Ativan, Valium, barbiturates)	Downers (barbiturates), sleeping pills	Oral	Sleepiness Relaxation Loss of motor coordination Loss of inhibition Dulled sensory experiences
Hallucinogens	LSD, PCP, peyote, mescaline, MDMA	Acid, window pane (LSD); angel dust (PCP); buttons (peyote); magic mushrooms	Oral; smoking (PCP)	Enhanced or altered perceptions Hallucinations Disorientation Psychosis
Narcotics	Heroin, morphine, opium, codeine	Smack, horse, H (heroin)	Injection, intranasal (heroin); oral (morphine, codeine, and related substances)	Euphoria Pain relief Sedation Slowed reaction time Impaired judgment

(continued)

393

Substance type	Specific substances	Slang words	Route of administration	Effects
Inhalants	Glue, aerosols, nitrous oxide (laughing gas), freon		Inhalation (includes sniffing)	Altered perceptions Disorientation
Over-the-counter medications	Antihistamines and related compounds (e.g., Benadryl, other cold tablets)		Oral	Sedation
Tobacco	Cigarettes, pipe tobacco, chewing tobacco, snuff	Casket nails, smokes, cigs, butts (cigarettes)	Smoking; under the tongue (chewing tobacco, snuff)	Alertness Relaxation
Caffeine	Coffee, tea, chocolate		Oral	Increased alertness
Antiparkinsonian agents	Cogentin, Artane, Symmetrel		Oral	Confusion Mild euphoria

INTERACTIONS BETWEEN SUBSTANCE USE AND MENTAL ILLNESS

Substances such as alcohol, marijuana, and cocaine can have a wide range of effects on people (see the table above). These and other substances can produce even more dramatic effects in persons with a mental illness. The key to understanding the interactions between substance use and mental illness lies in the stress–vulnerability model of psychiatric illness.

According to this model (see "The Stress–Vulnerability Model of Psychiatric Disorders," Handout B.10), psychiatric illnesses are caused by biological factors determined very early in life. Although this biological vulnerability must be present for a mental illness to develop, the severity of the illness and course of symptoms are influenced by other factors as well. One factor that can worsen vulnerability, leading to symptom relapses, is stress from the environment. On the other hand, if a person has good coping skills, he or she will be less vulnerable to the negative effects of stress.

In addition to stress and coping skills, medications and psychoactive substances can have an effect on vulnerability. Prescribed medications can help correct some of the chemical imbalances in the brain believed to cause mental illnesses. However, just as medications can reduce vulnerability, psychoactive substances, such as alcohol, marijuana, and cocaine, can increase vulnerability. These substances can have a negative effect on mental illness in two ways. First, they can directly affect the brain chemicals responsible for the illness, worsening the illness. Second, psychoactive substances can interfere with medications used to treat mental illness, making them less effective.

The stress–vulnerability model explains why persons with a mental illness are highly sensitive to the effects of psychoactive substances. These individuals have a biological vulnerability that is the cause of their mental illness. This vulnerability makes them highly sensitive ("supersensitive") to the effects of psychoactive substances such as alcohol and cocaine. This is the reason why people with a mental illness are often affected by even small quantities of alcohol or drugs.

> Persons with a mental illness are supersensitive to small amounts of substances.

(continued)

CONSEQUENCES OF SUBSTANCE USE IN MENTAL ILLNESS

Substance use can cause a variety of different negative effects in persons with mental illness. The specific consequences depend on the individual and the type of substance used. Some of the most common consequences experienced by persons with a mental illness include the following:

- Symptom relapses and rehospitalizations
- Depression and increased risk of suicide
- Housing instability and homelessness
- Family conflict
- Anger and violence problems
- Money difficulties
- Becoming a target for predators
- Legal problems
- Risky sexual behavior
- Infectious diseases

> Substance use can cause a variety of negative consequences for persons with mental illness.

SUMMARY AND CONCLUSIONS

Many different psychoactive substances are used in the general population. These substances can have a variety of different effects. People with mental illness are more sensitive to the effects of alcohol and drugs than the general population. Their higher sensitivity to the effects of these substances can be explained by their biological vulnerability to mental illness. Because of this vulnerability, they may experience consequences from using even very small amounts of alcohol and drugs.

Alcohol and Drugs: Motives and Consequences

Alcohol and drugs can have many different effects on people. Individuals with mental illness tend to be more sensitive to the effects of substances, due to their biological vulnerability. This handout focuses on understanding the reasons why people with mental illness use different substances, and it reviews some of the consequences of substance use.

> This handout discusses motives
> of substance use and the consequences of use.

COMMON MOTIVES FOR ALCOHOL AND DRUG USE

People with mental illness give a number of different explanations for their use of substances. Some of the most common reasons for using substances are described below.

Socializing

Individuals may feel that using drugs or alcohol helps their social interactions with others. People give several different reasons why they think using substances may be helpful. Some people report feeling less anxious around other people when they use alcohol or drugs. Others use substances with their acquaintances as a way of spending time together. Some people use substances because they feel pressured by others to use. Yet another reason why some persons use substances is that it helps them feel "normal" and "accepted" by others; sometimes people don't feel they have a mental illness or are different from others when they are using drugs or alcohol.

Self-Medication

Some people use substances in an attempt to *self-medicate* (reduce the effects of) unpleasant symptoms. Although efforts to self-medicate symptoms are usually unsuccessful in the long run, they may be temporarily effective. Here are some of the most common symptoms that people report using substances to self-medicate:

- Depression
- Anxiety
- Sleep problems
- Nervousness
- Tension
- Hallucinations
- Medication side effects
- Loss of interest

(continued)

Pleasure Enhancement

Some individuals use substances because it is one of the few sources of pleasure they experience. Sometimes people use substances because they believe it enhances other enjoyable activities. Using alcohol or drugs may be very tempting for some individuals, because it is so easy to get these substances and their effects are so rapid.

Habit or Routine

Some people who have used drugs or alcohol for a long period of time continue to use them simply because it has become part of their daily routine—a habit. For these people, substance use becomes second nature. They use substances automatically, without much thought, almost like brushing their teeth or taking a shower.

Relieving Cravings or Withdrawal Symptoms

Individuals who use larger quantities of substances may develop cravings for these substances, or they may experience withdrawal symptoms if they stop using suddenly. Substance use for these individuals may be primarily motivated by the desire to avoid the cravings or withdrawal symptoms.

> Common motives for using
> substances include:
> - Socializing
> - Self-medication
> - Pleasure enhancement
> - Habit or routine
> - Relieving cravings
>   or withdrawal symptoms

CONSEQUENCES OF SUBSTANCE USE

The consequences of substance use can be divided into two broad categories: *behavioral* and *physical* consequences. Examples of each category are provided below.

Behavioral Consequences

Social Relationships

Substance use may lead to conflicts in important relationships, such as with family members, a spouse, or friends. This can result in tension, arguments, or conflicts. For example, a person who frequently uses marijuana may have repeated arguments with relatives about often being high or having money problems.

(continued)

397

Work or Role Functioning

A person's substance use may interfere with his or her ability to fulfill important roles, such as worker, homemaker, or student. For example, a person may be repeatedly late to work because of drinking the night before, leading to job losses.

Money Problems

Substance use may lead to financial problems, such as not having enough money by the end of the month. For example, a person may use up all of his or her money for the month on a cocaine binge lasting only a few days.

Legal Problems

Substance use may lead to legal problems, such as being arrested for drunk and disorderly conduct or for possession of an illegal substance.

Housing Instability

People with substance use problems may experience problems maintaining stable housing. Housing difficulties are often the result either of conflicts with family members or of eviction from an apartment because of drug deals, loud parties, or inability to maintain the apartment properly. Many housing programs for persons with mental illness will not accept anyone who is using substances.

Dangerous Situations

Substances may be used in physically hazardous situations. Examples include driving under the influence of alcohol or operating heavy machinery after taking drugs. Such use of substances increases the risk of accidents and injuries.

> Common behavioral consequences
> of substance use include:
> - Poor social relationships
> - Poor work or role functioning
> - Money and legal problems
> - Housing instability
> - Exposure to dangerous situations

Physical Consequences

Symptom Relapses

Substance use may worsen psychiatric symptoms leading to relapses and rehospitalizations. For example, cocaine use may trigger psychotic symptoms, requiring hospitalization.

(continued)

Health Problems

Drugs and alcohol use can lead to a variety of health problems. For example, alcohol can damage the liver; marijuana can cause lung and respiratory problems; and intranasal use of substances (such as cocaine) can damage internal parts of the nose (such as the septum).

> Common physical consequences of substance use include symptom relapses and health problems.

SUBSTANCE ABUSE

A person who experiences negative consequences due to substance use has a *substance use disorder*. A *disorder* is just like a psychiatric diagnosis; it is a term used to describe common symptoms or problems. Individuals whose substance use results in problems in the areas described above (such as problems with social relationships, work, legal consequences, or use in dangerous situations) have a diagnosis of *substance abuse*. Substance abuse is simply a term describing people who experience negative consequences from their use of psychoactive substances.

> *Substance abuse* refers to experiencing common negative consequences from substance use.

LONG-TERM CONSEQUENCES OF SUBSTANCE USE

Individuals who use alcohol or other drugs over long periods of time sometimes experience other consequences as well. Two broad categories of these of consequences include *psychological* consequences and *physical* consequences. Examples of each category are discussed below.

PSYCHOLOGICAL CONSEQUENCES

Giving Up Important Activities

A person may give up activities he or she used to enjoy in order to spend more time using alcohol or drugs. For example, a person may spend less time playing sports or with family members, and more time drinking alcohol.

Spending Large Amounts of Time Getting or Using Substances

Over time, some people spend more and more of their time involved in substance-use-related activities. As an example, much of a person's day may be spent finding money (for instance, through panhandling), finding a person from whom to buy cocaine, and using the cocaine.

(continued)

Using More of a Substance Than Planned

A person may drink more alcohol or use a greater amount of drugs than he or she planned on using. For example, someone might go to a party planning on drinking just one beer, but end up drinking four or five beers.

Repeated Attempts to Cut Down or Quit

Someone who uses alcohol or drugs may attempt on several occasions to cut down on his or her use or to quit altogether, without success each time. This can be frustrating and lead to feelings of hopelessness. For example, an individual who smokes marijuana several times a week may have tried on many occasions to stop smoking altogether, but each time returns to his or her habit.

> Long-term psychological consequences
> of substance use include:
> - Giving up important activities
> - Spending large amounts of time getting or using substances
> - Using more of a substance than planned
> - Repeated attempts to cut down or quit

Physical Consequences

Tolerance

An individual may find that he or she needs to use larger quantities of a substance in order to achieve a desired effect. For example, an individual who used to feel a "buzz" after two or three beers may find over time that seven or eight beers is needed to experience the same "buzz."

Cravings

Individuals sometimes experience intense cravings or yearnings for alcohol or drugs. Some individuals may find that their desire for substances is so strong that it cannot be resisted. For example, a person who regularly uses crack cocaine may find that after several days of not using cocaine, he or she experiences strong cravings to use this drug.

Withdrawal Symptoms

People who use substances on a regular basis may experience unpleasant symptoms (such as nervousness, nausea, tremors, fatigue, agitation, or sleeping problems) if they stop using the substance. When the person uses the desired substance, these withdrawal symptoms go away. For example, someone who has drunk four to six beers per night for a long period of time may experience nausea or tremors if he or she stops drinking suddenly.

(continued)

> Physical consequences of long-term substance use include:
> - Tolerance
> - Cravings
> - Withdrawal symptoms

SUBSTANCE DEPENDENCE

Substance dependence is a term used to describe individuals who experience long-term consequences of substance use. An individual who experiences either the long-term psychological or physical consequences of using substances (described above) can be described as having substance dependence.

> *Substance dependence* refers to long-term psychological and physical consequences of substance use.

WHAT CAUSES ADDICTION?

A person who has a substance abuse or substance dependence diagnosis is said to have an *addiction*. (The term *substance abuse* is also used in the more general way, in addition to the diagnosis of substance abuse as described above.) People often ask about the causes of addiction. There is no simple answer to this question. Different causes may be responsible for addiction in different people. In addition, more than one factor can lead to an addiction in some individuals. Two important explanations for addiction in psychiatric clients are described below. However, other explanations are also possible.

Supersensitivity to Substances

People with psychiatric illness are more biologically vulnerable than other people. As a result of this, they are more sensitive to the effects of even small doses of psychoactive substances. The result of this vulnerability is that psychiatric clients are "supersensitive" to alcohol and drugs, even in small amounts. This may cause some of these individuals to have addiction problems, despite relatively low or infrequent use of substances.

Family History

Research has found that persons with substance use problems are more likely to have relatives with similar problems than individuals who do not have such problems are. This tendency is true even for those who are raised apart from their families. Many scientists believe that genetic factors play a role in increasing vulnerability to substance use problems. Therefore, if a psychiatric client has a relative who has had problems with substances, he or she may be more likely to experience similar problems.

> Two common causes of addiction in psychiatric clients are supersensitivity to substances and family history of addiction.

Treatment of Dual Disorders

People who have problems with both mental illness and substances can be described as having a *dual diagnosis*, *dual disorders*, or *co-occurring disorders*. There are many different ways of helping people with a dual diagnosis regain control over their lives and make progress toward important goals. Treatment strategies may involve self-help, working with professionals, and working with family members or other natural supports. This handout discusses some of the principles of treatment and common strategies for people with dual disorders.

> Many different treatments can help people
> with a dual diagnosis.

STAGES OF TREATMENT

Recovery from a substance use disorder occurs over a series of stages. Individuals progress from one stage to another as they recover. Sometimes people move back and forth between stages. Each stage is different in terms of the person's awareness of substance use as a problem and motivation to address it. Understanding the different stages of substance abuse treatment can be helpful in deciding what goals to be working toward. A brief description of each stage and the goal of each stage is provided in the table below.

Stage	Description	Goal
Engagement	The client does not see a professional on a regular basis and has no working relationship with a professional.	To establish a working alliance (therapeutic relationship) with a professional.
Persuasion	The client has a working alliance with a professional, but is not convinced that substance abuse is a problem.	To help the client view substance abuse as a problem that should be worked on.
Active treatment	The client is motivated to work on substance abuse and is decreasing use or has stopped briefly.	To help the client decrease (or stop) substance use so that it is no longer a problem.
Relapse prevention	The client has stopped using substances (or experiences no consequences from substance use) for a significant period of time.	To maintain awareness that relapse of substance abuse could happen, and to extend recovery to other areas (such as work).

(continued)

> Stages of recovery from substance abuse include:
> - Engagement
> - Persuasion
> - Active treatment
> - Relapse prevention

PRINCIPLES OF TREATMENT

The treatment of a person with a dual diagnosis is guided by five basic principles. Following these principles increases the chance that treatment will be successful. These principles are described below.

Medication Adherence

Medication for a psychiatric disorder can help to correct the imbalance in the brain chemicals responsible for the mental illness. Taking medication regularly can decrease symptoms and relapses, stabilizing a client's psychiatric illness. Encouraging medication adherence can decrease substance use that occurs as a result of problematic symptoms.

Decreased Stress

Stress resulting from tense relationships with others, upsetting life events, or other factors can worsen symptoms and lead to more severe substance abuse. Minimizing stress and bolstering clients' ability to manage stress are important goals of dual-diagnosis treatment.

Treatment of Both Mental Illness and Substance Abuse

Substance abuse often worsens mental illness and more severe symptoms sometimes lead to greater substance abuse. In order for dual-diagnosis treatment to be effective, both substance abuse *and* mental illness need to be addressed.

Individualized Treatment

Every client is a unique individual with personal strengths that are an important part of treatment. Understanding the individual strengths and needs of each client is important for developing a treatment plan that is specific for that person.

Collaboration

The lives of clients with dual disorders touch the lives of many other people, including their families, friends, and professionals. Collaboration and teamwork among clients, professionals, and other supportive persons is essential to meet the challenges of dual-disorder treatment.

(continued)

> The principles of dual-diagnosis treatment include:
> - Medication adherence
> - Decreased stress
> - Treatment of both mental illness and substance abuse
> - Individualized treatment
> - Collaboration

TREATMENT STRATEGIES

Many different strategies can be used in the treatment of dual disorders. The specific strategies used for a particular client will depend on that person's specific needs and goals. Several of the most commonly used strategies are described below.

Dual-Diagnosis Groups

Clients often find participating in groups with other people who have dual disorders helpful. These groups may focus on exploring the role that substance use has played in each person's life, and developing strategies for cutting down or stopping substance use. Important parts of these groups include social support, sharing personal experiences, and exchanging ideas about personal goals.

Increased Structure

Sometimes clients tend to use substances when they have nothing else to do. Increasing daily structure and meaningful activities can help clients decrease their opportunities to use substances. For example, working at a part-time job can decrease substance abuse and increase self-esteem.

Rehabilitation

Clients may use substances in order to achieve such goals as socializing, pleasure enhancement, or coping with symptoms. Participation in rehabilitation activities, such as social skills training, can help clients develop skills for achieving these goals in more effective ways than using substances.

Self-Help Groups

Self-help organizations, such as Alcoholics Anonymous or Double Trouble in Recovery, offer peer-supported sponsorship for individuals who wish to remain abstinent from alcohol and drug use. Self-help organizations have helped millions of people with addictive disorders, and are widely available in most communities. Self-help groups, such as Al-Anon, are also available for concerned family members of individuals with addictions.

(continued)

Motivational Strategies

Sometimes a client does not believe that his or her substance abuse is a problem, although other people think that it is a problem. With such clients, it is sometimes helpful to explore what their personal goals are, and to help them make progress toward achieving these goals. Often in this process, these clients become aware that their use of substances interferes with achieving goals that are important for them.

Family Support and Problem Solving

Family members (and other persons) can help clients with dual disorders by providing support, recognizing small positive steps, and engaging in problem solving about difficult issues. By working together, family members and clients can often come up with creative solutions for solving important problems or achieving desired goals.

Keeping Hope Alive

Some individuals with dual disorders feel discouraged about their chances for recovery. They may have battled their problems for many years and feel that there is little hope for improvement. However, there are good reasons for being optimistic about getting better. Research on the treatment of clients with a dual diagnosis indicates that most such clients *do* recover. Furthermore, once clients stop using substances, their outlook and their ability to pursue personal goals improve. For these reasons, optimism is warranted for clients with dual disorders who become involved in treatment.

Strategies for treating dual disorders include:
- Dual-diagnosis groups
- Increased structure
- Rehabilitation
- Self-help groups
- Motivational strategies
- Family support and problem solving
- Keeping hope alive

Communication Skills

Good communication skills are important to all families. There is a wide range of topics families discuss—such as running the household, meals, recreation, and money, as well as expressing feelings (happiness, sadness, anger, etc.). Effective communication can help families cope with day-to-day situations as they come up. Good communication can also help family members solve problems together and work toward goals.

> Good communication is helpful for families.

COMMUNICATION AND MENTAL ILLNESS

When a family member has a mental illness, the person may have trouble communicating because of difficulties with concentration, memory, or processing information. This can cause stress for everyone in the family. Stress can have a negative effect on the person with the mental illness by increasing symptoms. So improving communication skills in the family may decrease stress for the ill member, and for other family members as well.

> Good communication skills
> can decrease stress in families.

HOW TO IMPROVE COMMUNICATION

Many family members are good communicators, but almost everyone can benefit from reviewing and practicing the basics of effective communication. The following are specific suggestions to improve communication:

- *Get to the point*. People with mental illness sometimes get confused easily. It is best to avoid long-winded statements and to keep communications brief and to the point.
- *Keep communications focused*. When people have trouble concentrating, it is helpful to focus on one subject at a time.
- *Speak clearly*. The more specific the statement, the more likely it is to be understood by others.
- *Use feeling statements*. Let people know how you feel in a noncritical way. Using "I" statements ("I feel . . . ") and verbal feeling statements ("angry," "upset," "happy," "pleased," "concerned," "disappointed," "sad") can let other people understand your feelings.

(continued)

• *Speak for yourself, not others.* Family members sometimes speak for each other because they think they know how other persons think or feel. This can lead to confusion and misunderstandings. Speaking only for oneself can prevent the problems that occur when one person speaks for another.

• *Focus on behavior.* It is easier for a person to change a behavior than his or her personality, attitudes, or feelings. Focusing communications on behavior, especially when you are upset, can make it clear to the other person what you are talking about. Consider these examples:

Less specific	*More specific*
"I am concerned about your health."	"I am concerned about your health because you have been drinking a lot recently."
"You bothered me last night."	"I was annoyed when you woke me up last night coming home. Please be more quiet next time."
"That was thoughtful of you."	"I really liked that you remembered my birthday by getting me flowers."

Ways to improve communication:
• Get to the point.
• Keep communication focused.
• Speak clearly.
• Use feeling statements.
• Speak for yourself, not others.
• Focus on behavior.

OTHER COMMUNICATION TOOLS

How a person communicates can be just as important as what the person actually says. The following are some tools for improving communication:

• *Listening.* Use small comments like "uh-huh" or "okay" to let the person know you are listening. Repeating back what you heard shows the other person that you are paying attention.

• *Eye contact.* Look the person in the eye (or close to the eyes) when you talk, to focus his or her attention.

• *Tone of voice.* People respond better to a calm tone of voice. Your voice tone should be consistent with the feeling message you are communicating.

• *Facial expression.* Like voice tone, use a facial expression that matches the feeling message you are saying.

Other communication tools:
• Listening
• Eye contact
• Tone of voice
• Facial expression

(continued)

KEY COMMUNICATION SKILLS

Expressing Positive Feelings

It is always helpful to be able to tell a person in an effective way what the person did that pleased you. Follow these steps:

- Look at the person.
- Tell the person exactly what he or she did that pleased you—be specific.
- Tell the person how it made you feel—be specific.

Here is an example:

"I really enjoyed the meal you cooked tonight."

Making a Positive Request

It is important to be able to ask someone to do something for you in an effective and positive way. Follow these steps:

- Look at the person.
- Tell him or her what you are requesting—be specific.
- Tell the person how it would make you feel if the request were met—be specific.

Here are examples:

"I would appreciate it if you would cook dinner tonight."
"I would like it if you could come to my doctor's appointment with me next Monday, so you can help me talk with him about my medication side effects."

Expressing a Negative Feeling

It is helpful to express a negative feeling in a way that increases the chances that the person will hear what you have to say.

- Look at the person who displeased you.
- Tell the person exactly what he or she did to displease you—be specific.
- Tell the person how it made you feel—be specific.
- Make a positive request for change, if possible.

Here are examples:

"I am mad that you spent the money I gave you for clothes on alcohol. When you need clothes, perhaps we should go shopping together."
"I was worried when you didn't come home last night. The next time you are going to stay out I would appreciate it if you would give me a call."

(continued)

Compromise and Negotiation

When you would like someone to change something, it is important to have an effective way to discuss how it might work out.

- Look at the person.
- Explain your viewpoint.
- Listen to the other person's viewpoint.
- Repeat back what you heard.
- Suggest a compromise (more than one may be necessary).

Requesting a Time-Out

Sometimes when you are in a stressful situation, you need a break, and it is important to communicate that.

- Indicate that the situation is stressful.
- Tell the person that the stress is interfering with constructive communication.
- Say that you must leave temporarily.
- State when you will return and be willing to problem-solve.

Here is an example:

"I'm feeling stressed out by this conversation. I'd like to take a break now, and discuss this with you again later on when I'm feeling calmer."

Key communication skills:
- Expressing positive feelings.
- Making a positive request.
- Expressing a negative feeling.
- Compromise and negotiation.
- Requesting a time out.

SUMMARY

Communication is sometimes stressful in families. However, all family members need to be able to communicate with each other. By following the guidelines of good communication, family members can share their thoughts and feelings, and be effective in working together toward solving problems and achieving goals.

Infectious Diseases

Infectious diseases are illnesses that can easily be spread from one person to another. There are many different kinds of infectious diseases, and they can be spread in different ways. This educational handout describes three infectious diseases that are caused by viruses: the *hepatitis B virus*, the *hepatitis C virus*, and the *human immunodeficiency virus (HIV)*. These diseases are spread by contact with contaminated blood or other body fluids. Each of these diseases is serious, can harm a person's health and well-being, and can even result in death. This handout explains the following:

- How to avoid contact with these viruses
- Whether a person should be tested for the diseases
- The treatment options for the diseases
- If someone has a disease, how to avoid spreading it to others

> Infectious diseases are illnesses that can be easily
> spread from one person to another.

HOW COMMON ARE INFECTIOUS DISEASES?

Infectious diseases are more common in some places than others, and in some years compared to others. In the United States, about 5% of people are infected with hepatitis B virus, and about 2% have hepatitis C virus. HIV is less common; about 1 person in 200 (0.5%) is infected with HIV.

Some people are more likely to get infectious diseases than others. People who have severe mental illness and alcohol or drug problems (that is, dual disorders) are more likely to have an infectious disease than people who do not have dual disorders. Among people with dual disorders, almost 25% have hepatitis B virus, about the same percentage have hepatitis C virus, and about 5% have HIV.

> People with dual disorders are more likely to have
> hepatitis B virus, hepatitis C virus, or HIV.

HEPATITIS

Hepatitis hurts the liver. To understand hepatitis, it is helpful to know what the liver does. The liver is a very important organ of the body. The liver is part of the digestive tract. It helps filter out toxic materials; builds proteins for the body; and stores vitamins, minerals, and carbohydrates. A person needs a functioning liver to stay alive.

(continued)

When a person has hepatitis, the liver becomes sick or inflamed because it has been infected with a virus. This sickness or inflammation can cause more serious liver problems, including *cirrhosis* (permanent scarring of the liver reduces blood flow), *liver failure* (the liver is unable to function), and *liver cancer* (cancer cells attack the liver). Any of these diseases can make the person sick and cause him or her to die.

There are many kinds of hepatitis viruses, but the most common and most serious ones are hepatitis B and hepatitis C. Preventing hepatitis B virus and hepatitis C virus, or taking care of oneself if one has either virus, is important to prevent damage to the liver.

> - The liver is an important organ of the human body.
> - Hepatitis is a disease of the liver.
> - Hepatitis B virus and hepatitis C virus are the most common and serious types of hepatitis.

HIV AND AIDS

HIV is a virus that attacks and destroys special white blood cells in the body, called *T*-cells. T-cells are a part of the immune system, which helps the body fight infection and stay healthy. When HIV destroys these cells, the immune system breaks down and is unable to fight infections. This means that normally mild infections can grow to be very serious, causing the person to get very sick and even to die. *Acquired immunedeficiency syndrome (AIDS)* is the disease someone gets after HIV has destroyed the immune system and the body cannot fight infections.

> HIV is a virus that attacks the immune system,
> leading to AIDS.

TRANSMISSION OF HEPATITIS B VIRUS, HEPATITIS C VIRUS, AND HIV

All three of these viruses pass from one person to another through exposure to infected or contaminated blood. For an uninfected person to get hepatitis B virus, hepatitis C virus, or HIV, the blood of an infected person needs to enter his or her bloodstream. HIV can also be transmitted from the sex fluids (such as semen or vaginal secretions) of an infected person into the bloodstream of an uninfected person when the two people have sex.

Here are some of the ways people get exposed to the contaminated blood of other people and develop these infectious diseases:

- Sharing injection needles with other people
- Sharing a straw for snorting cocaine, amphetamine, or heroin with others
- Having unprotected sex (without a condom) with many partners or with people they do not know well
- Having had a blood transfusion, hemodialysis, or organ transplant from an infected source before 1992 (for hepatitis B virus or hepatitis C virus) or before 1985 (for HIV)
- Having body piercings or tattoos with improperly sterilized needles

(continued)

- Using personal articles (such as a razor, toothbrush, nail file, or nail clippers) that have been used by someone else with the infection
- Being born to a mother with the infection

None of these three viruses can be spread through insect bites, kissing, hugging, or using public toilet seats, unless there is direct contact with other people's body fluids.

> Hepatitis B virus, hepatitis C virus, and HIV are transmitted by exposure to infected blood.

TESTS FOR HEPATITIS B VIRUS, HEPATITIS C VIRUS, AND HIV

Most people who have one of these three viruses do not have symptoms until a long time after they get the virus. People who have chronic hepatitis B virus or hepatitis C virus infection may experience tiredness (fatigue), loss of appetite, abdominal pain, nausea or vomiting, dark urine, or jaundice (yellow skin). People who have early symptoms of AIDS may experience sores and difficulty fighting off infections, such as a cough that will not go away.

Blood tests can tell whether a person has hepatitis B virus, hepatitis C virus, or HIV. Since most infected people have no symptoms, who should be tested for the viruses? A person should get tested if he or she has had any of the risk factors listed in the previous section, such as sharing needles or having unprotected sex with multiple partners.

> Blood tests can detect hepatitis B virus, hepatitis C virus, and HIV.

TREATMENT

Hepatitis B Virus

A vaccine can prevent hepatitis B virus if the person gets the vaccine before he or she is exposed to the virus. This vaccine is free and widely available.

Most people who get hepatitis B virus recover on their own. However, about 1 in 10 people (10%) get a chronic illness. People who have chronic hepatitis B virus may improve from treatment with *interferon*, a medicine that boosts the body's ability to fight the infection. Interferon is given in a series of injections into the muscles over a 16-week period.

People infected with hepatitis B virus who are then infected with a different virus, the hepatitis A virus, can then get sick with *fulminant hepatitis*—a very serious disease that can be fatal. To prevent this, people with hepatitis B virus need to get a vaccination for hepatitis A.

> - A vaccine can prevent hepatitis B.
> - Most people with hepatitis B virus recover on their own.
> - Interferon treatment helps people infected with chronic hepatitis B virus.
> - Vaccination for hepatitis A can prevent fulminant hepatitis in people infected with chronic hepatitis B.

(continued)

Hepatitis C Virus

There is no vaccine that protects a person from getting hepatitis C virus, unlike hepatitis B virus. Another difference from hepatitis B virus is that about 85% of people with hepatitis C virus carry the virus for life unless they are treated.

Some treatments help people with hepatitis C. One treatment is taking interferon for up to 48 weeks. Another treatment is taking interferon with another medication (a combination of drugs called *Rebetron*) over 6 months. These treatments completely get rid of hepatitis C virus for some infected people (between 20% and 50%).

Treatments for hepatitis C virus can cause side effects, such as flu-like symptoms or depression. Therefore, the decision to treat hepatitis C virus is based on how sick someone is. Researchers are developing new medications for treating hepatitis C virus.

Similar to people with hepatitis B virus, people with hepatitis C virus who are then infected with the hepatitis A virus can develop *fulminant hepatitis*, a deadly disease. This can be prevented by taking a vaccine for hepatitis A.

- Most people with hepatitis C virus do not get well on their own.
- Treatment is helpful for hepatitis C virus.
- Vaccination for hepatitis A can prevent fulminant hepatitis in people infected with chronic hepatitis C.

HIV and AIDS

No vaccine or cure exists for HIV or AIDS. However, medications can slow down the illness. In addition, new medications are being developed and tested for HIV and AIDS that may help in the future.

- There is no cure for HIV or AIDS.
- Different medications are effective in managing HIV and AIDS.

TAKING CARE OF ONESELF

When a person has one of these viruses, good self-care can help the person stay well. Alcohol is toxic, or poisonous, to the liver. Since hepatitis also harms the liver, people infected with hepatitis B virus and hepatitis C virus should avoid drinking alcohol, or drink as little as possible.

There are several other things people with hepatitis B virus, hepatitis C virus, and HIV can do to help themselves:

- Getting a medical care provider (such as a doctor) who can monitor health and discuss treatment options
- Taking medication as prescribed
- Getting enough rest
- Eating healthy foods
- Avoiding using street drugs

(continued)

> - People with hepatitis B virus and hepatitis C virus should avoid alcohol.
> - Taking care of oneself can lessen the effects of all three viruses.

HOW TO AVOID SPREADING HEPATITIS B VIRUS, HEPATITIS C VIRUS, AND HIV TO OTHERS

There are several ways people can avoid spreading these infectious diseases:

- Not sharing needles with other people
- If a person *has* to share needles with other people, sterilizing the "works" by immersing them in bleach for 30 seconds at least three times
- Always using a latex condom when engaging in sexual relations
- Not sharing personal items (such as a razor, toothbrush, nail file, or nail clippers) with others

> People can take steps to avoid giving others hepatitis B virus, hepatitis C virus, or HIV.

APPENDIX C

Assessment Instruments and Other Forms

C.1. Dartmouth Assessment of Lifestyle Instrument (DALI)

C.2. Alcohol Use Scale—Revised (AUS-R)

C.3. Drug Use Scale—Revised (DUS-R)

C.4. Functional Assessment Interview

C.5. Drug/Alcohol Time-Line Follow-Back Calendar (TLFBC)

C.6. Payoff Matrix

C.7. Functional Analysis Summary

C.8. Substance Abuse Treatment Scale—Revised (SATS-R)

C.9. Individual Dual-Disorder Treatment Plan

C.10. Individual Treatment Review

C.11. Mental Illness Relapse Prevention Worksheet

C.12. Substance Abuse Relapse Prevention Worksheet

C.13. Pleasant Activities Worksheet

C.14. Recovery Mountain Worksheet

C.15. Orientation to Behavioral Family Therapy

C.16. Family Member Interview

C.17. Summary of Family Assessment

C.18. Family Treatment Plan

C.19. Family Treatment Review

C.20. Problem-Solving or Goal-Setting Sheet

Dartmouth Assessment of Lifestyle Instrument (DALI)

Client name: _____

Date: _____

INSTRUCTIONS

The DALI is a brief screening instrument, based on a client interview, for the detection of recent (past 6 months) substance use disorders in persons with severe mental illness. The DALI identifies three types of substance use disorders: alcohol, cannabis, and cocaine.

Reference: Rosenberg, S. D., Drake, R. E., Wolford, G. L., Mueser, K. T., Oxman, T. E., Vidaver, R. M., Carrieri, K. L., & Luckoor, R. (1998). The Dartmouth Assessment of Lifestyle Instrument (DALI): A substance use disorder screen for people with severe mental illness. *American Journal of Psychiatry, 155,* 232–238.

Circle the answer under each question as you ask it. At the end of the interview, select the corresponding DALI score and circle that on the right. List your scores on the last page and total them. (In the response options below, Ref = refused; NA = not applicable; DK = don't know.)

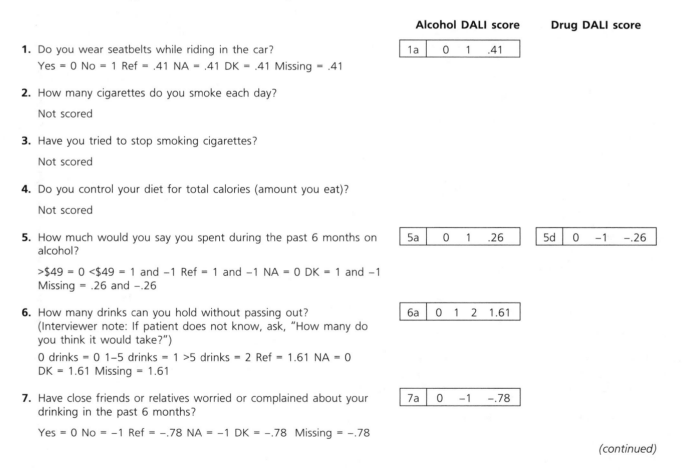

	Alcohol DALI score	Drug DALI score
1. Do you wear seatbelts while riding in the car? Yes = 0 No = 1 Ref = .41 NA = .41 DK = .41 Missing = .41	1a | 0 1 .41	
2. How many cigarettes do you smoke each day? Not scored		
3. Have you tried to stop smoking cigarettes? Not scored		
4. Do you control your diet for total calories (amount you eat)? Not scored		
5. How much would you say you spent during the past 6 months on alcohol? >$49 = 0 <$49 = 1 and −1 Ref = 1 and −1 NA = 0 DK = 1 and −1 Missing = .26 and −.26	5a | 0 1 .26	5d | 0 −1 −.26
6. How many drinks can you hold without passing out? (Interviewer note: If patient does not know, ask, "How many do you think it would take?") 0 drinks = 0 1–5 drinks = 1 >5 drinks = 2 Ref = 1.61 NA = 0 DK = 1.61 Missing = 1.61	6a | 0 1 2 1.61	
7. Have close friends or relatives worried or complained about your drinking in the past 6 months? Yes = 0 No = −1 Ref = −.78 NA = −1 DK = −.78 Missing = −.78	7a | 0 −1 −.78	

(continued)

	Alcohol DALI score	**Drug DALI score**

8. Have you ever attended a meeting of Alcoholics Anonymous (AA) because of your drinking?

| 8a | 0   –1   –.53 |

Yes = 0 No = –1 Ref = –.53 NA = –1 DK = –.53 Missing = –.53

9. Do you sometimes take a drink in the morning when you first get up?
(Interviewer note: If client asks, specify alcohol.)

| 9a | 0   –1   –.83 |

Yes = 0 No = –1 Ref = –.83 NA = –1 DK = –.83 Missing = –.83

10. How long was your last period of voluntary abstinence from alcohol (or most recent period when you chose not to drink)?
(Interviewer note: 2 weeks or more equals a month. Exclude periods of incarceration or hospitalization.)

| 10a | 0   1   .76 |

0–59 months = 1 >60 months = 0 Ref = .76 NA = 0 DK = .76 Missing = .76

11. How many months ago did this abstinence end for alcohol (or when did you start drinking again)?

| 11a | 0   1   .40 |

0 month = 0 >0 months = 1 Ref = .40 NA = 0 DK = .40 Missing = .40

12. Have you used marijuana in the past 6 months?

| 12a | 0   –1   –.70 | | 12d | 0   –1   –.70 |

Yes = 0 No = –1 Ref = –.70 NA = –1 DK = –.70 Missing = –.70

13. Have you lost a job because of marijuana use?

| 13d | 0   –1   –.93 |

Yes = 0 No = –1 Ref = –.93 NA = –1 DK = –.93 Missing = –.93

14. How much would you say you spent in the past 6 months on marijuana?

| 14d | 0   1   .18 |

$0 = 0 >$0 = 1 Ref = 1 NA = 0 DK = 1 Missing = .18

15. How troubled or bothered have you been in the past 6 months by marijuana problems?

| 15d | 0   1   .19 |

Not at all	Slightly	Moderately	Considerably	Extremely
1	2	3	4	5

1 = 0 2–5 = 1 Ref = 1 NA = 0 DK = 1 Missing = .19

16. Has cocaine abuse created problems between you and your spouse/partner or your parents?

| 16d | 0   –1   –.82 |

Yes = 0 No = –1 Ref = –.82 NA = –1 DK = –.82 Missing = –.82

17. How long was your last period of voluntary abstinence from cocaine (or most recent period when you chose not to use)?
(Interviewer note: 2 weeks equals a month. Exclude periods of incarceration or hospitalization.)

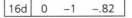

0–59 months = 1 >60 months = 0 Ref = .19 NA = 0 DK = .19 Missing = .19

18. Do you ever use cocaine when you're in a bad mood?

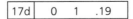

Yes = 0 No = 1 Ref = 0 NA = 1 DK = 0 Missing = 0

(continued)

The eight alcohol questions have possible scores ranging from –4 to +6. Anyone scoring +2 or higher on the Alcohol scale is at high risk for having a current alcohol use disorder. The six drug questions have possible scores ranging from –4 to +4. People scoring above –1 on the Drug scale are at high risk for cannabis and/or cocaine use disorders.

Alcohol scores		Drug scores	
1a	_____	5d	_____
5a	_____	12d	_____
6a	_____	13d	_____
7a	_____	14d	_____
8a	_____	15d	_____
9a	_____	16d	_____
10a	_____	17d	_____
11a	_____	18d	_____
12a	_____		

Total Alcohol score: _____   Total Drug score: _____

Alcohol Use Scale—Revised (AUS-R)

Client name: _____

Rater: _____

Date: _____

INSTRUCTIONS

This scale pertains to your client's use of alcohol over the past 6 months. Rate the *worst* period of alcohol use during this interval. If the client is in an institution, the reporting interval is the time period prior to institutionalization. Complete the information-gathering portion of this form, and then rate your client on the 5-point Rating Scale at the end of this form.

Use

Inquire whether the client has used alcohol over the past 6 months.

_____ No

_____ Yes

If no, give the client a 1 on the Rating Scale and complete the "Sources of Information" section at the end of this form. If yes, complete the rest of the form.

Abuse

Consequences of use in past 6 months. Check all recurrent problems related to the alcohol use that have persisted for *at least 1 month*. Use client report, plus any other sources of information (i.e., urine screens, collateral reports).

Social functioning and legal status

_____ Family problems

_____ Housing instability

_____ Social difficulties (e.g., arguments, threats of violence, or violent behavior)

_____ Social isolation

_____ Difficulty budgeting funds

_____ Prostitution

_____ Other legal problems

(continued)

Role functioning

____ Employment difficulties (e.g., loss of job, accidents on the job)

____ Difficulty attending or keeping up in school

____ Parenting difficulties (e.g., failure to care for children)

Physical status

____ Hygiene problems

____ Change in physical appearance

____ Health problems

____ Injuries

Psychiatric status

____ Treatment nonadherence

____ Suicidal thoughts

____ Cognitive impairment

____ Symptom relapses

____ Sudden mood shifts

____ Appearance of new symptoms

Use in dangerous situations

____ When driving

____ When operating machinery

If no problems are noted for abuse, stop here and rate client a 2 on the Rating Scale. If problems are noted, check for dependence (below).

Dependence

The client needs to have at least one symptom present in three out of the following seven categories to meet criteria for dependence. If not, rate the client a 3 on the Rating Scale for abuse.

1. Greater amounts or intervals of use than intended

____ Drinking more than planned

____ Drinking longer than planned

____ Repeated unsuccessful attempts to cut down

2. Frequent intoxication, or withdrawal, interferes with other activities

____ Spending most of the time drinking

____ Frequent hangovers

(continued)

3. Important activities given up because of alcohol use

____ Drinking instead of working

____ Drinking instead of spending time on leisure activities

____ Drinking instead of spending time with family or friends

4. Continued use despite knowledge of alcohol-related problems

____ Drinking is causing problems, but client continues to drink

5. Marked tolerance

____ Needing to drink a lot more to get high

____ Diminished effect with use of same amount of alcohol

6. Characteristic withdrawal symptoms

____ Sweating

____ Racing heart

____ Hands shaking

____ Trouble sleeping

____ Feeling nauseated or vomiting

____ Feeling agitated

____ Feeling anxious

7. Alcohol taken to relieve or avoid withdrawal symptoms

____ Drinking to keep from getting sick from withdrawal symptoms

____ Drinking to stop the shakes or other withdrawal symptoms

If the client meets the criteria for dependence, move on to see whether the client has severe dependence, where problems are so severe that living in the community is difficult.

DEPENDENCE WITH INSTITUTIONALIZATION

____ Psychiatric hospitalization(s)

____ Inpatient treatment(s) for substance abuse

____ Incarceration(s)

If the client has had more than one psychiatric hospitalization, inpatient treatment for substance abuse, or incarceration, or if the client has spent 3 or more months of the past 6 institutionalized, rate the client a 5 on the Rating Scale. If none of these apply, rate the client a 4.

(continued)

Rating Scale

Based on the information summarized on the previous pages, rate your client's use of alcohol during the worst period over the past 6 months, according to the following scale.

_____ **1 = Abstinence.** Client has not used alcohol over the past 6 months.

_____ **2 = Use without impairment.** Client has used alcohol over the past 6 months, but there is no evidence of persistent or recurrent problems in social functioning, legal status, role functioning, psychiatric status, or physical problems related to use, and no evidence of recurrent dangerous use.

_____ **3 = Abuse.** Client has used alcohol over the past 6 months, and there is evidence of persistent or recurrent problems in social functioning, legal status, role functioning, psychiatric status, or physical problems related to use, or evidence of recurrent dangerous use. For example, recurrent alcohol use leads to disruptive behavior and housing problems. Problems have persisted for at least 1 month.

_____ **4 = Dependence.** Client meets criteria for abuse, plus at least three of the following: greater amounts of use than intended; much of time spent obtaining or using alcohol; frequent intoxication or withdrawal interferes with other activities; important activities given up because of alcohol use; continued use despite knowledge of alcohol-related problems; marked tolerance; characteristic withdrawal symptoms; or alcohol taken to relieve or avoid withdrawal symptoms. For example, drinking binges and preoccupation with drinking have caused client to drop out of job training and non-drinking-related social activities.

_____ **5 = Dependence with institutionalization.** Client meets criteria for dependence, plus related problems are so severe that they make noninstitutional living difficult. For example, constant drinking leads to disruptive behavior resulting in incarceration.

Sources of Information

_____ Client self-report

_____ Observations by clinician(s)

_____ Lab tests

_____ Collateral sources (specify):

    _____ Mother

    _____ Father

    _____ Sibling

    _____ Spouse/boyfriend/girlfriend

    _____ Child

    _____ Other relative

    _____ Friend

    _____ Landlord

    _____ Police/probation/parole officer

    _____ Other (_____)

Drug Use Scale—Revised (DUS-R)

Client name: _____

Rater: _____

Date: _____

INSTRUCTIONS

This scale pertains to your client's drug use over the past 6 months. Rate the *worst* period of drug use during this interval. If the client is in an institution, the reporting interval is the time period prior to institutionalization. Complete the information-gathering portion of this form, and then rate your client on the 5-point Rating Scale at the end of this form.

Use

Inquire whether the client has used drugs (other than as prescribed) over the past 6 months.

____ No

____ Yes

If no, give the client a 1 on the Rating Scale and complete the "Sources of Information" section at the end of this form. If yes, complete the rest of the form.

Mark drugs used:

____ Sedatives/hypnotics/anxiolytics

____ Cannabis

____ Stimulants

____ Opioids

____ Cocaine

____ Hallucinogens

____ Over-the-counter (specify) _____

____ Other (specify) _____

_____

See last page of form for specific drugs within each category and slang words.

(continued)

Abuse

Consequences of use in past 6 months. Check all recurrent problems related to the drug use that have persisted for *at least 1 month*. Use client report, plus any other sources of information (i.e., urine screens, collateral reports).

Social functioning and legal status

____ Family problems

____ Housing instability

____ Social difficulties (e.g., arguments, threats of violence, or violent behavior)

____ Social isolation

____ Prostitution

____ Difficulty budgeting funds

____ Other legal problems

Role functioning

____ Employment difficulties (e.g., loss of job, accidents on the job)

____ Difficulty attending or keeping up in school

____ Parenting difficulties (e.g., failure to care for children)

Physical status

____ Hygiene problems

____ Change in physical appearance

____ Health problems

____ Injuries

Psychiatric status

____ Treatment nonadherence

____ Suicidal thoughts

____ Cognitive impairment

____ Symptom relapses

____ Sudden mood shifts

____ Appearance of new symptoms

Use in dangerous situations

____ When driving

____ When operating machinery

If no problems are noted for abuse, stop here and rate client a 2 on the Rating Scale. If problems are noted, check for dependence (below).

(continued)

425

Dependence

The client needs to have at least one symptom present in three out of the seven categories to meet criteria for dependence. If not, rate the client a 3 on the Rating Scale for abuse.

1. Greater amounts or intervals of drug use than intended

____ Using more drugs than planned

____ Using drugs longer than planned

____ Repeated unsuccessful attempts to cut down use of drugs

2. Frequent drug use or withdrawal interferes with other activities

____ Spending most of the time using drugs

____ Lengthy time spent recovering from effects

3. Important activities given up because of drug use

____ Using drugs instead of working

____ Using drugs instead of spending time on leisure activities

____ Using drugs instead of spending time with family or friends

4. Continued use despite knowledge of drug-related problems

____ Drug use is causing problems, but client continues to use

5. Marked tolerance

____ Needing to use a lot more drugs to achieve desired effect

____ Diminished effect with use of same amount of drug

6. Characteristic withdrawal symptoms

Sedatives/hypnotics/anxiolytics

____ Sweating or increased pulse rate

____ Increased hand tremor

____ Insomnia

____ Nausea or vomiting

____ Transient visual, tactile, or auditory hallucinations or illusions

____ Anxiety

____ Grand mal seizures

Stimulants/cocaine

____ Dysphoric mood

____ Fatigue

____ Vivid, unpleasant dreams

____ Insomnia or hypersomnia

____ Increased appetite

____ Psychomotor retardation or agitation

(continued)

Opiates

____ Dysphoric mood

____ Nausea or vomiting

____ Muscle aches

____ Pupillary dilation

____ Diarrhea

____ Fever

____ Insomnia

____ Sweating

7. Drug taken to relieve or avoid withdrawal symptoms

____ Use to keep from getting sick from withdrawal symptoms

____ Use when feeling sick with withdrawal symptoms

If the client meets the criteria for dependence, move on to see if the client has severe dependence, where problems are so severe that living in the community is difficult.

Dependence with Institutionalization

____ Psychiatric hospitalization(s)

____ Inpatient treatment(s) for substance abuse

____ Incarceration(s)

If the client has had more than one psychiatric hospitalization, inpatient treatment for substance abuse, or incarceration, or if the client has spent 3 or more months of the past 6 institutionalized, rate the client a 5 on the Rating Scale. If none of these apply, rate the client a 4.

Rating Scale

Based on the information summarized on the previous pages, rate your client's use of drugs during the worst period over the past 6 months according to the following scale.

____ **1 = Abstinence.** Client has not used drugs over the past 6 months.

____ **2 = Use without impairment.** Client has used drugs over the past 6 months, but there is no evidence of persistent or recurrent problems in social functioning, legal status, role functioning, psychiatric status, or physical status related to use, and no evidence of recurrent dangerous use.

____ **3 = Abuse.** Client has used drugs over the past 6 months, and there is evidence of persistent or recurrent problems in social functioning, legal status, role functioning, psychiatric status, or physical status related to use, or evidence of recurrent dangerous use. For example, recurrent drug use leads to disruptive behavior and housing problems. Problems have persisted for at least 1 month.

(continued)

____ **4 = Dependence.** Client meets criteria for abuse, plus at least three of the following: greater amounts of use than intended; much of time spent obtaining or using drugs; frequent intoxication or withdrawal interferes with other activities; important activities given up because of drug use; continued use despite knowledge of substance-related problems; marked tolerance; characteristic withdrawal symptoms; or drugs taken to relieve or avoid withdrawal symptoms. For example, binges and preoccupation with drugs have caused client to drop out of job training and non-drug-related social activities.

____ **5 = Dependence with institutionalization.** Client meets criteria for dependence, plus related problems are so severe that they make noninstitutional living difficult. For example, constant drug use leads to disruptive behavior resulting in incarceration.

Sources of Information

____ Client self-report

____ Observations by clinician(s)

____ Lab tests

____ Collateral sources (specify):

    ____ Mother

    ____ Father

    ____ Sibling

    ____ Spouse/boyfriend/girlfriend

    ____ Child

    ____ Other relative

    ____ Friend

    ____ Landlord

    ____ Police/probation/parole officer

    ____ Other (_____)

(continued)

DRUG NAMES AND SLANG WORDS

Sedatives/hypnotics/anxiolytics:

"Downers," Quaalude ("ludes"), Seconal ("reds"), Valium, Xanax, Librium, barbiturates ("barbs"), Miltown, Ativan, Dalmane, Halcion, Restoril, Klonopin, "Special K," "roofies," "tranks."

Cannabis:

Marijuana ("pot," "grass," "weed," "reefer," "smoke," "dope," "joint," "ganga," "doobie," "wacky tobacky," "Mary Jane"), hashish ("hash"), THC.

Stimulants:

"Uppers," amphetamine, "speed," "crystal meth," Dexedrine, Ritalin, "ice," "crank," "black beauties," "crosses," "hearts," STP, Ecstasy ("XTC," "X-file"), MDMA, MOA, DOM, DOB.

Opiates:

Heroin ("smack," "horse," "H"), morphine, opium (laudanum, paregoric, "Dover's powder"), methadone, Darvon, codeine, Percodan, Demerol, Dilaudid.

Cocaine:

"coke," "crack," "speedball," "freebase," "rock," "snow," "8-ball," "flake"

Hallucinogens ("psychedelics"):

LSD ("acid," "windowpane," "blotter," "microdot"), mescaline (peyote, "buttons," "cactus," "mesc"), psilocybin (mushrooms, "shrooms," "purple passion").

Over-the-counter:

Sleeping pills, diet pills, antihistamines.

Other:

PCP ("angel dust," "boat," "hog," "love boat"), steroids, "glue," ethyl chloride, paint, inhalants, nitrous oxide ("laughing gas"), amyl or butyl nitrate ("poppers"), White-Out, cough medicine.

Functional Assessment Interview

Client name: _____

Dates of assessment: _____

Check sources of information used. (*Note:* If respondent is someone other than the client, substitute the client's name for "you" in questions below.)

_____ Client

_____ Significant other (specify: _____)

_____ Treatment provider (specify: _____)

_____ Other informant (specify: _____)

_____ Medical records

I. Background information

A. Address _____

_____

_____

B. Telephone number: _____

C. Gender: _____ Male _____ Female

D. Date of birth: _____

E. Ethnicity: _____

F. Marital status: _____

G. Names and ages of siblings:

Name	Age

H. Children

   1. Do you have any children? _____ Yes _____ No

   2. Names and ages of children:

Name	Age

(continued)

    3.   Living situation for children: _____

_____

_____

    4.   Contact with children: _____

_____

_____

I.   Living situation

    1.   Where do you live (e.g., with relatives, supervised residence, independently)? _____

_____

    2.   Do you do your own:

        Cooking?   _____ Yes _____ No

        Cleaning?   _____ Yes _____ No

        Shopping?   _____ Yes _____ No

        Laundry?   _____ Yes _____ No

    3.   Are you satisfied with your living arrangement? _____ Yes _____ No

    4.   If no, why? _____

_____

    5.   If no, what other living arrangement would you prefer?

_____

_____

J.   Education

    1.   How far did you go in school? _____ years high school _____ High school diploma or (GED) _____ years college _____ College diploma

    2.   Are you interested in returning to school? _____ Yes _____ No

    3.   If yes, have you made previous efforts to return to school? _____ Yes _____ No

        If yes, describe: _____

_____

    4.   What would you like to do in school? _____

_____

_____

II. Psychiatric illness

    A.   DSM psychiatric diagnosis (from medical records or structured interview)

        1.   Axis I: _____

        2.   Axis II: _____

    B.   Understanding of psychiatric illness (from client self-report)

        1.   Do you think you have a psychiatric illness? _____

            Ask questions 2–6 if client either acknowledges having a psychiatric illness, or admits some kinds of difficulty (such as problems functioning, problems with "nerves," etc.).

(continued)

    2. What is it called? _____

_____

    3. What are some of the symptoms of the illness (problem)? _____

_____

_____

    4. What do you think caused this illness (problem)? _____

_____

_____

    5. What have you noticed makes your illness (problem) better? _____

_____

_____

    6. What have you noticed makes your illness (problem) worse? _____

_____

C. History of illness
    1. Age at illness onset (first symptoms): _____
    2. Age at first hospitalization: _____
    3. Number of psychiatric hospitalizations: _____
    4. Date and duration of most recent psychiatric hospitalization: _____
    5. Circumstances that led up to most recent hospitalization: _____

_____

_____

D. Medication
    1. Psychiatric medications and dosages: _____

_____

_____

    2. Do you take medications regularly? _____ Yes _____ No
    3. If no, why not? _____

_____

_____

Probe for client concerns about substance–medication interactions.
    4. Do your medications seem to help? _____ Yes _____ No
        Please specify: _____

_____

_____

    5. Side effects of medications: _____

_____

_____

_____

(continued)

6. How have you coped with these side effects?: _____

_____

_____

_____

Were these coping efforts effective? _____ Yes _____ No

E. Symptoms

Which of the following symptoms have you experienced over the past month? For each symptom, indicate how distressed you have felt by it, using the following scale: 1 = "not at all," 2 = "a little," 3 = "somewhat," 4 = "quite a bit," 5 = "extremely."

		Yes/no	Severity
1.	Depression (sadness, feeling blue, low self-esteem)	_____	_____
2.	Anxiety (worry, fear, panic attacks)	_____	_____
3.	Sleep problems (falling asleep, awakenings, nightmares, sleeping too much)	_____	_____
4.	Anger (irritability, outbursts)	_____	_____
5.	Cognitive problems (poor attention, memory problems)	_____	_____
6.	Apathy/anhedonia (not caring about anything, difficulty initiating action, lack of pleasure)	_____	_____
7.	Hallucinations (hearing or seeing things others don't)	_____	_____
8.	Delusions (unusual thoughts or ideas)	_____	_____
9.	Other symptoms (specify: _____)	_____	_____

III. Physical Health and Safety

A. Do you have any major physical illnesses that interfere with your life (e.g., diabetes, heart disease)? _____

B. When was the last time you saw a doctor for a physical reason, and what was the reason? __

_____

C. Do you take any medications on a regular basis for physical problems? _____ Yes _____ No

If yes, describe: _____

_____

D. Have you been physically assaulted over the past year? _____ Yes _____ No

If yes, describe: _____

_____

_____

E. Has anyone forced you or coerced you to have sexual relations against your will in the past year? _____ Yes _____ No

If yes, describe: _____

_____

(continued)

IV. Psychosocial Adjustment

A. Family functioning

1. Which members of your family do you have contact with (e.g., parents, siblings, spouse, children, grandparents, aunts, uncles)?

Relationship	Contact (daily, weekly, etc.)
_____	_____
_____	_____
_____	_____
_____	_____
_____	_____
_____	_____

2. What types of situations or problems are sources of conflict between you and your family members? Describe: _____
_____
_____

3. How do you and your relatives deal with these situations? Are you satisfied with how you cope with these stresses? _____
_____
_____
_____

4. Does anyone in the family yell, threaten, or hit each other during conflict?
_____ Yes _____ No
If yes, describe: _____
_____

5. What do you see as the major stressors that your family has to deal with?
_____
_____

6. What are some of the ways you help out in your family?
_____
_____

7. What do you see as the major strengths of your family?
_____
_____
_____

8. Overall, how satisfied are you with the support you receive from you family? _____
_____
_____

Which family members do you find most supportive? _____
_____

(continued)

Which family members are least supportive? _____

_____

How would you like things to be different? _____

_____

(Probe for desire for more contact with family.)

B. Friendship and romantic relationships
1. Whom do you consider your friends? _____

_____

2. How often do you get together with your friends? _____

_____

3. What do you like to do with your friends? _____

_____

4. Are you satisfied with your friends and the amount of contact you have with them?
_____ Yes _____ No
5. Do you have a romantic relationship? _____ Yes _____ No
6. If no, would you like one? _____
7. If yes, are you satisfied with it? _____

C. Leisure and recreation
1. How do you spend your free time? _____

_____

2. Whom do you spend it with? _____
3. Would you like to do more with your spare time? _____ Yes _____ No
4. If yes, what would you like to do? _____

_____

5. Are there activities you used to do but don't do any more? _____ Yes _____ No
If yes, describe: _____

_____

6. Would you like to start doing them again? _____

_____

7. What gets in the way of doing those activities? _____

_____

_____

D. Work
1. Are you working? _____ Yes _____ No
2. If yes, where and doing what? _____
3. How many hours per week? _____
4. If not working, are you interested in work? _____ Yes _____ No
5. Have you made any recent efforts to find work? _____ Yes _____ No
If yes, describe: _____

_____

(continued)

435

6. If no, what gets in the way of finding work? _____

_____

7. When was the last time you worked? _____

E. Spirituality
1. What are your spiritual beliefs? _____

_____

2. Are you involved with a religious group (e.g., church)? _____ Yes _____ No
3. Did you used to belong to a religious group that you are no longer an active participant in? _____ Yes _____ No
4. Do you seek more spiritual meaning in your life? _____ Yes _____ No
5. If yes, please explain: _____

_____

F. Financial matters
1. What are your sources of income (e.g., SSI, SSDI, family)? List all sources and approximate income from each.

Source	Monthly income
_____	_____
_____	_____
_____	_____
_____	_____

2. Who controls your money? _____

_____

3. How satisfied are you with this current arrangement?

_____

4. Have you experienced any problems when you control your own money?
_____ Yes _____ No

If yes, explain: _____

G. Legal problems
1. Have you ever been in trouble with the law? _____ Yes _____ No
2. Have you ever been arrested? _____ Yes _____ No
3. If yes, what were you arrested for? _____

_____

4. Are you awaiting charges, trial, or sentencing? _____ Yes _____ No
5. Have you ever spent time in jail? _____ Yes _____ No
6. Are you on probation or parole? _____ Yes _____ No

If yes, explain: _____

V. Substance Use

A. Alcohol
1. Do you drink alcohol? _____ Yes _____ No
2. If yes, what types of beverages? _____

_____

(continued)

436

How much at a time? _____

How often do you drink? _____

3. Complete the Drug/Alcohol Time-Line Follow-Back Calendar (Form C.5) for alcohol use.

4. In what situations do you drink (e.g., alone, with friends, etc.)?

_____

5. Motives for alcohol use

   a. What are the positive things you get from drinking?

   _____

   b. What do you like about the effects of alcohol?

   _____

   _____

   c. Which of the following is true about alcohol for you?

	Not true	Sometimes true	Often true
Drinking . . .			
• is important to socializing with friends	_____	_____	_____
• helps me meet and get to know people	_____	_____	_____
• lowers my anxiety when I'm with people	_____	_____	_____
• makes me feel less depressed	_____	_____	_____
• makes me feel less anxious	_____	_____	_____
• helps me forget my problems	_____	_____	_____
• helps me sleep better	_____	_____	_____
• helps reduce boredom	_____	_____	_____
• is an important source of pleasure to me	_____	_____	_____
• gives me something to look forward to	_____	_____	_____
• is one of the only things that makes me feel good	_____	_____	_____
• is chiefly a habit	_____	_____	_____

B. Drugs

   1. Which of the following drugs have you used?

	Ever	Recently (past 6 months)
Marijuana	_____	_____
Cocaine	_____	_____
Hallucinogens (e.g., LSD, PCP, mescaline)	_____	_____
Sedatives (not prescribed or misused, e.g., Klonopin, Valium)	_____	_____
Stimulants (e.g., amphetamines)	_____	_____
Opiates (e.g., heroin, Darvon)	_____	_____
Over-the-counter (specify: _____)	_____	_____
Other (specify: _____)	_____	_____

   Indicate with an asterisk (*) which substances are most preferred.

   2. How do you use those drugs (route of administration)? _____

   3. How often do you use them? _____

(continued)

4. How much do you use at a time? _____

5. Complete the Drug/Alcohol Time-Line Follow-Back Calendar (Form C.5) for drug use.

6. Motives for drug use

   a. What are the positive things you get from using drugs?

      _____

   b. What do you like about the effects of drugs?

      _____

      _____

   c. Which of the following is true about drugs for you?

	Not true	Sometimes true	Often true
Using drugs . . .			
• is important to socializing with friends	_____	_____	_____
• helps me meet and get to know people	_____	_____	_____
• lowers my anxiety when I'm with people	_____	_____	_____
• makes me feel less depressed	_____	_____	_____
• makes me feel less anxious	_____	_____	_____
• helps me forget my problems	_____	_____	_____
• helps me sleep better	_____	_____	_____
• helps reduce boredom	_____	_____	_____
• is an important source of pleasure to me	_____	_____	_____
• gives me something to look forward to	_____	_____	_____
• is one of the only things that makes me feel good	_____	_____	_____
• is chiefly a habit	_____	_____	_____

C. Problems and desire to change

   1. What problems have you had because of drinking/using drugs?

      _____

   2. What would happen if you stopped using alcohol/drugs?

      _____

   3. Has your use of alcohol or drugs led to any family problems or conflict?
      _____ Yes _____ No

      If yes, describe: _____

      _____

      _____

   4. Do you see your alcohol/drug use as a problem? _____

   5. Are you interested in stopping or cutting down on your alcohol/drug use?
      _____ Yes _____ No

   6. If yes, why? _____

   7. What do you think gets in the way of stopping or cutting down on your use of substances? _____

      _____

(continued)

438

VI. Goals

A. What would you like to see changed in your life? (Probe for work, school, social, leisure, living arrangements, independent living skills, coping with mental illness.)

_____

_____

_____

B. Is substance use something you need to work on? _____ Yes _____ No

If yes, why? _____

_____

C. What would you like to see changed in your relationships with your family members or others? _____

_____

_____

D. What things have you done to try to achieve these goals? _____

_____

What has worked? _____

_____

What has not worked? _____

_____

VII. Strengths

A. What do you see as your own personal strengths or abilities? _____

_____

_____

B. What things about yourself are you most proud of? _____

_____

_____

C. What do other people say are your positive qualities? _____

_____

_____

D. How have you used your personal strengths and abilities to achieve goals or deal with challenges in the past? _____

_____

_____

E. How do you think you could use your strengths to help you achieve your current goals?

_____

_____

FORM C.5

Drug/Alcohol Time-Line Follow-Back Calendar (TLFBC)

Client name: _____ Date : ___ / ___ / ___

Instructions to interviewers: The TLFBC summarizes the current month and the previous 6 months of the client's substance use. Start by asking about alcohol use, month by month, and then ask about drug use. Focus on an estimation of monthly use and the pattern of use. (More detailed instructions follow the chart below.)

Ask: For each month—(1) How many days have you used alcohol (or drugs)? (2) What kind of alcohol (or drugs) did you use? (3) How much did you use each day (on those days you drank or used drugs)? (4) What is the total number of days in _____ (month) that you drank (or used any drug at all)?

	Current month 1 (# days: ___)	Previous month 2	Previous month 3	Previous month 4	Previous month 5	Previous month 6	Previous month 7
Alcohol Kind							
How much (per day)							
How often (days/month)							
Total days/month alcohol used							
Drugs Kind (+ abused meds)							
How much (per day)							
How often (days/month)							
Total days/month drugs used							

FURTHER INSTRUCTIONS

First, fill in today's day and month, and each of the previous 6 months.
Make note of key events in client's life during these months, such as hospitalizations and jail time.

Alcohol Use

Start with the current month. Ask this series of questions for the current month:
1. "Today is September 15th." (First month is usually a *partial* month.)
2. "How many days, in the 15 days of September, did you use any alcohol?"
3. "What kind of alcohol did you use?" (Beer, wine, hard liquor?)
4. "How much did you drink each day, on the days you used?" (Ask for *each kind* used. If client used more than one kind per day, see notes on recording different kinds, below.)
5. "How many days in this month did you drink any kind of alcohol?" (Ask only if client used *more than one kind* of alcohol. You are looking for the total number of days of use.)

Then go back in time, month by month, using the technique described above for each month (except that questions should cover the whole month). Probe for *patterns* of use, particularly when going further back in time (when recall is more difficult). Ask: "Was your use this month the same as last month, or different?"

Drug Use

Start with the current month. Ask this series of questions for the current month:
1. "Today is September 15th."
2. "What kinds of drugs did you use in September?"
3. Ask the next questions for each kind used. (If client used more than one kind per day, see notes on recording different kinds, below.)
    *   "How many days, in the 15 days of September, did you use this drug?"
    *   "How much did you use each day you used?"
    *   "Were there any days this month when you took more of your medications than you were supposed to?"
    *   "What is the total number of days, this month, you took *any* kind of drug?"

Then go back in time, month by month, using the technique described above for each month (except that questions should cover the whole month). As for alcohol use, probe for *patterns* of drug use, particularly when going back in time (when recall is more difficult). Ask: "Was your use this time the same as last month, or different?"

OTHER NOTES

Recording different kinds of substances: For more than one kind of drug (or alcohol) used in the same month, you will need to divide up the available box and create a kind of code for each substance so you can keep track of each substance, differentiating it from the others, within the same month (see Figure 4.2 in Chapter 4).

When you are finished with the drug section, ask: "Was there any drug you used any time during the past 6 months—even once—that we haven't yet recorded here?" With drug use, also ask: "Was there any time you took more of your medications, even once, in the past 6 months?"

Nondirective questioning is useful when clients have a problem remembering their use over the past 6 months: "Did you use more than half the month or less than half the month?" will get you started.

Payoff Matrix

Client name: _____   Date: _____

Instructions: Instructions for completing each quadrant appear below. For all quadrants, please be as specific as possible about the consequences.

Advantages of Using Substances	**Advantages of <u>Not</u> Using Substances**
Consider possible motives for using substances, such as socializing; coping with symptoms or other problems; pleasure and recreation; or something to do.	Consider potential advantages of not using, such as less conflict with others; fewer symptoms and relapses; fewer money or legal problems; more stable housing; and improved ability to work, go to school, or parent.
Disadvantages of Using Substances	**Disadvantages of <u>Not</u> Using Substances**
Consider common negative consequences of using substances, such as more severe symptoms; more frequent relapses; conflict with others; money or legal problems; loss of housing; and problems with working, going to school, or parenting.	Consider the potential costs of becoming sober, such as more problems socializing; difficulties coping with symptoms or negative moods; lack of recreation and fun; or having nothing interesting to do.

Functional Analysis Summary

Client name: _____

Date: _____

    A.   Complete a Payoff Matrix (see Form C.6) that identifies the advantages and disadvantages of using substances, and the advantages and disadvantages of not using substances. For a client who is currently using substances, the perceived advantages of using substances (and disadvantages of not using substances) should *outweigh* the perceived advantages of not using substances (and the disadvantages of using substances). The short-term advantages of using substances (and disadvantages of not using) often maintain substance use behavior, despite the long-term disadvantages of using substances and (advantages of not using).

    B.   Based on the perceived advantages of using substances, and the disadvantages of not using substances, what factors seem to be most critical in maintaining the client's use of substances (or, if the client is not abusing substances, what factors pose the greatest risk for relapse)?

_____

_____

_____

    C.   What strategies might be used to *reduce* some of the negative consequences (or the "costs") of the client's not using substances? Consider rehabilitation-based interventions, such as teaching the client skills to cope with symptoms; providing social skills training to improve social competence and ability to make friends; assisting the client in developing new social outlets and new recreational activities; and helping the client find something meaningful to do (such as employment, supported education for school, or increased parenting responsibilities).

_____

_____

_____

    D.   What strategies might be used to *increase* the advantages of not using substances? Consider motivation-based interventions, such as motivational interviewing and contingency contracting.

_____

_____

_____

Substance Abuse Treatment Scale—Revised (SATS-R)

Client name: _____

Date: _____

Is client currently in an institution? _____ Yes _____ No

If yes, what institution? _____

Date of hospitalization or incarceration: _____

Instructions: This scale is for assessing a person's stage of substance abuse treatment, not for determining diagnosis. The reporting interval is the last 6 months. If the person is in an institution, the reporting interval is the time period prior to institutionalization. Check which stage of treatment the client is in.

_____ 1. *Preengagement.* The person (not yet a client) does not have contact with a case manager, mental health counselor, or substance abuse counselor, and meets criteria for substance abuse or dependence.

_____ 2. *Engagement.* The client has had only irregular contact with an assigned case manager or counselor, and meets criteria for substance abuse or dependence.

_____ 3. *Early Persuasion.* The client has regular contacts with a case manager or counselor; continues to use the same amount of substances, or has reduced substance use for less than 2 weeks; and meets criteria for substance abuse or dependence.

_____ 4. *Late Persuasion.* The client has regular contacts with a case manager or counselor; shows evidence of reduction in use for the past 2–4 weeks (fewer substances, smaller quantities, or both); but still meets criteria for substance abuse or dependence.

_____ 5. *Early Active Treatment.* The client is engaged in treatment and has reduced substance use for more than the past month, but still meets criteria for substance abuse or dependence during this period of reduction.

_____ 6. *Late Active Treatment.* The person is engaged in treatment and has not met criteria for substance abuse or dependence for the past 1–5 months.

_____ 7. *Relapse Prevention.* The client is engaged in treatment and has not met criteria for substance abuse or dependence for the past 6–12 months.

_____ 8. *In Remission or Recovery.* The client has not met criteria for substance abuse or dependence for more than the past year.

Individual Dual-Disorder Treatment Plan

Client: _____   Date: _____

Primary clinician: _____

Psychiatric disorder (Axis I): _____

Psychiatric disorder (Axis II): _____

Alcohol Use Scale—Revised: _____

Drug Use Scale—Revised: _____

Substance Abuse Treatment Scale—Revised: _____

Stage-Wise Goals

Problem	Goal	Intervention	Treatment modality	Responsible clinician(s)
1.				
2.				
3.				

Goals Based on Functional Analysis

Problem	Goal	Intervention	Treatment modality	Responsible clinician(s)
1.				
2.				
3.				

Date of treatment plan meeting with client: _____

Date of treatment plan meeting with family: _____

Date of next review of treatment plan: _____

Individual Treatment Review

Client: _____   Date: _____

A. Implementation of Planned Interventions

For each planned intervention, indicate whether the intervention was fully implemented, partially implemented, or not implemented.

	Fully implemented	Partially implemented	Not implemented
1. _____	☐	☐	☐
2. _____	☐	☐	☐
3. _____	☐	☐	☐
4. _____	☐	☐	☐

B. Implementation Obstacles or Problems

For each intervention not implemented or partially implemented, describe obstacles or problems encountered in attempting to implement it.

Intervention	Obstacle or problem
1. _____	_____
2. _____	_____
3. _____	_____
4. _____	_____

C. Goals Achieved

For each intervention that was implemented or partially implemented, indicate which of the goals (from prior Individual Dual-Disorder Treatment Plan) of that intervention were achieved.

Intervention 1

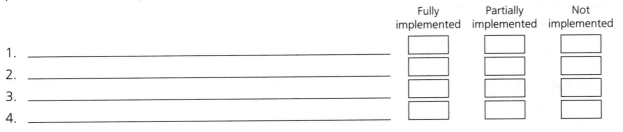

	Fully achieved	Partially achieved	Not achieved
Goals: 1. _____	☐	☐	☐
2. _____	☐	☐	☐
3. _____	☐	☐	☐

(continued)

Intervention 2

	Fully achieved	Partially achieved	Not achieved
Goals: 1. _____	☐	☐	☐
2. _____	☐	☐	☐
3. _____	☐	☐	☐

Intervention 3

	Fully achieved	Partially achieved	Not achieved
Goals: 1. _____	☐	☐	☐
2. _____	☐	☐	☐
3. _____	☐	☐	☐

Intervention 4

	Fully achieved	Partially achieved	Not achieved
Goals: 1. _____	☐	☐	☐
2. _____	☐	☐	☐
3. _____	☐	☐	☐

D. Changes in Substance Abuse

Briefly describe any changes in substance abuse since the last treatment plan. Describe which interventions seem to have worked and which ones seem not to have worked.

_____

_____

_____

_____

_____

Mental Illness Relapse Prevention Worksheet

A. Early warning signs that I may be about to experience a relapse of my mental illness (e.g., trouble sleeping, being isolated from others, confused thinking):

1. _____
2. _____
3. _____

B. Feelings I experience when I'm about to have a relapse of my mental illness (e.g., paranoia, nervousness, sadness):

1. _____
2. _____
3. _____

C. Plan to be implemented when early warning signs or feelings appear (e.g., call my doctor, call my case manager, call a support person, go to a Twelve-Step meeting):

1. _____
2. _____
3. _____

Doctor's name: _____ Phone number: _____

Therapist's/case manager's name: _____ Phone number: _____

Support person's name: _____ Phone number: _____

Support person's name: _____ Phone number: _____

Support person's name: _____ Phone number: _____

Substance Abuse Relapse Prevention Worksheet

A. Early warning signs that I may be about to experience a relapse of my substance abuse (e.g., going to places where I used to drink or use drugs, hanging out with people I used to drink or use drugs with, cravings, decreased need for sleep, becoming more isolated):

1. _____
2. _____
3. _____

B. Feelings I experience when I want to start using substances again (e.g., angry, sad, bored, nervous, anxious, guilty, excited, self-confident):

1. _____
2. _____
3. _____

C. Plan to be implemented when early warning signs or feelings appear (e.g., call my doctor, call my case manager, call a support person, go to a Twelve-Step meeting):

1. _____
2. _____
3. _____

Doctor's name: _____ Phone number: _____

Therapist's/case manager's name: _____ Phone number: _____

Support person's name: _____ Phone number: _____

Support person's name: _____ Phone number: _____

Support person's name: _____ Phone number: _____

Pleasant Activities Worksheet

1. List pleasant activities that do not depend upon others, are noncompetitive, and have some physical, mental, or spiritual value for you. You can improve your level of performance in these activities, and you can accept your level of performance without criticizing yourself.

   _____   _____   _____
   _____   _____   _____
   _____   _____   _____
   _____   _____   _____

2. Schedule 30–60 minutes of "personal time" at least three times per week to engage in these activities. Set aside the time each day. You do not have to select which activity you will do ahead of time. Select the activity from your list above.

	Appointment for personal time	Activity you choose to do
Monday	_____	_____
Tuesday	_____	_____
Wednesday	_____	_____
Thursday	_____	_____
Friday	_____	_____
Saturday	_____	_____
Sunday	_____	_____

3. At the end of the week, look back and note which activities you most enjoyed:

   _____
   _____
   _____

4. Are there any other activities not on your list that you would like to add to this list?

   _____
   _____
   _____

Recovery Mountain Worksheet

Instructions: Recovery from dual disorders is like climbing a mountain, *Recovery Mountain*. The process of recovery involves overcoming different obstacles and challenges, and dealing with various setbacks. You make progress on your personal journey of recovery by learning your warning signs of mental illness and substance abuse, and developing effective coping skills.

Use this worksheet to identify your warning signs and the coping skills you have found most helpful.

Warning signs of mental illness   Coping skills

_____   _____

_____   _____

_____   _____

_____   _____

_____   _____

_____   _____

Warning signs of mental illness   Coping skills

_____   _____

_____   _____

_____   _____

_____   _____

_____   _____

_____   _____

Recovery Mountain:
Health
Feeling good
Role functioning
Social relationships

Active dual disorders:
Alcohol abuse
Drug abuse
Severe mental
illness symptoms

Orientation to Behavioral Family Therapy

Role of the Therapist

- Coordinate, guide, and assist family members in learning new information and coping skills.

Goals

- Reduce tension in family relationships.
- Improve communications between family members.
- Increase the family's understanding and acceptance of the illness.
- Assist the family in developing more satisfactory problem-solving strategies.

Format of the Program

- Assessment of each individual family member.
- Assessment of the family's strengths and weaknesses as a unit.
- Education about the nature of the illness and its treatment.
- Communication skills training.
- Problem-solving training.
- Development of new strategies for specific problems.

What Is Expected of Family Members

- Regular attendance.
- A quiet working environment (if therapy is conducted at home).
- Active role playing.
- Completion of all homework assignments.
- Cooperation with each other and the therapist.

What the Family Can Expect the Therapist to Provide

- Regular attendance.
- A comfortable working environment (if therapy is conducted in clinic).
- Thoughtful, systematic intervention
- Strict confidentiality (except with treatment team and when obligated to report).
- Homework materials.
- Crisis counseling (if applicable).

Family Member Interview

Date: _____

I. Background Information

A. Name: _____

B. Relationship to client: _____

C. Age: _____

D. Marital status: _____

E. Address: _____

_____

_____

F. Telephone number: _____

G. How far did you go in school? _____

H. Occupation: _____

I. Have you ever had any psychiatric treatment? _____ Yes _____ No
    If yes, what? _____

II. Knowledge of Mental Illness

A. Do you think _____ has a mental illness? _____ Yes _____ No

B. If yes, what is it called? _____

C. What do you think caused it? _____

_____

D. Is there anything that makes it better? _____

_____

E. Is there anything that makes it worse? _____

_____

F. Does _____ take medication? _____ Yes _____ No

G. Do you know what he or she takes? _____

H. Is the medication helpful? _____ Yes _____ No
    How? _____

_____

(continued)

    I.   Does the medication have side effects? ____ Yes ____ No

        If yes, what are they? _____

        _____

        _____

    J.   Does _____ take the medication regularly? ____ Yes ____ No

        If no, is it a problem? _____

        _____

III. Problem Behaviors

    A.   How has _____'s disorder changed the family? _____

        _____

    B.   Has _____'s disorder caused any problems? ____ Yes ____ No

        If yes, what are they? _____

        _____

    C.   How do you cope with these problems? _____

        _____

    D.   What types of situations or problems are the source of conflict between you and

        _____? _____

        _____

        _____

    E.   How do family members deal with these situations? _____

        _____

        Are you satisfied with how you and other family members cope with these stresses?

        ____ Yes ____ No

        If no, why not? _____

        _____

    F.   What do you see as the family's major stressors? _____

        _____

IV. Substance Use

    A.   Does _____ use alcohol? ____ Yes ____ No

    B.   If yes, could you tell me a little bit about that (frequency, type, situation)? _____

        _____

    C.   If yes, is this a problem (for you or other relatives, for him or her, or for everyone)? _____

        _____

(continued)

D. If yes, what specific kinds of problems does it cause? _____
_____

E. Do you know whether _____ has used any of the following substances?

Substance	Ever	Recently (past 6 months)
Marijuana	_____	_____
Cocaine	_____	_____
Hallucinogens (e.g., LSD, PCP, mescaline)	_____	_____
Sedatives (not prescribed) (e.g., Valium)	_____	_____
Stimulants (e.g., amphetamines)	_____	_____
Opiates (e.g., heroin, Darvon)	_____	_____
Over-the-counter (specify: _____)	_____	_____
Other (specify: _____)	_____	_____

F. Do you use alcohol? _____ Yes _____ No

G. If yes, in what situations do you use alcohol? _____
_____

H. Do you use any of the other substances listed above? _____ Yes _____ No

I. If yes, in what situations have you used these substances? _____
_____

J. Have you experienced any problems related to your substance use (i.e., relationship, job, legal, financial)? _____
_____
_____

V. Leisure/Social Activities

A. How do you spend your free time? _____
_____

B. With whom do you spend it? _____

C. Would you like more activities? _____ Yes _____ No

D. If yes, what would you like to do? _____
_____

E. Are there activities you used to do but don't do any more? _____ Yes _____ No
If yes, describe: _____

F. Would you like to do them again? _____ Yes _____ No

G. What gets in the way of doing those activities? _____
_____

(continued)

VI. Goals

A. What would you like to see change? _____

_____

B. Name two things you would like to get out of these family meetings (for yourself):

_____

_____

C. What are obstacles to achieving these goals? _____

_____

D. What are supports to achieving these goals? _____

_____

_____

VII. Strengths

A. What do you see as your own personal strengths? _____

_____

B. What do you see as the major strengths of your family? _____

_____

C. In what ways does _____ help out the family? _____

_____

_____

D. How do you think your and your family's strengths can help you achieve your personal goals and the goals of your family? _____

_____

_____

VIII. Clinical and Other Observations

_____
_____
_____
_____
_____
_____
_____
_____
_____
_____
_____

Summary of Family Assessment

Client: _____

Date: _____

Instructions: Summarize and integrate the pertinent information from the functional assessment interview (with the client) and individual family member interviews on this form.

Description of family (e.g., living arrangement and family contacts):

Client's psychiatric disorder and substance abuse problems:

Impact of substance abuse on client and relatives:

Critical factors identified on functional analysis:

(continued)

Degree of supportiveness or tension among family members:

Client and relatives' motivation to improve management of psychiatric disorder:

Description of family's strengths (as gathered from individual interviews and observations of the family):

Client's stage of treatment (from the Substance Abuse Treatment Scale—Revised):

___ Preengagement   ___ Early Active Treatment

___ Engagement   ___ Late Active Treatment

___ Early Persuasion   ___ Relapse Prevention

___ Late Persuasion   ___ Remission/Recovery

Overall family stage of treatment (taking into consideration all family members):

___ Preengagement   ___ Early Active Treatment

___ Engagement   ___ Late Active Treatment

___ Early Persuasion   ___ Relapse Prevention

___ Late Persuasion   ___ Remission/Recovery

Family Treatment Plan

I. Client's Individual Goals

1.

2.

3.

II. Family Member 1's Individual Goals

1.

2.

3.

III. Family Member 2's Individual Goals

1.

2.

3.

IV. Family Member 3's Individual Goals

1.

2.

3.

V. Shared Family Goals

1.

2.

3.

VI. Factors Identified by Functional Analysis

1.

2.

3.

VII. Stage-Wise Treatment Goals

1.

2.

3.

Family Treatment Review

Client/family: _____ Date: _____

A. Implementation of Family Therapy Sessions

Were regular behavioral family therapy sessions fully implemented, partially implemented, or not implemented?

_____ Fully implemented

_____ Partially implemented

_____ Not implemented

B. Number of Family Sessions

How many family sessions were held since the last treatment plan? _____

C. Implementation Obstacles or Problems

Describe obstacles or problems encountered in attempting to implement family sessions.

_____

_____

_____

_____

D. Goals Achieved

Indicate goals achieved or progress made toward goals for each individual family member and the family as a unit.

		Successfully achieved	Partially achieved	Not achieved
Client Goals:	1. _____	☐	☐	☐
	2. _____	☐	☐	☐
	3. _____	☐	☐	☐

		Successfully achieved	Partially achieved	Not achieved
Family Member 1 Goals:	1. _____	☐	☐	☐
	2. _____	☐	☐	☐
	3. _____	☐	☐	☐

(continued)

		Successfully achieved	Partially achieved	Not achieved
Family Member 2 Goals:	1. _____	☐	☐	☐
	2. _____	☐	☐	☐
	3. _____	☐	☐	☐

		Successfully achieved	Partially achieved	Not achieved
Family Member 3 Goals:	1. _____	☐	☐	☐
	2. _____	☐	☐	☐
	3. _____	☐	☐	☐

E. Changes in Substance Abuse

Briefly describe any changes in substance abuse since the last treatment plan. Describe which interventions seem to have worked and which ones seem not to have worked.

_____

_____

_____

_____

_____

_____

Problem-Solving or Goal-Setting Sheet

1. **Discuss the problem or goal.** Get everyone's opinion. Try to reach agreement on exactly what the problem/goal is. Write down *specifically* what the problem/goal is.

_____

2. **Brainstorm at least three possible solutions.** Do not evaluate these at this time—wait till step 3.	3. **Briefly evaluate each solution.** List major advantages and disadvantages.

	Advantages	Disadvantages
(a) _____	_____	_____
	_____	_____
(b) _____	_____	_____
	_____	_____
(c) _____	_____	_____
	_____	_____
(d) _____	_____	_____
	_____	_____
(e) _____	_____	_____
	_____	_____

4. **Choose the best solution(s).** Consider how easy it would be to implement the solution, and how likely it is to be effective. _____

5. **Plan the implementation.** When will it be implemented? _____
What resources are needed ,and how will they be obtained? _____
Who will do what to implement the solution? _____
List what might go wrong in the implementation and how to overcome it. _____

_____

Practice any difficult parts of the plan.
Who will check that all the steps of the plan have been implemented? _____

6. **Review implementation at next family meeting.** (Date: _____) Revise as needed.

Index

Page numbers following by *f* indicate figure, *t* indicate table.